BIOLOGICAL PSYCHIATRY
Volume 1

BIOLOGICAL PSYCHIATRY

Volume 1

Proceedings of the 5th World Congress of Biological Psychiatry, Florence, 9–14 June 1991

Editors:

Giorgio Racagni, Ph.D.
Professor of Pharmacology
Director, Center of Neuropharmacology
Institute of Pharmacological Sciences
University of Milan, Milan, Italy

Nicoletta Brunello, Ph.D.
Assistant Professor of Pharmacology
Center of Neuropharmacology
Institute of Pharmacological Sciences
University of Milan, Milan, Italy

Tetsuo Fukuda, M.D., D.med.Sci.
Director, Osaka Institute of Clinical Psychiatry
Takatsuki, and Professor of Psychiatry and Mental Health
Doshisha University, Kyoto, Japan

1991

EXCERPTA MEDICA, AMSTERDAM, LONDON, NEW YORK, TOKYO

International Congress Series No. 968
ISBN 0 444 81410 8

This book is printed on acid-free paper.

Published by:
Elsevier Science Publishers B.V.
P.O. Box 211
1000 AE Amsterdam
The Netherlands

Sole distributors for the USA and Canada:
Elsevier Science Publishing Company Inc.
655 Avenue of the Americas
New York, NY 10010
USA

In order to ensure rapid publication this volume was prepared using a method of electronic text processing known as Optical Character Recognition (OCR). Scientific accuracy and consistency of style were handled by the author. Time did not allow for the usual extensive editing process of the Publisher.

Printed in The Netherlands

Preface

Six years have elapsed since the last World Congress held in Philadelphia in 1985, an unexpectedly long interval – the longest so far – between one congress and the next. This was however unavoidable in order not to interfere with other large scale international congresses being held in the same year.

Thus, the volumes now at the readers disposal comprise an essence, or resumé, of what was undertaken and/or achieved worldwide in the course of the past six years in the highly specialized research domain, biological psychiatry. For the high quality of the volumes, in terms of scientific and practical values, the Editors are indebted to the conscientious work of the Scientific Program Committee who made a selection of the symposia topics and competent experts for each topic. I would like to inform all readers that many of the Free Communications, oral and poster alike, were of an equally high level; exclusion of these from these volumes was warranted solely because of space limitation.

Speaking briefly of the World Federation of Societies of Biological Psychiatry (WFSBP), simple statistics in terms of member (national) societies show a sharp increase from 26 (September 1985) to 38 (June 1991), while the number of attenders to the congress grew from 2500 to 5000. This increase and growth may well be the result in part of the six years interval; colleagues worldwide could hardly wait to get together to learn and discuss what has been brought forward from various centers.

It might be timely to note here how the WFSBP started since only a few people who know of this are still living. Officially, it dates back from 1974 when the 1st World Congress of Biological Psychiatry was held in Buenos Aires. In actuality, however, it dates back even further, i.e. on the occasion of the 5th World Congress of World Psychiatry Association, Mexico City, 1971. I happen to be the person responsible for alluring some number of American biological psychiatrists into forming an international body for biological psychiatry, which was to be named three years later as the WFSBP. Dr. R. Mitsuda, Founder of the Japanese Society of Biological Psychiatry, was my strongest proponent and Dr. George A. Ulett, St. Louis, was also of great help. For further information a short remark can be found in the Preface of C. Shagaas et al. "Biological Psychiatry 1985". Therefore, taking into account the forming years, the WFSBP may now be looked at as twenty years old.

During all these years, and one way or another, I continuously had something to do with the WFSBP – as I do now – so that every phase of the development of the WFSBP has remained in my memory; the embryo to baby and further to adolescence.... Growth of the WFSBP has been, roughly speaking. proportional to that of biological psychiatry per se, particularly in terms of clinical science; it is best reflected in the issues of the criteria of diagnosis and classification from DSM-I, RDC, DSM-III, DSM-III R, and now DSM-IV. Needless to say, basic sciences are accordingly "growing up" along with the clinical moves, as they both have to be taken into account in our particular expertise.

The volumes that appear in the midst of such background will no doubt provide the readers with a wealth of knowledge and information in learning how far we have come, and which way we should better move, again roughly in proportion to the two decade growth of our discipline. Contributions made by biological psychiatry are now being more appropriately appreciated by fellow colleagues, whatever approaches they may prefer to choose, and general trends today are, unlike sometime ago, towards more cooperation and understanding of different approaches and/or discipline.

To this end, it is my duty to point out that this is the very first time the World Congress has been held outside the country of residence of the President. The two congress chairpersons had to communicate with each other by use of all available means of course, but the actual labor depended exclusively upon the Organizer and his crew. Moreover, the Organizer took care of the heavy work as Secretary-Treasurer of the WFSBP; to which I nominate myself as the best judge of the heavy workload since I myself carried out this task between 1982–1985. My sincere gratitude, therefore, goes to Professor Giorgio Racagni for his tireless work, both as the Congress Organizer and Secretary-Treasurer, and as my right hand of the WFSBP. To Dr. Nicoletta Brunello, my deepest appreciation is due; without her efficient assistance, the present volumes would not have seen the light of day.

I hope the volumes will be duly acknowledged worldwide and assume an important landmark in the history of biological psychiatry, and of psychiatry on the whole, for years to come; hopefully in someway comparable to what Florence, the congress site, and Renaissance have done to the world of art, science and humanity!

Tetsuo Fukuda
Past-President, World Federation of
Societies of Biological Psychiatry
Chairperson, 5th World Congress of
Biological Psychiatry

Introduction

The 5th World Congress of Biological Psychiatry took place in Florence from June 9th to 14th, 1991. It was attended by about 5,000 participants from 70 countries.

The congress included 120 symposia, 40 oral free communication sessions and 2,500 poster presentations. Moreover, 11 satellite symposia were organized.

These volumes contain the papers presented at the symposium sessions of congress.

Biological psychiatry represents a fusion of several scientific disciplines – pharmacology, neurobiology, biochemistry, genetics, physiology, anatomy, biophysics and psychology – all focused on acquiring an ultimate understanding of the relationships between brain and behaviour.

Psychiatric disorders include schizophrenia, affective disorders, the many forms of senile and presenile dementia including Alzheimer's disease, the anxiety disorders, childhood disorders and the variants of eating and sleeping dysfunctions. Each of these illnesses represents a complex interaction of biological, psychological and social variables.

The growing number of neuroscientists adopting the biological approach to neuropsychiatric diseases has resulted in a fast expanding body of knowledge regarding brain function and pathology. The field is exciting because we see complementary advances across a broad front of recently developed research areas.

Psychotherapeutic drugs used to treat psychiatric and neurologic disorders play a crucial role in elucidating the biological bases of these diseases.

Studying the mechanism of action of these compounds should give us important clues about the normal and pathological functioning of the brain.

The objectives of the effort are well reflected in the topics covered by the papers in these two volumes.

This book will be of interest to psychiatrists, neurologists, clinicians and neuropharmacologists.

The Editors

Acknowledgements

The editors acknowledge the following companies for their support in the publication of the proceedings:

Astra Research Centre, Sweden
Bayer A/G, Germany
Bristol-Myers Squibb Company, U.S.A.
Ciba-Geigy A/G, Switzerland
Duphar B.V., The Netherlands
Eli Lilly International Corporation, U.S.A.
FIDIA Research Laboratories, Abano Terme, Italy
Glaxo Holdings p.l.c., U.K.
F. Hoffmann-La Roche Ltd., Switzerland
H. Lundbeck A/S, Denmark
Janssen Pharmaceutica, Belgium
Laboratories Synthélabo, France
Menarini Industrie Farmaceutiche Riunite s.r.l., Italy
Pfizer International Inc., U.S.A.
Sandoz Pharma Ltd., Switzerland
SmithKline Beecham Pharmaceuticals, U.K.
Takeda Italia Farmaceutici, Italy
The Upjohn Company, U.S.A.
Wyeth-Ayerst, U.K.
Zambeletti S.p.A., Italy

The editors gratefully acknowledge the skilful assistance of Mrs. Carla Penza.

Contents

Volume 1

DIAGNOSIS AND CLASSIFICATION

Developing DSM IV: A preview of the future

Process and principles in the development of DSM IV
H.A. Pincus, A.J. Frances, N. Sydnor-Greenberg, W. Davis, M. First and T. Widiger 3
Schizophrenia and other psychotic disorders in DSM IV
N.C. Andreasen 6
DSM IV mood disorders
A.J. Rush 9

Classification of Depression: From biology to nosology

Psychopharmacology and the classification of depressive disorders
A. Dubini 12
Biological markers in nosology
B.J. Carroll 17
Distribution of morbidity risks in unipolar and bipolar mood disorders
B. Smeraldi and M. Gasperini 19
Classification of depression: From biology to functional psychopathology
H.M. van Praag 23
Nosology and the classification of depressive disorders
T.A. Ban 28

Diagnostic specificity – A useful guide to biological psychiatry?

Diagnostic specificity in twin studies
P. McGuffin and A. Farmer 31
Diagnostic unspecificity in family studies: The overlap of anxiety disorders and unipolar major depression
W. Maier, D. Lichtermann, J. Minges and R. Heun 34
Neuroendocrinological/sleep parameters and diagnostic distinctions
D.J. Kupfer 37
Drug response and the distinction between affective and schizophrenic disorders
E.C. Johnstone 40

Functional classification and the major/minor dichotomy of psychiatric disorders in 500 outpatients
O. Benkert, P. Winter, H. Gerbaldo and M. Philipp 43

AFFECTIVE DISORDERS: CLINICAL AND BIOLOGICAL RESEARCH

Clinical indices of vulnerability for depression

Stress and episode sensitization in recurrent depression
R.M. Post 49
The polysomnogram (PSG) as a vulnerability marker for depression
A.J. Rush, C.M. Gullion, R. Armitage and H.P. Roffwarg 52
An integrated view of vulnerability
D.J. Kupfer 55

Prophylaxis of affective disorders

Epidemiology and prognosis of depression
E.S. Paykel 57
Efficacy of maintenance therapy with TCAs and MAOIs: New findings
D.J. Kupfer and E. Frank 61
Long-term outcome of mood disorder on prophylactic lithium
M.T. Abou-Saleh and A.J. Coppen 64
The efficacy of prophylactic treatment with 5-HT reuptake inhibitors
S.A. Montgomery, D.B. Montgomery and M. Green 67

Biological markers in depression

Biological markers in depression: Introductory remarks
P.D. Hrdina 69
Platelet antidepressant sites and the serotonin transporter in depression
S.Z. Langer, M.F. Poirier, H. Loo and A.-M. Galzin 72
Antidepressant sites in human brain
J. Marcusson 75
Noradrenergic receptors in postmortem brains from depressed suicide victims
R.W. Horton, F. De Paermentier, J.M. King, M.R. Crompton and C.L.E. Katona 78
Status on amines in CSF in depression
A. Gjerris 81
Markers of hypothalamic-pituitary-thyroid axis dysfunction in depression
A.J. Prange Jr. 84

PET and SPECT studies of blood flow/metabolism in affective disorders

SPECT research in affective disorders
J.A. Schwartz and N.M. Speed 87
Amino acid pools, CBF and $CMRO_2$ in affective disorders
H. Kishimoto, H. Fujita, O. Takatsu, H. Takahashi, T. Maeda, T. Ishikawa, T. Hashimoto, K. Kosaka, F. Yokoi and M. Iio 91

Biological studies of suicide risk

CSF 5-HIAA predicts suicide risk after attempted suicide
P. Nordström 94
CSF studies and long-term suicidal behavior
A. Roy 97
CSF studies and long-term suicidal behavior
G. Regnéll, L. Träskman-Bendz, C. Alling and R. Öhman 100
Receptor studies in suicidal patients
A. Biegon 103
Serotonin system challenges in suicidal behavior
E.F. Coccaro and R.J. Kavoussi 106
Serotonin receptor sensitivity and aggression
S. Wetzler, R.S. Kahn, G. Asnis, M. Korn and H.M. van Praag 110

Neurobiology and pharmacotherapy of suicidal behaviour

Integration of neurobiology and psychopathology in a unified model of suicidal behavior
J.J. Mann 114
Neurochemical findings in the brain of suicide victims
V. Arango, M.D. Underwood and J.J. Mann 118
Prediction of suicidal behavior from biological tests
L. Träskman-Bendz, G. Regnéll, C. Alling, P. Simonsson, L. Oreland, E. Vinge and R. Öhman 121
Pharmacotherapy in the prevention of suicidal behaviour
D.B. Montgomery, D. Baldwin, M. Green, T. Bullock and S.A. Montgomery 124
Antidepressants and risk of suicide
A. Molcho and M. Stanley 126

Dysthymia and minor depressive disorder: Diagnosis and treatment possibilities

Evolution in the concepts of minor depressive disorders and unspecific somatic complaints
M. Linden 129

A prospective study of diagnostic change in dysthymic disorder
N. Seivewright and P. Tyrer 133
The pharmacological treatment of dysthymia
G.B. Cassano, M. Savino, G. Pervgi and P. Medda 136

Biological mechanisms in postpartum mental illness

Biochemical correlates of postnatal depression
V. Glover, P. Hannah, D. Adams, J. Littlewood and M. Sandler 142
Oestradiol in the treatment of postnatal depression
A. Gregoire, R. Kumar, A. Henderson and J. Studd 144
Prophylactic lithium in puerperal psychosis: Three centers' experience
D.E. Stewart, J.L. Klompenhouwer, R.E. Kendell and A.M. van Hulst 146
Dopamine receptor hypersensitivity precedes puerperal affective psychosis: A possible link with perinatal changes in oestrogen production
A. Wieck, A.D. Hirst, M.N. Marks, I.C. Campbell, S.A. Checkley and R. Kumar 149

Depression and stress: Pathophysiological and therapeutic aspects

Physiopathological and pharmacological aspects of the stress response
B. Silvestrini 152
Altered sleep, depression and antidepressant efficacy
M.B. Scharf 157
Antidepressants and sympatholytic activity: The case of etoperidone, a new triazolone derivative
J.P. Feighner and W.F. Boyer 161
Stress and aging brain: Markers of adaptation in dementia of the Alzheimer's type
G. Nappi, E. Martignoni, A. Costa, F. Petraglia, G. Bono and A.R. Genazzani 165

Second messenger transduction in the pathogenesis and treatment of affective disorders

Phosphodiesterase inhibitors as antidepressants
H. Wachtel 169
Effect of lithium on adenylate cyclase in rat brain
A. Mørk and A. Geisler 172
Lithium selective interaction with G proteins in the CNS
G. Schreiber and S. Avissar 173
Interaction of antidepressants with phosphoinositide turnover in rat brain and human platelets
G.M. Pandey, S.C. Pandey and J.M. Davis 177

ECS effect on second messengers in rat brain
J. Vetulani 181
Second messenger transduction associated with 5-HT in the pathogenesis and treatment of affective disorders
M.E. Newman, B. Shapira, P. Lichtenberg and B. Lerer 184
Effects of antidepressants and electroconvulsive shock on coupling of G protein to adenylate cyclase
H. Ozawa, S. Hatta, M.M. Rasenick, N. Takahata and T. Saito 188

The influence of mood stabilizing drugs on cerebral second messenger systems

Mechanisms of lithium in modulation of post receptor second messenger function in rat brain
A. Mørk and P. Hollund 192
Oral or ICV injection of compounds that reduce cyclic AMP affect rat behavior
O. Kofman and R.H. Belmaker 195
Lessons from the withdrawal of lithium prophylaxis
G.M. Goodwin, F.G.M. Souza and A.J. Mander 197
The influence of lithium and rubidium on cyclic AMP formation in vitro and ex vivo
A. Mørk and A. Geisler 200

Circadian rhythms in affective disorders: New concepts, novel therapies

Rapid re-entrainment of the circadian clock in "jet-lag" paradigm: Role for behavioral feedback
O. van Reeth, C. Wickland and F. Turek 202
Energy and metabolism in depression: A circadian link between synapse and symptom
J.L. Anderson 206

HPA regulation in depression

The role of HPA hormones in the neuroregulation of sleep in affective disorders
A. Steiger, U. von Bardeleben, J. Guldner, C. Lauer, B. Rothe and F. Holsboer 210
Pituitary changes in depression
K.R.R. Krishnan, P.M. Doraiswamy, D.A. Axelson, S.N. Lurie, G.S. Figiel, M.M. Husain, L. Patterson, O.B. Boyko, E.H. Ellinwood Jr, and C.B. Nemeroff 213

Aging and the canine hypothalamic-pituitary-adrenocortical (HPA) axis
J.M.H.M. Reul, J. Rothuizen and E.R. de Kloet 217
Glucocorticoid receptors in psychiatry: Clinical, functional and molecular aspects
R. Rupprecht, J. Kornhuber, N. Wodarz, P. Riederer, D. Spengler, K. Damm and F. Holsboer 222
Repression and differential regulation of the hCRH gene promoter through glucocorticoid receptors
D. Spengler, R. Rupprecht, K. Damm and F. Holsboer 225

Pain and depression

Does depression cause pain or pain cause depression?
H. Merskey 228
Chronic abdominal pain and depressive symptoms: An epidemiologic evaluation of the hispanic population in the United States
G. Magni, M. Merskey, M.R. Rossi and S. Rigatti-Luchini 231
Platelet [^{3}H]paroxetine binding in chronic pain patients
E.T. Mellerup, N.-H. Jensen, L. Lauritzen, M. Lunde and P. Plenge 234
Common pathogenetic mechanisms in chronic pain syndromes and in depressive disorders
L. von Knorring 237
Serotonergic agents in tricyclic non-responsive depressions
S.P. Roose 240
Lithium addition in treatment-resistant depression: Evidence for the involvement of the serotonin system
C. de Montigny 243
Monamine oxidase inhibitors in resistant major depression
W.A. Nolen, P.F. Bouvy and P.M.J. Haffmans 246
ECT in the treatment of medication-resistant depression
H.A. Sackeim 249
Psychotherapy of treatment-resistant depression
E. Frank, D.J. Kupfer and S. Johnson 253

Optimization of therapeutic outcome with ECT

Schedule of ECT administration: Implications for antidepressant efficacy and adverse effects
B. Shapira, J. Hadjez, A. Calev and B. Lerer 257
Effects of stimulus electrode placement on therapeutic outcome
R.D. Weiner and C.E. Coffee 260
Stimulus intensity and the efficacy of ECT
H.A. Sackeim 264

New insights into the neurobiology of ECT: Regionally selective alterations in noradrenaline release revealed by microdialysis
R.B. Holman, D.N. Thomas and D.J. Nutt 268
Neurobiological mechanisms of ECT: Clinical studies
J.J. Mann and S. Kapur 272

Serotonin uptake inhibitors in depression and other indications

Serotonin uptake inhibitors in depression and other indications
R. Fog 275
Psychiatric use of the selective serotonin reuptake inhibitors for indications other than depression
W.F. Boyer 276
Pharmacokinetics of antidepressants: Clinical relevance for citalopram and other 5-HT uptake inhibitors
P. Baumann 279
Citalopram in panic disorder: Short-term and long-term efficacy. Testing a 5-HT panic hypothesis
M. Humble, C. Koczkas, B. Norberg and B. Wistedt 282
New aspects in the treatment of depression
T. Silverstone 286
Citalopram in depression: Meta-analysis of intended and unintended effects
P. Bech and P. Cialdella 288
Treatment of depression in elderly patients with and without dementia disorders
C.-G. Gottfries and A.L. Nyth 291

Present status on the mode of action of antidepressant drugs

Antidepressant drugs acting on the serotonin transporter
S.Z. Langer, H. Esnaud and D. Graham 294
Adaptation of central 5-HT_{1A} receptors after chronic antidepressant treatment in rats
M. Hamon, L. Lanfumey, S. Haj-Dahmane, T. Jolas, E. Kidd, F. Bolaños and H. Gozlan 297
Enhancement of 5-HT synaptic efficacy by antidepressant treatments: A tenable unitary theory?
C. de Montigny and P. Blier 301
Distinct roles of 5-HT subsystems in panic, anxiety and depression
J.F.W. Deakin 305
Pilot studies in major depression of litoxetine: A selective 5-HT uptake inhibitor
M. Garreau, M. Bourgeois, M. Escande, J. Mendlewicz, M.F. Poirier and P. Legris 308

New antidepressants: Novel approaches and their implications

New antidepressants: Chemical diversity but unity of action?
B.E. Leonard 311
Subtypes of depression and serotonin function
J.A. den Boer, H.J.G.M. van Megen and H.G.M. Westenberg 315
Benzodiazepines in the treatment of depressive disorders: An updated review
A.F. Schatzberg and J.A. Posener 318
α_2-Adrenoceptor antagonists as antidepressants: New developments
R.M. Pinder 322
GABA ergic drugs as putative antidepressants: A review of available data
P.L. Morselli and M. Garreau 325

Onset of action of antidepressant activity: Biological and clinical aspects

Do pharmacokinetic factors affect the rapidity of antidepressant actions
A.C. Altamura and S.R. Bareggi 328
Some biological correlates of acute antidepressant activity in affective illness
P. Linkowski, M. Kerkhofs, P. Hubain and J. Mendlewicz 332
Pharmacological effects of antidepressants: Their chronology and potential clinical relevance
A.J. Puech 335
Strategies for confirming the rapid onset of antidepressants
J.P. Feighner and W.F. Boyer 338
Clinical aspects of onset of action of antidepressant efficacy
S.A. Montgomery and G. Magni 343
Venlafaxine: A new potent antidepressant agent with putative fast onset of action
K. Rickels 345

Lithium potentiation of tricyclic antidepressants: Clinical efficacy and basic mechanisms

Lithium enhancement of brain 5-HT function in resistant depression: Relation to clinical outcome
P.J. Cowen 347
Lithium supplementation therapy in refractory depression: Clinical aspects and neuroendocrine challenge effects
B. Shapira, M.J. Yagmur, M.E. Newman and B. Lerer 350
Lithium potentiation of bupropion and fluoxetine: Theory and practice
P.J. Goodnick 353

Effect of treatment with a lithium-imipramine combination on components of adenylate cyclase in the cerebral cortex of the rat
A. Mørk and A. Geisler 357

Pharmacokinetics of tricyclic antidepressants and MAO-inhibitors

Plasma/serum concentration of antidepressant and clinical response: State of the art
L.F. Gram 359

Plasma monitoring of antidepressants: Clinical relevance of the pharmacogenetic of metabolism and of α_1-acid glycoprotein binding
P. Baumann and C.B. Eap 362

Plasma levels of amitriptyline during treatment of depression: Influence of combined treatment with dibenzepine
A. Saria, R. Neumann, C. Humpel, F. Lieder, G. Dosser and H. Oberbauer 365

Pharmacokinetics of antidepressants: Fluoxetine and fluvoxamine in daily clinical practice
S. Vandel, S. Bouquet, B. Bonin, G. Bertschy and P. Baumann 368

Pharmacokinetics of reversible MAO-A inhibitors (RIMA)
G. Laux, M.P. Schoerlin, W. Classen, T. Becker, K.P. Lesch and G. Carl 372

Clinical utility of antidepressants' plasma level assessment: Methodical aspects
B. Müller-Oerlinghausen 375

Selective reversible MAO inhibitors as antidepressants

Direct and indirect actions of monoamine oxidase
K.F. Tipton, J.M. McCrodden and E.M. O'Brien 378

Comparison between the pharmacology of reversible and irreversible inhibitors of MAO-A
J.P.M. Finberg 380

Neurotransmitter turnover in neurodegenerative disorders of the CNS
P. Riederer, W. Gsell, C. Konradi, L. Käsbauer, E. Sofic, G. Moll, G. Hebenstreit and K. Jellinger 383

Effects of MAO inhibition on age-induced changes in tissue amino acid levels in mice and rats
M. Strolin Benedetti, P. Marrari, M. Cini, M. Da Prada and P. Dostert 386

Safety of the RIMA antidepressant moclobemide: Minimal interactions with dietary tyramine and 5-HT uptake blockers
E.P. Bonetti, R. Scherschlicht and M. Da Prada 390

Brofaromine and 5-HT uptake inhibition: Structure-activity relationship of congeners
P. Waldmeier, R. Bernasconi and W. Schilling 393

Modulatory actions of steroid hormones on MAO-A but MAO-B activities
M.B.H. Youdim 397

Renaissance of MAOIs: The new selective and reversible generation

The role of MAO inhibitors in the treatment of affective disorders
E.S. Paykel 400
Significance of reversibility as a safety factor of MAO-A inhibitors: Preclinical data
K.F. Tipton and M.C. Anderson 403
Clinical pharmacology of selective and reversible MAO-A inhibitors: Comparison with the first generation of MAO inhibitors
P.R. Bieck, K.-H. Antonin and R. Schulz 406
General efficacy and safety of brofaromine in depression
H.-J. Möller 410
Evaluation of brofaromine in geriatric depressed patients
P.A.F. Jansen and P.M.J. Haffmans 413

New findings in child psychiatry

New findings in child psychiatry
G. Nissen 416
Psychopharmacological treatment of stuttering in children
A. Rothenberger, H. Johannsen, H. Schulze and H. Amorosa 418
Pharmacotherapy of conduct disorders in children and adolescents
J.G. Simeon 423
Moclobemide, a new inhibitor in hyperkinetic children
G.E. Trott, H.J. Friese, M. Menzel and G. Nissen 425

SCHIZOPHRENIA AND RELATED DISORDERS: CLINICAL AND BIOLOGICAL STUDIES

Epidemiology of schizophrenia

Schizophrenia: Gender and age. Why is the onset of schizophrenia later in women?
H. Häfner, S. Behrens, J. de Vry and W.F. Gattaz 431
Molecular genetics and the epidemiology of schizophrenia: Emerging research issues
P. McGuffin 434
Certain aspects of epidemiology in biological schizophrenia research
F. Schulsinger 437

Long-term neuroleptic treatment of schizophrenia: A review of follow-up studies
C. Bellantuono 441
Schizophrenia and neuroleptic prescribing patterns: A survey on a representative sample of mental health services in Piedmont
C. Munizza, E. Pirfo, F. Punzo and G. Tibaldi 444

Clinical and neurobiological heterogeneity of schizophrenic psychoses

Clinical and neurobiological heterogeneity of schizophrenic psychoses
T. Fukuda 449
Multivariate analyses of brain imaging data from typical and atypical schizophrenic psychoses
T. Hatashi, H. Kitou, T. Kachi, H. Suga and M. Ohara 452
Clinical heterogeneity of schizophrenia: Perspectives from neuroimaging
N.C. Andreasen, M. Flaum, D. Miller, J. Ehrhardt, K. Rezai, G. Cohen and D.S. O'Leary 455
Long-term course in schizophrenia: Neurobiology and pscyhopathology
G. Gross and G. Huber 458
Different responsiveness of negative symptoms to pharmacotherapy
K. Inanaga and M. Kuniyoshi 461
Long-term course and outcome in delusional psychoses
N. Retterstøl and S. Opjordsmoen 464

Cognitive disturbance and cerebral dysfunction of schizophrenics

Schizophrenia viewed as a neurotransmitter imbalance syndrome, involving dysregulation of sensory input and arousal
A. Carlsson, M. Carlsson and A. Svensson 467
Cognitive science- and neuropsychological aspects of schizophrenia research
H.M. Emrich 469
Brain systems and abnormal word generation in schizophrenia
C. Frith 472
Event-related potentials in facial recognition task in schizophrenics
N. Tsuru, E. Minami and S. Genda 475

Cerebral blood flow or metabolic patterns (PET/SPECT) during cognition in schizophrenia

Brain glucose metabolism and clinical correlates in schizophrenia
F.-A. Wiesel and G. Wik 478

Postmortem brain studies in schizophrenia

Locomotion and behaviour: The interaction of loops and transmitter
P. Riederer and W. Berger 482
Pathomorphological aspects of schizophrenia
K.A. Jellinger, H. Beckmann and H. Heinsen 485
Markedly increased number of striatal D_2 dopamine receptors in human narcolepsy but without psychosis: Implications for the dopamine hypothesis of schizophrenia
S.J. Kish, M. Mamelak, A. Lewis, C. Slimovitch, L.M. Dixon, L. Distefano and O. Hornykiewicz 489
Amino acid transmitters and dopamine function in the brain in schizophrenia
G.P. Reynolds 491
Glutamate and schizophrenia
J. Kornhuber and P. Riederer 495
Postmortem investigations of sigma and PCP receptors in psychosis
A.D. Weissman and E.B. de Souza 498
Dopaminergic and glutamatergic abnormalities in postmortem schizophrenic brain
M. Toru, A. Kuramaji, S. Kumashiro, M. Ishimaru, I. Suga and T. Nishikawa 501

The neuroanatomy of schizophrenia

Entorhinal cortex pathology in schizophrenia and affective disorders
M. Casanova, R. Saunders, L. Altshuler, T. Goldberg, E. Armstrong, D. Weinberger and J. Kleinman 504
Postmortem brain morphology in schizophrenia: Studies from the new Düsseldorf brain collection
P. Falkai, B. Bogerts, S. David and B. Greve 507
Brain changes in schizophrenia and their meaning
T.J. Crow 511
The timing of morphological brain changes in schizophrenia: Do they progress?
L.E. DeLisi, P. Strizke, H. Riordan, V. Holan, M. Kushner, A. Boccio, O. van Eyl and A. Anand 515

Neurotransmitters in schizophrenia

Cholinergic activity and schizophrenic symptoms
R. Tandon, J. Greden, J. Shipley, N. Mann and W. Eisner 520
Experimental pharmacology in schizophrenia: Partial dopamine agonists
C.A. Tamminga, N.G. Cascella and R.R. Conley 523

Clinical pharmacology of clozapine
G.M. Simpson and J.B. Kessel 526

Serotonergic mechanisms in schizophrenia

Serotonergic receptor subsystems and their functional significance
R.W. Fuller 529
The MCPP challenge test in schizophrenia: Hormonal and behavioral responses
N. Iqbal, G.M. Asnis, S. Wetzler, R.S. Kahn, S.R. Kay and H.M. van Praag 532
5-HT_2 receptor antagonists in schizophrenia: Preclinical and clinical considerations
C.J.E. Niemegeers, F. Awouters, S.L.E. Heylen and Y.G. Gleders 535
5-HT_3 receptor antagonists: Preclinical and clinical considerations
B. Costall, A.M. Domeney, M.E. Kelly, R.J. Naylor and H.Y. Meltzer 538

Psychophysiological approaches to schizophrenia

Psychophysiological approaches to schizophrenia: Introduction and historical overview
C. Shagass 541
Computerized EEG in psychiatry
W. Günther, U. Klages, C. Haag, I. Bscheid and R. Riedel 544
Exploratory eye movements in schizophrenics: Comparison with temporal lobe epileptics and patients with frontal lobe lesions
T. Kojima, E. Matsushima, K. Nakajima, S. Ohbayashi, H. Ando, K. Ando and Y. Shimazono 547
Slow response-related negativities in chronic schizophrenics
R. Cohen, P. Berg and G. Hopmann 550

Modern trends in the treatment of chronic schizophrenia

Sertindole: A new concept in neuroleptic research
J. Hyttel 553
Depression in chronic schizophrenia
D.A.W. Johnson 556
Zuclopenthixol acetate and liquid oral haloperidol in the treatment of schizophrenic patients with acute exacerbation
G. Chouinard, G. Safadi and L. Beauclair 560
Zuclopenthixol decanoate versus haloperidol decanoate a could-blind comparative study
T. Koskinen, B. Wistedt and S. Thelander 563

Mechanism of action of atypical antipsychotic drugs

Dopamine modification and atypical neuroleptic properties
D.M. Coward, R. Markstein and A. Imperato 566
$5\text{-}HT_2$, $5\text{-}HT_{1C}$ and DA_2 receptors in the action of clozapine and other atypical antipsychotic drugs
H.Y. Meltzer and C.A. Stockmeier 570
Can the unique effect of clozapine on the functioning of midbrain dopamine neurons explain any of its special clinical properties?
B.S. Bunney 574
Amperozide, a putative antipsychotic drug with atypical properties
E. Christensson 577

Psychopathological side-effects of long-term administration of neuroleptics

CSF peptides and long-term neuroleptic treatment in schizophrenia: Effects of haloperidol withdrawal and relapse
D.P. van Kammen, J.L. Peters, D.T. O'Connor, J. Gelernter, R. Ekman, E. Widerlöv, A. Guidotti, J. Perel, M.E. Kelley, M. Beuger and J. Gurklis 580
Depressive symptoms in chronic schizophrenia: Clinical and pharmacological variables
C.A. Altamura, M.C. Mauri and P. Leva 583
Tardive dyskinesia: The long-term outcome
D.E. Casey 587
Subjective experiences of extrapyramidal side-effects in schizophrenia
S.R. Marder, T. van Putten, W.C. Wirshing, M. Aravagiri and T. Hicks-Gray 590
Side-effect profiles of atypical versus classical neuroleptics
J. Gerlach 593
Differential plasticity of dopamine receptors after pharmacological or functional deafferentation
P.F. Spano, M. Pizzi, A. Valerio, C. Missale and M. Memo 596

Tardive dyskinesia: Preclinical and clinical studies

Rodent models of tardive dyskinesia: Methodological considerations
G. Ellison 598
Continuous versus discontinuous neuroleptic treatment in an animal model of tardive dyskinesia
B. Glenthøj, T.G. Bolwig and R. Hemmingsen 602
Ultrastructural changes in rat CNS with typical and atypical neuroleptics
C.K. Meshul and D.E. Casey 605

D_1 dopamine hypothesis in tardive dyskinesia
J. Gerlach, L. Hansen and L. Peacock 609
Ageing and other determinants of baseline levels of spontaneous orofacial movement in rats during long-term neuroleptic treatment
J.L. Waddington 612
The reliability and significance of cognitive dysfunction in tardive dyskinesia
J.L. Waddington 615
Essential fatty and acids and α-tocopherol supplementation in tardive dyskinesia
K.S. Vaddadi 618
Nicotine and tardive dyskinesia
D.G. Kirch, L.L. Wing, R. Li and R.J. Wyatt 621
Diabetes mellitus and tardive dyskinesia
S. Mukheriee, R. Reddy and D.B. Schnur 624
The subjective awareness of movement disorders
P. Scapicchio, P. Decina and G. Caracci 628

STRESS, ANXIETY AND PERSONALITY DISORDERS: PATHOPHYSIOLOGY, BIOLOGY AND TREATMENT ISSUES

Post-traumatic stress disorder

A disorder of selective attention in post-traumatic stress disorder
A.C. McFarlane and C.R. Clark 635
Specific psychophysiological diagnosis in post-traumatic stress disorder
B. Raphael and D. Cumes-Rayner 639

Panic disorder: Controversies and consensus

Panic disorder: Diagnosis and course
R.M.A. Hirschfeld 646
The place of pharmacotherapy in the management of panic disorder
M. Roth 648

Biologic and therapeutic consideration in the long-term treatment of panic disorders

Cognitive therapy for panic disorder
M.G. Gelder, D.M. Clark and P. Anastasiades 654
Discontinuation and long-term follow-up of participants in a clinical drug trial for panic disorder
H. Katschnig, J.M. Stolk, G.L. Klerman, J.C. Ballenger, M. Amering, A. Briggs, R. Buller, G. Cassano, M. Garvey, M. Roth and C. Solyom 657

Rational pharmacotherapy in obsessive-compulsive disorders: From animal models to studies in man

What is obsessive-compulsive disorder: A review of the clinical syndrome
C.P. Freeman 661
Neurobiology of obsessive-compulsive disorder: A review
T.R. Insel and J.T. Winslow 664
Animal models of obsessive compulsive disorder
B. Olivier, M. Houben-Gelissen, J. Mos and G. van der Poel 668
Studies of fluvoxamine in OCD
C.J. McDougle and W.K. Goodman 671
How then should we treat OCD?
N. Fineberg, D.B. Montgomery and S.A. Montgomery 675

Clinical aspects of obsessive-compulsive disorder

Obsessive-compulsive disorder in different cultures: An Egyptian perspective
A. Okasha 677
Obsessive-compulsive related disorders
E. Hollander, D. Stein, C.M. Decaria, M. Frenkel, S. Trungold and M.R. Liebowitz 680

Imidazopyridines with selectivity for omega (BDZ) receptor subtypes: A novel approach in the pharmacotherapy of anxiety

Selectivity for ω-receptor subtypes as a strategy for a novel approach in the development of anxiolytic drugs
S.Z. Langer and S. Arbilla 683
Pharmacological and behavioural profile of alpidem as an anxiolytic
B. Zivkovic, G. Perrault and D.J. Sanger 686
Therapeutic activity of alpidem in anxious patients: An overview of European studies
M. Casacchia 689
Pharmacological treatment of anxiety in the elderly: New perspectives
P.L. Morselli 691
Anxiolytics and withdrawal signs: Comparatives studies of alpidem and benzodiazepines
M. Lader and S. Morton 693
Anxiolytic and dependence: Two double-blind studies of alpidem versus benzodiazepines
M. Garreau, J. de Wilde, L. Frattola, C. L'Heritier, P. Boval and P.L. Morselli 696

Benzodiazepine and the multiple forms of $GABA_A$ receptors

Independent cellular and ontogenetic expression of mRNAs encoding α polypeptides of the rat $GABA_A$ receptor
A.J. Tobin, K. Anderson, N. Brecha, M.-Y. Chiang, M. Khrestchatisky, M. Lai, A.J. MacLennan, R.W. Olsen, C. Sternini and N.J.K. Tillakaratne 699

^{3}H-propofol binding, a new tool to study the interaction of general anesthetics with the $GABA_A$ receptor complex
A. Concas, G. Santoro, M.P. Mascia and G. Biggio 702

Partial agonists at the benzodiazepine receptor

Pharmacology of partial agonists at the benzodiazepine receptor
W. Haefely 705

Clinical abuse liability of partial and full agonist benzodiazepines: A comparison of bretazenil, diazepam and alprazolam
E.M. Sellers, U. Busto and H.L. Kaplan 709

Attack-related treatment of panic disorder with bretazenil – A randomized placebo controlled clinical trial
H. Katschnig, W.A. Merz, P. Berger, D. Nutzinger, C. Alf, M. Kutzer and M. Amering 713

Pharmacological therapy of depression: Achievements and prospects
A. Delini-Stula 716

Beta carbolines: New trends in the treatment of anxiety disorders

Pharmacology of ß-carbolines
D.N. Stephens, M. Hillmann, R. Huba, H.H. Schneider, J.D. Turner and L. Turski 721

Abuse liability of benzodiazepine (BZ) receptor ligands: Abecarnil
N.A. Ator, R.R. Griffiths and C.A. Sannerud 724

Partial benzodiazepine agonists: New concepts in the treatment of panic disorder and schizophrenia
W. Merz 727

Problems in the diagnosis and treatment of anxiety disorders
M.H. Lader 732

Mitochondrial benzodiazepine receptors: Structure and function in CNS and peripheral organs

Gene structure and characterization of the mitochondrial benzodiazepine receptor
S.O. Casalotti, G. Pelaia, M. Whalin, D.R. Grayson and K.E. Krueger 735

Pharmacological, biochemical and endocrinological aspects of peripheral benzodiazepine receptors
M. Gavish 738
Hormone-stimulated steroidogenesis is coupled to mitochondrial benzodiazepine receptors
V. Papadopoulos 742
Molecular and functional characterization of peripheral-type benzodiazepine receptors in glial cells
K.E. Krueger and V. Papadopoulos 744
ω_3 (peripheral type benzodiazepine) binding sites as in vitro and in vivo markers of brain lesions
J. Benavides, S. Toulmond, P. Cornu and B. Scatton 747
Lymphocyte peripheral-type benzodiazepine receptors in neuropsychiatric diseases
L. Ravizza, P. Rocca and P. Ferrero 750

The rational use of benzodiazepines in the elderly

Neuropharmacology of benzodiazepines in aging
B. Vitiello and T. Sunderland 755
Relationship between anxiety and medical disorders
R.G. Kathol, T. Wald, R. Noyes and B. Carroll 757
Differential diagnosis of anxiety in later life
G.J. Maletta 761
Benzodiazepine treatment of late-life anxiety disorders
G.T. Grossberg 765

Benzodiazepines dependence

Patient characteristics in benzodiazepine abuse and therapeutic dependence
E.M. Sellers, U.E. Busto and M.K. Romach 767
Benzodiazepine abuse potential in normal and anxious individuals
H. de Wit and C.E. Johanson 771
Low-dose therapeutic benzodiazepine dependence: Are there differences between benzodiazepines?
M.H. Lader 775
Management of benzodiazepine discontinuation
K. Rickels, W.G. Case and E. Schweizer 778

HYPNOTICS AND SLEEP DISORDERS

Rhythm disorders and their novel treatment

Response of human sleep and melatonin secretion to changes in photoperiod: Implications for manic-depressive illness
T.A. Wehr 783
Delayed sleep phase syndrome: Clinical picture and treatment with light
N.E. Rosenthal, C.L. Cameron, S.H. Johnston, R.R. Joseph-Vanderpool, A.A. Levendosky and R. Allen 787
Resetting the sleep-wake cycle of schedule disorders and vitamin B_{12} treatment
T. Ohta, Y. Kayukawa, T. Okada, T. Iwata and M. Terashima 791
Vitamin B_{12} treatment for sleep-wake rhythm disorder
M. Okawa, K. Mishima, Y. Hishikawa and K. Takahashi 794

Clinical and biological issues of therapeutic sleep deprivation

Pathogenetic considerations on the antidepressant effect of sleep deprivation and the depressiogenic impact of daytime naps
M. Wiegand, D. Riemann and M. Berger 797
Therapeutic sleep deprivation and antidepressant medication
S. Kasper, S. Ruhrmann, G. Höflich and H.-J. Möller 800

Sleep EEG in depression and schizophrenia

REM sleep parameters and psychiatric diagnosis
C. Maggini, M. Guazzelli and A. Ciapparelli 804
Reduced REM latency in schizophrenia: Pathophysiological mechanisms
M.S. Keshavan, C.F. Reynolds, P. Houck and R. Ganguli 808
REM latency, eye movement density and slow wave sleep in schizophrenia and depression
K.L. Benson and V.P. Zarcone Jr. 811
REM latency in insomnia with depression
E.O. Bixler, A. Kales, A.N. Vgontzas, A. Vela-Bueno and R.L. Manfredi 814
Sleep EEG abnormalities in schizophrenia and depression are similar and not diagnostic of either condition
I. Feinberg 817

Recent studies on sleep wakefulness disorders and the hypnotic drug use

Insomnia: Biopsychosocial correlates
A. Kales 819

Macro- and micro-structure of sleep in insomniac patients under the influence of a benzodiazepine and a non-benzodiazepine hypnotic
H. Schulz, M. Jobert and P. Jähnig 823
Obstructive sleep apnea syndrome: Clinical, evolutive and epidemiological aspects
E. Lugaresi and E. Sforza 827
Oneiric behavior disorder in REM sleep without muscle atonia
Y. Hishikawa, T. Shimizu, N. Tachibana and Y. Sugita 831

Neurophysiological and sleep studies in aging and dementia

Effects of lecithin and physostigmine on REM sleep in Alzheimer's disease
H. Furuta, S. Yamamori, K. Nakagawa, Y. Maeda, N. Ishiguro, K. Ueno, J. Sano and N. Yamaguchi 833
Sleep-wake rhythm disorder and phototherapy in elderly patients with dementia
M. Okawa, Y. Hishikawa, S. Hozumi and H. Hori 837
Body temperature and sleep-wake rhythms of healthy elderly subjects
Y. Nakazawa, K. Nonaka, T. Kotorii, N. Uchimura and T. Sakamoto 841
Chronic insomnia in the elderly
G. Hajak, E. Rüther, A. Rodenbeck and V. Pudel 845
Longitudinal changes in REM sleep in Alzheimer's disease
C. Guilleminault, D. Bliwise and J.A. Yesavage 849
Information processing during sleep in brain damaged elderly
C. Cipolli and L. Murri 851

Hypnoselective imidazopyridins: A new generation of hypnotics

Rational approach to the treatment of insomnia
J.-M. Gaillard 854
Role of ω receptor subtypes in the action of hypnotic drugs
B. Zivkovic, S. Arbilla, D.J. Sanger, H. Depoortere, B. Scatton and S.Z. Langer 856
The therapeutic and safety profile of zolpidem
P. Attali and P.L. Morselli 860
Disturbances of cyclic alternating pattern in insomnia: Effect of hypnotics
M.G. Terzano and L. Parrino 863
Problems related to long-term use of hypnotics
J.M. Monti 867

Index of authors 871

Subject index 879

Diagnosis and classification

Biological Psychiatry, Volume 1. G. Racagni et al., editors.

Process and principles in the development of DSM IV

Harold Alan Pincus, Allen J. Frances, Nancy Sydnor-Greenberg, Wendy Davis, Michael First and Tom Widiger
Office of Research, American Psychiatric Association, 1400 K Street, N.W., Washington, D.C. 20005, U.S.A.

Introduction

There was a paradigm shift in DSM III toward descriptive psychiatric diagnosis meant to be neutral with regard to etiology and usable across theoretical orientations. Two methodological innovations explicit diagnostic criteria and the multiaxial system improved on the poor reliability achieved by previous systems and facilitated clinical communication and research. The manual has been widely used by clinicians, educators, trainees and researchers. DSM III was both a reflection of and a catalyst for the increased emphasis on empirical data in psychiatric practice and research.

In 1988, the board of trustees of the American Psychiatric Association (APA) appointed a task force to begin work on DSM IV. The major reason to begin work in preparation for DSM IV was the expected publication of the 10th edition of the *International Classification of Diseases* (ICD 10) in 1993. Early drafts of the Mental Disorders section of ICD 10 were quite different from that of ICD 10 and from DSM III-R. Since the United States is obliged to use ICD codes and since it is highly desirable to eliminate unnecessary differences between systems, it seemed crucial for the groups working on DSM IV and ICD 10 to have an opportunity for discussion and mutual influence. Indeed, the appointment of the task force on DSM IV was done with this in mind and repeated consultations have resulted in greatly increased compatibility between systems.

The most important result of this effort has been the simplification of the definitions in the ICD 10 short glossary to ensure that they are not overly specific and pseudo-precise. The success of this effort will make it easier for national systems of diagnosis to achieve code and construct equivalence with ICD 10, while allowing for those differences in the specific criteria that seem necessary and appropriate. The task force on DSM IV has also made many specific terminological and definitional suggestions which have been included in the ICD 10 clinical and research criteria.

Principles and methods of preparing DSM IV

The task force on DSM IV has 21 members, most of whom also chair a work group. There are 13 work groups, each of which is responsible for conducting a systematic empirical review that will result in the diagnostic criteria and accompanying text for a specific group of DSM IV disorders. Each work group draws on the expertise of between 50 and 100 advisors, including many international advisors. We also have an international advisory board, consisting of members drawn from around the world. The emphasis on empirical review and the large number and diversity of advisors is meant to establish an open process to ensure that DSM IV will be applicable in the wide variety of settings in which it will be used.

Work on the development of DSM IV has been divided into three separate steps. Initially each work group considered each of the diagnostic categories within its purview and agreed on a series of issues requiring review and resolution in DSM IV. Issues included problems with some aspect of the DSM III or the DSM III-R definitions, differences between the DSM system and the ICD 10, important developments in the research literature, input from clinical perspectives and other specific issues that had been identified by advisors. In the first step of empirical review, the work groups conducted 150 extensive literature reviews applying a uniform, systematic and detailed methodology. Initial drafts of literature reviews have been circulated to advisors for their comment. Suggestions and additional data that advisors share with members of the work groups are incorporated into the successive drafts of these literature reviews which will be published as the first volume of the *DSM IV Sourcebook* to document the empirical data on which decisions have been based.

While many issues have been satisfactorily answered by reviews of the available published literature, other questions have required the reanalysis (funded by the John D. and Catherine T. MacArthur Foundation) of previously collected, but unpublished or incompletely analyzed, data sets. For each issue, a variety of sites, including many international sites, have participated in the reanalysis of existing data sets.

There are some issues which cannot be completely resolved by literature reviews and unpublished data analysis. It is also important to test the implications of possible changes in DSM IV through field trials. We have selected 12 such issues which are the focus of field testing sponsored by the U.S. National Institute of Mental Health. These field trials will be the most carefully designed and monitored of any field trials conducted to date, with several of the field trials including extensive international participation. The field trials will compare DSM III, DSM III-R, ICD 10 research criteria, and proposed DSM IV criteria items in terms of their impact on reliability, prevalence, performance characteristics, and validity.

Issues and options

This process has resulted in the development of a range of options for resolution of the nosological questions identified by the work groups cutting across the following paradigmatic issues in each major category: adding or deleting categories; subtyping; revising criteria; and placement issues. These options are being made available in a *DSM IV Options Book*, which will be made immediately available to the field for comment. Work groups will use the results of the field trials and the data reanalyses along with recommendations from literature reviews and commentary from the field to make final decisions about DSM IV criteria.

We hope that this presentation will itself facilitate international communication and that many readers will write to us with their thoughts and suggestions on the issues raised and with their more specific concerns related to, or desire to participate in the development of, DSM IV. Readers interested in learning more about and participating in the process for developing DSM IV, in obtaining the Options Book, or in joining the mailing list for the twice yearly DSM IV Update should write to Harold Alan Pincus, M.D., American Psychiatric Association, 1400 K Street, N.W., Washington, D.C. 20005. Recent developments in psychiatric diagnoses have greatly contributed to international communication and have benefited from it. Our efforts on DSM IV are intended to further this process.

References

1. American Psychiatric Association, Committee on Nomenclature and Statistics (1987) Diagnostic and Statistical Manual of Mental Disorder, Revised. 3rd ed. American Psychiatric Association, Washington D.C.
2. Frances AJ, Widiger TA and Pincus HA (1989) Arch. Gen. Psychiatry 46: 373–375.
3. Frances AJ, Pincus HA, Widiger TA, Davis WW and First MB (1990) Am. J. Psychiatry 147: 11.

Biological Psychiatry, Volume 1. G. Racagni et al., editors.

Schizophrenia and other psychotic disorders in DSM IV

Nancy C. Andreasen
The University of Iowa, Department of Psychiatry, 500 Newton Road, Iowa City, IA 52242, U.S.A.

As with the other disorders to be included in DSM IV, the development of text and criteria for schizophrenia and other related disorders is following a 3-stage process: literature reviews in order to identify key issues and problems; analyses of existing data sets in order to partially address these issues and problems (funded by the McArthur Foundation); and the conduct of field trials to focus on specific issues that cannot be addressed by the previous 2 methods (funded by NIMH).

At present, literature reviews have been completed, and key areas of controversy have been identified. These include the following: boundary issues and breadth of the construct of schizophrenia; consonance with ICD 10; complexity of the algorithm used to define schizophrenia; reliability of symptoms; coverage of symptoms; emerging emphasis on negative symptoms; and the educational role of DSM [1–10].

Literature reviews have indicated that DSM III and III-R markedly narrowed the concept of schizophrenia, making it currently among the narrowest in the world. Its relationship to other systems needs further examination, particularly its relationship to ICD 10. ICD 10 is due to be published in 1993 and it will become the standard operational system throughout the world. It is important, therefore, to ensure that the DSM definition resembles the ICD definition as closely as possible. The literature reviews have also indicated a strong resurgence of interest in negative symptoms, suggesting that these should perhaps be given greater prominence in the DSM-IV definition of schizophrenia. In addition, some of the symptoms used to define schizophrenia appear to be somewhat unreliable. The concept of bizarre delusions, which plays a particularly important role in DSM III-R since it marks the boundary with paranoid disorders, may lack reliability. Because DSM plays an important educational role, often providing beginning students with their first introduction to the definition of mental illnesses, attention is also being given to evaluating the utility of the definition for teaching purposes. In this context, concerns have been raised about the algorithm used to define schizophrenia, since it tends to be very difficult to learn. In addition, concerns have been raised about coverage of symptoms, since the current definition places a strong emphasis on some symptoms that have a relatively low base rate (e.g. first-rank symptoms), while de-emphasizing symptoms that are especially common (e.g. negative symptoms).

One major difference between DSM III-R and ICD 10 is the duration criterion used to define schizophrenia. ICD 10 requires only 1 month of symptoms, but specifies that psychotic symptoms must be present during this duration, while III-R requires only 1 week of psychotic symptoms, but an overall duration of the syndrome for 6 months. DSM III-R includes the concept of prodromal and residual symptoms, while ICD does not. There are also several other differences between ICD 10 and DSM III-R. For example, ICD includes the construct of simple schizophrenia, groups non-psychotic spectrum conditions with schizophrenia (e.g. schizotypal disorder) and includes several types of reactive psychoses of short duration.

McArthur analyses completed to date have raised additional issues or provided some support for concerns suggested by the literature reviews. For example, McArthur analyses have indicated that both bizarre delusions and first-rank symptoms tend to be more unreliable than simpler constructs (persecutory delusions, auditory hallucinations, etc.). They have also indicated that negative symptoms are common in both first-episode and chronic patients and that negative symptoms in fact tend to have a higher base rate than positive symptoms of psychosis. Catatonic symptoms appear to be quite rare. These results have suggested the importance of re-evaluating the symptoms that are included in the DSM III-R A criterion.

Based on this work, a decision was made to compare 5 alternative approaches to defining schizophrenia in the field trials. These include: ICD 10, DSM III, and III-R; Option 1 (minor modifications of III-R); Option 2 (a new definition that includes a 1-month duration criterion and symptoms and algorithms similar to those used in III-R and ICD 10); and Option 3 (a 1-month duration criterion, simplified symptoms and definitional algorithm). These alternative definitions are currently being explored in field trials in 7 sites: Arkansas, Columbia, Long Island – Hillside Jewish Hospital, University of Virginia, Yale, University of Iowa, and Harvard. A total of 350 patients will be evaluated in these sites, with more than two-thirds being included in reliability studies. Data from field trials will be used to make decisions about the final criteria and classification system for DSM IV. Criteria that will be used to assess field trial data include diagnostic reliability, item reliability, base rate, caseness, and user-friendliness. Because of the importance of maintaining continuity with existing research and clinical data, the DSM IV definition will emphasize maintaining similar boundaries to those that currently exist in III-R. Within the constraint of maintaining a conservative approach to caseness, approaches that have improved reliability, symptoms with high base rate and user-friendliness will be considered to be more desirable.

References

1. Amador XF, Strauss DH, Yale SA and Gorman JM (1991) Schizophr. Bull. 17: 113–132.
2. Andreasen NC and Flaum M (1991) Schizophr. Bull. 17: 27–49.
3. Flaum M and Andreasen NC (1991) Schizophr. Bull. 17: 133–142.
4. Kane JM and Selzer J (1991) Schizophr. Bull. 17: 69–73.

5. Keith SJ and Matthews SM (1991) Schizophr. Bull. 17: 51–67.
6. Siris SG (1991) Schizophr. Bull. 17: 75–98.
7. Szymanski S, Kane JM and Lieberman JA (1991) Schizophr. Bull. 17: 99–111.
8. American Psychiatric Association (1980) DSM III: Diagnostic and Statistical Manual of Mental Disorders, 3rd Edition. The Psychiatric Association, Washington D.C.
9. American Psychiatric Association (1987) DSM III-R: Diagnostic and Statistical Manual of Mental Disorders, 3rd Edition, Revised. The Psychiatric Association, Washington D.C.
10. World Health Organization (1973) The International Pilot Study of Schizophrenia. WHO, Geneva.

Biological Psychiatry, Volume 1. G. Racagni et al., editors.

DSM IV mood disorders

A. John Rush

Mental Health Clinical Research Center and Department of Psychiatry, University of Texas Southwestern Medical Center, 5323 Harry Hines Blvd., Dallas, TX 75235, U.S.A.

The Diagnostic and Statistical Manual of Mental Disorders, Fourth Edition (DSM IV) [1]: Work Group on Mood Disorders (Chaired by A. John Rush, M.D.) includes David Dunner, M.D., Ellen Frank, Ph.D., Martin Keller, M.D. and Donald F. Klein, M.D. Various options for DSM IV are currently under consideration.

The major DSM III-R [2] categorical divisions will be retained. These include bipolar disorder, cyclothymia, bipolar disorder, not otherwise specified (NOS), major depression, dysthymia and depression, NOS. Organic mood disorders will likely be renamed secondary mood disorders and moved into the mood disorders section in order to facilitate clinical use.

Bipolar disorder may be further divided into bipolar I (recurrent episodes of mania, with or without hypomania, and major depression) and bipolar II (recurrent hypomania and major depressive episodes but without manic episodes). As an alternative, bipolar II may be listed as major depression, recurrent with hypomanic episodes. DSM III-R criteria for bipolar I disorder will be retained, except that a minimal time period for a manic episode (e.g. seven days) may be added.

Course modifiers for bipolar I and II disorder would include “with seasonal pattern” (as phototherapy may be indicated), “with postpartum onset,” as this may be the first clue to an ultimate bipolar disorder and such postpartum episodes likely repeat in subsequent postpartum periods and “rapid cycling pattern,” which may have prognostic and treatment selection implications. A course modifier to designate either antecedent and/or inter-episode symptoms may be considered, as antecedent symptomatology may predict subsequent inter-episode recovery and the level of residual inter-episode symptomatology may have prognostic value.

Bipolar I disorder, mixed phase may require revision if a “rapid cycling” course modifier is adopted. “Mixed phase” refers both to patients who switch quickly between short, severe depressive and manic poles without euthymic intervals, and those who meet criteria for both manic and major depressive episodes simultaneously without clear-cut polarity shifts. If both “rapid cycling” and the duration criterion for a manic episode are adopted, “mixed phase” would refer only to the case of simultaneous presentation of both manic and major depressive symptoms.

Major depression will continue to be designated as single or recurrent. There are no symptom or duration criteria changes planned for major depression, except that the mood item may be expanded to include irritability. An ongoing field trial to evaluate the reliability of diagnosing dysthymia and major depression may lead to a higher symptom number threshold (e.g. 6 or 7 of the 9 DSM III-R criterion symptoms to diagnose a major depressive episode) compared to the DSM III-R requirement of 5 of the 9 criterion symptoms.

Psychotic, melancholic or atypical symptom feature modifiers can be specified for major depressive episodes seen in the course of either bipolar I or II or major depressive disorder, as treatment selection is particularly affected by some of these feature modifiers. Psychotic features have treatment selection and prognostic implications. In addition, major depression with psychotic features appears to be familial and associated with marked laboratory abnormalities. Melancholic features will likely be retained, as they usefully predict ECT response and predict tricyclic response in some but not all studies. The definition of melancholic criteria may return to DSM III [3] or continue with DSM III-R.

The "atypical symptom features" modifier designates the weight gaining, over-eating, oversleeping depressed patients who may also demonstrate interpersonal rejection sensitivity, and a feeling of leadened weight or paralysis in their limbs, but who continue to demonstrate mood reactivity. This modifier may apply to major depression, bipolar disorder, depressed phase and dysthymia. The possible inclusion of atypical symptom features is based on the suggestion that such patients may respond better to monoamine oxidase inhibitors (MAOIs) than to tricyclic antidepressants, although both medications appear more effective than placebo in this group.

For major depression, "with seasonal pattern," "with postpartum onset," and "with antecedent/inter-episode symptoms" course modifiers may be allowed.

Dysthymic disorder may be narrowed so that if major depressive episodes occur in the course of a chronic "dysthymic level" of symptoms, then major depression with antecedent dysthymia could be diagnosed.

Depression, NOS, may be expanded by either text examples or by additional categories to include minor depression, recurrent brief depression and mixed anxiety/depression. Minor depression presents with symptoms of major depression and other symptoms that are not strictly part of major depression, that come and go over time, but which are present for at least two weeks at a time. Recurrent, brief depression features recurrent (6–10 times/year), brief (3–7 days) episodes that meet full symptomatic but not duration criteria for major depression). Mixed anxiety/depression is characterized by both depressive and anxious symptoms, neither of which meet criteria for any other formal mood or anxiety disorder.

Other mood disorder syndromes include those caused by Axis III disorders (secondary mood disorders), and those induced by intoxication or withdrawal from substances of abuse or by medication (substance-induced mood disorders). Both will be listed with the etiologic agent to be specified.

The views expressed in this article are those of the authors and do not represent the official positions of the DSM IV Task Force or the American Psychiatric Association.

Acknowledgements

The author would like to express his appreciation to David Savage for secretarial assistance and to Kenneth Z. Altshuler, M.D., Professor and Chairman, for his administrative support. Preparation of this report was supported in part by a Mental Health Clinical Research Center Grant (MH-41115) to the Department of Psychiatry, University of Texas Southwestern Medical Center at Dallas.

References

1. American Psychiatric Association (1980) Diagnostic and Statistical Manual of Mental Disorders, Third Edition (DSM III). American Psychiatric Association.
2. American Psychiatric Association (1987) Diagnostic and Statistical Manual of Mental Disorders, Third Edition-Revised (DSM III-R). American Psychiatric Association.
3. American Psychiatric Association (in preparation) Diagnostic and Statistical Manual of Mental Disorders, Fourth Edition (DSM IV). American Psychiatric Association.

Biological Psychiatry, Volume 1. G. Racagni et al., editors.

Psychopharmacology and the classification of depressive disorders

Adriana Dubini
Farmitalia Carlo Erba R & D, CNS Department, Via Imbonati 24, 20159 Milan, Italy

Introduction

Depressive disorders are recognised to be undoubtedly heterogeneous in terms of response to treatment [1].

Response to pharmacologic agents, used either as a challenge or as a treatment, has been extensively explored, trying to identify subgroups of patients with a common response, which then could be employed to classify the disorders. Final goal of this type of research is to find leads to underlying mechanisms [2], or empirical criteria of predictive significance [3].

The present overview will be restricted to the investigations carried out evaluating response in terms of modification of clinical symptoms: modification of biochemical or neurophysiological parameters will be discussed by other authors during the symposium.

Within this frame of reference, classification implies the description of a "responder" group to drug treatment, by difference in comparison with non-responders, or by characterizing different subgroups in terms of responsiveness. The aim of this overview is to look at the field in search for possible hints useful for psychopharmacological research.

However, there is considerable difficulty in deriving meaningful results in such research, because of the different experimental conditions and study designs (well reviewed in [2–5]): first of all, admission criteria, particularly diagnostic criteria and their reportedly non-uniform application [6,7]. In addition, of obvious relevance is the source of variability deriving from the factors known to bear an influence on response, or lack of response: pharmacokinetics [8], inadequate dosage [9] or treatment duration [10], spontaneous remission, placebo response [11] and the definition of response itself (response vs. remission vs. recovery) [12]. As to the latter aspects, usefulness of a concurrent treatment with placebo is suggested as negative control [3], response pattern analysis [13] being probably more useful than end treatment analysis to identify true drug response.

Response to pharmacologic challenge

The proposed differential mood response to short-term administration of stimulant drugs, usually amphetamine, has been consistently verified in the studies carried out with similar experimental procedure [14]. Mood brightening has been consistently reported to identify imipramine and desipramine responders [15], whereas a dysphoric or no response has been associated with subsequent therapeutic response to amitriptyline [16] and nortriptyline [17]. Differential response to different antidepressant has been recently challenged [14]. In any case the initially-derived implications in terms of classification, i.e. the proposed "noradrenergic" vs. "serotoninergic" depression, appear little supported. On the other hand, selectivity of presynaptic action of uptake inhibitors has been demonstrated to be of limited relevance, when their long-term effects and interactions at the receptor level are considered [19,20].

The differential anxiogenic response to lactate infusion and fenfluramine administration has been reported to differentiate major depressive disorders (MDD) with history of panic attacks from MDD with negative history, thus identifying a subgroup within MDD. Possible implications in terms of treatment strategies are questionable [21].

Clinical response to antidepressant drug treatment

Has clinical response to antidepressant drugs been shown to identify homogeneous subgroups of patients? The matter has been dealt with in most of the available recent reviews [3–5] in the opposite way: do existing nosological categories identify subpopulations differentially responsive to treatment?

The bipolar depression category is reported to be particularly responsive to lithium [22,23] and to bromocriptine [24] than the unipolar category. On the other hand, possible differential response of the unipolar vs. bipolar depression to monoamine oxidase inhibitors and to monoamine uptake inhibitors has not been adequately studied: therefore the homogeneity of the bipolar category is supported, but no link between the pharmacological activity of antidepressants and the pathological process behind the disorder is possible.

The atypical depression category – not homogeneously defined by the different groups, but generally characterized by presence of mood reactivity, reverse functional shift and hysteroid features [25], suggested to include distinctive forms of personality disorders [26] – has been reported to be more frequently responsive to MAOIs than to tricyclics. Longitudinal studies have found consistency of response to either MAOIs or tricyclics within patients and family members [27]. Also in the case of the most extreme results [25], the extent of the overlap between tricyclic and MAOI response makes it very difficult to hypothesize working models relating differences to pharmacological mechanisms.

The depression with psychotic features category has been reported by several authors to be associated with poor response to tricyclics [e.g. 28], particularly in the elderly [29], though the severity of the disorder [30] and the consequent need of adequate therapy in terms of doses and treatment duration [31] could represent the key issue. Increased likelihood of response to the combined antipsychotic/antidepressant therapy of up to 80% is reported [29], the mechanism of which (pharmacokinetic and/or pharmacodynamic interaction, additive vs. synergistic) has not been elucidated. Implications for psychopharmacology are therefore difficult to define.

The non-psychotic, non-bipolar major depression appears to be the most heterogeneous in terms of drug response. Conflicting results have been reported when endogeneity has been considered, either in favour [32] or not [33] of the hypothesis of higher response to tricyclics, possibly connected with the positive correlation between endogeneity and severity. Endogenomorphic depressives were also separated as a more responsive population from a therapeutically less responsive one (dysthymic or disappointment reactions) [34]. As to symptom profiles, a cluster analytic method [32] allowed differentiation of anxious depressives, depressives characterized by "hostility" and "self-pity" and depressives with associated personality disorders as groups with lower response to amitriptyline than the classical endogenous ones. In an extensive review [35], the "retarded anhedonic" has been differentiated from the "agitated delusional" endogenous depression, with a strong association of retardation and a moderate association of loss of interest/emotional withdrawal with tricyclic response. Published data are often difficult to reconcile: in any case, differences in treatment response/non-response are minor; therefore, of difficult pharmacological interpretation.

The chronic depression category is obviously very heterogeneous, being "a priori" described only by course. Treatment response has been initially suggested to be lower with respect to acute depressions, though difference in outcome vs. placebo is similar to the acute conditions when the early onset cases are considered [5]. Treatment resistant depression, when properly identified, could be the most interesting in terms of pharmacological implications [36]. Instead the only indication deriving from literature is related to evidence, mainly anecdotal, on the increased likelihood of response with combination therapies (TCA/MAOI, TCA/lithium, TCA/T3, TCA or MAOI/stimulant, TCA or MAOI/L-tryptophan) [5], compatible with either higher efficiency of a multiple site of action toward the same end-point or with the permissive effect at one site of action in the cascade of events linked with antidepressant efficacy.

Comment

Treatment response per se does not seem to identify homogeneous subpopulations within depressive illness. These negative findings could be related to the absence of a link between the pharmacological activities of available antidepressant agents and the clinical entities they are expected to modify. If this is the case, either unspecificity of the mechanism of action of these molecules, or specificity with respect to psychological dysfunctions [37], not to disease entities, should be envisaged. Alternatively the negative findings could be related to the scarce discriminative power of the nosological instruments adopted. In the latter case, the clinical prerequisite [1] has to be faced. In any case, proper models have to be tested with proper methodology, if we wish to understand the relevance of the specific pharmacological activities of the supposedly effective antidepressant compounds presently under development and provide the "psychopharmacology in transition" [38] of these years with this piece of information.

References

1. Ban T (1987) Prog. Neuro-Psychopharmacol. Biol. Psychiatry 11: 527–580.
2. Insel TR and Murphy DL (1984) In: Post RM, Ballenger JC (eds.) Neurobiology of Mood Disorders. Williams & Wilkins, Baltimore, pp. 854–865.
3. Joyce PR and Paykel ES (1989) Arch. Gen. Psychiatry 46: 89–99.
4. Brotman AW, Falk WE and Gelenberg AJ (1987) In: Meltzer HY (ed.) Psychopharmacology: the Third Generation of Progress. Raven Press, New York, pp. 1031–1040.
5. Kocsis JH (1990) Psychopharmacol. Bull. 26: 49–53.
6. Hirschfeld RMA and Cross CR (1987) In: Meltzer HY (ed.) Psychopharmacology: the Third Generation of Progress. Raven Press, New York, pp. 1021–1029.
7. Zimmerman M, Coryell WH and Black DW (1990) Am. J. Psychiatry 147: 1173–1179.
8. Preskorn SH and Mac DS (1984) Psychiatr. Dev. 3: 201–222.
9. Lydiard RR (1985) J. Clin. Psychiatry 46: 412–417.
10. Quitkin FM, Rabkin JG, Ross D and McGrath PG (1984) Arch. Gen. Psychiatry 41: 238–245.
11. Edwards JG (1989) Human Psychopharmacol. 4: 235–236.
12. Montgomery SA (1990) In: Hindmarch I and Stonier PD (eds.) Human Psychopharmacology. Measures and Methods, Vol. 1. John Wiley and Sons, pp. 73–87.
13. Quitkin FM, Rabkin JD, Markowitz JM, Steward JW, McGrath PJ and Harrison W (1987) Arch. Gen. Psychiatry 44: 259–264.
14. Goff DC (1986) J. Clin. Psychiatry 47: 538–543.
15. Fawcett J and Siomopoulos V (1971) Arch. Gen. Psychiatry 25: 247–255.
16. Brown P and Brawley P (1983) Am. J. Psychiatry 140: 990–993.
17. Sabelli HC, Fawcett J, Javaid JJ and Bagri S (1983) Am. J. Psychiatry 140: 212–214.
18. Kravitz HM, Edwards JH, Fawcett J and Fogg L (1990) J. Affective Disord. 20: 121–128.
19. Brunello N, Barbaccia ML, Chuang DM and Costa E (1982) Neuropharmacology 21: 1145–1149.
20. Tassin JP (1986) Psychiatr. & Psychobiol. 1: 62–72.
21. Targum SD (1990) Biol. Psychiatry 28: 21–34.
22. Goodwin FK, Myrphy DL, Dunner DL and Bunney WE (1972) Am. J. Psychiatry 129: 44–47.
23. Carroll BJ (1979) Arch. Gen. Psychiatry 36: 870–878.
24. Silverstone T (1984) Lancet i: 903–904.
25. Quitkin FM, McGrath PJ, Stewart JW, Harrison W, Tricamo E, Wager SG, Ocepek-Welikson K, Nunes E, Rabkin JG and Klein DF (1990) Arch. Gen. Psychiatry 47: 935–941.
26. Roth SM and Mountjoy CQ (1990) Drugs Today 26: 315–328.
27. Pare CMB and Mack JW (1971) J. Med. Genet. 8: 306–309.
28. Spiker DG, Weiss JC, Dealy RS, Griffin SJ, Hanin I, Neil JF, Perel JM, Rossi AJ and Soloff PH (1985) Am. J. Psychiatry 142: 430–436.
29. Baldwin RC (1988) Br. Psychiatry 152: 39–44.
30. Kocsis JH, Croughan JL, Katz MM, Butler TP, Secunda S, Bowden CL and Davis JM (1985) Arch. Gen. Psychiatry 42: 1145–1147.
32. Paykel ES (1972) Br. J. Psychiatry 120: 147–156.
33. Simpson GM, Lee HL, Cuche Z and Kellner R (1976) Arch. Gen. Psychiatry 33: 1093–1102.
34. Guy W, Ban TA and Shaffer JD (1982) In: Barrett JE and Clayton P (eds.) Treatment of Depression: Old Controversies and New Approaches. Raven Press, New York.

35. Nelson JC, Charney DS and Quinlan DM (1981) Arch. Gen. Psychiatry 38: 555–559.
36. Garattini S (1988) Br. J. Psychiatry 152: 140–141.
37. Van Praag HM, Kahn RS, Asnis GM, Wetzler S, Brown SL, Bleich A and Korn ML (1988) In: Briley M and Fillion G (eds.) New Concepts in Depression (Pierre Fabre Monograph Series, Vol. 2). Macmillian Press, pp. 96–119.
38. Sulser F (1989) Hum. Psychopharmacol. 4: 1–2.

Biological Psychiatry, Volume 1. G. Racagni et al., editors.

Biological markers in nosology

Bernard J. Carroll

Department of Psychiatry, Box 3414, Duke University Medical Center, Durham, NC 27710, U.S.A.

Current classifications of depressive subtypes are based solely on clinical features (e.g. DSM III). Evidence of the validity of DSM III melancholia vis-à-vis alternative definitions is lacking and the reliability (Kappa) coefficients for these diagnoses are only modest (about 0.6). Even the clinical features used in the diagnostic algorithms show weak individual discriminating power [1]. Because of these problems in the "gold standard", biologic markers and other external validators in nosology will often appear weaker than they really are, and their potential contributions may be overlooked. Three strategies are recommended to assist progress in this area.

The iterative strategy

Only an iterative approach can establish the value of laboratory measures. By alternately regarding the clinical diagnosis as the independent, then the dependent variable in relation to other data, can our nosology be refined. A good example of this strategy is the genetic study of Pauls et al. [2], which concluded that Tourette's syndrome, multiple tics and obsessive-compulsive personality disorder are equivalent manifestations of a genetic diathesis within affected pedigrees even though the three conditions would be regarded as quite separate by strict (clinical) nosologic constructionists.

The triangulation strategy

In the iterative strategy discussed above, the clinical classifications are evaluated with reference to a single putative external validator (natural history, genetics, specific treatment response or biologic marker). The triangulation strategy takes this approach a step further by employing two putative external validators simultaneously. An example of this approach with the dexamethasone suppression test [DST] has been described [1]. Abnormal DSTs associate significantly with ICD 9 rather than DSM III-defined endogenous major depression, and also the cases with abnormal DST results have a very low rate (< 5%) of response to treatment with placebo. In contrast, the cases with normal DST results have over a 50% rate of response to placebo. In this example the placebo-controlled treatment outcome data add a new dimension to the clinical classification-neuroendocrine test association. In the eventual development of construct validity additional convergent evidence is sought, e.g. persistent abnormal DSTs predict poor prognosis and apparently false-positive DSTs may predict diagnostic change on blind follow-up [3,4].

Combining clinical and laboratory features

Laboratory markers do not have to stand alone but can be combined with clinical signs or symptoms in new diagnostic algorithms for depressive subtypes. Indeed, there is now evidence that laboratory measures like the DST are superior in discriminating power to any of the individual clinical features used in DSM III or the Newcastle I Index for the endogenous-non-endogenous distinction [1].

A good model of this process can be found in the diagnostic criteria of the American Rheumatism Association (ARA) for systemic lupus erythematosus (SLE). Like Kraepelin's manic-depressive disorder, SLE is a pleomorphic condition with variable clinical manifestations and a moderately large degree of unreliability for the clinical diagnosis. In 1971 the ARA proposed *clinical* criteria for the diagnosis [5] even though "it was apparent ... that newer laboratory data such as antinuclear antibodies and complement would (sooner or later) have to be considered for inclusion" [6]. The updated criteria were published in 1982 [7]. According to the new criteria, 11 possible groups of signs or symptoms are included, of which 7 are traditional clinical features and 4 are laboratory data. Only four of the eleven criteria are required for a diagnosis of SLE to be made. Thus, the ARA has moved from a purely clinical set of criteria to a mixed set of clinical and laboratory criteria. Data-based studies of putative biologic markers of endogenous depression, comparing their performance to standard clinical features, are now required.

References

1. Carroll BJ (1989) In: Robins LN and Barrett JE (eds.) The Validity of Psychiatric Diagnosis. Raven Press, New York, pp. 229–245.
2. Pauls DL, Towbin KE, Leckman JF et al. (1986) Arch. Gen. Psychiatry 43: 1180–1182.
3. Coryell W (1990) J. Affective Disord. 19: 163–169.
4. Coryell W, Zimmerman M, Winokur G and Cadoret R (1988) Eur. Arch. Psychiatry Neurol. Sci. 237: 197–199.
5. Cohen AS, Reynolds WE, Franklin EC et al. (1971) Bull. Rheum. Dis. 21: 643–648.
6. Cohen AS (1982) Current Contents/Clinical Practice 10(11): 24.
7. Garfield E (1989) Current Contents/Life Sciences 32(2): 3–8.

Biological Psychiatry, Volume 1. G. Racagni et al., editors.

Distribution of morbidity risks in unipolar and bipolar mood disorders

B. Smeraldi and M. Gasperini
Milan, Italy

In aggregation studies of mood disorders polarity was focused upon as a possible criterion for identifying homogeneous groups of the disease and according to 2 alternative hypotheses, unipolar (UP) and bipolar (BP) forms could represent different degrees of severity of the same disorder or discrete entities. BP and UP subjects showed different levels of familial load as measured by more or less morbidity risks (MR) in their first and second degree relatives [1–4].

Homotypical transmission for secondary cases in BP and UP was not found but the variability of age at onset [5] and the instability of the diagnosis of polarity did not allow any conclusive finding to be reached.

The outcome of pharmacological treatments seemed to be useful to identify homogeneous subgroups of affective disease, since poor responders on lithium and tricyclics showed different segregation patterns in families when compared to good responders [6]. Nevertheless, the distinction was not yet sufficiently unequivocal, even for the complexity in defining the correct criteria to strictly identify biological parameters of non-responsiveness.

A segregation analysis of familial data on mood subjects divided into responder/ non-responders on tricyclics and with and without coexisting Axis II disorders confirmed that the presence of personality disorder (PD) conditions the differential model of transmission with more severe susceptibility and penetrance [7]. The hypothesis that personality disorders could be included as subclinical manifestations in the liability spectrum of mood disorders has been suggested, especially for BDL PD [8–12].

BDL PD is strongly associated in affective disorder patients and when it is co-present in subjects with mood disorders appears to add severity in the familial risks for mood illness. In addition, BDL PD without mood disorder is reported to have MR for affective illness which are not significantly different from those of mood disorders. This occurred independently of the presence of histrionic and narcissistic associated PD [13]. This study sample included 139 mood subjects (81 female and 48 male): 89 with major depression (77 recurrent, 12 single episodes) and 50 with bipolar disorders, all referred to our in- outpatient unit.

All subjects were diagnosed on Axis II using SIDP-R [14]. The distribution of PD was not significantly different according to polarity and sex. The more frequent were the histrionic and dependent PD (30%). The mean ± S.D. age of BP vs. UP

Table 1. Late and early onset unipolar personality profile according to canonical discriminant function

Early onset	Late onset
PARA1	SCHIZOID6
PARA2	HIST8
PARA5[a]	DEPN2
COMP7[a]	DEPN6
HIST1[a]	MAS4
HIST2[a]	
HIST4[a]	
DEPN3[b]	
DEPN9	
BDL2[b]	
BDL6[a]	
NARC1	
NARC5	
NARC8[a]	
AVOI5[b]	
PASS-AGGR3[b]	

[a] $P = 0.03$; [b] $P = 0.0001$.

overlapped (40.9 ± 13.07 vs. 42.7 ± 12.6) as did their mean ± S.D. age of onset (30.96 ± 10.67 vs. 33.6 ± 12.4).

We revised the MR for secondary cases of affective illness in first degree relatives of our patients, estimating the 2 separate rates for UP and BP forms. We considered affected the relatives with a diagnosis of major depression and dysthymic disorders and bipolar and cyclothymic disorders. Data for unaffected relatives were age-corrected [15]. The overall risks of UP and BP were 21.4% and 36.4% in UP and BP ($P = 0.006$). More specifically, UP and BP subjects did not significantly differ in their risk for UP disease (24.9% vs. 25.9%) but their risks for BP disorder were significantly different (1.4% vs. 10.5%, $P = 0.0001$). These findings confirmed marked homotypical components for the disorder transmission.

Any of the specific PD except the BDL did not condition higher risks for the disease. BDL UP vs. BP without and with BDL PD showed increasing risks for bipolar illness (3% vs. 9.2% vs. 29% N.S.) which were higher than non-BDL UP. The bimodal distribution of age of onset in UP patients appeared to identify at least 2 separate groups of subjects, one with early and another with late mode of onset. However, the age at onset in BP subjects was normally distributed.

BDL PD subjects in our sample had a younger age at onset both in the group of UP and BP subjects. Nevertheless, BDL PD accounted for 10% and 14.6% in BP and UP subjects; thus we realized that the presence of BDL PD could not explain per se earlier age at onset in the unipolar group.

In addition, BDL traits and disorders are often accompanied by traits and disorders also different from cluster B. In the aim of better characterizing the 2 unipolar groups we tentatively applied to their personality traits a discriminant analysis [16] using early (less than 25) and late (more than 26) onset criterion as group variable.

We tested 60 personality traits selected for their higher frequency (cut-off: 15%). We obtained a high degree of separation, as indicated by the final Wilk's lambda (0.34) and canonical correlation (0.81) for the discriminant function. The discriminant analysis provided a satisfactory proportion of correct classification (92.1%) for UP subjects in the 2 onset classes.

According to the size of their correlation within the canonical function, 22 personality traits were selected in the analysis, 9 of them being significantly higher in the early vs. late onset UP group and not different from those of the bipolar subjects (Table 1).

We supposed the first unipolar group with early age of onset could share with BP subjects higher rates of MR in agreement with previous reports [17].

Early UP had identical overall risks when compared to BP subjects and significantly different from that of late onset UP group ($P = 0.02$). This latter group was also significantly different from the bipolars ($P = 0.02$). Specific MR for bipolar forms accounted for 10% and 6.6% of the risks in the early and late onset unipolar groups. That was much more higher (50% and 24%) in the 2 groups of bipolar patients, suggesting some as yet unexplained heterogeneity.

In conclusion, even if only segregation analyses and then recombinant DNA studies could clarify the problem of the differential pathogenesis of UP and BP, we suggest that both personality and early onset are important contributing factors in the susceptibility to mood disorders.

References

1. Nurnberger JI and Gershon ES (1982) In: Paykel ES (ed.) Handbook of Affective Disorders. Churchill Livingstone, Edinburgh, pp. 126–145.
2. Reich T, Rice J and Von Eerdewegh P (1986) The Familial Association of Bipolar and Non-Bipolar Affective Disorders. National Institute of Mental Health Workshop on Family and Genetic Studies of Affective Disorders, Bethesda, MD.
3. McGuffin P and Katz MM (1986) Nature, Nurture and Affective Disorders. In: Deakin JFW (ed.) The Biology of Affective Disorders. Royal College of Psychiatrists, Gaskell Press, London.
4. Gershon ES, Hamovit J, Guroff JJ, Dibble E, Leckman JF, Sceery W, Targum SD et al. (1982) Arch. Gen. Psychiatry 39: 1157–1167.
5. Smeraldi E, Gasperini M, Macciardi F, Bussoleni C and Morabito A (1983) J. Psychiatr. Res. 17(3): 304–317.
6. Orsini A (1986) In: Racagni G and Smeraldi E (eds.) Antidepressant Responses and Segregation Analyses in Affective Families. Workshop on Anxious Depression: Assessment and Treatment. Raven Press, New York.
7. Smeraldi E, Gasperini M, Macciardi F, Orsini A, Provenza M and Sciuto G (1987) Segregation Analysis in Families of Affective Patients Subdivided According to Treatment Outcome and Personality Disorders. In: Lerer B and Gershon S (eds.) New Directions in Affective Disorders. Springer-Verlag, New York.
8. Gasperini M and Provenza M (1986) The Relationship between Affective Illness and Personality Disorders: Preliminary Reports. In: Racagni G and Smeraldi I (eds.) Anxious Depression Assessment and Treatment. Raven Press, New York.

9. Baron M, Gruen R, Asnis L et al. (1985) Am. J. Psychiatry 142: 827–834.
10. Gunderson JG and Eliot GR (1985) Am. J. Psychiatry 142: 277–288.
11. Loranger AW, Oldham JM and Tulis EH (1982) Arch. Gen. Psychiatry 39: 785–798.
12. Pope HG Jr, Jonas JM, Hudson JI et al. (1983) Arch. Gen. Psychiatry 40: 23–30.
13. Gasperini M, Battaglia M, Scherillo P, Sciuto G, Diaferia G and Bellodi L (1991) J. Affective Disord. 21: 265–272.
14. Pfohl B, Blum N, Zimmerman M et al. (1989) Structured Interview for DSM III-R Personality. SIDP-R. The University of Iowa, Iowa City.
15. Crowe RR and Smouse PE (1979) J. Psychiatr. Res. 13: 273–285.
16. Klecka WR (1975). Discriminant Analysis. In: Nie NH, Hull CH, Jenkinson JG, Steinbrenner K and Bent DH (eds.) Statistical Package for the Social Sciences (SPSS), 2nd edition. McGraw Hill.
17. Weissmann MM, Gershon ES, Kidd KK et al. (1984) Arch. Gen. Psychiatry 41: 13–21.

Biological Psychiatry, Volume 1. G. Racagni et al., editors.

Classification of depression: From biology to functional psychopathology

Herman M. van Praag

Albert Einstein College of Medicine/Montefiore Medical Center, Department of Psychiatry, New York, NY 10467, U.S.A.

How to systematize psychopathology for biological psychiatric research

Biological psychiatry studies the interrelation between brain dysfunctions and abnormal behavior and the means to correct abnormal behavior via direct interference in the brain. What is the most sensible way to systematize abnormal behavior in order to study its biological roots? The most obvious and most current conceptual framework is the nosological. Within that frame of reference psychiatric disorders are conceived as discrete entities, each with their own typical symptomatology, causation, treatment and prognosis. The search is for biological markers and eventually causes of a disease entity, such as schizophrenia, major depression or panic disorder. If a biological variable does not significantly correlate with a particular disease entity, it is (dis-)qualified as non-specific.

From its very beginnings nosology has been biological psychiatry's major lead. This comes as no surprise. Its first heyday was in the second part of the 19th century and (neuro-) pathology was its major partner at the time. Pathology had provided major building blocks for Virchov's attempts to classify physical disorders categorically and Kraepelin in his conceptualization of mental disorders was deeply influenced by the developments in medicine. It was no more than natural that uncovering the (neuro-) pathological roots of the entities delineated by Kraepelin was to become the major focus of biological psychiatric research of the day.

In the fifties, a renaissance of biological research in psychiatry set in. Nosology retained its predominant position, not because logical reasoning had irrevocably supported that position, but out of sheer habit. The nosological tradition was strong, particularly in European psychiatry and had been passed on unquestioned from generation to generation of psychiatrists.

In the U.S.A., it was the publication of the DSM III that strongly reinforced a nosological orientation not only in biological psychiatry, but in clinical practice as well.

Nosological organization of psychopathology

The core idea underlying nosological taxonomy is the classical Kraepelinian assumption that psychiatric disorders can be classified on more axes than symptomatology alone; that a predictable relation exists between syndrome on the one hand, and such variables as duration, severity, concomitant personality disorder on the other and that, therefore, mental disorders can be divided in discrete entities of which the underlying brain dysfunctions can be meaningfully explored.

Though its position seems almost unassailable, nosological taxonomy is, I would like to submit, an unreliable partner for biological psychiatric research. A siren, who can be held responsible for the fact that though a lot of "biology" has been uncovered in mental disorders, most of it seems to be without any (nosological) specificity to speak of. The major reason for the stalemate in which we find ourselves today is that the disease entities that are being explored are, for the most part, pseudo-entities. It would be little less than a miracle if a single cause, or even a single marker would be found identifying such an "entity".

Let me briefly clarify that statement with one example: schizophrenia [1]. Kraepelin [2] distinguished five subgroups in terms of symptoms as disparate as anemia and jaundice. Kleist described 21 subforms [3]. The DSM III employs the choice principle – to qualify for a particular syndromal diagnosis the presence of x out of y symptoms suffice, no matter which one. Hence, one label covers a multitude of syndromes.

Is outcome determined by the syndromal diagnosis of schizophrenia, or severity, or treatment response or concomitant personality disorder? By no means; even within one and the same syndromal cluster, these variables vary. Take paranoid schizophrenia as an example. This condition may lead to chronicity or it may remit; it may hamper someone's social functioning entirely or the symptoms can only be established in a careful and pointed interview; the premorbid personality disorder may be schizotypal, more paranoid or signs of disordered personality may be only minimal. Neuroleptics sometimes eliminate the paranoid symptoms fully; rapid or more protracted. In other cases the symptoms stubbornly resist all pharmacotherapeutic efforts. Schizophrenia is in this context only a paradigm. Much of the above is applicable to most of the entities we distinguish in the psychiatric vernacular [4]. They are in truth no more than broad umbrellas for a range of loosely related syndromes that differ in most other respects which are considered clinically relevant. Again, it is unlikely that those entities are being carried by a single pathology and hence, can hardly be considered as an appropriate focus for biological research. The nosological tradition I dare say, is largely a construct of wishful thinking, not of empirical data. It is kept alive by the ineradicable hope that mental pathology is organized in neat "packages", practically handy and aesthetically pleasing.

Syndromal organization of psychopathology

A second level of organization of psychopathological phenomena is the syndromal. A mental disorder is typified by a cluster of symptoms that usually go together.

That is a diagnostic approach I favor in biological research [5]. The patient's diagnosis is, for instance, the syndrome of major depression, melancholic type, or that of paranoid schizophrenia, or of obsessive compulsive disorder. Other variables, such as severity, duration, recurrency, prognosis, treatment outcome and concomitant personality disorder are assessed separately and scored on independent axes. Syndromal typology is a much better starting point for biological psychiatry than (present day's) nosology is. Yet, this system too, is seriously flawed as far as biological research is concerned. Syndromes seldom occur in isolation. The same patients often presents (parts of) several syndromes. For instance, depression and various forms of anxiety; schizophrenic syndromes and various clinical manifestations of mood disorder; addiction disorder and personality disorder, and so forth. In actual practice it is virtually impossible to decide to which syndrome a given biological variable might relate.

Symptomatological/dimensional/functional organization of psychopathology

A third level of organization of psychopathological phenomena is the one that could be named symptomatological, dimensional, or functional; terms that, though related are not identical or interchangeable.

One could dissociate oneself entirely from the larger psychopathological constructs – nosological entities or syndromes – and search for correlations between biological variables and individual psychopathological symptoms. A psychopathological symptom is seldomly an all or nothing phenomenon. It occurs in all measures of severity and blends almost imperceptibly into normality. Many phenomena familiar in psychopathology occur in normal individuals as well; anxiety, depressed mood, suicidal ideation, perceptual disturbances, overvalued thoughts bordering on delusions, to mention only a few examples [6]. They are, however, of short duration, surmountable without treatment and not seriously intervening with normal life. For those reasons, I prefer the term dimension to symptom: it expresses more clearly the gradual transition from outright pathology to (sub)normality.

Few if any psychopathological dimensions are specific for a given syndrome or nosological entity. If a biological variable could be coupled to a particular psychopathological dimension, one would expect that variable to be non-specific on a syndromal and nosological level. Dimensional specificity would, in most cases, exclude syndromal or nosological specificity.

Psychopathological symptoms or dimensions are not entities sui generis. They are the behavioral manifestations of an underlying psychological dysfunction. For instance, the phenomenon the patient experiences as an hallucination presupposes a perceptual dysfunction; the thought disorder we diagnose as a delusion is a consequence of a damaged critical function: the patient is unable to screen thoughts for probability and to drop those that available evidence screens out as highly unlikely; insufficiently bridled (auto) aggressivity manifests disordered aggression regulation or, more generally, disordered impulse control.

A psychological dysfunction may occur at a certain point in life, transient or lasting, or it may be present during the entire lifespan. In the first case it forms a component of a psychopathological syndrome, in the second case of a disordered personality structure. For example, sadness, pessimism, dependency can be part of a depressive syndrome, or of a particular personality disorder.

Rather than nosological entities or syndromes, I consider psychological dysfunctions as the elementary units of classification in psychopathology. In biological psychiatry, however, they have not been given serious consideration. That is a serious omission, particularly since other classificatory systems lack, as we saw, precision and reliability and since their application in biological psychiatry has so far barely yielded diagnostic relevant information [7,8]. Moreover, several lines of evidence indicate that at least some biological variables, originally introduced as markers of disease entities, but which turned out to possess disappointingly low diagnostic specificity, relate quite strongly to particular psychopathological dimensions or psychological dysfunctions [9].

For a functional psychopathology

This plea for a functional psychopathology does not imply rejection of nosological taxonomy, however imprecise the latter may be. We need a categorical diagnostic system as a language for easy professional communication, though research to enhance the informative value of that language is urgently needed. The plea does imply that I consider a nosological diagnosis as incomplete and that psychiatry should pursue a two-tier diagnostic approach. Tier-one marks the nosological diagnosis, that is the broad, general diagnostic framework, Major depression would be an example. The tier-two diagnosis depicts the dissection of the syndrome into its component parts: the psychological dysfunctions and would, in the case of major depression entail a detailed depiction of, amongst many others, disturbances in mood-, anxiety- and aggression-regulation, in drive and in hedonistic functioning. I use the word depiction, not description, to indicate that many psychological (dys-)functions are measurable quantitatively, and that with great precision; at least in principle, that is if the patient is willing to collaborate with the experimental psychologist. This is in striking contrast to syndromes or nosological entities, whose presence can only be estimated and expressed in such terms as mild, moderate or severe or anywhere in between. Two-tier diagnosis, then, will not only refine the diagnostic process but will bring psychopathology onto a true scientific footing.

Functional psychopharmacology

Another consequence of two-tier diagnosis, I foresee, is a move of psychopharmacology from a nosological to a functional orientation. The indication of a particular psychotropic drug will no longer be based primarily on the tier-one diagnosis, for instance, schizophrenia or major depression, but chiefly on the functional disturbances that are the manifestations of that illness. Drugs will be prescribed that correct, for instance, particular disturbances in perception, in cognition, in impulse control, in mood regulation, and will be dispensed simultaneously, i.e. goal-directed, dysfunction-oriented polypharmacy. Two-tier diagnosing would thus redeem the maligned concept of polypharmacy. The development of a functional psychopharmacology is predicated on the development of drugs with great selectivity on the biochemical level. In the field of 5-HT drugs with representatives influencing for example, very particular subpopulations of 5-HT receptors, the process is already ongoing.

A two-tier diagnostic system with a corresponding functional pharmacology is not a chimera. Cardiology, for one, provides a telling example. In that specialty, two-tier diagnosis is the rule. Myocardial infarction, for instance, would be a tier-one diagnosis, always complemented with a tier-two analysis stating explicitly the functional sequelae, in terms of rhythm, conduction, frequency, etc. Drugs are dispensed on the basis of the tier-two, not the tier-one diagnosis; drugs often administered simultaneously.

In conclusion, then, functional psychopathology could be to psychiatry what physiology is to medicine: a level of organization of psychopathology fundamental for the understanding of abnormal behavior. Functional psychopathology is not an alternative for nosological/categorical classification, but its complement. A two-tier diagnostic system for mental disorders to be developed in close collaboration with experimental clinical psychologists, seems to me an indispensable precondition for the scientific maturation of psychiatry.

References

1. van Praag NM (1976) Compr. Psychiatry 17: 481–497.
2. Kraepelin E (1899) Psychiatrie II Band: Sechste Auflage. Verlag von Johann Ambrosius Barth, Leipzig.
3. Leonhard K (1960) In: NW Gruhle, Jung R, Mayer-Gross W and Muller M (eds.) Psychiatrie der Gegenwart Band II: Klinische Psychiatrie. Springer-Verlag, Berlin.
4. van Praag NM (1989) Psychiatr. Dev. 4: 375–394.
5. van Praag NM and Leijnse B (1965) Psychiatr. Neurol. Neurochir. 68: 50–66.
6. Posey TB and Losch ME (1983) Imag. Cogn. Personal. 2: 99–113.
7. van Praag NM, Korf J, Lakke JPWF and Schut T (1975) Psychol. Med. 5: 138–146.
8. van Praag HM, Kahn R, Asnis GM, Wetzler S, Brown S, Bleich A and Korn M (1987) J. Affective Disord. 13: 1–8.
9. van Praag HM, Asnis GM, Kahn RS, Brown SL, Korn M, Harkavy Friedman JM and Wetzler S (1990) Br. J. Psychiatry 157: 723–734.

Biological Psychiatry, Volume 1. G. Racagni et al., editors.

Nosology and the classification of depressive disorders

Thomas A. Ban
Department of Psychiatry, Vanderbilt University, A-2215 Medical Center North, Nashville, Tennessee, U.S.A.

Unipolar depression in psychiatric nosology

It was not before the description of "la folie circulaire" in the 1850s by Jean-Pierre Falret [1] that development which led to the nosologic concept of unipolar depression began. In "la folie circulaire" a naturally occurring category of mental illness was identified for the first time in which the psychopathologic process, without identifiable neuropathologic changes, did not follow a continuous-deteriorating course, but was characterized by a discontinuous episodic course with full or partial remissions between episodes. In subsequent years, however, based on their different contents, numerous episodic-recurrent syndromes had been described. From this multitude of syndromes, Emil Kraepelin [2], in the first edition of his textbook, recognized six different subforms of "melancholia", i.e., simple, gravis, stuporous, paranoid, fantastic and delirious. However, by adopting the first organizing principle of psychiatric nosology, Kraepelin [3] in the fifth edition of his textbook, pooled together all these different morbid states in the nosologic category of "manic-depressive insanity".

From the time of its inception, Kraepelin's [3] unitary nosologic concept of manic-depressive insanity has been challenged. Nevertheless only with the adoption of "polarity", as an (second) organizing principle in psychiatric nosology by Karl Leonhard [4] was manic-depressive insanity separated into bipolar (polymorphic or multiform) and unipolar (monomorphic or simple) forms, i.e., in terms of depression, into a bipolar and a unipolar form of depressive illness.

Independent of psychiatric nosology, during the past 30 years a wide variety of techniques, borrowed from several other disciplines, (e.g., genetics, biochemistry), have been employed in attempts to subdivide unipolar depression into clinically meaningful categories. As a result, we are today confronted with a large number and wide variety of classifications of unipolar depression, which will need to be validated by nosologic research.

The code system

At present it is not known which, if any of the many classifications proposed, will provide a nosology with a high predictive validity of unipolar depressive disorders. Since the same applies also to other diagnostic categories, a methodology was developed for the study of relationships between different classifications of mental illness. The methodology is referred to as the CODE, or Composite Diagnostic Evaluation System.

The prototype of all CODE's is CODE-DD, the Composite Diagnostic Evaluation for Depressive Disorders [5], which can provide diagnoses within 25 diagnostic systems.

Preliminary findings with code-DD

Preliminary analyses of data on 230 newly admitted patients with a DSM III-R clinical diagnosis of major depression (single episode or recurrent) revealed a similar CODE-DD (DSM III-R) diagnosis in 229, i.e., in 99.6 percent of patients. In the same study 230, i.e., 100 percent of the patients with a DSM III-R diagnosis of major depression fulfilled ICD 10 criteria of depressive episode or recurrent depressive disorder indicating a 100 percent overlap in spite of the differences in diagnostic criteria.

Investigations with CODE-DD revealed that approximately 1/3 (32.61%) of patients with a depressive diagnosis in the DSM III-R, do not fit the Vienna Research Criteria of depression; approximately 1/6th (17.8%) do not fit Leonhard's Criteria of pure depression or pure melancholia; and approximately 1/8th (13.5%) do not fit any of the Research Diagnostic Criteria of depressive disorder.

The steadily accumulating information obtained by CODE-DD indicates that the different phenotypic syndromes do not represent nosologically meaningful groups of depression. In fact, of 87 patients identified as depressed on the basis of Leonhard's Criteria [4], 53 fit the diagnosis of pure melancholia, whereas the other 34 fit more than one subform of pure depression. On the other hand, there are some indications that pure depression regardless of subform represent a nosologically distinctive category from pure melancholia.

Finally, looking at the data of one clinical drug trial CODE-DD did not succeed in identifying the treatment responsive depressive group. On the other hand, the CODE-DD data suggest that there is a linear relationship between responsiveness to treatment with an inactive placebo, a standard antidepressant and an investigational antidepressant drug.

Concluding remarks

In the foregoing, development of the diagnostic concept of unipolar depression within the frame of reference of psychiatric nosology has been briefly outlined.

The presentation was based on the assumption that a valid psychiatric nosology is an essential prerequisite for the interpretation of contributions from the neurosciences with possible relevance to mental illness and for the identification of treatment responsive populations to antidepressant drugs; that unipolar depression is a valid, but probably a biologically heterogeneous nosologic category; and that by employing CODE-DD, i.e., by applying a method of psychiatric nosology, clinically and heuristically important forms and subforms of unipolar depression could be identified.

One might argue, however, that none of these preconceptions are correct and that any attempt to identify clinically and/or heuristically important forms and subforms of depression by employing a nosologic method, such as CODE-DD would remain in vain, because unipolar depression is not a legitimate nosologic concept, (i.e., depression is the content and not the form of the episodically recurring and remitting change in the perception of experience).

Pursuing further the same line of thinking, one may consider the possibility of employing a psychopharmacologic method, in identifying an antidepressant responsive population (which extends far beyond the boundaries of unipolar depression) instead of a nosologic method in identifying an antidepressant responsive population within unipolar depression. To be considered as meaningful, however, the diagnosis identified by responsiveness to antidepressants must be of predictive validity. Probably even more important is that by employing different psychopharmacologic means the patient belonging to the new category should be attributable to only one class, i.e. unresponsive to drugs other than antidepressants. Todate, no such diagnostic category has been identified.

References

1. Falret JP (1854) Bull. Acad. Méd. (Paris) 19: 382–400.
2. Kraepelin E (1883) Lehrbuch der Psychiatrie. 1. Aufl. Barth, Leipzig.
3. Kraepelin E (1896) Lehrbuch der Psychiatrie. 5. Aufl. Barth, Leipzig.
4. Leonhard K (1957) Aufteilung der endogenen Psychosen. Akademie, Berlin.
5. Ban TA (1989) Composite Diagnostic Evaluation of Depressive Disorders. J.M. Productions, Nashville, Tennessee.

Biological Psychiatry, Volume 1. G. Racagni et al., editors.

Diagnostic specificity in twin studies

Peter McGuffin and Anne Farmer

Department of Psychological Medicine, University of Wales College of Medicine, Cardiff CF4 4XN, U.K.

Introduction

It is now virtually mandatory to apply operational definitions of disorders such as schizophrenia or depression in studies aimed for publication in peer-reviewed journals. The great advantage offered by operational definitions is that because they are clear and explicit, they afford good inter-rater reliability and hence improve the chances that a set of research findings in one site can be replicated elsewhere. One of the main drawbacks is that there exists not one but many different systems of diagnosis both for depression [1] and for schizophrenia [2]. Furthermore, these various definitions do not always match each other so the same patient might be classified as schizophrenic under one system but receive some other diagnosis under another. Faced with these difficulties, the researcher needs to make the difficult decision about which system of operational definitions to choose.

Probably the best established aetiological clue both for affective disorders and for schizophrenia is that there is a substantial genetic component. Therefore one way to select useful operational definitions for biological and genetic studies is to discover which definition provides the greatest difference in monozygotic vs. dizygotic concordance rates and which maximizes the heritability (h^2) of the disorder.

Schizophrenia

So far there are no completed data sets resulting from twin studies which have been "purpose-built" to examine the question of phenotypic definition. However, one of the larger series from the preoperational criteria era, that of [3], has proved sufficiently robust to withstand "recycling". Using detailed case abstracts we applied a variety of operational definitions to a series of 22 monozygotic (MZ) twin pairs (26 probands) and 21 dizygotic (DZ) pairs (34 probands) [4,5]. We worked blindly in that abstracts were identified only by a code number so that the zygosity and identity of the co-twin were unknown. Some of the more important results are summarized in Table 1.

As we see, DSM III and its predecessors [6,7] define highly heritable syndromes. Against expectation, a definition based on the first rank symptoms [9]

Table 1. Probandwise twin concordance and heritabilities of operational criteria for schizophrenia (data from [4,5])

Definition	MZ concordance (1%)	DZ concordance (1%)	h^2
RDC narrow [6]	52.6	9.5	0.83
Feighner definite [7]	47.4	11.1	0.72
DSM III [8]	47.6	9.5	0.85
Schneider [9]	22.2	50.0	0.0

gave a heritability estimate of zero. All the listed definitions were show to have satisfactory inter-rater reliability, and indeed Schneider's definition gave perfect agreement between 2 blind raters. The clear lesson therefore is that high reliability is no guarantee of validity.

We went on to scrutinise the validity of the DSM III definition [5], and tried to discover whether the criteria could be "improved" by repositioning the boundaries of the disorder. To do this we examined the effect of subsuming other categories within the definition of "schizophrenia". Because of difficulties in defining population base rates, different definitions were compared using the MZ/DZ concordance ratio. This is considerably cruder than heritability, but still provides some indicator of the degree of genetic determination. Broadening the definition of schizophrenia to include schizotypal personality disorder and atypical psychosis as well as affective disorder with mood incongruent delusions produced the highest MZ/DZ concordance ratio. However, further broadening of the definition appeared merely to add "noise", so that when any Axis I one diagnosis was included, there was nearly a 4-fold drop in the ratio.

Depression

A recently completed twin study, again using the Maudsley Hospital register in London, was designed to address diagnostic issues more specifically [10]. Of a total of 408 probands with a primary diagnosis of depression, 177 probands fulfilled blindly applied DSM III-R criteria for at least one episode of major depression. A variety of definitions to define concordance were employed and the results of using two of these, the broadest and narrowest, are shown below.

We fitted a simple path model using the FORTRAN programme TWIN D to obtain maximum likelihood estimates of the model parameters, the heritability, h^2 and the proportion of phenotypic variance contributed by common family environment, c^2. The full model was compared with reduced models (e.g. no additive gene effects, no shared environment) using likelihood ratio tests and the most parsimonious model was selected. As seen in Table 2, the favoured model for the broad definition of depression based on hospital-treated cases required both genes and common environment to explain familial transmission. By contrast, the narrow

Table 2. Probandwise twin concordance and best-fit models for a broad (hospital-treated, any CATEGO class) and narrow (blind DSM III-R) definition of depression

Definition	MZ twins		DZ twins		h^2	c^2	χ^2
	n	Concordance (%)	n	Concordance (%)			
Broad	66	62	109	46	0.39	0.46	0.0
Narrow	68	46	109	22	0.79	0.0	0.9

definition based on strictly applied DSM III-R criteria yielded a phenotype with heritability close to 80% and no effect from common family environment.

Conclusions

Twin data on schizophrenia even when not originally collected for this purpose provide important leads on the definition of disorder which is "most valid" from the viewpoint of genetic research. In particular our results underline the fact that an operational definition may have high reliability but show zero heritability. The results of unipolar depression are intriguing. Both broad and narrow definitions delineate phenotypes with a substantial genetic contribution. However, the broader phenotype in which hospital treatment is included in the definition has a lower heritability and the effect of common family environment is significant. The transmission of the narrow version can be explained purely in terms of additive gene effects. This suggests that the narrowly-defined syndrome of major depressive disorder is largely genetically determined, but that seeking hospital treatment is substantially influenced by non-genetic familial factors.

References

1. Farmer AE and McGuffin P (1989) Br. J. Psychiatry 155: 437–443.
2. Berner P, Gabriel E, Katschnig H et al. (1983) In: Diagnostic Criteria for Schizophrenia and Affective Psychoses. World Psychiatric Association, American Psychiatric Press Inc.
3. Gottesman II and Shields J (1972) In: Schizophrenia and Genetics: A Twin Study Vantage Point. Academic Press, New York.
4. McGuffin P, Farmer AE, Gottesman II, Murray RM and Revely A (1984) Arch. Gen. Psychiatry 41: 541–545.
5. Farmer AE, McGuffin P and Gottesman II (1987b) Arch. Gen. Psychiatry 44: 634–641.
6. Spitzer RL, Endicott J and Robins E (1978) Arch. Gen. Psychiatry 35: 773–782.
7. Freigner JP, Robins E, Guze SB, Woodruffe RA, Winokur G and Munoz R (1972) Arch. Gen. Psychiatry 26: 57–63.
8. American Psychiatric Association (1980) Committee on Nomenclature and Statistics. Diagnostic and Statistical Manual of Mental Disorders, 3rd Edn. American Psychiatric Association.
9. Schneider K (1959) Hamilton MW (trans.) Clinical Psychopathology. Grune and Stratton, London.
10. McGuffin P, Katz R and Rutherford J (1991) Psychol. Med. (Vol.2) 20: 329–335.

Biological Psychiatry, Volume 1. G. Racagni et al., editors.

Diagnostic unspecificity in family studies: The overlap of anxiety disorders and unipolar major depression

W. Maier, D. Lichtermann, J. Minges and R. Heun
Department of Psychiatry, University of Mainz, Untere Zahlbacher Straße 8, D-6500 Mainz, Germany

Introduction

Diagnostic specificity of the familial transmission of disorders running in families is defined by the familial pattern of breeding true conditions; these are met if the familial cross prevalence of two disorders (i.e. prevalence of disorder B in families of probands with disorder A and vice versa) do not indicate an increased familial risk as compared with healthy controls. Family studies including probands with various disorders either as pure or as combined conditions and preserving the blind for probands' diagnoses when interviewing relatives are required in order to examine these conditions.

In several family studies, both anxiety disorders and unipolar depression have been reported to run in families. In spite of the great number of family studies in the literature, there is none which includes probands with both unipolar depression and anxiety disorders (mainly panic disorder) either as comorbid ("MDD+PD") or as pure conditions ("MDD-PD" or "PD-MDD"). Consequently, the diagnostic specificity of the familial transmission of anxiety disorders and unipolar depression is widely unknown. The present study examines the diagnostic specificity of major depressive disorder and panic disorder by their cross-prevalence rates in families of all three index proband types as postulated above.

Material and Methods

A sample of 230 consecutively admitted psychiatric inpatients with a lifetime diagnosis of unipolar major depression or panic disorder or both, but without any other axis I diagnosis according to DSM III-R were personally interviewed with the Schedule for Affective Disorders and Schizophrenia (lifetime version, modified for the study of anxiety disorders – SADS-LA [1]). Likewise, 598 (i.e. about 80%) of their first-degree relatives could be rated blindly to the index subjects' diagnoses. In the same fashion, a control sample of 109 families of the general population was investigated, to whom we matched a random subsample of patient families. "Best estimate" psychiatric lifetime diagnoses [2] were agreed upon for all of them by reconsideration of the interviews, case records and family history information. Lifetime morbid risk figures for unipolar major depression without

Table 1.

	First degree relatives' lifetime morbid risk of:		
	MDD-PD (%)	PD+MDD (%)	PD-MDD (%)
Patient subtype			
MDD-PD	18.7	0.9	3.2
PD+MDD	24.1	3.8	6.1
PD-MDD	18.1	2.5	4.6
Healthy controls	9.8	0.7	1.4

panic disorder (and vice versa) as well as for the comorbidity of both conditions in the patients' and controls' families were calculated following the Strömgren-Weinberg algorithm (see [3]) for the age at onset correction.

Results

In Table 1, the age-corrected lifetime morbid risks of comorbid or single DSM III-R diagnoses of major depressive disorder (MDD) or panic disorder (PD) in first-degree relatives are demonstrated by the index subjects' diagnoses.

Two patterns of lacking specificity emerge. The familial risk of panic disorder plus major depression is increased in probands showing panic disorder/agoraphobia alone. However, unipolar depression, even without associated panic disorder/agoraphobia, is also more frequent in families of probands with "pure" panic disorder (18.1% versus 9.8% in control families; $P = 0.05$). Furthermore, there is a tendency towards an increased risk of "pure" panic disorder in the relatives of probands with major depression, but without panic disorder. Consequently, neither unipolar depression nor panic disorder breed true.

Discussion

Both panic disorder and unipolar depression aggregate in families as predicted by previously published family studies [4–6]. However, the familial pattern of illness observed showed a high degree of diagnostic heterogeneity; there was no apparent pattern of "breeding true" or homotypia that emerged.

The distinction between "pure" and "combined" disorders has given the opportunity to test the hypothesis that the comorbidity of anxiety and depressive disorders in probands explains the diagnostic heterogeneity; depression in families of panic disorder probands, for instance, might be due to secondary depression in these probands which also segregates in families. However, the results as presented in Table 1 have rejected this hypothesis.

In conclusion, diagnostic distinctions of anxiety and mood disorder are not able to establish a homotypal pattern of familial aggregation; the high degree of overlap of both disorders in families proposes the hypothesis that both disorders define separate or even overlapping intervals on an underlying common variable which may be termed as "anxiety-depression-continuum" that is transmitted in families. A test of this hypothesis is provided by biometric model fitting.

References

1. Mannuzza S, Fyer AJ, Klein DF and Endicott J (1986) J. Psychiatr. Res. 20: 317–325.
2. Leckman JF, Sholomskas D, Thompson WD, Belanger A and Weissman MM (1982) Arch. Gen. Psychiatry 39: 879–883.
3. Gershon ES, DeLisi LE, Hamovit J, Nurnberger JI, Maxwell ME, Schreiber J, Dauphinais D, Dingman CW II and Guroff JJ (1988) Arch. Gen. Psychiatry 45: 328–336.
4. Cloninger CR, Martin RL, Clayton P and Guze SB (1981) In: Klein DF and Rabkin J (eds.) Anxiety: New Research and Changing Concepts. Raven Press, New York, pp. 137–150.
5. Crowe RR, Noyes R Jr, Pauls DL and Slymen DJ (1983) Arch. Gen. Psychiatry 40: 1065–1069.
6. Noyes R Jr, Crowe RR, Harris EL, Hamra BJ, McChesny CM and Chaudhry DR (1986) Arch. Gen. Psychiatry 43: 227–232.

Biological Psychiatry, Volume 1. G. Racagni et al., editors.

Neuroendocrinological/sleep parameters and diagnostic distinctions

David J. Kupfer

Department of Psychiatry, University of Pittsburgh School of Medicine, Western Psychiatric Institute and Clinic, 3811 O'Hara Street, Pittsburgh, PA 15213, U.S.A.

The advent of psychobiology as applied to psychiatric disorders has inaugurated a new era of investigative efforts to develop objective criteria for such disorders and to apply biological measures to elucidate several key "boundary" issues. The first application has been to study the longitudinal course of selected disorders and their subtypes. In this regard, depression has received considerable attention especially in relation to the onset and offset of specific individual episodes, as well as specifying episode correlates. Over the last 20 years, an array of biologic changes have been proposed as potential episode or more persistent trait markers of a depressive illness. Our own pragmatic view is that episode correlates are worth studying if they are easier to identify and quantitate as indicators of an episode than are clinical changes in symptoms or social/work impairments either of the index episode or the onset of the new episode. Furthermore, alterations that may persist beyond the episode could serve as important residual or trait markers during the phase of clinical remission. Thus, one underlying aim in biological psychiatry has been the hope that biological indicators may ultimately represent the gold standard to delineate the boundaries (onset and termination) of an episode.

The second application of biological correlates has proceeded parallel with the increasing interest in nosology and diagnostic distinctions. It has been expected that biological correlates will provide the refinements in criteria necessary to discriminate various subtypes of affective disorders. While the particular choice of which biological correlates to study is not easy, it is now widely recognized that depression is associated with definite biological changes. Moreover, since the major affective disorders are characterized by a variety of disturbances in physiological functioning (including sleep, motor activity, appetite and libido), the pursuit of studies of potential biologic correlates is conceptually appealing. Finally, evidence of the efficacy of anti depressants for the major affective disorders strengthens the intuitive and conceptual appeal of the role of biological factors in these conditions.

Rather than attempt to review in a systematic fashion all the proposed biological "markers" suggested for boundary distinctions in depression, the intent of this selective review is to demonstrate current research efforts as examples in a few specific domains that appear most promising. Specifically, we will mention some of the most recent work in the following 2 domains: neuroendocrine/neuropeptide studies and aspects of neurophysiology/electrophysiology. While there have been many proposed subtypes of depression, we would like to specify only several dichotomous types and then point by example of the type of investigative activity proceeding in each of these areas. The 5 diagnostic distinctions include the following: delusional versus non-delusional; bipolar versus unipolar; melancholia (endogenous) versus non-endogenous; major depression versus minor/brief depression; and single episode versus recurrent depression. While results are uneven in these groups, these 5 subtypes represent comparisons consistent with differences in clinical course, treatment and prognosis, family history and possibly different genetic bases.

All-night electroencephalographic sleep investigations have received considerable attention as possible biological "markers" for depressive states. Such studies initially were utilized to document the characteristic sleep disturbances of depressed individuals. Despite the proliferation of studies in this area, there is still controversy about the sensitivity and specificity of the REM and NREM sleep changes observed in the state of depression [1]. It is still not understood why some patients do not display the "classic" sleep stigmata during depression or, conversely, why some patients with other psychiatric or medical disorders display some of the sleep features associated with depression. Hudson et al. [2] have also reported shortened REM sleep latency during the manic phase of bipolar illness, while Thase et al. [3] reported normal REM sleep latency during the depressive phase of bipolar illness. Thase et al. [4] have also shown distinct sleep features in delusional depression.

Studies on the HPA axis have pointed to the increased level of HPA abnormalities in delusional depression, as well as melancholic states. Nemeroff and Bissette [5] concluded that neuropeptide approaches have revealed hypersecretion of corticotropin-releasing factor (CRF) in the HPA axis as evidenced by increased CSF CRF concentrations, decreased CRF receptor number in frontal cortex of suicide victims and a blunted adrenocorticotropin hormone (ACTH) response to CRF. Considerable evidence exists that this CRF hypersecretion, like the associated hypercortisolemia, is state-dependent; as suggested earlier, a blunted TSH response to TRH is found in depression, often associated with hypersecretion of TRH (increased CSF TRH concentrations). Finally, reduced CSF concentrations of somatostatin (SRIF) have been found in individuals with major depression.

Other neuroendocrine parameters which have received less extensive study include regulation of growth hormone secretion, prolactin regulation and study of the pineal hormone, melatonin. While some evidence of disturbances in each of these systems in major depression has been reported, none of these findings has been consistently replicated or is robust enough to meet the criteria for either a state or trait marker. Recently, Jarrett et al. [6] reported systemic reduction in sleep-related growth hormone (GH) secretion in recurrent major depression. The reduction in sleep-related GH secretion found in depressed patients persisted during treatment and was also present in a period of drug-free clinical remission.

It would have been expected in 1991 that research investigators would be able to routinely apply biological markers for clinical studies and for improved diagnostic differentiation. It would have been hoped that operational criteria for the DSM IV nosology of affective disorders would have included specific laboratory methodology as part of the diagnostic criteria. Unfortunately, we have not yet achieved a sufficient level of sophistication with respect to the application of newer technology. More importantly, we have not been able to conduct a sufficient number of studies that apply techniques that derive from more than one domain at a time. Over the next decade the combined application of neurochemical, neuroendocrine, neurophysiological and imaging techniques should provide the necessary studies to lead to a more routine application of such tools as markers. Our major caveat concerning such investigative activities focuses on the need to employ rigorous criteria in establishing the evidence for biologic "markers". We need to couple our enthusiasm with systematic verification by multiple settings prior to concluding that we have succeeded in doing for affective disorders what is being done in other medical disorders. Finally, we need to realize that it is very unlikely that one marker will emerge; more probably we can expect a profile of biologic and clinical correlates from diverse domains to provide the markers of depressive illness.

References

1. Buysse DJ and Kupfer DJ (1990) J. Nerv. Ment. Dis. 178: 405–414.
2. Hudson JI, Lipinski JF, Frankenburg FR, Grochocinski VJ and Kupfer DJ (1988) Arch. Gen. Psychiatry 45: 267–273.
3. Thase ME, Himmelhoch JM, Mallinger AG, Jarrett DB and Kupfer DJ (1989) Am. J. Psychiatry 146: 329–333.
4. Thase ME, Kupfer DJ and Ulrich RF (1986) Arch. Gen. Psychiatry 43: 886–893.
5. Nemeroff CB and Bissette G (1990) Neuropeptide alterations in major depression: State or trait markers? Presented at the 1990 Annual ACNP Meeting, December 10–14, 1990, San Juan, Puerto Rico.
6. Jarrett DB, Miewald JM and Kupfer DJ (1990) Arch. Gen. Psychiatry 47: 113–118.

Biological Psychiatry, Volume 1. G. Racagni et al., editors.

Drug response and the distinction between affective and schizophrenic disorders

Eve C. Johnstone
University Department of Psychiatry, The Kennedy Tower, Royal Edinburgh Hospital, Morningside Park, Edinburgh EH10 5HF, Scotland, U.K.

Introduction

Functional psychosis is conventionally subdivided into schizophrenia and manic depressive psychosis [1]. Response to treatment has been assumed to be a validating criterion for these diagnoses and this assumption has been tested in the present study which has two phases: Phase I – concerned with the treatment of acute psychotic episodes; and Phase II – concerned with continuation treatment intended as a prophylaxis against relapse.

Phase I

Method and Results

The efficacy of pimozide (a D_2 dopamine antagonist), lithium and their combination was blindly compared with that of placebo in a four-week trial of 120 functionally psychotic patients selected from 326 consecutive admissions of possibly psychotic patients to a psychiatric unit in North London [2]. Before and twice weekly during the study each patient was assessed for positive and negative psychotic symptoms using the Krawiecka [3] Scale, manic symptoms using the Bech-Rafaelsen [4] Scale and depressive symptoms using the Montgomery and Asberg [5] Scale. The sample was subdivided into patients with predominantly elevated mood, predominantly depressed mood and those with no consistent mood change. Pimozide showed a significant ($P < 0.0001$) effect in reducing positive psychotic symptoms in all three subgroups of patients. The only significant effect of lithium was to reduce elevated mood ($P < 0.02$). Thus D_2 dopamine receptor blockade, the principal action of pimozide, appeared relevant to the improvement of psychotic symptoms in all types of "functional" psychosis, while the effective mechanisms of action of lithium in the treatment of acute psychotic patients appeared only to concern mood.

Phase II

Method and Results

After the 28 days of Phase I, patients were classed as recovered or non-recovered and patients in the recovered category who were able to participate in a maintenance study were blindly continued on the medication of pimozide, lithium, the combination of both or placebo that they had had in Phase I until the point of relapse, and were assessed every 4 weeks during that period using the Krawiecka [3], Bech-Rafaelsen [4] and Montgomery and Asberg [5] Scales. Thirty patients entered the maintenance phase and their allocation to treatment and stratification in terms of mood change is shown in Table 1.

Pimozide was significantly more effective than placebo pimozide in preventing relapse ($P = 0.01$). No significant effect for lithium was found.

Table 1. Allocation and stratification in terms of symptoms of the 30 patients who entered Phase II

	Delusions or hallucinations	Delusions or hallucinations and thought disorder	Thought disorder without delusions
Elevated mood	AL/PL (3) PP/PL (1) PP/AL (1)	AP/AL (2)	
Depressed mood	AP/AL (3) AP/PL (2) PP/AL (1)	AP/AL (1)	
Neither consistently present	AP/AL (5) AP/PL (2) PP/PL (1) PP/AL (1)	AP/PL (2) AP/AL (2) PP/PL (1)	AP/PL (2)

AP = active pimozide; AL = active lithium; PP = placebo pimozide; PL = placebo lithium; figures in brackets refer to numbers of patients.

Conclusion

The results of Phase I of the study suggest that at least two processes are involved in functional psychoses – one concerned with dopaminergic mechanisms and positive symptoms but not mood change, and the other not demonstrably associated with positive symptoms but concerned with the stabilisation of elevated mood and related to a mechanism which lithium has and pimozide has not.

The results of Phase II emphasise the importance of dopaminergic mechanisms in a rather different way. Patients who were on placebo pimozide in Phase II had reached the recovery standard on that medication in Phase I. It may be concluded that prophylactic medication with dopamine-blocking agents is of value even in patients who have recovered from an acute episode of psychosis without active neuroleptics. Such an acute response does not identify a group of patients who can be predicted to do well without the continued administration of dopamine-blocking agents.

References

1. Kraepelin E (1899) Psychiatrie, Ein Lehrbuch fur Studenende und Arzte. 6th Edition. Barth, Leipzig.
2. Johnstone EC, Crow TJ, Frith CD and Owens DGC (1988) Lancet ii: 119–126.
3. Krawiecka MA, Goldberg D and Vaughan M (1977) Acta Psychiatr. Scand. 55: 299–308.
4. Bech P, Rafaelsen OJ, Kramp P and Bolwig T (1978) Neuropharmacology 17: 430–431.
5. Montgomery SA and Asberg M (1979) Br. J. Psychiatry 134: 382–389.

Biological Psychiatry, Volume 1. G. Racagni et al., editors.

Functional classification and the major/minor dichotomy of psychiatric disorders in 500 outpatients

O. Benkert, P. Winter, H. Gerbaldo and M. Philipp
Department of Psychiatry, University of Mainz, Untere Zahlbacher Straße 8, 6500 Mainz, Germany

Recently, strategies of denosologization of psychiatric disorders have been outlined, especially by Buchsbaum and Haier [1] and van Praag [2]. This approach has been further developed to a functional classification [3]. We still adhere to a nosological classification but are aiming for a biological classification by pursuing the functional classification in the meantime. The relation between the 3 different types of classification is demonstrated in Fig. 1.

Functional classification will lead to a typology which presently is essentially oriented by therapy response. Functional classification does not propose diagnostic dogmas but represents a set of variable constructions adaptable to new empirical findings. Therefore, functional classification represents an open system. It is not a concept which is trying to grasp the essence of a hypothetical illness but an auxiliary conceptual frame putting therapeutical possibilities in a practical order. Practical means manageable, based on experience yet possibly provisional.In the framework of functional classification we can take 2 strategic approaches: one is a select-by-marker and the other is a select-by-diagnosis strategy. This wide and pluralistic position is highly desirable and more advantageous than a one-sided one.

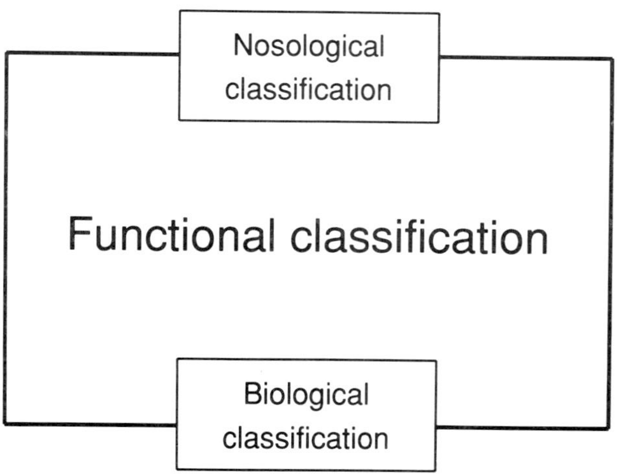

Fig. 1. Relationship between nosological, functional and biological classification.

It is possible that the *major/minor dichtomy* will replace the endogenous/neurotic dichtomy. A distinct and clear major/minor concept appears to be important, because the theoretical assumptions on biological parameters, the evaluation of specific therapeutic responses and the validation of the course of disorders are more likely to be corroborated in major than in minor psychiatric disorders.

Until now, the criteria for the severity of DSM III-R disorders are very heterogeneous and poorly operationalized. Severity criteria are explicitly defined for 6 diagnostic categories only.

There is some empirical evidence that biological variables may be more reliably identified in a major than in a minor depression. Furthermore, the consideration of severity in studies of therapeutical response has contributed significantly to the knowledge about specific or non-specific therapeutical effects. Paykel et al. [4] could not find any therapeutical response to TCA in depressed patients with a Hamilton score below 13. Elkin et al. [5] demonstrated that in mild depressions there is no significant difference between response to a variety of biological and psychological therapies, whereas in severe depressions with a Hamilton score of at least 20 points imipramine and interpersonal psychotherapy are significantly superior to placebo. In the Cross-National Collaborative Panic Study, Maier et al. [6] demonstrated the efficacy of imipramine and alprazolam in panic disorder, mainly in the subgroup of agoraphobic patients but less so in the subgroup without avoidance behaviour, i.e. less severely ill patients.

The major/minor concept of psychiatric disorders is also relevant for family studies. McGuffin [7] showed that the genetic contribution appears to be greater in more severe depressive disorders while it is likely that environmental conditions play a more prominent role in milder depressive disorders.

In a diagnostic study we evaluated the prevalence of psychiatric disorders in *500 adult outpatients* seeking professional advice in a primary care setting. We hypothesized a large percentage of patients with “minor psychiatric disorders” and many patients that acquire ill-defined diagnoses. The interview applied was the Polydiagnostic Interview (PODI) [8] which enables us to establish computerized diagnoses for a variety of operational diagnoses in competing classification systems such as RDC, DSM III-R, ICD 10.

DSM III-R diagnoses not otherwise specified (NOS) appeared in 42% of the cases; 20.6% were diagnosed as having both anxiety NOS and depression NOS, 9.2% received the diagnosis of depression NOS. We analyzed what percentage of the subsample with NOS depression would meet specific Research Diagnostic Criteria and found that more than 70% of the patients with ill-defined diagnoses in DSM III-R can be classified more specifically according to RDC [9]. This indicates that Research Diagnostic Criteria leave fewer patients in a residual category. On the one hand this phenomenon can be explained by the use of less strict time criteria in RDC (fulfillment of time criteria is not required for every single symptom), on the other hand by the provision of the subtype “minor” depression to which there is no equivalent in DSM III-R. Furthermore, 57% of the patients with NOS depression reached a score of 13 or higher on the 17-item-

HAM-D when DSM III-R original time criteria for major depression were applied and the symptom cut-off of 5 relevant symptoms was simultaneously lowered. When looking at the number of relevant symptoms for establishing a DSM III-R diagnosis and applying the time criterion in analogy to RDC, 72% of the subjects with a major depression (5–9 symptoms) and 33% of the subjects with a minor depression (3 or 4 symptoms) had a HAM-D score of 13 and above. According to recent findings these cases will profit from psychopharmacological treatment [4]. The duration of the depression in our NOS subsample was more than one year for 27%, between 2 weeks and 1 year for 56% of the sample; 17% had suffered for less than 2 weeks.

With regard to *DSM IV* we therefore propose the introduction of a "*minor depressive disorder*" with a minimum duration of 2 weeks but only 3 or 4 relevant symptoms in agreement with research diagnostic criteria.

References

1. Buchsbaum MS and Haier RJ (1983) Ann. Rev. Psychol. 34: 401–430.
2. Praag van HM, Kahn RS, Asnis GM, Wetzler S, Brown SL, Bleich A and Korn ML (1987) J. Affective Disord. 13: 1–8.
3. Benkert O (1990) Functional classification and response to psychotropic drugs. In: Benkert O, Maier W and Rickels K (eds.) Methodology of the Evaluation of Psychotic Drugs. Springer-Verlag, Berlin.
4. Paykel ES, Hollyman JA and Freeling P (1988) J. Affective Disord. 14: 83–95.
5. Elkin I, Shea MT, Watkins JT, Imber SD, Sotsky SM, Collins JF, Glass DR, Pilkonis PA, Leber WR, Docherty JP, Fiester SJ and Parloff MB (1989) Arch. Gen. Psychiatry 46: 971–982.
6. Maier W, Argyle N, Buller R, Roth M and Benkert O (1991) Vehaltenstherapie 1: 26–33.
7. McGuffin P and Katz R (1989) Br. J. Psychiatry 155: 294–304.
8. Philipp M and Maier W (1986) Psychopathology 19: 175–185.
9. Winter P, Philipp M, Buller R, Delmo C, Schwarze H and Benkert O (1991) Identification of minor affective disorders and implications for psychopharmacotherapy. J. Affective Disord. (in press).

Affective Disorders: Clinical and biological research

Biological Psychiatry, Volume 1. G. Racagni et al., editors.

Stress and episode sensitization in recurrent depression

R.M. Post

Biological Psychiatry Branch, National Institute of Mental Health, 9000 Rockville Pike, Bethesda, MD 20892, U.S.A.

Numerous studies detailing the longitudinal course of recurrent affective disorders document two types of sensitization phenomena – episode sensitization and sensitization to the effects of psychosocial stressors as precipitants of the episodes. Initial episodes of affective disorders may be followed by long well-intervals but with successive recurrences, there is a tendency for episodes to occur with greater rapidity [1]. At the same time, a critical role for psychosocial stressors as precipitants of subsequent episodes may become less evident. Clinicians have long noted that first episodes of major affective illness may be highly associated with psychosocial stressors but with successive recurrences, episodes begin to appear more autonomously. Twelve systematic studies document an approximate 60% incidence of psychosocial precipitants with the first episode compared with 36% in the second or successive episodes [2]. This process may be analogous to that observed in kindling where initial stimulations are not sufficient to induce full-blown episodes, but with successive repetitions of stimulations, full-blown seizures emerge and eventually seizures begin to occur spontaneously. In this fashion the kindling model provides an analogy for considering how early events (psychosocial stressors, losses, etc.) in development could provide a substrate for subsequent precipitation of full-blown episodes upon recurrence of stressors. Then, with subsequent repetition of precipitated episodes, the role of the psychosocial stressors becomes less important and episodes emerge autonomously. In behavioral sensitization to stimulants a prominent conditioned component is evident in that animals show greater reactivity to a cocaine challenge administered in the same environment where they were pretreated compared with pretreatment with either saline or cocaine in a different environment [3]. Since stimulant sensitization shows cross-sensitization to some stressors, it is possible that conditioned components of stressors become increasingly capable of precipitating some episodes, resulting in apparent autonomy of episodes.

While the biological mechanisms underlying behavioral sensitization to psychomotor stimulants (and stressors) and kindling evolution have not been definitively elucidated, new evidence implicates alterations at the level of gene expression. Not only do alterations in neurotransmission lead to short-term adaptations in neurotransmitter and receptor function, but also changes in the level of the nucleus are now demonstrated that could convey long-lasting alterations in responsivity and "memory" functions by inducing immediate early oncogenes such as c-fos, which then initiate a cascade of events which unfold in a spatio-temporal pattern. For example, mRNA for c-fos is translocated to the ribosomes where Fos protein is synthesized and Fos and another oncogene, Jun, dimerize with a "leucine zipper" motif and translocate back to the nucleus, where they activate AP-1 binding sites on DNA leading to transcription of mRNAs for peptides, neurotransmitters, receptors, enzymes, and growth factors [4]. Thus, long-term changes in neurotransmitters, peptides and receptors may be achieved by an initial stressor event and these changes may become greater in magnitude or more sustained with repetition of that event, as in kindling or sensitization. In the kindling model repeated stimulations can lead to increases in mRNA and levels of a variety of neuropeptides including somatostatin, TRH, CRH, and enkephalin, as well as decreases in dynorphin. In a parallel fashion it is possible that appropriate psychosocial stressors, upon repetition, could lead to long-lasting alterations in neuropeptide levels and function (such as TRH and CRH hypersecretion and somatostatin decrements) that are associated with acute episodes of depression. With each successive recurrence of a depressive episode this biochemical pathway may become progressively facilitated or sensitized, providing the neurobiological substrate for recurrence vulnerability and autonomy from psychosocial stressors. In this fashion, stressors provide one type of trait vulnerability to the development of full-blown episodes and the occurrence of episodes themselves additionally enhances vulnerability to further recurrences. Both processes may be encoded at the level of gene expression and occupy pathways involved in other types of neuroplasticity, learning and memory.

This data base and its associated conceptual models suggesting that "episodes beget episodes" highlights the importance of early intervention in the course of illness to prevent episode sensitization and highlights the importance of maintenance of pharmaco-prophylaxis. In several cases of discontinuation of long-term and effective lithium maintenance treatment, we have observed not only the occurrence of new episodes, but the induction of a state of lithium-refractoriness once treatment has been resumed. We raise the question whether an analogous process might occur in some patients with recurrent depressions adequately treated with tricyclics, where treatment discontinuation might not only be associated with the occurrence of new episodes, but with the possibility of drug refractoriness as well.

A substantial database now documents the marked efficacy of maintenance of antidepressant treatment with imipramines [5,6], fluoxetines [7], maprotiline [8], and other agents in preventing recurrences of affective episodes compared with placebo substitution. There is an extremely high rate of relapse on placebo within the first year (over 50% in many studies of patients with just two or three prior depressive episodes). All of these studies have been conceptualized from the perspective of the importance of preventing episodes themselves and their associated severe morbidity and potential mortality via suicide. In addition, we suggest the importance of prophylaxis from the perspective that it might also prevent episode sensitization, the transition to a more autonomous course (independent of psychosocial stressors) and even the (virtually unstudied) potential for drug-refractoriness. In this fashion we conceptualize recurrent affective disorders as a process not unlike that of cancer evolution involving multiple induction and suppression of oncogenes with the potential for malignant transformation if not adequately treated. Attention to the long-term and potentially evolving and progressive course of recurrent affective disorders may help engender greater respect for the possibility of malignant transformation and its prevention with early treatment and institution and maintenance of long-term prophylaxis.

References

1. Post RM, Rubinow DR and Ballenger JC (1986): Br. J. Psychiatry 149: 191–201.
2. Post RM (1991) The transduction of psychosocial stress into the neurobiology of recurrent affective disorder (unpublished manuscript).
3. Weiss SRB, Post RM, Pert A, Woodward R and Murman D (1989) Pharmacol. Biochem. Behav. 34: 655–661.
4. Morgan JI and Curran T (1989) Trends Neurosci. 12: 459–462.
5. Frank E, Kupfer DJ, Perel JM, Cornes C, Jarrett DB, Mallinger AG, Thase ME, McEachran AB and Grochocinski VJ (1990) Arch. Gen. Psychiatry 47: 1093–1099.
6. Prien RF, Kupfer DJ, Mansky PA, Small JG, Tuason VB, Voss CB and Johnson WE (1984) Arch. Gen. Psychiatry 41: 1096–1104.
7. Montgomery SA, Dufour H, Brion S, Gailledreau J, Laqueille X, Ferrey G, Moron P, Parant-Lucena N, Singer L, Danion JM, Beuzen JN and Pierredon MA (1988) Br. J. Psychiatry 153: 69–76.
8. Rouillon F, Phillips R, Serrurier D, Ansart E and Gerard MJ (1989) Encéphale 15: 527–534.

Biological Psychiatry, Volume 1. G. Racagni et al., editors.

The polysomnogram (PSG) as a vulnerability marker for depression

A. John Rush, Christina M. Gullion, Roseanne Armitage and Howard P. Roffwarg
Mental Health Clinical Research Center and Department of Psychiatry, University of Texas Southwestern Medical Center, 5323 Harry Hines Blvd., Dallas, TX 75235, U.S.A.

A "vulnerability marker" associated with a disorder may indicate any of several aspects of its expression: a) increased lifetime risk of expression; b) heightened risk of having a recurrent form of the disorder; or c) reduced treatment responsiveness (e.g. failure to respond or symptomatic breakthrough during treatment). From both etiological and public health perspectives, the lifetime risk of expression of the disorder is clearly the most important. However, the definitive prospective study remains to be completed.

Logically, a vulnerability marker for lifetime risk must be observable prior to first clinical expression of the disorder (i.e. the first episode in an episodic disorder such as major depression). A vulnerability marker may also be present after the first episode, though this is not essential, since treatment or the disorder itself may obscure the marker. Conversely, a vulnerability marker to a recurrent form of the disorder might not be observable prior to the first episode. However, to be clinically useful, it should be present thereafter, and it should be relatively persistent upon repeated assessment, regardless of whether or not the patient is currently in an episode. This kind of marker would have both clinical and scientific value in predicting prognosis (i.e. long-term course of illness).

We have recently completed a longitudinal follow-up study of 42 (major depression: n = 41; bipolar II disorder: n = 1) formerly depressed patients who were assessed both when symptomatic and when clinically remitted. These data provide a useful illustration of how an analysis might identify a putative vulnerability factor. These patients were treated in the acute phase with tricyclic medication (n = 23), cognitive therapy (n = 10), the combination in sequence (n = 7), or they were followed without treatment into remission (n = 2). All subjects had identical pretreatment diagnostic evaluations.

A 17-item HRS-D score of ≥14 was required for entry into the acute phase. The pretreatment mean HRS-D score was 20.2 (S.D. = 7.0). For medication-treated patients, all received 6 months of continuation treatment, followed by medication tapering over 2–4 weeks. For those in cognitive therapy, 20 sessions over roughly 12 weeks was used acutely. No continuation treatment was provided. Thereafter, subjects were followed monthly in a drug- and psychotherapy-free state with polysomnographic (PSG) studies and symptom severity ratings. All PSG's were conducted for 2 consecutive nights in the sleep laboratory.

In this outpatient sample (n = 42), 38% were RDC endogenous, 95% were RDC primary, 29% were in their first episode of depression, 50% had recurrent depressive episodes with complete interepisode recovery, while 21% were recurrent with incomplete interepisode recovery. Family history was distributed as follows: familial pure depressive disorder (36%); depressive spectrum disease (29%); sporadic depressive disorder (24%); bipolar (5%); unknown (7%).

The primary focus of the analysis was whether features of the PSG were stable characteristics of the patient regardless of change in state, and thus might be a candidate vulnerability marker. We selected data for occasions when patients were either clearly depressed (HRS-D $\geq$ 14) or clearly remitted (HRS-D < 7), and not in treatment. In subjects for whom we found more than 10 occasions, we dropped occasions beyond the tenth. This yielded a total of 168 measurements for the 42 cases in the "remitted" state, with an average HRS-D score of 3.7 (S.D. = 2.0). For the "symptomatic" state, there were 52 measurements in the 42 subjects (some became depressed during treatment-free follow-up), with a mean HRS-D score of 20.8 (S.D. = 6.3).

We conducted an analysis of variance using all of the measurements with state (ill vs. well), subject, and state + subject to examine the contribution of each to rapid eye movement (REM) latency. If state contributed significantly to the variance in REM latency, the "trait-like" nature of REM latency as a marker would be cast in doubt.

Results revealed that state accounted for only 0.1% of the variance in REM latency (N.S.), 2.7% of the variance in REM density for REM period 2 and 1.9% of the variance in % stage 4. These results suggest that state per se did little to account for these PSG parameters. Conversely, these measures are far from fixed. The intraclass correlations (on repeated measures while remitted) were 0.47 for REM latency, 0.34 for REM density #2, and 0.59 for % stage 4. Other unknown factors (e.g. life events, instability of underlying pathophysiological processes, measurement error, etc.) likely affect these variables. This finding is consistent with our own initial [1] and more recent reports [2].

In addition to being a stable "trait-like" characteristic, a vulnerability marker for a particular aspect of the disorder should have substantial predictive value to that aspect. For instance, a marker for recurrent illness should predict subsequent course of illness (i.e. who will have a recurrence). In this sample, a lower ratio of delta wave zero cross in non-REM period 1 vs. non-REM period 2 [3], or those with pretreatment reduced REM latency [4], respectively, in the symptomatic state had earlier relapses once treatment was discontinued. Therefore, aspects of the PSG may be predictive of the course of illness.

A "vulnerability" marker might also predict treatment efficacy, either in obtaining an acute response or in maintaining the response in an asymptomatic state during continuation. Specifically, if a factor predicts poor treatment response, those with it should be less likely to respond or may respond more slowly (possibly being titrated to a higher dose), while those without it would respond more frequently and/or rapidly. With regard to continued treatment efficacy, one might speculate that the effect of this factor would be seen in a similar pattern (i.e. those with it might have "breakthrough" symptoms, while those without it would be easily maintained in the asymptomatic state while on medication).

To examine this notion, outpatients with either major depression or bipolar II disorder, depressed phase were treated acutely with tricyclics for 6–9 weeks. Those who responded (end of acute phase HRS-D score usually ≤10) were continued with the same treatment for 6–7 months. Symptom measures and medication visits were conducted monthly. The continuation dosage was kept at the acute phase level, unless a lowering was necessitated by significant side-effects. The preliminary data reported here evaluate the relationship between pretreatment REM latency (drug-free state) and the level of symptomatology during the continuation phase.

Acknowledgements

Appreciation is expressed to Laurie Arnold for secretarial assistance and to Kenneth Z. Altshuler, M.D., Professor and Chairman, for administrative support. Preparation of this report was supported in part by a Mental Health Clinical Research Center Grant (MH-41115) to the Department of Psychiatry, University of Texas Southwestern Medical Center at Dallas.

References

1. Rush AJ, Erman MK, Giles DE, Schlesser MA, Carpenter G, Vasavada N and Roffwarg HP (1986) Arch. Gen. Psychiatry 43: 878–884.
2. Thase ME and Simons AD (1990) Biol. Psychiatry 27: 92A.
3. Kupfer DJ, Frank E, McEachran AB and Grochocinski VJ (1990) Arch. Gen. Psychiatry. 47: 1100–1105.
4. Giles DE, Jarrett RB, Roffwarg HP and Rush AJ (1987) Neuropsychopharmacology 1: 33–39.

Biological Psychiatry, Volume 1. G. Racagni et al., editors.

An integrated view of vulnerability

David J. Kupfer
Department of Psychiatry, University of Pittsburgh School of Medicine, Western Psychiatric Institute and Clinic, 3811 O'Hara Street, Pittsburgh, PA 15213, U.S.A.

It is now obvious that both the knowledge base and interest of scientists to integrate various domains are fostering attempts to establish the interrelationships of diverse clinical, biological and psychosocial factors as they contribute to vulnerability and to increased risk of developing depression. In order to most appropriately carry out this overall goal, it is also clear that several issues must be more precisely understood in order to provide conceptual clarity to address the overall goal. Such issues include the following: the state-trait issue; the integration of biological and psychosocial domains; the appropriate use of vulnerability and protective factors; and finally, aging or differential levels of vulnerability across the life cycle.

In attempting to reach such an integrated view, we need to understand that, by-and-large, depression is an episodic illness and not a chronic one. Most individuals recover but they become ill again at some point in their life with the likelihood of a second lifetime episode ranging from 50–80%. Each time an individual has a new episode the risk for suicide, marital and social disruption increase as does the likelihood that an individual will go on to develop chronicity (an episode of depression lasting at least 2 years). In short, if we are to examine issues relating to vulnerability, we need to set up longitudinal designs since they represent the best shot at examining risk factors and elucidating the road to the first onset of disorder.

In examining the first onset, we must realize that the most relevant domains include the following: biological genetic, psychosocial (including personality) and also the larger context of environment and culture. We suggest that specific risk factors will have a differential weight at various points in the life cycle and are more or less prominent depending on when the first onset of disorder occurs. For example, in childhood and adolescence, an increased family history of depression is more strongly associated with onset than in later life. If we understand that there may be a differential weight for risk factors leading to first onset and that they may be different from risk for subsequent onset, then one can begin to develop a series of paradigms in order to examine issues of vulnerability and protection. But before we investigate those particular issues, we also need to see what role recovery from the episode plays since most of the previous scientific investigations have been primarily concerned with onset of episode. We know that recovery from the episode may be related to such factors which represent early intervention for psychopharmacologic agents, and on the negative side such factors as inadequate tricyclic dose with a reduction in the drug dosage prematurely or the solitary use of psychological treatments for severe depression. Moderating factors with respect to faster recovery may also include the lack of comorbid conditions, the lack of Axis II (personality) disorders, adequate social support systems, positive self-esteem and finally, the reduction in difficulties in fresh starts.

The models that relate to first-episode onset and subsequent onset may be considered significantly different in that with first onset much more attention is given to basic endowment and developmental processes. From a tactical point of view, research in this area is complicated because first onsets of depression will include both the initial episode of a recurrent illness and single lifetime episodes. Most researchers have attempted to deal with risk/vulnerability factors and predictors of second episodes. Subsequently, the search for a more homogenous route to the onset of episode is an important one. For example, if we were to just focus on the first onset of recurrent illness, we would likely propose the following factors. In a childhood/adolescent onset it appears that increased family history, developmental issues (such as repeated separation or abandonment) and in adolescents increased drug and alcohol use, as well as the presence of medical illness, provide important vulnerability factors for an early onset of depression. During the adult period of time, first onset may very well be associated with increased stressful life events, especially among women, as compared to those individuals who do not have an onset of depression, increased drug and alcohol use and increased medical illness. It also appears that in adult onset disorder, negative environmental factors such as negative interaction with children or husband (if married) or interaction with children or lack of a very close tie for a single mother is important. This negative environmental factor plus a negative psychological factor, such as low self-esteem or chronic subclinical conditions and childhood sexual abuse provide important vulnerability factors for adult onset. In late life onset, it appears that increased medical illness is clearly a vulnerability factor.

As another example of various integrated approaches, recently Dr. Marjorie Klein et al. have proposed a model of personality and depression relationships (personal communication) which differentiate a pathway to a first episode versus subsequent episode. In such a model, they provide differential weights between certain basic environments, baseline states and mediators of stress and buffers of such stress. In examining the model for recurrent episodes, which represents an integrated model of personality and depression for subsequent episodes, it would appear that less attention is provided with respect to basic environment and, indeed, the first episode itself becomes one of the key vulnerability factors in developing a subsequent episode. In many cases, it is proposed that the outcome of the first episode may effect stability and rhythmicity. It may also provide a continued environment in which attachment conflicts, interpersonal patterns and social support systems may be sufficiently disturbed to continue to provide sufficient stress that a subsequent episode of depression occurs.

Biological Psychiatry, Volume 1. G. Racagni et al., editors.

Epidemiology and prognosis of depression

E.S. Paykel
Professor of Psychiatry, University of Cambridge, Addenbrooke's Hospital, Cambridge CB2 2QQ, U.K.

This paper will discuss the epidemiology and prognosis of depression, as a brief introduction to what will follow.

Epidemiology

There are now good data available regarding rate and of depression [1]. Using admission statistics, about 1 per 1,000 of the general population are admitted to hospital annually with depression [2]. Better figures for psychiatric care of all kinds come from case register studies, particularly from Scandinavia [3,4] and England [5,6]. These show that about 3 per 1,000 are seen annually by psychiatrists, including those admitted. These figures are a little outdated; there may now be more outpatients seen.

In the U.K. only a relatively small proportion of psychiatric problems are referred to psychiatrists. In national morbidity surveys about 3% of the general population are diagnosed as depressed by general practitioners annually [7]. Probably equal numbers are unrecognized [8]. Freeling et al. [9] found that missed depressions showed less overt and less typical symptoms, and more links with physical illness.

In the long run, enumeration of all cases in the general population ought to provide the best information. Epidemiological studies require some definition of a disorder. In Britain, the PSE and ID/CATEGO have been used [10], and in the U.S.A., the DIS and DSM III [11]. Studies using these methods from London, Edinburgh, Canberra, Athens, several American cities and Puerto Rico give 6-month prevalences which average to approximately 5% overall: 6% in women and 3% in men [1]. Essentially this is disorder satisfying clinical criteria, but it is skewed toward the milder and less biological range [12].

Few community studies have attempted to estimate episode rates rather than prevalences. Surtees et al. [13] found an annual inception rate in women for all disorders of 12.6%; about half was due to major depression.

Attempts to estimate lifetime risk of unipolar depression from single retrospective interviews are risky, because of poor recall and failure of recognition. A more prospective attempt came from the Swedish Lundby study, in which a sample was interviewed in 1957 and re-interviewed in 1972 [14]. The lifetime incidence figures for cases of mild or greater impairment were 49% in women and 28% in men: for medium and severe impairment they were 17% and 32%. Even mild cases had to have definitely pathological symptoms requiring intervention, with reduced capacity to function of 50%. There are also figures suggesting that rates are increasing, at least for younger males, although findings are not yet conclusive. Good lifetime figures are available for bipolar disorder, since most subjects present for treatment. The morbid risk is around 0.7% [4].

Demographic associations are now fairly clear [1]. Although severe hospitalized samples tend to be older, community and outpatient samples show that milder disorder is common in the 20s and 30s. The female predominance ranges from 2:1 to 3:1, both in treated and community samples, except for bipolars. The explanation is probably complex [15], and may include hormonal influences, psychosocial effects and differential acknowledgement and direction of distress.

Prognosis

If the message from epidemiology is that depression is much more common than we thought, the message from follow-up studies is that, even with the availability of modern treatments, it is still more recurrent than we had hoped. Coryell and Winokur [16] have recently reviewed studies. Bipolar disorder is more recurrent than unipolar. I will concentrate on unipolar disorder and on a small number of particularly informative studies. It is useful to differentiate between "relapse" or early return of symptoms which may be regarded as reappearance of a recent episode and later "recurrence" which might be regarded as a new episode (Klerman and Paykel, 1976).

The most informative recent short-term follow-up is that from the NIMH Psychobiology Study [17–20]. Although episode length was protracted if taken from onset, the outcome for remission from the time of treatment was moderately good; 63% of patients recovered within the first 4 months, after which recovery rates declined markedly and 26% of patients still had not recovered at 1 year. When patients were followed beyond the point of remission, outcome was not so good. Twenty-four percent of patients relapsed within the 3 months after recovery, and 36% in the first year. Some relapses became chronic and there was often under-treatment [20]. In general, poor outcome was associated with more previous episodes, slower onset, greater severity, a dysthymic pattern and older age of onset. These relapse figures are consistent with those which emerged from the studies of drug continuation vs. withdrawal undertaken in the 1970s which showed relapse rates reduced to about half by drug continuation but not usually eliminated. Symptom return is highest in the first year after remission [21].

Longer-term follow-up studies show substantial relapse rates. Until recently, most samples who had received long-term follow-up had been treated in a previous era, and it was difficult to know if findings applied in modern circumstances. However, at the end of 1988 two long-term follow-up studies were published, one of depressives admitted to the Maudsley Hospital in 1965–1966 [22]; the other of

Australian admissions between 1966–1970 [23]. Like the NIMH Study, the samples may have been biased to treatment resistance by coming from special university treatment centers. Outcomes were poor in both studies. Over approximately 16 years, 60% and 56% respectively were readmitted at least once: this applied to 51% and 47% of those who were first admissions at index episode. Readmission was more common in endogenous depressives and where there had been a previous episode. Among those readmitted, some showed very recurrent illnesses. Among those not readmitted, 22% and 16% showed either mild/moderate chronic illness, or very slow recovery from index episode. Overall, in the 2 studies respectively 25% and 11% showed very poor outcomes with chronic severe disorder and handicaps. Suicide and overall mortality rates were increased compared with the general population. An 11-year follow-up of a Canadian sample produced comparably poor outcome [24]. The classic review of suicide in affective disorders by Guze and Robins [25] suggested that 15% of deaths are by suicide, and there is good evidence that mortality rates have increased [16].

Long-term outcome in outpatients, general practice patients and subjects in the community is not known, but is likely to be better. It is noteworthy from the 2 inpatient follow-ups that, among first-episode patients, half had at least 1 further episode requiring admission, i.e. of comparable intensity, and half did not; a smaller number had very recurrent episodes; some additional subjects had at least 1 further milder recurrence not requiring admission. An estimate would be that whatever the severity and intensity of care: community, general practice, outpatient, inpatient, about 50% have at least one further episode at that level and 50% do not, although they may have another milder episode. This is not very well informed guesswork, however: it needs testing properly.

References

1. Paykel ES (1989) Br. J. Psychiatry 155: 754–763.
2. Bebbington PE (1978) Cult. Med. Psychiatry 2: 297–341.
3. Juel-Neilsen N, Bille M, Flygenring J and Helgason T (1961) Acta Psychiatr. Scand. 162: 69–80.
4. Boyd JH and Weissman MM (1982) In: Paykel ES (ed.) Handbook of Affective Disorders. Churchill Livingstone, Edinburgh, pp. 106–152.
5. Grad de Alarcon J, Sainsbury P and Costain WR (1975) Psychol. Med. 5: 32–54.
6. Wing JK and Fryers T (1976) Psychiatric Services in Camberwell and Salford: Statistics from the Camberwell and Salford Psychiatric Registers 1964–1974. MRC Social Psychiatry Unit, London.
7. HMSO (1986) Morbidity Statistics from General Practice: Third National Study. HMSO, London.
8. Goldberg D and Huxley P (1980) Mental Illness in the Community: The Pathway to Psychiatric Care. Tavistock Publications, London, pp. 57–107.
9. Freeling P, Rao BM, Paykel ES, Sireling LI and Burton RH (1985) Br. Med. J. 290: 1880–1883.
10. Wing JK, Mann SA, Leff JP and Nixon JN (1978) Psychol. Med. 8: 203–217.
11. Robins LN, Helzer JE, Croughan J and Ratcliff KS (1981) Arch. Gen. Psychiatry 38: 381–389.
12. Sireling LI, Freeling P, Paykel ES and Rao BN (1985) Br. J. Psychiatry 147: 119–126.
13. Surtees PG, Sashidharan SP and Dean C (1986) Br. J. Psychiatry 148: 176–186.
14. Rorsman B, Gräsbeck A, Hagnell O, Lanke J, Öhman R, Öjesjo L and Otterbeck L (1990) Br. J. Psychiatry 156: 336–342.

15. Paykel ES (1991) Br. J. Psychiatry 158(10): 22–29.
16. Coryell W and Winokur G (1992) In: Paykel ES (ed.) Handbook of Affective Disorders, 2nd Edition. Churchill Livingstone, Edinburgh.
17. Keller MB, Shapiro RW, Lavori PW and Wolfe N (1982a) Arch. Gen. Psychiatry 39: 905–910.
18. Keller MB, Shapiro RW, Lavori PW and Wolfe N (1982b) Arch. Gen. Psychiatry 39: 911–915.
19. Keller MB, Lavori PW, Lewis CE and Klerman GL (1983) J. Am. Med. Assoc. 250: 3299–3304.
20. Keller MB, Lavori PW, Rice J, Coryell W and Hirschfeld RMA (1986) Am. J. Psychiatry 143: 24–28.
21. Lavori PW, Keller MB and Klerman GL (1984) J. Psychiatr. Res. 18(1): 13–25.
22. Lee AS and Murray RM (1988) Br. J. Psychiatry 153: 741–751.
23. Kiloh LG, Andrews G and Neilson M (1988) Br. J. Psychiatry 153: 752–757.
24. Lehmann HE, Fenton FR, Deutsch M, Feldman S and Engelsmann F (1988) Acta Psychiatr. Scand. 78: 57–65.
25. Guze SB and Robins E (1970) Br. J. Psychiatry 117: 437–438.
26. Bebbington PE, Hurry J, Tennant C et al. (1981) Psychol. Med. 11: 561–579.

Biological Psychiatry, Volume 1. G. Racagni et al., editors.

Efficacy of maintenance therapy with TCAs and MAOIs: New findings

David J. Kupfer and Ellen Frank

Department of Psychiatry, University of Pittsburgh School of Medicine, Western Psychiatric Institute and Clinic, 3811 O'Hara Street, Pittsburgh, PA 15213, U.S.A.

The need to successfully treat individuals who develop repeated episodes of depression has become a pressing public health issue. While more sophisticated diagnostic criteria have made the identification of the recurrent patient less difficult once the individual presents for treatment in a medical setting, many persons with recurrent depression accept their frequent episodes as their natural seasonal mood variation or "plight", never thinking to seek treatment. Still others are seen in a variety of health settings, treated for each acute episode, and sent on their way only to suffer another recurrence. Such "strategies" underscore the point that the longitudinal nature of the illness must be considered when evaluating the effectiveness of long-term prophylaxis.

Several recent studies reflect the improving picture for long-term treatment. In one study, Robinson et al. [1] investigated the effectiveness of maintenance treatment with phenelzine in which patients with major depression were randomized to 2-year double-blind treatment with phenelzine 60 mg/day, phenelzine 45 mg/day, or placebo if they responded initially to non-blind phenelzine treatment and sustained remission for 16 weeks. Both doses of phenelzine were significantly better than placebo in preventing relapse/recurrence of depression. Forty-seven patients were randomly assigned to double-blind treatment. Sixteen patients experienced early return of depression (<3 months after randomization) and were categorized as relapsers (with respect to the index episode). The 6 patients who had late-occurring (3 to 16 months) exacerbations of depression were considered to have experienced a new episode of major depression. This study has raised questions concerning the rate at which MAOIs should be tapered, both in controlled trials and in clinical practice. Since the authors included a defined symptom-free period before maintenance treatment, the issue of whether the re-emergence of the syndrome following drug withdrawal represents a relapse or a recurrence is not resolved. They pointed out that depressive episodes can exist for a period greater than a year in many individuals, suggesting that relatively abrupt discontinuation may serve as an important "probe" to test the need for long-term active drug maintenance treatment.

In a second study, Frank et al. [2] concluded a randomized 3-year maintenance trial in 128 patients with recurrent depression who had responded to combined short-term and continuation treatment with imipramine and interpersonal psychotherapy (IPT). A 5-cell design was used to determine whether a maintenance form of interpersonal psychotherapy (IPT-M), alone or a combination with medication, could play a significant role in the prevention of recurrence. A second question was whether maintaining antidepressant medication at the dose used to treat the acute episode rather than decreasing to a "maintenance" dose would provide prophylaxis superior to that observed in earlier trials in which a maintenance dose strategy (lower than acute dose) was employed. Survival analysis demonstrated a highly significant prophylactic effect for active imipramine maintained at an average dose of 200 mg and a modest prophylactic effect for monthly IPT-M which appears to lengthen the time between episodes in patients not receiving active medication.

The study by Frank et al. [2] is an outgrowth of the earlier Prien et al. [3] study and offers an opportunity to make some comparisons with the results of that investigation. The greatest comparability between the 2 investigations occurs in the medication clinic and placebo conditions where results for 2-year survival were virtually identical in the 2 studies. In each instance, only 20% of patients survived 2 years without recurrence of illness. In contrast, the medication clinic and active imipramine cell was associated with considerably better median survival in the Frank et al. [2] investigation than in the investigation of Prien et al. [3] It should be noted, however, that while the mean daily dose of imipramine hydrochloride at the start of the maintenance phase was 137 mg/day (range 75–150 mg/day) in the Prien et al. [3] protocol, in the Frank et al. [2] investigation patients were continued at their acute treatment dose throughout the maintenance phase, resulting in an average maintenance dose of 208 ± 65 mg/day (range 50–350 mg/day) and a median of 200 mg/day.

Studies such as the Frank et al. [2] and Montgomery et al. [4] investigations point to the impact of maintenance pharmacotherapy on the likelihood of recurrence; however, several methodological points remain to be addressed. Montgomery et al. [4] found a 50% placebo recurrence rate at the end of a 1-year prophylactic study versus a 26% rate of recurrence with fluoxetine. In a randomized clinical trial to evaluate the relative efficacy of treatments in the prevention of a recurrent disorder, we believe that it is essential to admit patients to the study during an acute episode of the illness so that patients are roughly comparable with respect to the timing of the "natural" cycle of their illness. Furthermore, in any prospective study patients will withdraw or drop out for various reasons, often for reasons related to the treatment they are receiving. If maintenance therapy trials suffer from methodological flaws that confound our ability to answer the question of what is the best treatment for preventing or delaying the recurrence of depression following an acute episode, then perhaps this question is unanswerable. How, then, can a maintenance therapy trial be conducted which minimizes potential sources of bias? A possible solution suggested by Greenhouse et al. [5] is to design a study in which patients in an acute episode are randomized from the first day of the study to an acute, continuation and maintenance treatment strategy.

Clearly, further studies examining other tricyclics and MAOIs are necessary to extend these findings. A number of issues relating to discontinuation patterns, total length of maintenance treatment, role of psychotherapy in combination with medication and biological and clinical correlates of maintenance treatment are still largely unanswered.

References

1. Robinson DS, Lerfald SC, Bennett B, Laux D, Devereaux E, Kayser A, Corcella J and Albright D (1991) Psychopharmacol. Bull. (in press).
2. Frank E, Kupfer DJ, Perel JM, Cornes C, Jarrett DB, Mallinger AG, Thase ME, McEachran AB and Grochocinski VJ (1990) Arch. Gen. Psychiatry 47: 1093–1099.
3. Prien RF, Kupfer DJ, Mansky PA, Small JG, Tuason VB, Voss CB and Johnson WE (1984) Arch. Gen. Psychiatry 41: 1096–1104.
4. Montgomery SA, Dufour H, Brion S, Gailledreau J, Laqueille X, Ferrey G, Moron P, Parant-Lucena N, Singer L, Danion JM, Beuzen JN and Pierredon MA (1988) Br. J. Psychiatry 153: 69–76.
5. Greenhouse JB, Stangl D, Kupfer DJ and Prien RF (1991) Arch. Gen. Psychiatry 48: 313–318.

Biological Psychiatry, Volume 1. G. Racagni et al., editors.

Long-term outcome of mood disorder on prophylactic lithium

M.T. Abou-Saleh[1] and A.J. Coppen[2]

[1]University Department of Psychiatry, Royal Liverpool Hospital, Liverpool; and [2]MRC Neuropsychiatry Laboratory, West Park Hospital, Epsom, Surrey, U.K.

Introduction

In the present open prospective study we have explored the predictive value of the clinical and personality characteristics in determining long-term clinical outcome over many years of lithium therapy. Moreover, we have studied biological correlates of response including the dexamethasone suppression test (DST), electrodermal activity and measures of thyroid and renal functions. Initial response over the first 6 months and first year was also studied as an empirical predictor of long-term response to lithium.

Patients and Methods

The present cohort of patients was studied in 1981 prior to starting a double-blind study of reduced lithium dosage/levels. The clinic had a very low drop-out rate of 3–5% per annum and the cohort studied is a representation of the population of affectively ill patients attending the lithium clinic including patients who have not responded to lithium, i.e. who have experienced relapses and recurrences of illness.

All patients were followed up for the whole time they had lithium, which varied between 2–12 years (mean 5.9, S.D. 2.7 years).

The cohort consisted of bipolar and unipolar patients whose episodes met appropriate criteria for primary depression or mania. There were 41 male and 73 female patients whose ages ranged between 22 and 83 years (mean 56.8, S.D. 12.1 years). They all received lithium carbonate in the form of sustained-release tablets in a once daily dosage regime to achieve plasma lithium levels of 0.6–1.2 mmol/l 12 h later.

Patients who suffered relapses or recurrences received ad hoc appropriate treatment. Relapse or recurrence was defined as the occurrence of depressive or manic symptoms that warranted treatment as in-patients or out-patients with antidepressants, neuroleptics, anxiolytics or ECT as appropriate. This extra indication was discontinued upon recovery and patients remained on lithium only.

Clinical outcome of prophylactic treatment was measured using the Affective Morbidity Index (AMI) [1]. The AMI is a measure related not only to the severity of an episode of affective illness, but also the duration of such an episode. AMI score, therefore, indicates the average level of morbidity throughout the year. AMI was calculated for each patient for the whole time spent on prophylactic lithium. For purposes of this investigation response to lithium was classified as excellent if the patient suffered no relapses/recurrence and as fair if relapse/s or recurrence/s were experienced for the whole time on lithium. According to this classification there were 60 patients who had an excellent response and 56 who had a fair response to lithium and/or other psychotropic medication.

Unipolar patients were classified on the ICD-9 Diagnostic Scale and in accordance with Winokur's genetic types [2]. Personality characteristics were measured during an euthymic phase of illness. Unipolar and bipolar patients completed four personality questionnaires, the Eysenck Personality Questionnaire which measures extraversion-introversion, neuroticism, and psychoticism; Foulds' Personality Deviance Scale, the Marke-Nyman Temperament Scale, the Crown-Crisp Experiential Index (CCEI).

Patients were administered the overnight DST during lithium therapy. A total of 62 patients had their electrodermal activity in accordance with the method described by Mirkin and Coppen.

Ninety-one patients had their thyroxin levels determined and 87 of these patients also had their thyrotropine plasma concentrations estimated. Urine volume (mean of 2 24-h volumes) and osmolality were measured in 78 of these patients. Initial response (AMI) was determined for the first 6 months from starting lithium for the clinical subgroups of unipolar/bipolar, endogenous/non-endogenous, Winokur's genetic types and excellent/fair responders.

Results

Bipolar patients showed more favourable long-term responses to lithium than did unipolar patients ($P < 0.05$). Among unipolars, those with endogenous illness as defined by the Newcastle Index, but not by ICD, showed more favourable responses than those with non-endogenous depression for their initial response over the first 6 months ($P < 0.01$) and their whole time on lithium ($P < 0.05$) within the unipolar group, those with pure familial depressive disorder (PFDD) had similar long-term response to bipolars. The bipolar group, however, showed better response than the sporadic depressive (SDD) ($P < 0.05$) and depression spectrum disorder (DSD) ($P < 0.04$) groups for the whole time on lithium.

Comparisons between excellent and fair responders in the combined group unipolar and bipolar patients showed several significant differences in personality characteristics, with fair responders showing more abnormality than was shown by excellent responders.

There were no associations between the response to lithium and any of the biological variables investigated. Excellent responders compared to fair and poor responders had similar DST results: they had similar mean post-dexamethasone cortisol concentrations. The 2 groups had similar means for T_4, TSH, urine volume and urine osmolality. Patients who were hyper-responders, habituators and non-responders to electrodermal stimuli had similar AMI for the whole time on lithium.

Excellent responders had significantly lower AMI in the first 6 months than did fair responders ($P < 0.0001$).

Discussion

The results of the present investigation, however, do not confirm our previous findings of an association between response to lithium over 2 years and Winokur's genetic types [3]. Worthy of note, however, is that bipolar patients had better responses than patients with SOD and DSD for the first 6 months and the whole time, with a similarity in outcome to patients with PFDD.

Excellent responders showed less personality disturbance than did fair responders. Moreover, excellent responders had better responses for the first 6 months and the first year of treatment. These results confirm our previous findings in a 2-year follow-up study [1], in which patients were sub-divided into responders and non-responders on the basis of the presence or absence of a recurrence in their illness. Response to prophylactic lithium was not associated with biological markers of depression, including DST and electrodermal activity. Moreover, failure to respond to lithium was not related to thyroid or renal dysfunctions. While it could be argued that greater endogenicity and the presence of a family history of depression but not of alcoholism or sociopathy and the relative absence of personality disturbance might be correlates of a biological component of the illness, this was not consistent with the absence of an association between response and biological markers such as DST and electrodermal activity. The most useful predictor of response to prophylactic lithium is, however, an empirical one: a trial of lithium over 6 months appears to determine the likelihood of the patients responding to it in the years to come.

References

1. Coppen A, Peet M and Bailey J (1973) Psychiatr. Neurol. Neurochir. (Amst.) 76: 501–510.
2. Winokur G (1979) Am. J. Psychiatry 136: 911–913.
3. Abou-Saleh MT and Coppen A (1986) J. Affective Disord. 10: 9–13.

Biological Psychiatry, Volume 1. G. Racagni et al., editors.

The efficacy of prophylactic treatment with 5-HT reuptake inhibitors

S.A. Montgomery, D.B. Montgomery and M. Green
St. Mary's Hospital, London, U.K.

The regulatory authorities in Europe now require that the evidence of long-term efficacy of antidepressants should be established in properly conducted long-term studies independently of the efficacy demonstrated in acute studies. If an antidepressant is discontinued shortly after symptomatic response is registered, rather a high proportion of patients suffer a relapse. This propensity to relapse is seen over the subsequent 4 or 6 months with a high proportion occurring in the first 2 months.

The placebo controlled studies of relapse prevention over a 4- to 6-month period provide consistent evidence of the efficacy of antidepressants over this period, and this is seen even in quite small studies. The implication is that antidepressants given for the acute treatment course should be given for a further 4 to 6 months following symptomatic response. In those studies which have included a mixed population of first-time and recurrent depressives, the relapse rate is seen to be equally high in both groups and this suggests that the symptomatic response of the acute depression is incomplete and that the reappearance of symptoms does not represent a new episode since this would be unlikely to occur so soon in first-time depressives.

One early study suggested a higher relapse rate might occur if the response to acute treatment is not properly established in that residual symptoms were associated with early relapse. However, this is not confirmed in the recent large sertraline placebo relapse prevention study where the relapse rate appeared to be equal in patients with more or fewer residual symptoms. Nevertheless, an adequate response needs to be documented before a relapse prevention study is undertaken.

Prophylactic studies of longer-term efficacy are aimed at the prevention of new episodes of depression, and these studies therefore need to be undertaken in those suffering from recurrent depressions, whether major depression or recurrent brief depression. The prophylactic design is at present the only feasible way of demonstrating the efficacy of any treatment for recurrent brief depression. Recurrent brief depression (ICD10 38.10) is a common, dangerous disorder where quite profound depressions lasting mostly 2 to 4 days recur erratically some 20 times a year. The prophylactic design is used in this case to test efficacy in reducing the severity, duration or recurrence rate.

Prophylactic studies in unipolar depression are more likely to demonstrate efficacy if a criterion of previous frequent recurrence is used. Studies using the criteria of either 2 previous episodes or, more commonly, 1 previous episode in the last 5 years have been able to demonstrate the prophylactic efficacy of antidepressants. Prophylactic studies should document the index depressive episode and its response and should also establish that the depressive episode continues to respond during a symptom-free period of at least 4 months before entering the placebo controlled prophylactic study proper.

The power calculations for these studies require that for any meaningful result a comparison against placebo is necessary, since the numbers required to demonstrate equivalent efficacy of 2 active drugs are so large. Four serotonin reuptake inhibitors (SRI) have been shown to have prophylactic efficacy, zimelidine, fluoxetine, sertraline and paroxetine.

The evidence in favour of SRIs as a group is now stronger than the evidence for tricyclic antidepressants where many of the studies have been variable in quality. The evidence of efficacy is good for imipramine and may probably be accepted for maprotiline. For amitriptyline, however, an adequate prophylactic study has still not been carried out. For nortriptyline there is evidence of lack of effect. With maprotiline, despite the long-term efficacy, there is evidence of the provocation of suicide attempts which were significantly higher in the maprotiline-treated group than in the placebo group.

There are no studies comparing different doses of SRIs in prophylactic treatment. However, the studies of zimelidine and fluoxetine used relatively high doses and the study of sertraline used a low dose which did not appear to compromise efficacy. It would seem wise to use the dose that is established as effective in acute treatment until studies comparing different doses have been undertaken.

The SRIs appear to be well tolerated, which has advantages in terms of compliance particularly in long-term treatment. There is evidence that some SRIs are associated with significantly less manic episodes than conventional tricyclic antidepressants and this is important in long-term treatment of major depression where some patients are likely to be undetected bipolars.

With effective prophylactic treatment the recurrence rate of new episodes appears to be halved. It is also clear from the survival curves in the studies that the prophylactic efficacy is maintained over time, and patients with highly recurrent depression should therefore continue with long-term treatment probably indefinitely.

Biological Psychiatry, Volume 1. G. Racagni et al., editors.

Biological markers in depression: Introductory remarks

Pavel D. Hrdina

Departments of Pharmacology and Psychiatry, University of Ottawa, 451 Smyth Rd, Ottawa, Ontario, K1H 8M5, Canada

One of aims of biological psychiatry has been to use the advances of biological sciences in investigation and treatment of psychiatric disorders. Regulatory mechanisms, feedbacks, new set points all reflect the adaptability of the organism, its ability to cope with perturbations and maintain a state of functional equilibrium. Failure of these mechanisms, from molecular to organ level, results in dysregulations expressed as symptoms of abnormal behaviour, syndromes or a defined illness entity. The reasons for dysregulation may lie at different levels, from receptor protein malfunction to lack of specific enzymes or abnormal neuronal response. Despite dramatic recent advances in neurosciences including the successful cloning of many neurotransmitter receptor subtypes and biogenic amine transporters, identification of intracellular signalling pathways and novel potential endogenous ligands, the biological basis or correlates of mental disorders are far from being understood. The search for biological markers in psychiatry has therefore been a part of the research of functional changes or responses (e.g. receptor sensitivity, components of the signalling system, enzyme synthesis, disposition of neurotransmitters) that would be associated with the diseased state in a hope that some of these alterations will be proven to be reliable markers of diseased state (state markers) or of vulnerability to the illness (trait markers). Another aim of this search is to detect symptomatologically silent prodromal phase of the illness and devise means to prevent a full-blown episode.

A variety of biological measures have been assessed for their possible causal or at least associative relationship to symptoms or syndromes of main psychiatric disorders such as depression or schizophrenia. The tools being used are biochemical, genetic, neurophysiological, molecular, pharmacological, imaging and psychometric. Most studies of biological markers in depression have been related to the currently prevailing neurotransmitter-hormonal dysregulation hypothesis of this disorder and have aimed at direct or indirect demonstration of central or peripheral neurotransmitters or hormonal function abnormalities in the course of the illness.

The main neurotransmitter systems implicated in the pathogenesis of depressive disorder are the serotonergic [1] and noradrenergic [2]. Consequently, many studies have investigated the levels of serotonin or norepinephrine and their metabolites, in blood, cerebro-spinal fluid and postmortem brain samples from patients with depression. The only well-documented finding has been a decreased level of the main serotonin metabolite, 5-HIAA, in a subgroup of depressed patients with suicidal behaviour [3]. Serotonin uptake by platelets was found to be significantly decreased in depression [4] but also in mania and schizo-affective disorder [5]. Some but not all studies have also reported a reduced density of [^{3}H]imipramine binding, presumably to serotonin transporter, in platelets from depressed patients [viz. 6]. Other reported changes in serotonergic system in depression include increased density of 5-HT_2 receptors in both postmortem brain tissue [7] and platelets [8]. Results of studies on the status of α_2 adrenergic receptors in platelets of depressed patients remain inconclusive, but several studies have found decreased density and functional responses of β-adrenergic receptors on mononuclear leukocytes isolated from depressed subjects [viz. 9]. Findings on α_2 and β-adrenoceptor changes in postmortem brain samples of depressed suicide victims are reviewed by Horton et al. (this volume) and the potential significance of [^{3}H]antidepressant binding sites in human brain is discussed by Marcusson (this volume).

One of most widely documented findings in depression are the abnormalities in the function of hypothalamo-pituitary-adrenal axis most likely related to changes in central neurotransmitter function. Decreased sensitivity to dexamethasone suppression, to TRH stimulation of TSH secretion, adrenergic stimulation of GH, tryptophan stimulation of prolactin release and adrenergic stimulation of melatonin secretion all presumably reflect altered neurotransmitter interaction with the hypothalamo-pituitary axis. This area of research is reviewed in detail by Prange (this volume).

So far, none of these putative biological markers has been found to be entirely selective for depression. It would be, however, unrealistic to expect that a single biological marker will characterize a multifaceted and heterogeneous disorder such as depression. It is likely that certain biochemical abnormalities (e.g. serotonergic deficiency) will be associated with certain types of behaviour or function (e.g. aggressivity, sleep) regardless of given diagnostic entity (e.g. depression, anxiety etc.). A more rewarding approach may be to cross the defined boundaries of structured diagnostic categories and to tie together the biological variables with the symptoms (e.g. insomnia) or altered behaviours (e.g. aggressivity) they are associated with. This approach might yield markers of partial dysfunction that will correlate with cluster of symptoms or specific symptoms across nosological units and help more in our understanding of the biological basis of altered behaviour. Tools of molecular biology and DNA hybridization technique offer novel approaches in the search for unique illness-specific mRNAs in postmortem brain tissue of psychiatric patients. Furthermore, new techniques of in vivo brain receptor imaging by positron emission tomography can now be used to define dynamic alterations in neurotransmitter, hormonal and peptidergic systems thought to be involved in various types of behaviour.

References

1. Coppen A (1967) Br. J. Psychiatry 113: 1237–1264.
2. Siever LJ and Davis KL (1985) Am. J. Psychiatry 142: 1017–1031.
3. Asberg M, Traskman L and Thoren P (1976) Arch. Gen. Psychiatry 33: 1193–1197.
4. Tuomisto Z and Tukiainen E (1976) Nature (Lond.) 262: 596–598.
5. Meltzer H (1989) Br. J. Psychiatry 155: 25–31.
6. Mellerup ET and Plenge P (1988) Acta Psychiatr. Scand. (Suppl. 345) 78: 61–98.
7. Yates M, Leake A, Candy JM, Fairbaim AF, McKeith IG and Ferrier IN (1990) Biol. Psychiatry 27: 489–496.
8. Biegon A, Weizman A, Karp L, Ram A, Tiano S and Wolff M (1987) Life Sci. 41: 2485–2492.
9. Werstiuk ES, Steiner M and Burns T (1990) Life Sci. 47: 85–105.

Biological Psychiatry, Volume 1. G. Racagni et al., editors.

Platelet antidepressant sites and the serotonin transporter in depression

Salomon Z. Langer, Marie France Poirier, Henri Loo and Anne-Marie Galzin
Department of Biology, Synthélabo Recherche (LERS), 58 rue de la Glacière, 75013 Paris, France

Introduction

It is now well established that serotonin (5-hydroxytryptamine, 5-HT) plays a major role in the etiology of depression. In particular, it has been reported that 5-HT uptake V_{max} values are significantly reduced in platelets of untreated depressed patients [1–3]. Active transport systems for 5-HT play an important physiological role in the homeostasis of this biogenic amine [4]. Among the various pathologies in which 5-HT seems to be involved (obesity, alcoholism, memory deficit), it is in depression that 5-HT uptake inhibitors have been used with the most clearly established efficacy [5]. Two classes of drugs can be distinguished: the tricyclic antidepressants (imipramine, cyanoimipramine and chlorimipramine) and recently introduced non-tricyclic antidepressant drugs such as fluoxetine, citalopram, sertraline, paroxetine and litoxetine (SL 81.0385) [6]. All these drugs, which are 5-HT uptake inhibitors, have been proven to be effective in the management of depression.

The advantage of the non-tricyclic antidepressant drugs is that they limit the appearance of a large number of the undesirable side-effects noted upon tricyclic antidepressant treatments, such as sedation, fatigue, orthostatic hypotension, dry mouth, constipation, blurred vision and urinary retention resulting from interactions of tricyclic drugs at α-adrenergic, histaminergic and cholinergic receptors. In addition, these new selective 5-HT uptake inhibitors do not produce arythmias, tachycardia or cardiac toxicity. In this context, the existence of high affinity binding sites in brain and blood platelets for radiolabeled antidepressant drugs has been an important step in our understanding of the mechanism of action of these compounds.

Pharmacology of the 5-HT transporter

Radiolabelled forms of 5-HT uptake inhibitors have been used extensively in in vitro membrane binding assays to study the sodium-coupled 5-HT transporter [4]. In initial studies, [^{3}H]-imipramine was used and more recently, [^{3}H]-paroxetine, a non tricyclic 5-HT uptake inhibitor [7]. Both radioligands label with high affinity binding sites in both platelet and cerebral cortical membrane preparations from several mammalian species [8]. Moreover, the potencies of a number of compounds to inhibit [^{3}H]-imipramine or [^{3}H]-paroxetine binding and [^{3}H]-5-HT uptake in both brain and platelets show an excellent correlation [7,9,10]. These results indicate the suitability of both radioligands as specific probes of the sodium-coupled 5-HT transporter.

The platelet 5-HT transporter as a biological marker of depression

Clinical research has centered almost exclusively on [^{3}H]-imipramine binding to platelets as a potential biological marker in depression (for review, see [7,11]). The first clinical investigation reported that platelets isolated from untreated depressed patients contained smaller amounts of [^{3}H]-imipramine binding sites than platelets from control subjects [12]. This was followed by numerous others, and so far more than 50 studies have analyzed platelet imipramine binding in depressed patients and healthy controls. Around two-thirds of the reports showed decreased platelet imipramine binding in depressed patients, whereas one-third found no differences between depressed patients and controls (for review, see [5,8,13]). Methodological differences or clinical factors might to some extent explain these conflicting results. Recent results obtained in a WHO collaborative study between 9 centers all around the world emphasized the methodological difficulties concerning membrane preparation, measurement of protein concentration or estimation of K_d values (see [11] for review).

Another important parameter to be considered to explain discrepancies among clinical studies is the circadian variation reported for serotonin uptake in human blood platelets [14] and for imipramine or paroxetine binding in rabbit blood platelets [15,16]. The existence of such circadian variations for imipramine binding in human blood platelets remains to be demonstrated.

Conclusions

The validity of imipramine platelet binding sites as a biological marker of endogenous depression remains an open question. Evidence currently available does not exclude the possibility that differences in the number of binding sites may exist among subgroups of depressed patients. On the other hand, it is now clearly established that the sodium-dependent 5-HT transporter, labelled with [^{3}H]-imipramine or [^{3}H]-paroxetine, is the target of 5-HT uptake inhibitors currently used or developed as antidepressant drugs.

Recent development in our knowledge of molecular mechanisms of amine transport should contribute in a near future to gain more insight into the functioning of the 5-HT transporter macromolecule and clarify the involvement of this system in the pathophysiology of depression.

References

1. Born GVR, Grignani G and Martin K (1980) Br. J. Clin. Pharmacol. 9: 321–325.
2. Coppen A, Swade C and Wood K (1980) Br. J. Psychiatry 136: 235–238.
3. Le Quan-Bui KH, Plaisant O, Leboyer M, Gay C, Kamal L, Devynck MA and Meyer P (1984) Psychiatr. Res. 13: 129–139.
4. Graham G and Langer SZ (1988) In: Osborne NN and Hamon M (eds.) Neuronal Serotonin. Wiley, Chichester, pp. 367–391.
5. Langer SZ, Galzin AM, Poirier MF, Loo H, Sechter D and Zarifian E (1987) J. Rec. Res. 7: 499–521.
6. Scatton B, Claustre Y, Graham D, Dennis T, Serrano A, Arbilla S, Pimoule C, Schoemaker H, Bigg D and Langer SZ (1988) Drug Dev. Res. 12: 29–40.
7. Langer SZ and Galzin AM (1988) Experientia 44: 127–130.
8. Langer SZ and Schoemaker H (1988) Prog. Neuro-Psychopharmacol. Biol. Psychiatry 12: 193–216.
9. Habert E, Graham D, Tahraoui L, Claustre Y and Langer SZ (1985) Eur. J. Pharmacol. 118: 107–114.
10. Langer SZ, Moret C, Raisman R, Dubocovich ML and Briley M (1980) Science 210: 1133–1135.
11. Mellerup ET and Langer SZ (1990) Pharmacopsychiatry 23: 113–117.
12. Briley MS, Langer SZ, Raisman R, Sechter D and Zarifian E (1980) Science 209: 303–305.
13. Bech P, Eplov L, Gastpar M, Gentsch C, Mendlewicz J, Plenge P, Rielart C and Mellerup E (1988) Pharmacopsychiatry 21: 147–150.
14. Galzin AM and Langer SZ (1987) Naunyn-Schmiedeberg's Arch. Pharmacol. 336: 464–466.
15. Rocca P, Galzin AM and Langer SZ (1989) Naunyn-Schmiedeberg's Arch. Pharmacol. 340: 41–44.

Biological Psychiatry, Volume 1. G. Racagni et al., editors.

Antidepressant sites in human brain

Jan Marcusson

Department of Geriatric Medicine, University of Linköping, Vallavägen 13, S-582 46 Linköping, Sweden

Introduction

It is now more than 10 years since the important discovery was made that the antidepressant agent imipramine binds with high affinity to platelet plasma membranes and membrane fragments of brain [1]. Since the antidepressant action of imipramine and other tricyclic agents has been suggested to be at least partly due to the inhibition of the re-uptake of 5-HT into the nerve terminals, the high affinity binding of [^{3}H]imipramine to brain membranes became a new technique to study the 5-HT transporter. Over the last few years, several new data have emerged not only from studies on the [^{3}H]imipramine binding but also from those using more selective 5-HT uptake inhibitors as ligands. In the following sections data from our own laboratory and from other research groups are discussed.

The uptake site for 5-HT has been studied in binding experiments with several different radioligands, which are believed to bind to the exterior part of the 5-HT transporter. In addition to the radioligands reviewed below, i.e. [^{3}H]imipramine, [^{3}H]paroxetine and [^{3}H]citalopram, the 5-HT uptake site has been studied in binding experiments with [^{3}H]norzimeldine, [^{3}H]cyanoimipramine, [^{3}H]cocaine, [^{3}H]indalpine and [^{125}I]iodoimipramine.

[^{3}H]Imipramine binding

Both high and low affinity [^{3}H]imipramine binding sites exist and only the high affinity sites are related to the 5-HT uptake system [2,3]. Inhibition studies with 5-HT and 5-HT uptake inhibitors have confirmed the heterogeneity of [^{3}H]imipramine binding [4]. The heterogeneity of the binding appears to be due to at least two separate binding sites; one high affinity (1 nM) site of protein nature that correlates with the regional distribution of 5-HT uptake and one low affinity (>100 nM) site that is not of protein nature and does not correlate with the regional distribution of 5-HT uptake [5]. Only the high affinity [^{3}H]imipramine binding site is sodium-dependent and located on serotonergic nerve terminals [6–8].

A proper pharmacological definition of the specific [^{3}H]imipramine binding is of course crucial. High-affinity binding of [^{3}H]imipramine can be distinguished by using non-tricyclic selective 5-HT uptake inhibitors as displacing agents (e.g. paroxetine, citalopram, norzimeldine) [6,9] or 5-HT itself [6,10]. The use of desipramine-sensitive [^{3}H]imipramine binding, however, will result in binding not only to 5-HT uptake sites, but also to non-specific binding sites that may represent 40–50% in rat cortex and 80–90% in human cortex of the binding regarded as "specific" [6,10]. This may sometimes result in erroneous results in applied studies. For example, desipramine-defined [^{3}H]imipramine has been found to show a marked age-related increase [11,12], whereas 5-HT sensitive [^{3}H]imipramine binding remains unaltered or decreases with age [12].

Since the high affinity fraction of [^{3}H]imipramine binding was competitively inhibited by 5-HT and 5-HT uptake inhibitors, it was suggested that this fraction represents binding to the substrate recognition site for 5-HT uptake and a "single-site model" of the [^{3}H]imipramine binding and 5-HT uptake site was proposed [6].

In human brain tissue, the initial studies also pointed to a homogenous population of [^{3}H]imipramine binding sites [13,14]. However, more recent studies have demonstrated both high and low affinity sites where only the high affinity sites are related to the 5-HT uptake site [10,12,15,16].

[^{3}H]Paroxetine binding

In contrast to [^{3}H]imipramine binding, most of the [^{3}H]paroxetine binding is abolished after destruction of 5-HT terminals, suggesting a selective localization to 5-HT neurites [17,18]. Drug competition studies using 5-HT and 5-HT uptake inhibitors produced competitive inhibition patterns [18,19].

In the human brain, [^{3}H]paroxetine binding exhibits the same pharmacological characteristics as in rat brain [19,20]. The potencies of various compounds in inhibiting [^{3}H]paroxetine binding in human brain seem to correlate with their potencies in inhibiting 5-HT uptake in rat brain [21]. However, the amount of specific binding is lower, for example in cortical areas the specific binding represents about 40% of total binding in human brain in comparison with 90% in rat brain [18,20]. In a recent report on human brain tissue by Plenge et al. [16], it was concluded that [^{3}H]paroxetine and [^{3}H]citalopram in comparison with [^{3}H]-imipramine allowed a more precise determination of 5-HT uptake sites [16].

[^{3}H]Citalopram binding

The [^{3}H]citalopram binding in human brain tissue is different from the [^{3}H]-paroxetine binding on one important aspect: the 5-HT-sensitive [^{3}H]citalopram binding in human cortex represents 80%, whereas that of [^{3}H]paroxetine only about 40–50% [20,22]. This suggests that [^{3}H]citalopram may be a better radioligand for studying the 5-HT uptake site.

Summary and Conclusion

In summary, when considering the most recent studies on [^{3}H]imipramine, [^{3}H]-paroxetine and [^{3}H]citalopram binding, the radioligand binding to the 5-HT uptake site is consistent with a single-site binding model. Of course, this requires an adequate definition of the specific binding. The single-site model of the 5-HT uptake site proposes a common binding site for 5-HT and its uptake inhibitors. But the 5-HT uptake inhibitors probably have additional bonds outside the substrate recognition site, contributing to their uptake inhibiting properties. The 5-HT uptake site is subject to allosteric alterations during the translocation of 5-HT. 5-HT uptake inhibitors at high concentrations may cause allosteric alterations of the 5-HT uptake site. Whether these alterations involve a separate low-affinity site for 5-HT and 5-HT uptake inhibitors or non-specific membrane effects remains to be clarified.

References

1. Marcusson J and Ross SB (1990) Psychopharmacology 102: 145–155.
2. Reith MEA, Sershen H, Allen H et al. (1983) J. Neurochem. 40: 389–395.
3. Hrdina PD (1984) Eur. J. Pharmacol. 102: 481–488.
4. Sette M, Briley MS and Langer SZ (1983) J. Neurochem. 40: 622–628.
5. Marcusson J, Fowler CJ, Hall H et al. (1985) J. Neurochem. 44: 705–711.
6. Marcusson J, Bäckström I and Ross SB (1986) Mol. Pharmacol. 30: 121–128.
7. Severson JA, Woodward JJ and Wilcox RE (1986) J. Neurochem. 46: 1743–1754.
8. Hrdina P (1987) Can. J. Physiol. Pharmacol. 65: 2422–2427.
9. Mellerup E and Plenge P (1986) Psychopharamcology 89: 436–439.
10. Bäckström IT and Marcusson J (1987) Brain Res. 425: 128–136.
11. Severson JA, Marcusson JO, Osterburg H et al. (1985) J. Neurochem. 45: 1382–1389.
12. Marcusson J, Alafuzoff I, Bäckström IT et al. (1987) Brain Res. 425: 137–145.
13. Rehavi M, Paul SM, Skolnick P and Goodwin FK (1980) Life Sci. 26: 2273–2279.
14. Langer SZ, Javoy Agid F, Raisman R, Briley M et al. (1981) J. Neurochem. 37: 267–271.
15. Cash R, Raisman R, Ploska A and Agid Y (1985) Eur. J. Pharmacol. 117: 71–80.
16. Plenge P, Mellerup ET and Laursen H (1990) Prog. Neuro-Psychopharmacol. Biol. Psychiatry 14: 81–72.
17. Habert E, Graham D, Tahraoui L et al. (1985) Eur. J. Pharmacol. 118: 107–114.
18. Marcusson J, Bergström M, Eriksson K and Ross SB (1988) J. Neurochem. 50: 1783–1790.
19. Marcusson J, Andersson A and Bäckström I (1989) Psychopharmacology 99: 17–21.
20. Bäckström I, Bergström M and Marcusson J (1989) Brain Res. 486: 261–268.
21. Laruelle M, Vanisberg M-A and Maloteaux J-M (1988) Biol. Psychiatry 24: 299–309.
22. D'Amato RJ, Zweig RM, Whitehouse PJ et al. (1987) Ann. Neurol. 22: 229–236.

Biological Psychiatry, Volume 1. G. Racagni et al., editors.

Noradrenergic receptors in postmortem brains from depressed suicide victims

R.W. Horton[1], F. De Paermentier[1], J.M. King[1], M.R. Crompton[2] and C.L.E. Katona[3]

[1]Departments of Pharmacology and Clinical Pharmacology; [2]Forensic Medicine, St. George's Hospital Medical School, London SW17 ORE; and [3]Department of Psychiatry, University College and Middlesex School of Medicine, London W1N 8AA, U.K.

Introduction

Chronic administration of antidepressant treatments to animals results in adaptive changes in several classes of monoamine receptors, including α_2- and β-adrenoceptors. There has been much speculation that such effects are critical to antidepressant action and also that depression is associated with abnormalities in monoamine receptors. Studies in drug-free depressed patients, using peripheral receptor models and neuroendocrine challenge tests, provide some support for this latter view. We now provide further evidence of altered monoamine receptors in depression from studies of postmortem brain tissue.

Materials and Methods

Subject selection

Confirmed suicide deaths were subjected to retrospective diagnosis using hospital and coroner's records and interviews with the subjects' medical practitioner. Only subjects with a firm diagnosis of depression and who had not received antidepressant treatment in the 3 months prior to their deaths were included in this study. Suicides died by hanging (8), carbon monoxide poisoning (5), drug overdose (4), self-inflicted wounding (2) and jumping (2). Control brains were from subjects dying suddenly from causes not involving the CNS and were without evidence of mental or significant physical illness. Causes of death were acute myocardial infarction (17), road traffic accident (1), fall (1) and acute asthma (n = 1).

Radioligand binding assays

Binding assays were performed in well-washed membrane suspensions using coded samples. β-Adrenoceptors were labelled with [^{3}H]CGP 12177 (0.03–1 nM), defined with 200 μM (–) isoprenaline or 500 nM CGP 20712A (β_1). α_1-Adreno-

Table 1. Noradrenergic binding sites in suicides (C) and controls (S)[a]

Brain area	β-NA		α_1-NA		α_2-NA	
	C	S	C	S	C	S
Frontal cortex	67 ± 2	60 ± 2	95 ± 6	80 ± 5	233 ± 13	260 ± 13
Occipital cortex	65 ± 3	55 ± 3	110 ± 13	123 ± 13	279 ± 10	314 ± 14
Temporal cortex (Ba 21/22)	61 ± 2	58 ± 2	115 ± 7	104 ± 8	255 ± 13	316 ± 22[b]
Temporal cortex (Ba 38)	72 ± 4	59 ± 2[c]	138 ± 10	139 ± 10	292 ± 12	281 ± 14
Caudate	103 ± 5	92 ± 4	33 ± 1	33 ± 1	94 ± 6	97 ± 5
Putamen	134 ± 9	123 ± 7	26 ± 2	31 ± 3		
Hypothalamus			123 ± 4	122 ± 5	260 ± 15	274 ± 14
Thalamus	44 ± 3	45 ± 2	88 ± 4	93 ± 4	91 ± 6	81 ± 5
Hippocampus	61 ± 3	57 ± 3	234 ± 21	232 ± 20	354 ± 13	325 ± 13
Amygdala	44 ± 2	42 ± 3			147 ± 8	156 ± 6

Bmax values (means ± S.E.M.) fmol/mg protein;
Significant differences from controls denoted by $^aP < 0.05$ and $^bP < 0.01$.

ceptors were labelled with [^{3}H]prazosin (0.06–1 nM) and α_2-adrenoceptors with [^{3}H]rauwolscine (0.125–4 nM), defined with 100 μM phentolamine.

Results

Suicides (15 M, 6 F) and controls (15 M, 5 F) were well-matched for age (mean ± S.E.M.; controls 43 ± 3 years, suicides 42 ± 2 years) and postmortem delay (controls 40 ± 3 h, suicides 35 ± 4 h).

In cortical areas the number of β- and β_1-adrenoceptors (Table 1) were generally lower in suicides than controls. The differences were statistically significant for β-adrenoceptors in temporal cortex (Brodmann area (Ba) 38, lower by 19%) and for β_1-adrenoceptors in temporal cortex (Ba 21/22, lower by 17%).

The number of α_1-adrenoceptors did not differ significantly between suicides and controls (Table 1). The number of α_2-adrenoceptors was significantly higher (by 24%) in temporal cortex (Ba 21/22) of suicides than controls (Table 1); significant differences were not seen in other brain regions, although there was a trend to higher α_2-adrenoceptor binding in frontal and occipital cortex of suicides.

Twelve of the suicides died by violent means. Violent suicide was associated with lower numbers of β- and β_1-adrenoceptors in frontal cortex (by 23% and 25%) and lower β_1-adrenoceptors (by 16%) and higher numbers of α_2-adrenoceptors (by 39%) in temporal cortex (Ba 21/22) than matched controls. Nine suicides died by non-violent means. Non-violent suicide was associated with lower numbers of total β- and β_1-adrenoceptors (by 27 and 24%) in temporal cortex (Ba 38), lower

β-adrenoceptors (by 24%) in occipital cortex and lower α_2-adrenoceptors (by 17%) in hippocampus compared with controls.

Discussion

The present study provides evidence that depression in suicide victims is associated with altered cortical monoamine receptors; reduced β-adrenoceptors in frontal and temporal cortex and increased α_2-adrenoceptors in temporal cortex. The findings are in contrast to previous reports of increased β-adrenoceptors in frontal cortex of suicides [1,2]. This apparent discrepancy may relate to methodological differences or subject selection [3]. The higher α_2-adrenoceptor binding in temporal cortex is in broad agreement with higher frontal cortical [^{3}H]clonidine binding in a small group of depressed suicides [4]. The present findings contrast with our previous reports of lack of differences in cortical 5-HT_1, 5-HT_{1A} and 5-HT_2 binding sites in drug-free depressed suicides selected by the same criteria [5–7].

Acknowledgement

We thank The Sir Jules Thorn Charitable Trust for financial support.

References

1. Mann JJ, Stanley M, McBride PA and McEwan BS (1986) Arch. Gen. Psychiatry 43: 954–959.
2. Biegon A and Israeli M (1988) Brain Res. 442: 199–203.
3. De Paermentier F, Cheetham SC, Crompton MR, Katona CLE and Horton RW (1990) Brain Res. 525: 71–77.
4. Meana JJ and Garcia-Sevilla JA (1987) J. Neural Transm. 70: 377–381.
5. Cheetham SC, Crompton MR, Katona CLE and Horton RW (1988) Brain Res. 443: 272–280.
6. Cheetham SC, Crompton MR, Katona CLE and Horton RW (1990) Psychopharmacology 102: 544–548.
7. Lowther S, De Paermentier F, Cheetham SC, Crompton MR, Katona CLE and Horton RW (1990) Second IUPHAR Satellite Meeting on Serotonin, Basel, Switzerland, p. 164.

Biological Psychiatry, Volume 1. G. Racagni et al., editors.

Status on amines in CSF in depression

Annette Gjerris
St. Hans Psychiatric Hospital and Research Laboratory, Roskilde, Denmark

The amine system

The pharmacological bridge between the possible pathophysiology of an illness and the action of drugs that treat it has given rise to fundamental discoveries and developments in the understanding of a variety of disorders. The discovery that reserpin in some cases provokes depression and the findings of imipramine and also monoamineoxydase inhibitors (MAO-I) having an antidepressant effect led to the amine hypothesis. This hypothesis, in its simplest form, suggesting that the amount of amine available in the synaptic cleft is reduced in depression, has encouraged extensive research on amines in depression.

The discussion about the existence of serotonin or noradrenalin specific depressions has flourished for almost 30 years. However, the lack of consistency of results in studies attempting to verify this variation of the amine hypothesis, as well as the somewhat disappointing results in the efficacy studies of the selective serotonin reuptake inhibitors in treatment of depression, force us to reconsider the hypothesis.

A review of the literature on baseline studies of amines, their metabolites and peptides in cerebrospinal fluid CSF in depression has been compiled by Gjerris [1]. This review indicates, including all studies from the period 1966–1987 (Table 1) irrespective of subclassification of depression, that in 8 out of 24 studies CSF

Table 1. Baseline studies comparing concentrations of CSF 5-HIAA, CSF HVA and CSF MHPG in depressed patients and in controls (1966–1987)

Neurotransmitter	Number of studies	Change in neurotransmitter in depression
CSF 5-HIAA	8	↓
	1	↑
	15	↔
CSF HVA	4	↓
	1	↕
	13	↔
CSF MHPG	2	↓
	1	↑
	9	↔

Table 2. Baseline studies comparing amine metabolite concentration in patients with *major* depression and in controls (1966–1987)

Neurotransmitter	Number of studies	Changes in neurotransmitter in major depression
5-HIAA	1	↓
	1	↑
	7	↔
HVA	3	↓
	6	↔
MHPG	7	↔
	1	↑

concentrations of the serotonin metabolite 5-HIAA were low in depressed patients when compared to those of controls. For CSF concentrations of the dopamine metabolite HVA and the noradrenaline metabolite MHPG, the numbers were 4 out of 18 studies and 2 out of 12, respectively.

By including only those studies in which patients could be classified as having major depression, the hypothesis of CSF concentrations of 5-HIAA, HVA and MHPG being low in depression were actually weakened (Table 2). Except for noradrenaline (NA), the parent amines have been measured in only few studies (Table 3). These results seem to confirm that CSF concentrations of NA apparently are not affected in depression, whereas there might be disturbances in CSF concentrations of serotonin (5-HT), dopamine (DA) and adrenaline (A).

Although many lines of evidence support the hypothesis of an involvement of biogenic amines in the biology of depression, we have not yet succeeded in identifying a specific dysfunction in one of the amine systems as pathogenetic for depression. The theory of the existence of an amine-specific subgroup of depression has not gained convincing support, either in research into the biology of depression or in clinical experience with new antidepressant-specific 5-HT re-uptake inhibitors.

In future research we will have to abandon the very simplistic models and, to a greater extent, take into account the complexity and interactions of the different

Table 3. Baseline studies comparing CSF NA, serotonin, adrenaline and dopamine (1978–1987) in depressed patients and in controls

Amine	Number of studies	Change in neurotransmitter in depression
NA	5	↔
A	2	↓
5-HT	1	↑
DA	1	↑
	1	↔

neurotransmitter systems [2], including amines as well as peptides. Moreover, we have to consider the large variety of methodological problems including the possible consequences of the rostro-caudal gradients found for several transmitter substances when it comes to interpretation of data [1,3,4].

References

1. Gjerris A (1988) Acta Psychiatr. Scand. 78: 5–35.
2. Ågren H, Mefford IN, Rudorfer MV, Linnoila M and Potter WZ (1986) J. Psychiatr. Res. 20: 175–193.
3. Gjerris A, Gjerris F, Sørensen PS, Sørensen EB, Christensen NJ, Fahrenkrug J and Rehfeld JF (1988) Acta Neurochir. 91: 55–59.
4. Gjerris A, Werdelin L, Gjerris F, Sørensen PS, Rafaelsen OJ and Alling C (1987) Acta Psychiatr. Scand. 75: 619–628.

Biological Psychiatry, Volume 1. G. Racagni et al., editors.

Markers of hypothalamic-pituitary-thyroid axis dysfunction in depression

Arthur J. Prange Jr.

Department of Psychiatry, University of North Carolina School of Medicine, Chapel Hill, North Carolina, U.S.A.

There are many markers of dysfunction of the hypothalamic-pituitary-thyroid (HPT) axis. Signs and symptoms are well known, and the psychiatrist does well to bear them in mind. However, when they are obvious, one is usually confronted with a frank endocrinopathy, and while these are important, subtle degrees of dysfunction are more frequent in psychiatric patients. To recognize subclinical dysfunction one must rely on biochemical tests. It is markers of this sort and their significance that will be discussed below.

The HPT axis, like the adrenal axis and the gonadal axis, is organized in hierarchical fashion. Thyrotropin-releasing hormone (TRH), a tripeptide, is elaborated in the hypothalamus. Via the portal venous system it reaches the anterior pituitary gland, where it causes the release of thyroid stimulating hormone (TSH), which in turn enters the general circulation and causes the thyroid gland to secrete thyroxine (T_4) and a small amount of triiodothyronine (T_3). Most T_3 comes from the deiodination in tissues of T_4. Both hormones are tightly bound to serum proteins; it is their free fraction that is active. T_3 is more potent than T_4. So-called reverse T_3 (rT_3) also comes from the deiodination of T_4. It is metabolically inert, though not without significance.

All five hormones mentioned above can be readily assayed in serum. This fact, plus the availability of TRH for administration to test the TSH response of the pituitary, has allowed the definition of several HPT axis syndromes, at least five of which are of significance in depressed patients. In another place we have offered a detailed account of thyroid hormones, their measurement and the significance of their alterations in depression [1].

In overt hypothyroidism, thyroid hormones are diminished. Basal TSH is very high, due to diminished feedback inhibition by thyroid hormones of the pituitary, and for the same reason TSH response to TRH administration is grossly exaggerated. Most patients with overt hypothyroidism show prominent elements of depression, but drug treatment of depression is useless until the thyroid condition is corrected, as by the administration of T_4. When a depressed patient shows a poor response to an antidepressant drug, the possible presence of hypothyroidism, overt or subclinical, should be considered.

In subclinical hypothyroidism, levels of thyroid hormones are in the normal range, but either basal TSH is elevated or the TSH response to TRH is exaggerated or both. The significance of this condition is uncertain, though some evidence suggests that it can lower the threshold for the occurrence of depression [2] and presumably can impoverish the response to an antidepressant drug.

In the so-called euthyroid sick syndrome (ESS), values for T_3 are low while values for rT_3 are elevated. Thus, there is a paucity of the potent hormone and an abundance of the impotent one. Whether this occurs in depression or in some other chronic condition, it is usually understood as representing an effort of the organism to conserve energy. The syndrome is probably adaptive at the outset but may then become maladaptive. It is for this reason that many endocrinologists treat the ESS with T_4.

In the blunted TSH response to TRH, one encounters a syndrome that is now familiar to most psychiatrists. It occurs in some 30% of depressed patients. Its frequency, of course, depends on its definition. Usually one gives 500 μg of TRH i.v. and then observes that half an hour later the peak response of TSH is less than 5 IU above basal levels. There are almost certainly several ways for patients to come to the common endpoint of a blunted TSH response. One is hyperthyroidism, or even hyperthyroxinemia (see below); another is hypercortisolemia. While both of these conditions can occur in depressed patients, they do not seem to account for more than a few of the blunted responses that are seen. Not all aspects of the significance of a blunted response are known, but it is clear that if a blunted response persists into remission from depression, then depressive relapse within a few months is more likely.

In hyperthyroxinemia, T_4 is elevated but other HPT markers are generally normal. It may indicate the presence of a central command for more activity in the thyroid axis but the absence of peripheral compliance. The elevated T_4 does not result in the elevated T_3 that would come from enhanced (peripheral) deiodination. This syndrome may foretell an excellent response to an antidepressant drug [3].

There are no set rules concerning when to determine which marker of HPT activity in a depressed patient. Nevertheless, the following might be a useful guide. All depressed patients should have a determination of basal TSH and a so-called thyroid panel, in which total T_4 is measured, the residual binding space for T_4 is measured (by using radioactive T_3 as an in vitro reagent) and the free thyroxine index is calculated. This index is proportional to actual levels of T_4 over a broad range. If the above is done, very few cases of frank HPT axis disorder will be missed, and hyperthyroxinemia, if present, will be identified. If the patient, even with normal values, responds poorly to medication, one can then do a TRH test. It may be exaggerated even if the basal TSH was (and remains) in the normal range. This concatenation of results indicates a subtle degree of subclinical hypothyroidism, more subtle than the degree to which thyroid hormones are normal but basal TSH is elevated. It probably has the same significance (see above). Another possible result of the TRH test is that, in the face of all other markers being normal, the TSH response will be blunted. It is this result that augurs badly for depressive relapse. Usually, the TRH test is used for research rather than ordinary clinical purposes.

In most clinical settings the determination of the HPT markers described above can be accomplished for a fraction of the cost of one day of hospitalization. Thus, it is probably cost-efficient to obtain them. Even slight degrees of HPT dysfunction, especially in the direction of hypothyroidism, can contribute to the occurrence of depression, impair recovery and contribute to relapse.

References

1. Prange AJ Jr, Mason GA and Garbutt JC (1989) In: Amsterdam JD (ed.) Pharmacotherapy of Depression: Applications for the Outpatient Practitioner, Marcel Dekker, Inc., New York, pp. 35–55.
2. Prange AJ Jr, Haggerty JJ Jr, Browne JL and Rice JD (1990) In: Bunney WE Jr, Hippius H, Laakmann G and Schmauss M (eds.) Neuropsychopharmacology. Springer, Berlin-Heidelberg, pp. 353–361.
3. Whybrow PC, Coppen A, Prange AJ Jr, Noguera R and Bailey JE (1972) Arch. Gen. Psychiatry 26: 242–245.

Biological Psychiatry, Volume 1. G. Racagni et al., editors.

SPECT research in affective disorders

Joseph A. Schwartz and Nancy M. Speed
Department of Psychiatry, University of Michigan School of Medicine 1500 E. Medical Center Dr, Ann Arbor, MI 48109-0020, U.S.A.

Introduction

To date only a few investigations of affective disorder patients with single photon emission computed tomography (SPECT) have been reported. Studies have looked for differences in regional cerebral blood flow (rCBF) between normals and depressed patients and between depressed and recovered patients. An increased understanding of normal variations in blood flow on the basis of gender and mental activity makes interpretation of the findings difficult. To date the most striking findings have involved abnormalities of cortical activation with perceptual and motor tasks and the effect of treatment (i.e. ECT, antidepressants) on rCBF. Other observations have suggested a relationship between changes in mood and rCBF in patients with organic mental disorders such as epilepsy, dementia and stroke.

Depression and CBF

The majority of studies comparing rCBF in normals and depressed patients utilize xenon inhalation methods. Most of the xenon CBF work has used a surface detection system, though xenon SPECT has also been utilized. The results of these CBF studies are somewhat contradictory. Some studies show no differences between normal and depressed patients [1–4] while others suggest that depression is associated with a decrease in global CBF [5,6] or perhaps a more specific frontal flow diminution [7,8]. The single study utilizing ^{195}Au shows lowered global CBF in the subgroup exhibiting endogenous depression [7]. Two studies found higher CBF values in the depressed group [2,9]. Both involved patients approved of ECT. The one published study using IMP shows a globally decreased cortical to cerebellar ratio in depressed patients [10]. The currently available data suggest that patients with unipolar endogenous subtype depression appear to have global reductions in CBF and a loss of the normal hyperfrontal ratio. The apparent heterogeneity of the findings may reflect different subtypes in the pathophysiology of depressive symptoms. For example, in a study which evaluated dexamethasone suppression, it was the normally suppressed subgroup that exhibited abnormal CBF [11]. This difference was not confirmed by Delvenne [3].

The overall picture these studies provide is that if there are differences in CBF in depression, the changes are either subtle, or confined to particular groups of patients. Though these studies were well designed, the evolution of our understanding of CBF now allows a more critical assessment of the findings. We now know the influence of age [12,13] (resting CBF declines with age), medications [7,14] (most psychotropics reduce CBF acutely), as well as caffeine [15] and nicotine intake on CBF. Women have lower hemoglobin than men and, for this reason exhibit higher CBF [1]. Mental activity can lead to significant and lateralized changes in CBF [10]. For example, visual and auditory input increase CBF [16]. Thinking about moving one's hand increases CBF, more so when it is the non-dominant hand. In normals, hand movements are associated with a 25% increase in rCBF in the contralateral motor cortex, while patients with severe depression show only a modest, diffuse increase in CBF with this activation procedure [17].

Evaluation of patients while manic is difficult. The available data [2] shows no difference between manic patient and controls. Most of the patients were medicated with lithium or antipsychotics at the time of the scan.

Symptom severity and CBF

Several investigators have reported significant negative correlations between Hamilton Depression Ratings and global CBF, regardless of depressive subtype [2,5,6]. Lower global CBF has also been reported to be associated with BPRS severity, especially the factor of emotional withdrawal [7]. Silfverskiold [2] is alone in his observation of a significant positive relationship between depressive symptom severity and CBF.

Treatment effects

Paradoxically, treatment of depression has been consistently associated with a decrease in CBF [9,18,19]. Several studies show acute and late effects of ECT to be diminished global and frontal blood flow. This is true for unilateral and bilateral treatment. Antidepressants (chlomipramine and maprotiline) have been associated with decreased global blood flow [7]. HMPAO studies show significant decreases in rCBF in bilateral frontal regions when OCD patients are treated with high-dose fluoxetine [14]. There appears to be a dose-related decline in CBF for patients on antipsychotics [2].

Organic mood disorders

A particularly interesting line of investigation has pursued the relationship between depressive symptoms and CBF in depression secondary to neurologic illness. Clear abnormalities will be present in most cases and therefore recognizable changes in

CBF can be analyzed. Patterns of association may then have a useful theoretical implication which could be tested in primary affective illness. Studies of HMPAO CBF in post-stroke depression show a relationship between severity of asymmetry and depression [20]. Late onset depression seems to be associated with focal CBF defects.

Future directions

Improved scan resolution and the development of receptor labels may focus SPECT research on the clinical problems of treatment matching for patients with affective disorders. Quantitative studies using multiple activation methods would be better done with PET. SPECT will be most effective psychiatrically in evaluating the utility of iodine-labeled receptor molecules for classifying depressive subtypes [21]. The evaluation of the clinical and prognostic significance of these subtypes will require the study of large patient samples. The development of uniform scan procedures will advance SPECT research in psychiatric disorders to its full potential.

References

1. Gur RE, Skolnick BE, Gur RC, Caroff S, Rieger W, Obrist WD, Younkin D and Reivich M (1984) Arch. Gen. Psychiatry 41: 695–699.
2. Silfverskiold P and Risberg J (1989) Arch. Gen. Psychiatry 46: 253–259.
3. Delvenne V, Delecluse F, Hubain P, Schoutens A, DeMaertelaer V and Mendlewicz J (1990) Br. J. Psychiatry 157: 359–365.
4. Reischies FM, Hedde J and Drochner R (1989) Psychiatry Res. 29: 323–326.
5. Mathew RJ, Meyer JS, Francis DJ, Semchuk KM, Mortel K and Claghorn JL (1980) Am. J. Psychiatry 137: 1449–1450.
6. Sachkeim HA, Prohovnik I, Moeller JR, Brown RP, Apter S, Prudic J, Devanand DP and Mukherjee S (1990) Arch. Gen. Psychiatry 47: 60–70.
7. Schlegel S, Aldenhoff, Eissner D, Lindner P and Nickel O (1989) J. Affective Disord. 17: 211–218.
8. Charbol H, Guell A, Barrere M, Dupui P, Bes A and Moron P (1985) Encéphale 11: 207–208.
9. Rosenberg R, Vorstrup S, Anderson A and Bolwig TG (1988) Convulsive Ther. 4: 62–73.
10. O'Connell RA, Van Heertum R, Billick SB, Holt AR, Gonzalez A, Notardonato H, Luck D and King LM (1989) J. Neuropsychiatry 1: 145–153.
11. Charles G, Uytdenhoef P, Portelange P, Wilmotte J, Mendlewicz J and Jacquy J (1983) Biol. Psychiatry 18: 1336–1338.
12. Devous MD, Stokely EM, Chehabi NH and Bonte FJ (1986) J. Cereb. Blood Flow Metab. 6: 95–104.
13. Helsey JH, Blauenstein UW, Wilson EM and Wills EH (1979) Neurology 29: 21–28.
14. Hoehn-Saric R, Pearlson GD, Harris GJ, Machlin SR and Camargo EE (1991) Am. J. Psychiatry (in press).
15. Mathew RJ and Wilson WH (1985) Stroke 16: 814–817.
16. Woods SW, Hegeman IM, Zubal G, Krystal JH, Koster K, Smith EO, Heninger GR and Hoffer PB (1991) J. Nucl. Med. 32: 210–215.
17. Guenther W, Moser E, Mueller-Spahn F, von Oefele K, Buell U and Hippius H (1986) Biol. Psychiatry 21: 889–899.

18. Silfverskiold P, Gustafson L, Risberg J and Rosen I (1986) Ann. N.Y. Acad. Sci. 462: 236–249.
19. Prohovnik I, Sackeim HA, Decina P and Malitz S (1986) Ann. N.Y. Acad. Sci. 462: 249–262.
20. Schwartz JA, Speed NM, Mountz JM, Gross MD, Modell MD and Kuhl DE (1990) Am. J. Psychiatry 147: 242–244.
21. Mertens J, Bossuyt-Piron C, Guns M, Bossuyt A and Leysen J (1989) J. Nucl. Med. 30: 741.

Biological Psychiatry, Volume 1. G. Racagni et al., editors.

Amino acid pools, CBF and $CMRO_2$ in affective disorders

Hideji Kishimoto[1], Haruhiro Fujita[1], Osamu Takatsu[1], Hideo Takahashi[1], Tadashi Maeda[1], Takashi Ishikawa[1], Taiko Hashimoto[1], Kenji Kosaka[1], Fuuji Yokoi[2] and Masaaki Iio[2]

[1]Department of Psychiatry, Yokohama City University School of Medicine, Minami, Yokohama 232; and [2] Nakano National Hospital, Nakano, Tokyo 160 Japan

Introduction

To examine the relationship between amino acid and functions of the brain in affective disorders, the authors used positron emission tomography (PET). Also the authors determined the plasma amino acid concentrations.

Subjects and Methods

Fourteen patients with unipolar depression (10 men and 4 women; age range 26–56 years; mean age 45 years), 4 fully manic patients (2 men and 2 women; age range 40–54 years; mean age 45 years) and 6 patients in remission from depression (4 men and 2 woman; age range 36–63 years; mean age 48 years) were studied. All were outpatients at the Yokohama City University Hospital. Ten normal subjects (8 men and 2 women; mean age 46 years) were used as controls. All the patients and control subjects were in good physical health and showed no abnormalities in neurological examinations or laboratory tests, which included electroencephalography, skull X-ray and computed tomography (CT).

Diagnoses were based on the DSM III criteria (American Psychiatric Association, 1980) and were agreed upon by at least 2 psychiatrists. The 14 patients with unipolar depression met the criteria for major depressive disorder and had no personal or family history suggestive of hypomanic episodes. None were receiving medication. Scores on the 21-item Hamilton Rating Scale for Depression (Hamilton, 1960) ranged from 21–36, with a mean of 29, indicating moderate levels of depression.

A slight modification of the method of Lifton et al. (1971) was used to prepare ^{11}C-glucose. Previous studies by our group had shown an 85.6% distribution to amino acids, 6.3% to pyruvic acid and 8.1% to glucose 20 min after oral administration of ^{11}C-glucose and an 87.0% distribution to amino acids, 6.9% to pyruvic acid and 6.1% to glucose 30 min after oral administration of ^{11}C-glucose in rat brain (Hara and Izuchi, 1983; Iio et al., 1983). Jones et al. (1983) obtained data similar to ours, using ^{11}C-glucose as a tracer. Regional cerebral blood flow (rCBF), regional cerebral metabolic rate for oxygen ($rCMRO_2$) and oxygen extraction ratio (OER) were measured by inhalation of C1502 and 1502 in a steady state.

The subjects lay down on a PET bed in a darkened room. An i.v. line with a 0.9% saline solution drip for the ^{11}C-glucose study and an i.a. line for C1502, 1502 study were inserted into the right arm for blood sampling. Subjects were allowed to relax; 10 min before radionuclide administration, the room lights were turned off and the subjects were asked to close their eyes. No talking was allowed during the test and all subjects remained quiet and cooperative. Ten minutes after oral administration of ^{11}C-glucose (about 20 mCi) and inhalation of C1502, 1502 (about 10 mCi), 3–10 scans parallel to the orbital meatal (OM) line were done as quietly as possible. One to 6 series of PET images were taken every 10 min up to 65 min from the start of the procedure. The PET scanner was a Headtome-IV (Shimazu, Japan) and had a resolution of 4.5 mm in the horizontal plane and 8 mm in the axial direction. For the present analysis, slices at 40, 49, 58, 67, 75, 84, 93 and 102 mm above the OM line were chosen. CT scans at the same levels as the PET slices were obtained. Each part of the brain was evaluated using the human brain atlas of Matsui and Hirano (1978) for computed tomography. Each pixel (3.2 × 3.2 mm) count in each part of the brain was used for statistical analysis (two-tailed Student's *t*-test). Blood ^{11}C and 150 were counted with a well counter.

The blood samples for plasma amino acids were obtained from both patients and control subjects between 10–11 a.m. Five ml of blood was collected into a syringe with sodium heparin (2 I.U./ml) and centrifuged immediately at 1500 × g for 10 min at 20°C. The 1.5 ml of plasma were deproteinized by the modified picric acid precipitation procedure of Hamilton. The residual picric acid was removed by use of Dowex 2 × 8 Cl (200–400 mesh) columns. The eluates from the column were lyophilized in lyophilizer VirTis Uni-Trap Model 10-100 and the samples were dissolved in 1.0 ml of 0.01 N NaOH and made up to 1.5 ml with citrate buffer (pH 2.2). Aliquots were analyzed with a Hitachi KLA-5 amino acid auto-analyzer using the modified gradient elution system of Piez and Morris.

Results

Manic patients

One patient showed normal CBF (cerebral blood flow), but amino acid pools were increased in both hemispheres. The other 3 patients showed normal CBF, but amino acid pools were increased in the left hemisphere and decreased in the right.

Depressed patients

The PET images of patients with unipolar depression indicated decreased amino acid pools, compared with controls. Results from patients in remission were equivalent to those in normal controls. The CBF, $CMRO_2$ and OER in depressed patients were normal, compared with controls, in the cortex and subcortical areas. Certain amino acids (leucine, isoleucine, lysine, histidine, phenylalanine, alanine, methionine and ornithine) in plasma in both depressed patients and manic patients were significantly lower ($P < 0.01–0.05$).

Discussion

It is important to note that certain amino acids in plasma were decreased in both depressed patients and manic patients. It is also interesting that bipolar manic patients showed increased cortical amino acid pools, especially in the left hemisphere, whereas unipolar depressed patients showed reduced cortical amino acid pools, although regional cerebral blood flow (rCBF), regional cerebral metabolic rate for oxygen ($rCMRO_2$) and oxygen extraction ratio (OER) were normal. Flor-Henry reported that euphoric reactions are correlated with disturbance in the right anterior location and our results support this view. Anyway, the disturbance of amino acid metabolism was found both in plasma and cortical area of the brain, indicating new direction for the study for affective disorders.

References

Available from author upon request.

Biological Psychiatry, Volume 1. G. Racagni et al., editors.

CSF 5-HIAA predicts suicide risk after attempted suicide

Peter Nordström

Department of Psychiatry, Karolinska Hospital, S-104 01 Stockholm, Sweden

An association has repeatedly been reported between attempted suicide and low concentrations of the serotonin metabolite 5-hydroxyindoleacetic acid (5-HIAA) in the cerebrospinal fluid (CSF) [1,2]. Åsberg et al. [3] first reported in 1976 that depressed patients with low CSF 5-HIAA attempted suicide significantly more often and with more violent means. Several studies [1,2] have replicated the finding of an association between low CSF 5-HIAA and different measures of past suicidal behavior. Results from postmortem biochemical and receptor studies [4–7] of brains from suicide victims lend further support to the serotonin hypothesis of suicide.

However, as yet only few studies have addressed the specific hypothesis suggested by Åsberg [3] that CSF 5-HIAA might be a biochemical suicide predictor. Originally this idea was based on their report of two subsequent suicides occurring in the low CSF 5-HIAA mode and none in the high mode. To further address this question, Träskman et al. [8] performed a follow-up study and reported that the suicide risk was highest among the 46 depressed patients who had made an index episode suicide attempt. A 5-HIAA level below the median (92.5 nM) of the entire sample was associated with a higher suicide risk. Within the group of suicide attempters, 30 patients had a 5-HIAA level below 92.5 nM. All 6 suicide attempters who died of subsequent suicide belonged to this group, i.e. a 20% mortality by suicide among low CSF 5-HIAA suicide attempters within a year after lumbar puncture. Similar findings have been reported by Roy et al. [9]. In their sample of 27 depressed patients, 4 committed suicide within the 1-year follow-up period and all of these suicides occurred among the 19 patients with prior suicide attempts. Two out of 8 patients with a prior suicide attempt and a low CSF 5-HIAA (<75 nM) committed suicide, i.e. a 25% 1-year mortality from suicide. Roy et al. [10] also carried out a 5-year follow-up telephone interview study of suicidal behavior among depressed patients who earlier had had determinations of CSF monoamine metabolites. They concluded that the 7 patients who attempted suicide before the index admission and who reattempted suicide during the follow-up had significantly lower CSF levels of 5-HIAA. Particularly, 3 (25%) of the 12 depressed patients who had made a past suicide attempt and who had a CSF level of 5-HIAA below 80 nM committed suicide during the first year of follow-up.

The aim of the present study was to investigate retrospectively the suicide risk among psychiatric patients hospitalized after an index episode suicide attempt, and to further explore whether CSF 5-HIAA was a suicide predictor after attempted suicide.

Patients and Methods

Included in this follow-up study were 92 psychiatric mood disorder patients admitted from 1973 to 1987 after an index episode suicide attempt shortly prior to hospitalization. The CSF 5-HIAA concentrations were determined by mass fragmentographic methods. All patients were searched in January 1988 on line in the Stockholm County Council database to identify those who had died. The reported causes of deaths were then obtained from the causes of death register at the National Central Bureau of Statistics. Suicide was defined as reported by the forensic medical pathologist in all cases.

Results

During follow-up 14 patients committed suicide, 11 during the first year of observation after the index suicide attempt.

The mean CSF 5-HIAA was 91 ± 35 nM (median 87). The mean 5-HIAA among the 14 suicide attempters who later committed suicide (85 ± 18 nM) was not statistically significantly lower than among the 78 patients who survived (92 ± 38 nM). However, when studied by median split subgrouping and comparison of the incidence of completed suicide in the two 5-HIAA modes the suicide risk within the first year of follow-up after the index suicide attempt among patients with low, i.e. below the median CSF 5-HIAA was 17% (8/46) as compared with 7% (3/46) in the high CSF 5-HIAA mode.

Conclusion

These results lend further support to the serotonin hypothesis of suicide risk. Crude baseline CSF 5-HIAA level seems to be a predictor of short-term suicide risk, i.e. death by suicide within 1 year after attempted suicide among psychiatric inpatients. The magnitude of the association between CSF 5-HIAA and short-term suicide risk points to the possibility to use low CSF 5-HIAA concentration as a criterion for defining a high suicide risk target group for future treatment studies. However, the clinical value of 5-HIAA determinations as an indicator of suicidal potential still remains to be proven.

References

1. Åsberg M, Nordström P and Träskman-Bendz L (1987) In: Mann JJ and Stanley M (eds.) Psychobiology of Suicidal Behavior. Ann. N.Y. Acad. Sci. 487: 243–255.
2. Åsberg M and Nordström P (1988) In: Möller HJ, Schmidtke A and Weltz R (eds.) Current Issues of Suicidology. Springer-Verlag, Berlin, pp. 221–241.

3. Åsberg M, Träskman L and Thorén P (1976) Arch. Gen. Psychiatry 33: 1193–1197.
4. Åsberg M, Schalling D, Träskman-Bendz L and Wägner A (1987) In: Meltzer HM (ed.) Psychopharmacology: The Third Generation of Progress. Raven Press, New York, pp. 655–668.
5. Stanley M and Stanley B (1989) In: Lann IS, Moscicki EK and Maris R (eds.) Strategies for Studying Suicide and Suicidal Behavior. The Guilford Press, New York, pp. 30–42.
6. Mann JJ, Arango V, Marzuk PM, Theccanat S and Reis DJ (1989) Br. J. Psychiatry 155(8): 7–14.
7. Mann JJ, Arango V and Underwood MD (1990) In: Whitaker-Azmitia PA and Peroutka SJ (eds.) The Neuropharmacology of Serotonin. Ann. N.Y. Acad. Sci. 600: 476–485.
8. Träskman L, Äsberg M, Bertilsson L and Sjöstrand L (1981) Arch. Gen. Psychiatry 38: 631–636.
9. Roy A, Ågren H, Pickar D, Linnoila M, Doran AR, Cutler NR and Paul SM (1986) Am. J. Psychiatry 143: 1539–1545.
10. Roy A, De Jong J and Linnoila M (1989) Arch. Gen. Psychiatry 46: 609–612.

Biological Psychiatry, Volume 1. G. Racagni et al., editors.

CSF studies and long-term suicidal behavior

Alec Roy
Hillside Hospital, P.O. Box 38, Glen Oaks, NY 11004, U.S.A.

In 1976 Asberg et al. [1] reported a bimodal distribution of levels of the serotonin metabolite 5-hydroxyindoleacetic acid (5-HIAA) in the lumbar cerebrospinal fluid (CSF) of 68 depressed patients. Asberg et al. noted that significantly more of the depressed patients in the "low" CSF 5-HIAA group had attempted suicide in comparison with those in the "high" CSF 5-HIAA group. Such data, along with those from post-mortem neurochemical and receptor studies, have subsequently led to the suggestion that reduced central serotonin metabolism may be associated with suicidal behavior.

We measured CSF levels of 5-HIAA and the dopamine metabolite homovanillic acid (HVA) among 27 depressed patients [2]. We present here the results of a 5-year follow-up study of suicidal behavior in relationship to CSF levels of 5-HIAA and HVA among these depressed patients. This data has been previously published [3].

Results

Before their index NIMH admission, 19 of the 27 depressed patients (70.4%) had made a suicide attempt at some time. Seven (36.8%) of these 19 patients reattempted suicide during the mean (± S.D.) 57.4 ± 9.0 months of follow-up. They made nine further attempts, four of them successful suicides.

First, we compared patients who reattempted suicide during follow-up (n = 7) with the rest of the patients (n = 20). Patients who reattempted suicide showed significantly lower CSF levels of both 5-HIAA (mean, 66.9 ± 28.8 vs. 98.7 ± 32.6 pmol/ml; $t = 2.28$; $df = 25$; $P < 0.03$) and HVA (mean, 83.1 ± 51.4 vs. 151.5 ± 76.7 pmol/ml; $t = 2.18$; $df = 25$; $P < 0.04$).

Melancholics who reattempted suicide (n = 6), compared with the rest of the melancholics (n = 16), also showed significantly lower CSF levels of both 5-HIAA (mean, 57.2 ± 14.4 vs. 99.5 ± 32.4 pmol/ml; $t = 3.06$; $df = 20$; $P < 0.006$) and HVA (mean, 65.2 ± 21.4 vs. 144.2 ± 69.7 pmol/ml; $t = 2.69$; $df = 20$; $P < 0.01$).

Then, we examined the three groups that did (n = 7) or did not (n = 13) reattempt suicide during follow-up and that never attempted (n = 7). There was a significant difference between the three groups for CSF levels of HVA (ANOVA, $F(2,24) = 3.36$, $P < 0.052$; ANCOVA, $F(2,22) = 3.55$, $P < 0.046$). Patients who reattempted suicide had significantly lower CSF levels of HVA than patients who never attempted suicide (mean, 83.1 ± 51.4 vs. 180.4 ± 76.6 pmol/ml; $P < 0.05$). There was a trend for a significant difference between the three groups for CSF levels of 5-HIAA (ANOVA, $F(2,24) = 2.68$, $P < 0.09$; ANCOVA, $F(2,22) = 3.00$, $P < 0.07$).

Next, we examined only the melancholic patients in each of the 3 groups. There were significant differences between the 3 groups for CSF levels of both 5-HIAA (ANOVA, $F(2,19) = 6.11$, $P < 0.009$) and HVA (ANOVA, $F(2,19) = 7.56$, $P < 0.004$). Melancholic reattempters had significantly lower CSF levels of both 5-HIAA and HVA than melancholics who never attempted suicide ($P < 0.01$ and $P < 0.01$, respectively) and lower CSF levels of 5-HIAA than melancholics who did not reattempt suicide ($P < 0.05$). The ANCOVAs showed the same pattern of results, as did analysis with only female melancholics.

Comment

We carried out a 5-year follow-up study of suicidal behavior among depressed patients in relationship to CSF levels of monoamine metabolites. We found that patients who attempted suicide before the index admission and who reattempted suicide during the follow-up had significantly lower CSF levels of 5-HIAA or HVA.

Striking findings were obtained when only depressed patients with melancholic episodes were examined. For example, 11 (91.7%) of 12 melancholics with a CSF level of 5-HIAA below 80 pmol/ml had attempted suicide before their index admission; 6 (54.5%) of these 11 reattempted suicide during follow-up. Nine (90%) of the 10 melancholics with a CSF level of HVA below 100 pmol/ml had attempted suicide before their index admission; 6 (66.6%) of these 9 reattempted suicide during follow-up.

There were also striking findings in relationship to committing suicide during the follow-up. Three (25%) of the 12 depressed patients who had made a past attempt and who had a CSF level of 5-HIAA below 80 pmol/ml committed suicide during the first year of follow-up. In the present study, the percentages of patients who committed suicide were higher when we examined subgroups of past suicide attempters with a CSF level of 5-HIAA below 80 pmol/ml: 3 (27.3%) of 11 melancholics and 3 (33.3%) of 9 female melancholics. Also, the percentage of patients committing suicide was higher when we examined past attempters with a CSF level of HVA below 100 pmol/ml: 3 (30%) of 10, 3 (33.3%) of 9 melancholics, and 3 (37.5%) of the 8 female melancholics.

We reported similar CSF HVA findings in our initial report about suicide behavior occurring before the index admission in these patients [2]. Others have also reported a more strongly significant relationship between suicidal behavior and low CSF levels of HVA. 5-HIAA and HVA have a high degree of covariance and invariably show a strong positive correlation.

In summary, we carried out a 5-year follow-up study of suicidal behavior among depressed patients. Patients who reattempted suicide during the follow-up had significantly lower CSF levels of 5-HIAA and HVA. These follow-up results suggest that among depressed patients who have previously attempted suicide, these measures may be predictive markers of an increased risk of further suicidal behavior.

References

1. Åsberg M, Traskman L and Thoren P (1976) Arch. Gen. Psychiatry 33: 1193–1197.
2. Roy A, Agren H, Pickar D, Linnoila M, Doran A, Cutler N and Paul S (1986) Am. J. Psychiatry 143: 1539–1545.
3. Roy A, DeJong J and Linnoila M (1989) Arch. Gen. Psychiatry 46: 609–612.

Biological Psychiatry, Volume 1. G. Racagni et al., editors.

CSF studies and long-term suicidal behavior

Göran Regnéll, Lil Träskman-Bendz, Christer Alling and Rolf Öhman
Departments of Psychiatry and Neurochemistry, University Hospital, S-221 85 Lund, Sweden

Introduction

A suicide/suicide attempt is a multifactorial event, where psychiatric, psychological, social and biochemical conditions interact as predisposing/triggering factors.

Since the findings by Åsberg et al. in the mid-seventies [1], an ever-increasing interest has emerged in the field of biological markers of suicidal behavior, and especially studies of monoamine metabolites, particularly the serotonin metabolite 5-hydroxyindoleacetic acid (5-HIAA) in the cerebrospinal fluid (CSF). Most research has been performed as comparisons of various groups of patients/subjects in a wash-out situation. Some studies, though, have been carried out with a longitudinal design, e.g. Träskman et al. [2], Roy et al. [3].

The aim of this study has been to follow, for at least one year, the course of events in a group of suicide attempters in respect of various biochemical factors with concomitant clinical-psychiatric ratings. We were interested, on the one hand, to investigate correlations between biochemical and clinical measures (e.g. "degree of suicidality") in individual patients over time. On the other hand, we wanted to learn about the characteristics of the group of patients that could be expected to repeat self-destructive behavior during the follow-up period.

Patients and Methods

Eighteen patients have so far been followed for at least one year, taking part in the complete research program (yet another 7 patients accepted repeated clinical rating and the sampling of blood and urine, but not a spinal tap).

There were 5 males and 13 females. According to the DSM III-R Axis I [4] more than half of the patients were diagnosed as affective disorders. Sixteen of the patients met the criteria of a personality disorder (Axis II).

The great majority of subjects made the suicide attempt by means of tablet intoxication.

Rating scales

Shortly after the suicide attempt we administered the Suicidal Intent Scale, SIS [5] and the Karolinska Scales of Personality, KSP [6].

Biochemistry

A spinal tap under standardized conditions was made after wash-out, and every third month thereafter. Analyses were made for the monamine metabolites 5-hydroxyindoleactic acid (5-HIAA), homovanillic acid (HVA), and 4-hydroxy 3-methoxy phenyl glycol (HMPG).

Results

Repeaters

Eleven patients (1 male, 10 females) repeated their self-destructive behavior after the index attempt. Clinically they were characterized by less often than the non-repeaters, carrying a DSM III-R diagnosis of major depression and all of them met the criteria of a personality disorder.

The intent to die (as scored on the SIS) was lower, and the impulsivity score (KSP) higher in the repeater group.

At wash-out there was a tendency for the repeaters to be higher in CSF HMPG (7/11 vs. 2/7 above the median) and lower in the CSF HVA/5-HIAA ratio (7/11 vs. 2/7 below the median).

Repeated measurements in individual patients

We found no clear-cut pattern of correlation between the CSF amine metabolite levels and time of the year, and also no correlations with sex, age or height.

Treatment with antidepressants tended to lower CSF 5-HIAA and CSF HMPG. Patients with high initial CSF 5-HIAA values tended to stay in the higher range during the follow-up period, and those with low initial values generally remained low.

Discussion

The advantage of a longitudinal study design is that patients serve as their own controls. The disadvantage is, however, confounding factors such as drug-treatment. Other investigators claim that there are seasonal variations of CSF monoamine metabolite levels [7]. In our sample, such variations are not evident.

Our findings indicate that longitudinally, CSF 5-HIAA remain within the same concentration range, and thus give support to earlier studies of repeated CSF samples from drug-free patients and controls [8]. The present results give further evidence of CSF 5-HIAA being a trait marker.

Acknowledgements

The assistance of Margot Alsén, RN, is greatly acknowledged. Our studies were supported by the Bank of Sweden Tercentenary Foundation, the Swedish Medical Research Council, the Söderström Köning Foundation, and funds from Lund University, and Malmöhus County.

References

1. Åsberg M, Träskman L and Thorén P (1976) Arch. Gen. Psychiatry 33: 1193–1197.
2. Träskman L, Åsberg M, Bertilsson L and Sjöstrand L (1981) Arch. Gen. Psychiatry 38: 631–636.
3. Roy A, De Jong J and Linnoila M (1989) Arch. Gen. Psychiatry 46: 609–612.
4. Diagnostic and Statistic Manual of Mental Disorders, 3rd Edn., Revised (1987) The American Psychiatric Association, Washington D.C.
5. Beck A, Herman I and Schuyler D (1974) In: Beck AT, Resnik HLP and Lettieri D (eds.) The Prediction of Suicide. Chales Press, Bowie, MD, pp. 45–46.
6. Schalling D, Åsberg M, Edman G and Oreland L (1987) Acta Psychiatr. Scand. 76: 172–182.
7. Åsberg M, Bertilsson L, Rydin E, Schalling D, Thorén P and Träskman-Bendz L (1981) In: Angrist B, Burrows GD and Lader M (eds.) Recent Advances in Neuro-Pharmacology. Pergamon Press, New York, pp. 257–271.
8. Träskman-Bendz L, Åsberg M, Bertilsson L and Thorén P (1984) Acta Psychiatr. Scand. 69: 333–342.

Biological Psychiatry, Volume 1. G. Racagni et al., editors.

Receptor studies in suicidal patients

Anat Biegon
Research Medicine and Radiation Biophysics, Lawrence Berkeley Laboratory, Berkeley, CA 94720, U.S.A.

Introduction

Biological studies of suicidal patients have repeatedly demonstrated decreased levels of the serotonin (5-HT) metabolite, 5-hydroxy indole acetic acid (5-HIAA) in cerebrospinal fluid [1]. These findings imply abnormal serotonergic neurotransmission in such patients, which may in turn result in adaptive changes in post-synaptic receptors, of a type known to occur in monoaminergic systems [2]. There are several subtypes of 5-HT receptors which have been characterized to date [3]. Of those, the 5-HT_2 receptors, found in the brain as well as on blood platelets [4], respond to tricyclic antidepressants [4,5] and electroconvulsive therapy [6] in humans and experimental animals. Since platelets are readily accessible and often used as a model for the serotonergic neuron, the platelet 5-HT_2 receptors appeared to be an attractive marker for study in the context of suicidality and depression. Suicide risk also varies with age, sex and hormonal state, suggesting the effect of these variables on 5-HT_2 receptors may also be of interest. The results of several studies of 5-HT_2 receptors on platelets of suicide attempters, patients with major depressive disorder and normal high school students are described below.

Serotonergic as well as other neurotransmitter receptors can be examined in the brains of suicide victims postmortem to gain insight into the possible involvement of specific receptors and brain regions in suicide. The results of quantitative autoradiographic studies of serotonin, noradrenaline and acetylcholine receptors in brains of suicide victims are briefly summarized as well.

Materials and Methods

Subjects

All subjects included in the platelet studies described below were drug and medication free for at least 3 weeks prior to determination of baseline 5-HT_2 receptor binding. The only diagnosis included was major depressive disorder. Controls were age- and sex-matched with patients and had no significant medical or psychiatric history. Brains of suicide victims and age- and sex-matched controls were obtained from the medical examiners' offices in N.Y. and Jaffa. The same inclusion and exclusion criteria were used in postmortem studies, in which toxicological examination by the medical examiners' laboratory was used to exclude presence of drugs and medication. Blood was collected from all subjects and processed for 5-HT_2 receptor binding on platelet membranes as previously described [4,7,8]. Tritiated ketanserine was routinely used as a ligand at a concentration of 3.0 nM, with excess mianserine included in half of the assay tubes to assess non-specific binding. Brains were collected at autopsy, frozen, sectioned and incubated with appropriate radioactive ligands for quantitative receptor autoradiography as previously described [9–13].

Results

Quantitative autoradiography of several receptors for aminergic transmitters revealed a pattern of pharmacologically as well as anatomically specific changes. Within the serotonergic system, we found no changes in 5-HT_{1A} receptors, while 5-HT_2 receptors were affected in prefrontal cortex and hippocampus. Both receptors showed a negative dependence on age, which was, however, especially pronounced for 5-HT_2 receptors over the second and third decades of life [9–11]. Noradrenergic receptors of the β type were increased and α_1 receptors were decreased in suicide victims [12,13]. The regions most implicated were the dorsolateral portion of the prefrontal cortex and the hippocampus. No change was observed in cholinergic muscarinic M_1 receptors.

Platelet 5-HT_2 receptors were found to be significantly elevated in a group of young suicide attempters [7]. However, when the suicide attempters and controls were grouped by diagnosis rather than by the presence or absence of a suicide attempt, it turned out that suicide attempters with no depressive symptoms had normal receptor levels; while elevated receptor binding was repeatedly observed in 2 groups of older patients with major depressive disorder who had not attempted suicide [4,8]. Interestingly, though, suicidality was the only single symptom significantly correlated with changes in 5-HT_2 receptor binding in these patients. This was also true for overall depression scores measured by the Hamilton or Beck Scales but not for sleep, appetite, agitation or any other symptom or cluster of symptoms.

In addition, we found that 5-HT_2 receptor binding was significantly increased in women during the premenstrual period [14]. This is the period associated with the highest incidence of suicide attempts in women. Platelet 5-HT_2 receptors, like brain receptors, decrease sharply with age during the second and third decade of life (Table 1). Boys and girls appear to have similar receptor levels up to the age of onset of menstruation (14 years in our sample). From that age on, girls show a trend towards higher levels of receptors than age-matched boys, but this difference has not reached statistical significance (Table 1).

In summary, 5-HT_2 receptors are increased in depressed and suicidal patients. They are also increased in those segments of the population known to be most at risk for suicidal behavior, e.g. people in the second and third decade, women

Table 1. Age-related changes in platelet 5-HT_2 receptor levels

Age (years)	^{3}H-ketanserin specifically bound (fm/mg)		
	All (n)	Males (n)	Females (n)
13–14	38.3 ± 14.7 (57)	37.4 ± 15.0 (31)	39.4 ± 14.2 (26)
15–16	37.2 ± 14.2 (36)	36.0 ± 11.0 (23)	39.3 ± 18.4 (13)
17–18	24.2 ± 13.7 (37)	21.5 ± 9.0 (22)	28.2 ± 17.9 (15)

Blood was taken from healthy high school students as part of a study on plasma lipoproteins (Gruener et al., submitted). The platelets were used for 5-HT_2 receptor assay. Two-way ANOVA of the data reveals a non-significant effect of sex (F = 2.3, $P = 0.13$) a significant effect of age (F = 11.75, $P < 0.0001$) and a non-significant interaction term ($P = 0.75$). Post hoc analysis (Duncan's, α preset at 0.05) shows that the oldest group is significantly lower than the younger groups (13–14 and 15–16 year olds), which are not different from each other.

during the premenstrual period and teenage girls. These observations suggest that platelet 5-HT_2 receptors may be a promising peripheral marker for suicidal depression.

References

1. Åsberg M, Traskman L and Thoren P (1976) Arch. Gen. Psychiatry 33: 1193–1197.
2. Sporn JR, Wolfe BB, Harden TK and Molinoff PB (1977) Mol. Pharmacol. 13: 1170–1180.
3. Bradley PB, Engel G, Feniuk W et al. (1986) Neuropharmacology 25: 563–576.
4. Biegon A, Weizman A, Karp L, Ram A, Tiano S and Wolff M (1987) Life Sci. 41: 2486–2492.
5. Begstrom DA and Kellar KJ (1979) J. Pharmacol. Exp. Ther. 209: 256–261.
6. Bergstrom DA and Kellar KJ (1983) Nature 278: 464–466.
7. Biegon A, Grinspoon A, Blumenfeld B, Bleich A, Apter A and Mester R (1990) Psychopharmacology 100: 165–167.
8. Biegon A, Essar N, Israeli M, Elizur A, Bruch S and Barnathan A (1990) Psychopharmacology 102: 73–75.
9. Gross-Isseroff R, Salama D and Biegon A (1990) Brain Res. 519: 223–227.
10. Gross-Isseroff R, Salama D and Biegon A (1990) Brain Res. 507: 208–215.
11. Dillon KA, Gross-Isseroff R, Israeli M and Biegon A (1991) Brain Res. 554: 56–64.
12. Biegon A and Israeli M (1988) Brain Res. 442: 199–203.
13. Gross-Isseroff R, Dillon HA, Fieldust SJ and Biegon A (1990) Arch. Gen. Psychiatry 47: 1049–1053.
14. Biegon A (1990) Ann. N.Y. Acad. Sci. 600: 427–434.

Biological Psychiatry, Volume 1. G. Racagni et al., editors.

Serotonin system challenges in suicidal behavior

Emil F. Coccaro and Richard J. Kavoussi
Clinical Neuroscience Research Unit, Department of Psychiatry, Medical College of Pennsylvania at EPPI, 3200 Henry Avenue, Philadelphia, Pennsylvania, U.S.A.

Central serotonin in suicidal behavior

The role of central serotonergic (5-HT) system in suicidal behavior is one of the most researched areas in biological psychiatry. The vast majority of studies involving both central and peripheral indices of 5-HT system function suggest an abnormality in patients displaying suicidal behavior [1]. Abnormalities reflected by these indices suggest widespread alterations in the 5-HT system at pre-synaptic, post-synaptic, and possibly both locations within the 5-HT synapse. Reduced brain concentrations of 5-HT or its metabolite (5-hydroxyindolacetic acid: 5-HIAA), or of tritiated imipramine in suicide victims clearly suggest a reduction in pre-synaptic 5-HT system function; due either to a loss of 5-HT neurons or of 5-HT synthesis and release. Conversely, increased numbers of 5-HT_2 receptors in the brains of suicide victims suggest an upregulation of receptor numbers, if not sensitivity at post-synaptic 5-HT sites in suicide victims. Whether this combination of a reduction in pre-synaptic 5-HT innervation and/or turnover with a possible increase in post-synaptic 5-HT receptor function results in reduced, normal, or increased overall 5-HT system function, however, is unclear from current studies of suicide brains. Studies of cerebrospinal fluid (CSF) 5-HIAA concentrations, platelet 5-HT uptake, platelet tritiated imipramine, or platelet 5-HT_2 receptor binding in suicide attempters are similarly unrevealing in this regard. This is because none of these indices assess functional aspects of the central 5-HT system as occur in vivo where the result of endogenous pre- and post-synaptic 5-HT system factors can be assessed simultaneously.

Relevance of the pharmacochallenge strategy in the study of suicidal behavior

Unlike the 5-HT indices described above, the 5-HT pharmacochallenge strategy offers the opportunity to assess physiologic function within the central 5-HT synapse [2]. This method typically assesses the neuroendocrine or behavioral responses to single doses of 5-HT active agents. Interpretation of these responses to 5-HT challenge depends upon the pharmacologic properties of the agent and the role of pro and/or post-synaptic receptors within specific brain regions mediating the response. Indirect 5-HT agonists (i.e., releasing agents, uptake inhibitors, and precursors) may reflect both pro and/or post-synaptic aspects of 5-HT function in the relevant areas of the brain. In addition, by utilizing the endogenous 5-HT contained within the terminal and the synaptic cleft, these agents (e.g., releasing agents, especially) may yield information about receptor stimulation by 5-HT itself rather than by an exogenous 5-HT-like agent. In contrast, direct 5-HT receptor agonists (i.e., m-CPP, MK-212, buspirone, gepirone, ipsaperone) have the potential capability to assess post-synaptic 5-HT receptor and/or receptor subtype, sensitivity specifically. Pharmacologic dissection of specific 5-HT receptor subtypes involved in suicidal behavior is an evolving science, however, and should occur in conjunction with other studies which can also assess overall 5-HT system function. Finally, in contrast to cerebrospinal fluid studies of 5-HT metabolites (i.e., CSF 5-HIAA, which probably reflects the integrity of central 5-HT neurons in general; [2]), pharmacochallenge studies have the potential to localize a potential abnormality of central 5-HT system function in the brain (e.g. neuroendocrine responses may be localized to the limbic-hypothalamic-pituitary axis).

5-HT pharmacochallenge studies in suicidal behavior

Despite the wealth of data regarding the neurochemistry of suicidal behavior in psychiatric patients, there have been few investigations utilizing 5-HT pharmacochallenge agents. To date, only two full reports have been published in the literature [3,4]; see Fig. 1.

The first study reported increased cortisol (CORT) responses to 5-HT precursor

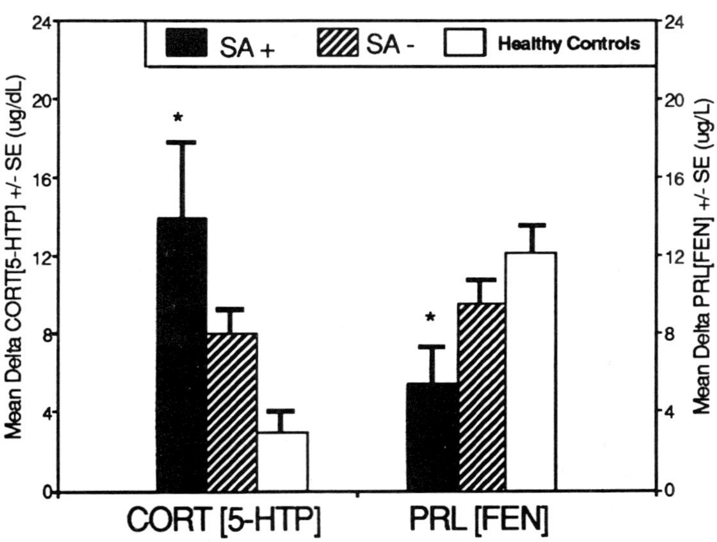

Fig. 1. Mean δ CORT responses to 5-HTP challenge (CORT[5-HTP]) and mean PRL responses to fenfluramine challenge (PRL[FEN]) in MAD and PD patients with (SA+) and without (SA–) history of suicidal behavior compared to healthy controls. Asterisk: $P < 0.05$ for SA+ difference from SA– and from healthy controls. Data adapted from Meltzer et al. [3] and Coccaro et al. [4].

5-HTP challenge (i.e., CORT[5-HTP]) in major affective disorder (MAD) patients who had attempted suicide (n = 7) compared with those who had not (n = 33) and healthy controls (n = 15; [3]). This finding was interpreted as consistent with the finding of increased 5-HT_2 receptor binding previously reported in the brains of suicide victims. This interpretation was supported by two additional observations. First, the CORT[5-HTP] responses were correlated inversely with CSF 5-HIAA concentrations (i.e., a putatively "pre-synaptic" index) in a subgroup of these patients [5]. Second, CORT[5-HTP] responses could be blunted by the 5-HT_2 ($/5\text{-HT}_{1C}$) receptor antagonist ritanserin [6]. The second study, in contrast, reported decreased prolactin responses to 5-HT releaser/uptake inhibitor fenfluramine challenge (i.e., PRL[FEN]) in MAD and/or personality disorder (PD) patients with a life history of suicide attempt (n = 14), regardless of diagnosis, compared with MAD/PD patients without this history (n = 31) or healthy controls (n = 18; [4]). History of impulsive aggressive behavior in PD, but not MAD, patients accounted for nearly all the variance in PRL[FEN] values associated with past history of suicidal behavior. This was because history of suicidal behavior correlated directly, and PRL[FEN] responses correlated inversely, with dimensional indices of impulsive aggression in these PD patients. These interrelationships were absent in MAD patients because there was no significant relationship between PRL[FEN] values and indices of impulsive aggression in these patients. These findings suggested that overall 5-HT system function in the limbic-hypothalamic-pituitary system was inversely related to impulsive aggressive behavior, and thereby reduced, in PD patients with history of suicidal behavior (i.e., in turn, a manifestation of a lifelong personality trait characterized by impulsive aggressive behaviors). The difference between MAD and PD patients was interpreted as reflective of fundamental biological differences between the groups [4].

Specific aspects of 5-HT system function reflected by pharmacochallenge studies

Both studies suggest an abnormality in central 5-HT system function in MAD and/or PD patients as a function of suicidal behavior. However, the directionality of the putative abnormality is different. Meltzer et al. [3] suggest hypersensitivity of post-synaptic $5\text{-HT}_2(/5\text{-HT}_{1C}$; n.b.: 5-HT_{1C} receptors are now thought to be more 5-HT_2-like than 5-HT_1-like; [7]) receptors, while Coccaro et al. [4] suggest a reduction in overall 5-HT system function. These two interpretations are not mutually exclusive, however. One, heightened sensitivity of $5\text{-HT}_2(/5\text{-HT}_{1C})$ receptors could exist in the presence of reduced overall 5-HT system function. 5-HT_2 ($/5\text{-HT}_{1C}$) receptor upregulation may be inadequate to compensate for reduced 5-HT output (as might be suggested by brain 5-HT and CSF 5-HIAA studies; [1]). Conversely, $5\text{-HT}_2(/5\text{-HT}_{1C})$ receptor upregulation may be pathological (i.e., not compensatory) and regulated in an inverse fashion ([8]; if not independent) relative to 5-HT_1 receptor regulation. If the latter is true, P[FEN] responses could be low in suicidal patients if it largely reflects 5-HT activity at post-synaptic 5-HT_1-like (i.e., 5-HT_{1A} and/or 5-HT_{1D}) receptors. Evidence supporting this hypothesis comes from studies in progress which demonstrate a high positive correlation between PRL[FEN] and PRL[m-CPP] values and inverse relationships between PRL[m-CPP] and PRL[buspirone] responses and indices of impulsive aggression in PD patients [9,10].

These, along with animal study [11], data suggest that PRL[FEN] responses may largely reflect the sensitivity of 5-HT_1-like receptors. Since 5-HT_1-like (i.e., 5-HT_{1A}/5-HT_{1D}) receptors tend to hyperpolarize (i.e., inhibit), and 5-HT_2(/5-HT_{1C}) receptors tend to depolarize (i.e., excite), neuronal membranes [12], it is possible that suicidal behavior could arise from a reduction in 5-HT mediated inhibition, and/or enhancement, of aggressive responses to noxious (i.e., triggering) stimuli. Under this model, reduced function of 5-HT_1-like receptors would disinhibit aggressive responding directly, while heightened function of 5-HT_2(/5-HT_{1C}) receptors would enhance aggressive responding through excitation of neurons distal to the relevant 5-HT synapse. Further research will be required to test these hypotheses.

References

1. Coccaro EF and Astill JL (1990) Prog. Neuro-Psychopharmacol. Biol. Psychiatry 14:663–674.
2. Murphy DL, Mellow AM, Sunderland T et al. (1990) In: Coccaro EF and Murphy DL (eds.) Serotonin in Major Psychiatric Disorders. American Psychiatric Press, Washington D.C.
3. Meltzer HY, Perline R, Tricou BJ et al. (1984) Arch. Gen. Psychiatry 41: 379–387.
4. Coccaro EF, Siever LJ, Kiar HM et al. (1989) Arch. Gen. Psychiatry 46: 587–599.
5. Koyama T, Lowy MT and Meltzer NY (1987) Am. J. Psychiatry 144: 334–337.
6. Lee MA, Nash JF, Barnes M et al. (1991) Psychopharmacology 103: 258–264.
7. Hoyer D (1988) Trends Pharmacol. Sci. 9: 89–94.
8. Lahorski JM and Aghajanian GK (1985) Neuropharmacology 24: 265–273.
9. Coccaro EF, Siever LJ, Kavoussi R and Davis KL (1989) Biol. Psychiatry 25(7): 86A.
10. Coccaro EF, Gabriel S and Siever LJ (1990) Psychopharm. Bull. 26: 393–405.
11. Willoughby JO, Menadue MF and Liebelt HJ (1988) Neuroendocrinology 47: 83–87.
12. Andrade R and Araneda R (1989) Proc. 29th ACNP Ann. Scientific Meeting, p. 137.

Biological Psychiatry, Volume 1. G. Racagni et al., editors.

Serotonin receptor sensitivity and aggression

Scott Wetzler, Rene S. Kahn, Gregory Asnis, Martin Korn and Herman M. van Praag
Albert Einstein College of Medicine/Montefiore Medical Center, New York, NY 10467, U.S.A.

Signs of serotonin (5-hydroxytryptamine; 5-HT) dysfunction have been found in several psychiatric disorders, including major depression [1] and obsessive-compulsive disorder [2]. An alternative approach is to identify the brain/behavior relationships between 5-HT dysfunction and particular psychopathological dimensions, irrespective of psychiatric diagnosis [3–6]. For example, abnormal 5-HT function has been related to anxiety and aggression. This study focuses on the relationship between 5-HT dysfunction and aggression, and uses the challenge test with m-chlorophenylpiperazine (MCPP) as a strategy [7].

Methods

To determine the effects of MCPP in outwardly directed aggression, 42 psychiatric patients volunteered for the study including 22 patients with major depression (MD) (8 men and 14 women; 10 outpatients, 12 inpatients; mean age: 34.3 ± 2.2 years) and 20 outpatients with panic disorder (PD) (8 men and 12 women; mean age: 35.0 ± 2.2 years). To determine the effects of MCPP on inwardly directed aggression, 11 psychiatric patients with a recent (n = 6) or past (n = 5) suicide attempt (4 men and 7 women; 8 outpatients, 3 inpatients; mean age: 28.6 ± 1.8 years), including 8 patients with major depression (1 bipolar depression, 1 psychotic depression), 2 patients with adjustment disorder, and 1 patient with mixed personality disorder, and 19 normal control subjects (9 men and 10 women; mean age: 30.0 ± 2.6 years) volunteered for the study.

All subjects were given a Schedule for Affective Disorders and Schizophrenia (SADS) interview. The MD and PD patients met Research Diagnostic Criteria (RDC) [8] for major depression and panic disorder respectively and completed the Buss Durkee Hostility Inventory (BDHI) [9]. The normal subjects met RDC for "never mentally ill". All subjects were within 25% of their ideal body weight, had normal laboratory and physical exams, had been free of drug and alcohol use for at least 2 weeks before the study and gave written informed consent prior to participation. The *procedure* of the MCPP test was described in Kahn et al. [10].

Five kinds of *data analysis* were performed. Analysis #1 compared the psychiatric patients' (n = 42) level of induced anger (δ: peak-minus-baseline) on MCPP and on placebo using a t-test. Analyses #2 and #3 compared cortisol and prolactin release of aggressive patients with that of non-aggressive patients. Patients (n = 42) were classified as aggressive/non-aggressive using cut scores of >2 ("Slight and of doubtful clinical significance") on two SADS items (#332 – "Overt expression of irritability, annoyance and anger..." and #330 – "Subjective feeling of anger, resentment, or annoyance (directed externally) whether expressed overtly or not"). Analysis #$ compared cortisol and prolactin release of patients with a (recent or past) history of suicide attempt (n = 11) to normal subjects (n = 19). For analyses #2–4, the two groups were compared using t-tests for the area-under-the-curve of placebo-corrected change-from-baseline. For analysis #5, correlations were calculated between δ (peak-minus-baseline) hormone (cortisol, prolactin) release on MCPP and scores on the BDHI scales among the MD and PD patients (n = 36). Considering the number of correlations, a significance level of $P < 0.01$ was used.

Results

Induced anger

Across psychiatric patients, MCPP did not induce significantly more or less anger than did placebo (paired t-test = 1.60, df = 36, $P = 0.12$). However, within the PD group alone, there was a non-significant trend ($P < 0.10$) for greater induced anger on MCPP than on placebo (placebo: 1.39 ± 5.89; MCPP: 11.90 ± 25.20). Furthermore, induced anger on MCPP was uncorrelated with peak MCPP blood level in the psychiatric patients (r = –0.03). In contrast, delta cortisol on MCPP was significantly correlated to peak MCPP blood level (r = 0.44).

Overt irritability

As described in Methods, PD and MD patients were classified as aggressive/non-aggressive on the basis of the SADS item concerning overt irritability. MCPP blood levels for these two groups were comparable (low hostile: 16.1 ± 2.2 ng/ml; high hostile: 19.1 ± 3.9 ng/ml; t = 0.72, $P = 0.48$). As Fig. 2 indicates, the high hostile patients (n = 16) and the low hostile patients (n = 26) did not have significantly different cortisol (t = –0.89, $P = 0.38$) or prolactin (t = –0.90, $P = 0.37$) release.

Subjective anger

The same patients were also classified as aggressive/nonaggressive on the basis of the SADS item concerning subjective anger. MCPP blood levels for these two groups were comparable (low hostile: 17.8 ± 3.2 ng/ml; high hostile: 17.0 ± 2.7 ng/ml; t = 0.18, $P = 0.86$). The high hostile patients (n = 25) and the low hostile (n = 17) did not have significantly different cortisol (t = 0.38, $P = 0.71$) or prolactin (t = 0.62, $P = 0.54$) release.

Suicide attempts

Patients with a recent or past history of suicide attempt were contrasted with normal control subjects. MCPP blood levels for these two groups were comparable (suicide attempters: 17.3 ± 5.5 ng/mg; normal controls: 16.3 ± 3.8 ng/ml; $t = -0.15$, $P = 0.88$). There were no significant differences in cortisol ($t = 0.13$, $P = 0.90$) or prolactin ($t = -1.17$, $P = 0.25$) release.

Hostility as a dimension

δ Cortisol and δ prolactin on MCPP were not significantly related to scores on any of the BDHI scales from 36 MD and PD patients. The correlation between δ cortisol and suspiciousness ($r = -0.31$) showed a non-significant trend ($P < 0.05$).

Discussion

This study reports consistently negative results regarding the expected association between increased 5-HT receptor sensitivity and aggression: 1) MCPP 0.25 mg/kg p.o. did not induce or reduce anger in psychiatric patients; 2) MD and PD patients with clinically significant levels of aggression had similar MCPP-induced cortisol and prolactin release to patients who were non-aggressive; 3) patients with a history of suicide attempts had similar MCPP-induced hormone release to normal controls; and 4) MCPP-induced cortisol and prolactin release was not related to levels of hostility in MD and PD patients as measured by the BDHI.

Thus, contrary to our predictions, we did not find evidence of *increased* 5-HT receptor sensitivity in patients with inwardly or outwardly directed aggression, nor did the administration of a 5-HT agonist influence hostility levels. Aggression dysregulated patients are known to have consistently low levels of CSF 5-HIAA – a deficit which we expected to be associated with 5-HT receptor *hyper*sensitivity. However, as measured by the MCPP challenge paradigm, there was no evidence of increased 5-HT receptor sensitivity. This study design does not rule out the possibility that these patients exhibit 5-HT receptor *hypo*sensitivity, which would need to be evaluated in future research using higher doses of MCPP. In humans, MCPP seems to have a predominant effect on 5-HT_{1C} and 5-HT_3 receptors [11]. The negative results of this study could be explained by assuming that other 5-HT receptor systems are involved in aggression regulation.

References

1. Kalus O, Asnis GM and van Praag HM (1989) Psychiatr. Ann. 19: 348–353.
2. Zohar J, Mueller EA, Insel TR, Zohar-Kadouch RC and Murphy DL (1987) Arch. Gen. Psychiatry 44: 946–951.

3. van Praag HM, Korf J, Lakkee JPWF and Schut T (1975) Psychol. Med. 5: 138–146.
4. van Praag HM, Lemus CZ and Kahn RS (1987) Biol. Psychiatry 22: 86–98.
5. van Praag HM, Asnis GM, Kahn RS, Brown SL, Korn M, Friedman JM and Wetzler S (1990) Br. J. Psychiatry 157: 723–734.
6. Wetzler S, van Praag HM and Katz M (1991) In: Feighner J (ed.) Diagnosis of Depression. John Wiley, New York.
7. Wetzler S, Kahn RS, Asnis G, Korn M and van Praag HM (1991) Psychiatr. Res. (submitted).
8. Endicott F and Spitzer RL (1978) Arch. Gen. Psychiatry 35: 837–844.
9. Buss A and Durkee A (1957) J. Consult. Psychol. 21: 343–349.
10. Kahn RS, van Praag HM, Wetzler S, Asnis GM and Barr G (1988) Biol. Psychiatry 23: 189–208.
11. Murphy DL (1990) Neuropsychopharmacology 3: 457–471.

Biological Psychiatry, Volume 1. G. Racagni et al., editors.

Integration of neurobiology and psychopathology in a unified model of suicidal behavior

J. John Mann

Western Psychiatric Institute and Clinic, 3811 O'Hara Street, Pittsburgh, PA 15213, U.S.A.

Risk factors for suicide originate from a number of domains which include psychiatric [1], psychological [2], genetic [3], familial [3], demographic, psychosocial [4] and biological. The development of an explanatory or predictive model of suicidal behavior must take into account the relative contribution of factors from all of these domains. Most studies have investigated only a single domain of risk and thus the relationship between domains of risk are largely unknown and remain a major research priority. A hypothetical model or integration will be discussed.

Defining suicidal behavior

Suicidal behavior ranges from ideation to completed suicide. One must distinguish self-destructive behavior from behavior that has overt suicidal intent. It is important to distinguish those patients who carry out a so-called failed suicide attempt versus parasuicide or suicide gesture. There are clinical and demographic group differences between the failed suicide and the suicide-gesture groups. The failed suicide is generally characterized by careful planning and a highly lethal method and the suicide gesture by impulsivity and the use of a low lethality method.

Biology of completed suicide

Levels of 5-HT and 5-HIAA are reduced in the brain stem but not in cortical regions of the brain in the suicide group compared to non-psychiatric controls [5–9]. Although early studies [10,11] showed a reduction in the number of presynaptic imipramine binding sites in the prefrontal cortex of suicide victims, subsequent studies have been less consistent [12]. It will be important to consider differences in brain regions in studying the biological correlates of suicide and other psychiatric conditions [12]. Imipramine binds to receptors other than the serotonin receptor and changes in these other receptor populations may account for discrepant results. Postsynaptic serotonin 5-HT_2 receptors number is increased in the prefrontal cortex of suicide victims [13–16]. There are other serotonin receptor populations in human brain including the 5-HT_{1A}, 5-HT_{1C}, 5-HT_{1D}, and 5-HT_3 receptor populations. These represent an area of future research. β-adrenergic receptors are generally reported to be increased in some brain regions in suicide victims [15,17,18]. The direction of change in β-adrenergic binding and 5-HT_2 receptor binding is the opposite to that observed in animals that receive anti-depressants chronically. Muscarinic cholinergic receptors assayed by ^{3}H-QNB do not appear to be altered in the brain of suicide victims [19].

Studies of the biology of suicide attempters

Studies by many research groups indicated that patients with an affective disorder [20–23], schizophrenia [24–26], or a personality disorder [22], and characterized by serious suicidal behavior had low levels of CSF 5-HIAA compared to diagnostically matched patients who had not made a suicide attempt. There are no differences in CSF 5-HIAA between suicide attempters and non-attempters with bipolar disorder [27,28]. Low levels of CSF 5-HIAA may predict future suicidal behavior rather than the primary psychiatric disorder [20,29]. CSF 5-HIAA may be a trait characteristic of the individual that predicts susceptibility or predisposition towards suicidal behavior [30]. The prolactin response to the serotonin agonist fenfluramine is blunted in patients who have carried out suicide attempts [31,32]. It is difficult to know whether the relationships observed are due to the suicidal behavior, depression, or the personality disorders. One study [33] has found that the cortisol response to 5-HTP is increased in patients who have a history of suicidal behavior. Studies using l-tryptophan have found blunting in depressed patients compared to non-psychiatric controls, but the relationship to suicidal behavior remains to be determined [34]. Studies of the hypothalamic-pituitary-adrenocortical axis and cortisol regulation have yielded conflicting results with regard to prediction of suicide risk [35], and appear more closely related to type or severity of depression.

Genetics of suicide

There appears to be a genetic component involved in suicide risk [3]. Trait-dependent changes may be phenotypic expressions of the genetic predisposition towards suicide risk.

The integration of biological findings into a comprehensive explanatory model of suicidal behavior

Clinical, demographic and familial characteristics distinguish patients at high risk for suicide or attempted suicide. How biological findings may be integrated into a model that explains suicidal behavior is an important theoretical and practical question. One possible formulation is that the biological findings represent a combination of state and trait-related effects. The trait-related effects may represent genetic or early life experience factors. The state-dependent effects may reflect acute psychiatric conditions, the impact of alcohol or substance abuse, or interpersonal or social stressors of other kinds. Since, there is a poor relationship between the severity of the acute psychiatric condition or psychosocial stressors and suicide risk, one is forced to conclude that constitutional factors may play an important role in determining whether or not someone who feels suicidal carries out a suicidal act. The measurement of biological factors such as those described above may allow assessment of the constitutional susceptibility for suicide or the level of the suicide threshold for the individual. Patients with a low suicide threshold are more likely to act than those with a high suicide threshold. A combination of clinical and pharmacological interventions may help to by relieving the acute stressor as well as raising the suicide threshold and thereby placing the patient at lower risk.

Acknowledgement

This work was supported by the NIMH Clinical Research Center for the Study of Suicidal Behavior (MH46745).

References

1. Miller F and Chabrier LA (1987) Suicide Life-Threatening Behav. 17(1): 13–17.
2. Minkoff K, Bergman E and Beck A (1973) Am. J. Psychiatry 130: 455–459.
3. Roy A (1983) Arch. Gen. Psychiatry 40: 971–974.
4. Durkheim E (1951) In: Spaulding JA and Simpson G (translators) Suicide, 897th edition. Free Press, New York.
5. Shaw DM, Camps FE and Eccleston EG (1967) Br. J. Psychiatry 113: 1407–1411.
6. Bourne HR, Bunney WE Jr, Colburn RW, Davis JM, Shaw DM and Coppen AJ (1968) Lancet ii: 805–808.
7. Pare CMB, Yeung DPH, Price K and Stacey RS (1969) Lancet ii: 133–135.
8. Beskow J, Gottfries CG, Roos BE and Winblad B (1976) Acta Psychiatr. Scand. 53: 7–20.
9. Lloyd KG, Farley IJ, Deck JHN and Hornykiewicz O (1974) Adv. Biochem. Psychopharmacol. 11: 387–397.
10. Stanley M, Virgilio J and Gershon S (1982) Science 216: 1337–1339.
11. Rehavi M, Skolnick P and Paul SM (1985) Proc. 3rd Int. Meeting Clin. Pharmacol. Psychiatry. Macmillian Press, London, pp. 846–853.
12. Gross-Isseroff R, Israeli M and Biegon A (1989) Arch. Gen. Psychiatry 46: 237–241.
13. Mann JJ, Arango V, Marzuk PM, Theccanat S and Reis DJ (1989) Br. J. Psychiatry (Suppl.) 155: 7–14.
14. Stanley M and Mann JJ (1983) Lancet i: 214–216.
15. Mann JJ, Stanley M, McBride PA and McEwen BS (1986) Arch. Gen. Psychiatry 43: 954–959.
16. Ferrier IN, McKeith IG, Cross AJ, Perry EK, Candy JM and Perry RH (1986) Ann. N.Y. Acad. Sci. 487: 128–142.
17. Meyerson LR, Wennogle LP, Abel MS, Coupet J, Lippa AS, Rauh CE and Beer B (1982) Pharmacol. Biochem. Behavior 17: 159–163.

18. Biegon A and Israeli M (1988) Brain Res. 422: 199–203.
19. Stanley M (1984) Am. J. Psychiatry 141: 1432–1436.
20. Åsberg M, Nordström P and Träskman-Bendz L (1986) Ann. N.Y. Acad. Sci. 487: 243–255.
21. Ågren H (1980) Psychiatr. Res. 3: 225–236.
22. Träskman-Bendz L, Åsberg M and Schalling D (1986) Ann. N.Y. Acad. Sci. 487: 168–174.
23. Träskman-Bendz L, Åsberg M, Bertilsson L and Sjöstrand L (1981) Arch. Gen. Psychiatry 38: 631–636.
24. van Praag HM (1983) Lancet ii: 977–978.
25. Ninan PT, van Kammen DP, Scheinin M, Linnoila M, Bunney WE Jr and Goodwin FK (1984) Am. J. Psychiatry 141: 566–569.
26. Pickar D, Roy A, Breier A, Doran A, Wolkowitz O, Colison J and Ågren H (1986) Ann. N.Y. Acad. Sci. 487: 189–196.
27. Secunda SK, Cross CK, Koslow S, Katz MM, Kocsis J, Maas JW and Landis H (1986) Biol. Psychiatry 21: 756–767.
28. Berrettini WH, Nurnberger JI and Narrow W (1986) Ann. N.Y. Acad. Sci. 487: 197–201.
29. Roy A, Ågren H, Pickar D, Linnoila M, Doran A, Cutler N and Paul SM (1986) Am. J. Psychiatry 143: 1539–1545.
30. Träskman-Bendz L, Åsberg M and Bertilsson L (1984) Acta Psychiatr. Scand. 69: 333–342.
31. Coccaro EF, Siever LJ, Klar HM, Maurer G, Cochrane K, Cooper TB, Mohs RC and Davis KL (1989) Arch. Gen. Psychiatry 46: 587–599.
32. De Meo M, McBride PA, Mann JJ and Keilp J (1988) 141st Annual Meeting of the American Psychiatric Association 1991 (Abstr.).
33. Meltzer HY, Perline R, Tricou BJ, Lowy M and Robertson A (1984) Arch. Gen. Psychiatry 41: 379–387.
34. Heninger GR, Charney DS and Sternberg DE (1984) Arch. Gen. Psychiatry 41: 398–402.
35. Targum SD, Rosen L and Capodanno AE (1981) Am. J. Psychiatry 140: 877–879.

Biological Psychiatry, Volume 1. G. Racagni et al., editors.

Neurochemical findings in the brain of suicide victims

Victoria Arango, Mark D. Underwood and J. John Mann

Laboratories of Neuropharmacology, Biomedical Science Tower W1645, Western Psychiatric Institute and Clinic, 3811 O'Hara Street, Pittsburgh, PA 15213, U.S.A.

Introduction

Alterations in the serotonergic system have been associated with suicidal behavior. Lower levels of serotonin and its metabolites have been found in the cerebrospinal fluid of suicide attempters than in non-attempters in groups with different psychiatric diagnoses [1–3]. Postmortem studies have largely confirmed these findings in that levels of 5-HT and 5-HIAA are lower in the brainstem of suicide victims (see [4] for review). Neurotransmitter receptors are more stable after death and studies in brain homogenates have revealed that 5-HT_2 binding sites are increased in the prefrontal cortex (PFC) of suicide victims [5,6]. In addition, β-adrenergic binding is substantially increased in the PFC of suicide victims [5] However, measurements in brain homogenates do not allow for the precise anatomical localization of where the changes are occurring and therefore provide little insight into the organization and interactions of different pre- and postsynaptic receptors.

Quantitative autoradiographic analysis of receptor binding provides the opportunity of analyzing, with high anatomical resolution, the precise localization of changes in receptor populations in the brain of suicide victims. Using quantitative autoradiography we sought to determine the localization of 5-HT_2 and β-adrenergic receptor binding changes in the PFC and temporal cortex (TC) of suicide victims compared to controls.

Materials and Methods

Brain samples from suicide victims and controls were obtained at autopsy. Toxicological screens were performed on blood, bile, urine and in many cases, brain. Only those cases with negative screens entered the study. Suicide victims were matched with controls based on postmortem interval (±5 h, range 5–23 h), age (±5 years, range 15–81 years), sex and race. All pairs were assayed together and exposed to the same sheet of ^{3}H-sensitive film in order to reduce variance.

Quantitative autoradiography of 5-HT_2 and β-adrenergic binding was performed by modifying previously published methods using ^{125}I-lysergic acid diethylamide (^{125}I-LSD) [7] and ^{125}I-pindolol (^{125}I-PIN) [8] respectively. Autoradiograms were analyzed using a computerized image analysis system as previously described [9,10].

Results

5-HT_2, binding in both suicides and controls was highest within the intermediate cortical layers (III and IV) in both PFC and TC and lowest in the inner (V and VI) cortical layers. In the PFC 5-HT_2 binding was increased in all cortical layers of the suicide group, ranging from 49 to 73% of control ($P < 0.05$), but not in the white matter. ^{125}I-LSD binding in the TC of suicide victims did not differ from that of controls ($P > 0.05$ all layers).

In contrast to the laminar distribution of 5-HT_2, binding sites, β-adrenergic binding appeared uniformly distributed across cortical layers in the 2 areas studied. Binding was increased in all layers of the PFC (37 to 41%, $P < 0.05$) of suicide victims, but not in the TC ($P > 0.05$).

Discussion

Increased 5-HT_2 binding has been reported in membrane homogenates from the PFC of suicide victims in some [5,6,11] but not all [12–14] studies. To address the question of whether the receptor changes are regionally selective and anatomically specific, we have employed quantitative autoradiography in brain tissue from drug-free, carefully-matched suicide victims and controls with a short postmortem interval. Another study [15] used quantitative autoradiography to examine 5-HT_2 receptor changes in the brain of suicide victims and found, in contrast with our findings, decreased binding in the suicide group under the age of 50 years. Since antidepressants and antipsychotics reduce 5-HT_2 binding, differences with our study [11] may be due to drug effects, use of different ligands, longer postmortem intervals, or the heterogeneity of psychiatric illnesses associated with suicide.

Previous studies of β-adrenergic binding in membrane homogenates, using mostly ^{3}H-dihydroalprenolol (^{3}H-DHA), are also divided in that some investigators report increased binding in the PFC of the suicide group [5,11,16] and some do not [17,18]. However quantitative autoradiographic studies from 2 laboratories [11,16] using ^{125}I-PIN found increased β-adrenergic binding in the PFC of suicide victims compared to controls.

The observed increases in 5-HT_2 [5,6,11], 5-HT_{1A} [19] and β-adrenergic receptors [5,11,16,20] may represent compensatory upregulation of postsynaptic elements in response to deficiencies in the presynaptic neurons innervating cortical targets. Further support for this hypothesis can be found in the finding that serotonin uptake sites are decreased in suicide victims [6,21]. It remains unclear whether the total extent of neurochemical changes in the brain of suicide victims is restricted to the serotonergic and noradrenergic systems. Recent evidence suggests that μ-opioid receptors are increased in the brain of suicide victims [22], but GABA receptors are not [23]. It may be that it is the interaction of all these neurotransmitter systems which is important in the pathogenesis of suicide.

Acknowledgement

This work was supported by PHS Grant MH40210.

References

1. Träskman L, Åsberg M, Bertilsson L et al. (1981) Arch. Gen. Psychiatry 38: 631–636.
2. Ågren H (1980) Psychiatry Res. 3: 225–236.
3. Träskman-Bendz L, Åsberg M and Schalling D (1986) Ann. N.Y. Acad. Sci. 487: 168–174.
4. Mann JJ, McBride PA and Stanley M (1986) Ann. N.Y. Acad. Sci. 487: 114–121.
5. Mann JJ, Stanley M, McBride PA et al. (1986) Arch. Gen. Psychiatry 43: 954–959.
6. Stanley M and Mann JJ (1983) Lancet i: 214–216.
7. Nakada MT, Wieczorek CM and Rainbow TC (1984) Neurosci. Lett. 49: 13–18.
8. Rainbow TC, Parsons B and Wolfe BB (1984) Proc. Natl. Acad. Sci. U.S.A. 81: 1585–1589.
9. Arango V, Ernsberger P, Reis DJ et al. (1990) Brain Res. 516: 113–121.
10. Ernsberger P, Arango V and Reis DJ (1988) Neurosci. Lett. 85: 179–186.
11. Arango V, Ernsberger P, Marzuk PM et al. (1990) Arch. Gen. Psychiatry 47: 1038–1047.
12. Owen F, Chambers DR, Cooper SJ et al. (1986) Brain Res. 362: 185–188.
13. Cheetham SC, Crompton MR, Katona CLE et al. (1988) Brain Res. 443: 272–280.
14. Owen F, Cross AJ, Crow TJ et al. (1983) Lancet ii: 1256.
15. Gross-Isseroff R, Salama D, Israeli M et al. (1990) Brain Res. 507: 208–215.
16. Biegon A and Israeli M (1988) Brain Res. 442: 199–203.
17. Stockmeier CA and Meltzer HY (1991) Biol. Psychiatry 29: 183–191.
18. De Paermentier F, Cheetham SC, Crompton MR et al. (1990) Brain Res. 525: 71–77.
19. Arango V, Miller WE, Miller ML et al. (1991) Soc. Neurosci. Abstr. (in press).
20. Arango V, Ernsberger P, Marzuk P et al. (1988) Soc. Neurosci. Abstr. 14: 171.
21. Henteleff RA, Arango V and Mann JJ (1991) Soc. Neurosci. Abstr. (in press).
22. Gross-Isseroff R, Dillon HA, Israeli M et al. (1990) Brain Res. 530: 312–316.
23. Cross JA, Cheetham SC, Crompton MR et al. (1988) Psychiatry Res 26: 119–129.

Biological Psychiatry, Volume 1. G. Racagni et al., editors.

Prediction of suicidal behavior from biological tests

Lil Träskman-Bendz, Göran Regnéll, Christer Alling, Per Simonsson, Lars Oreland, Ellen Vinge and Rolf Öhman

Departments of Psychiatry, Neurochemistry, Clinical Pharmacology (Uppsala and Lund), University Hospital, S-221 85 Lund, Sweden

Introduction

Patients, who repeat self-destructive behavior (repeaters) are well-known consumers of psychiatric resources. We and others have found that these patients often have personality disturbances and problems in the use of alcohol and drugs. Furthermore, they often have weak social support. As a part of their self-destructive life-style, they often harm themselves without excessive planning [1].

Biochemical studies of suicide attempters have dealt with patients with recent or life-time suicide attempts, or patients who later completed suicide. Both monoaminergic measures and corticosteroids have been suggested as predictors of suicidal behavior [2].

The present investigation deals with patients who have made suicide attempts before and/or after an index attempt, at which time they were studied comprehensively as inpatients.

Material and Methods

Patients

Until April 1990, complete cerebrospinal fluid (CSF) and urinary biochemical information was available in 61 patients, who were hospitalized on a research ward after a suicide attempt. They were subgrouped according to method into violent (n = 18) and nonviolent attempters, and into those who had or had not made attempts before (n = 35), or after (n = 17) the index attempt.

Ratings

Shortly before transferring the patient to psychiatric care, psychiatrists and social workers rated the patients according to the Suicidal Intent Scale (n = 52) [3].

Biochemical variables

CSF. The monoamine metabolites 5-hydroxyindoleacetic acid (5-HIAA), homovanillic acid (HVA) and 4-hydroxy 3-methoxy phenyl methods.

Blood. In the present calculations we used the 16 h post dexamethasone (DST) plasma cortisol.

Blood samples for platelet monoamine oxidase (MAO)-activity (n = 53) and serotonin 5-HT_2-receptor function in platelets (n = 17) were drawn before the lumbar punctures, and the latter were also studied in outpatients on drugs.

Urine. Cortisol, noradrenaline (Na) and adrenaline (A) were measured in 24-h urinary samples, which were collected shortly before the lumbar puncture.

Results

Patients who made violent suicide attempts often had CSF 5-HIAA below the median of 95 nmol/l ($\chi^2 = 4.68$, $P < 0.05$) and CSF HMPG above the median of 41 nmol/l ($\chi^2 = 6.56$, $P < 0.02$). They also tended to have post DST cortisol above the median.

Patients who repeated their suicidal behavior after the index attempt had CSF HMPG and MAO-activity in the high range, and low urinary cortisol levels (N.S.).

Four patients who later committed suicide had high CSF HMPG levels, and 3 of these had high Na/A and high cortisol levels in urine. Platelet MAO was available in 3 suicides, and all had high activity.

Changes of phosphatidyl-inositolbisphosphate (PIP)-2 hydrolysis after 5-HT-stimulation (platelet 5-HT_2 function) were significantly greater in patients than in matched healthy controls (Wilcoxon, $P < 0.01$). In patients, there was no significant correlation between CSF 5-HIAA and 5-HT_2 receptor function (r = 0.20).

Discussion

Our findings indicate that both the serotonergic and the noradrenergic systems have some relationship with suicidal behavior. Low CSF 5-HIAA has been regarded as a possible suicide predictor [2] and a predictor for future suicide attempts [4]. In this study 2 of 4 patients who committed suicide had low CSF 5-HIAA levels, and one had a median value. These 3 patients committed suicide by violent means, while the fourth died from an overdose.

In contrast to findings in depressed patients by Roy et al. [4], repeated suicidal behavior after the index attempt was not prominent in low CSF 5-HIAA subjects. One reason could be that we in fact are responsible for the after care of most of these patients.

In this study we found more violent attempters and somewhat more repeaters among high CSF HMPG subjects. Furthermore, all committed suicides had CSF HMPG in the high range. Like us, Roy et al. recently reported that (depressed female) violent attempters had high CSF HMPG levels [5].

If findings in this study hold true, it is evident that we need to consider the relative balances between neurotransmitter functions in future studies of violent, aggressive and impulsive behavior.

Acknowledgements

The assistance of Margot Alsén, RN, is greatly acknowledged. Our studies were supported by the Bank of Sweden Tercentenary Foundation, the Swedish Medical Research Council, the Söderström König Foundation, and funds from Lund University and Malmöhus County.

References

1. Öjehagen A, Regnéll G and Träskman-Bendz L (1991) Acta Psychiatr. Scand. (in press).
2. Åsberg M, Schalling D, Träskman-Bendz L and Wägner A (1987) In: Meltzer HY (ed.) Psychopharmacology: The Third Generation of Progress. Raven Press, New York, pp. 655–668.
3. Beck AT, Herman I and Schuyler D (1974) In: Beck AT, Resnik HLP and Lettieri D (eds.) The Prediction of Suicide. Charles Press, Bowie, MD, pp. 45–46.
4. Roy A, De Jong J and Linnoila M (1989) Arch. Gen. Psychiatry 46: 609–612.
5. Roy A, Pickar D, De Jong J, Karoum F and Linnoila M (1989) Biol. Psychiatry 25: 341–350.

Biological Psychiatry, Volume 1. G. Racagni et al., editors.

Pharmacotherapy in the prevention of suicidal behaviour

D.B. Montgomery, D. Baldwin, M. Green, T. Bullock and S.A. Montgomery
Department of Psychiatry, St Mary's Hospital Medical School, London, U.K.

Investigations into possible treatments for suicidal behaviour have seldom paid sufficient attention to the basic methodological issues to ensure the validity of the results. The failure of studies to demonstrate differences between treatments may therefore reflect inadequate trial methodology. The most common error has been to include a group of patients who did not have sufficient predicted morbidity in the trial period to provide an adequate test.

In major depression it has been assumed that antidepressants reduce the suicide risk. Since suicide attempts are comparatively rare, large numbers of patients observed for a long period are needed in order to test the validity of this assumption. The recent placebo controlled study of the long-term efficacy of 2 doses of the antidepressant maprotiline was large enough (1141 patients included) and continued long enough (1 year) to test the hypothesis. Maprotiline was shown to be clearly effective in reducing relapse or new episodes of depression but was nevertheless associated with a higher rate of suicide attempts than placebo. There were 14 suicide attempts in the maprotiline-treated group, 5 of which were fatal, compared with 1 attempt in the placebo group which was fatal and the difference was significant ($P < 0.01$) [1]. The lower dose of maprotiline was significantly less effective than the higher dose, although still significantly better than placebo, but was also associated with an increased number of suicide attempts.

The rate of suicide attempts on maprotiline in this study was higher than that reported in other long-term treatment studies in major depression and the conclusion that maprotiline provokes suicide cannot be avoided. The assumption that an effective antidepressant cannot provoke suicide appears to be unfounded.

Suicide attempts are relatively uncommon events during follow-up of patients whose depression has responded to treatment. Our approach to determining the effect of pharmacotherapy on suicidal behaviour has been to focus on suicidal behaviour in the absence of major depression. In order to ensure sufficient morbidity during the studies, a high-risk group characterised by a history of 2 or more suicide attempts was included. In these studies major depression and schizophrenia were excluded, but brief depression was permitted [2]. In our earlier 6-month placebo controlled prophylactic study, low-dose neuroleptic was found to be effective in reducing suicidal behaviour compared with placebo ($P < 0.01$) [3]. In a parallel study, the antidepressant mianserin was not significantly different to placebo in its effect on the suicide attempt rate [4]. There was, however, some effect and it is possible that the study had insufficient power for a proper test of efficacy.

In a similar design to the earlier studies of prophylactic treatment of suicidal behaviour, 107 patients with a history of 2 or more episodes of suicidal behaviour were treated double-blind with fluoxetine or placebo for 6 months or until they had a further suicide attempt. Patients with major depression or schizophrenia were excluded, but patients with brief episodes of depression lasting less than 2 weeks were included. Preliminary analysis of the results shows that 18 of the 54 patients treated with fluoxetine and 18 of the 53 patients treated with placebo had a suicide attempt during the study, demonstrating that fluoxetine had no advantage over placebo in protecting against subsequent suicidal behaviour. There is no evidence that fluoxetine provokes suicidal attempts.

The preliminary results of this prophylactic study of a 5-HT reuptake inhibitor do not show an advantage for the antidepressant compared with placebo and demonstrate the necessity for carrying out carefully-conducted placebo controlled studies with sufficient power to investigate the effect of antidepressants on suicidal behaviour.

References

1. Roulillon F, Phillips R, Serrurier D, Ansart E and Gerard MJ (1989) Encéphale XV: 527–534.
2. Montgomery SA, Montgomery D, Baldwin D and Green M (1989) Neuropsychobiology 22: 128–134.
3. Montgomery SA, Montgomery D, McAuley R et al. (1979) Proc. 10th Int. Congr. Suicide Prevent. Crisis Intervent. pp. 227–229.
4. Montgomery SA, Roy D, McAuley R et al. (1983) Br. J. Clin. Pharmacol. 15: 183S–188S.

Biological Psychiatry, Volume 1. G. Racagni et al., editors.

Antidepressants and the risk of suicide

Avi Molcho[1,3] and Michael Stanley[1,2,3]
[1]*Departments of Psychiatry and* [2]*Pharmacology, College of Physicians and Surgeons, Columbia University; and* [3]*The Division of Neuroscience, New York State Psychiatric Institute, 722 West 168th, New York, NY 10032, U.S.A.*

Introduction

Depression, which is a common illness, severely compromises quality of life and is associated with excessive mortality. A great proportion of deaths are due to suicide. The quality of life of depressed patients has been significantly improved since the introduction of antidepressants. However, reports of lethal antidepressant overdoses started appearing as early as 1959. In addition to their therapeutic effect, these agents may be a risk for life through their toxicity. The American Association of Poison Control Centers reported antidepressants as the most frequent cause of death from drug ingestion in the years 1983–1984. Thus, the clinician faces a dilemma in the treatment of depression, since many of the drugs in the treatment of the illness can result in as fatal an outcome as the disease itself.

Two main hypotheses have been suggested to explain the association of antidepressant agents with suicide. It is possible that the association of these agents with suicide reflects their toxicity and the increased risk for suicide in those who require antidepressant treatment. Alternatively, it has been suggested that certain antidepressants may increase the risk for suicide by inducing this behaviour.

Toxicity of antidepressants

The life-threatening effects of cyclic antidepressant poisoning are related to cardiovascular disturbances, mediated by the drugs' quinidine-like effect and central nervous system manifestations. The mechanism of MAOI toxicity is complex and in severe cases of intoxication the manifestations include hyperpyrexia, hypo- or hypertension, cardiorespiratory arrest, convulsion and coma.

Several authors have calculated a fatal toxicity index (FTI), expressed as number of the deaths per million prescriptions as way to compare the relative risk associated with different drugs [1]. Using the FTI, Cassidy and Henry [1] have found that the TCAs appearing before 1970 have been reported to have a higher ratio of deaths per million prescriptions than the mean for all antidepressants marketed in the United Kingdom between 1975–1984, while MAOIs, when grouped, are not significantly different. The drugs introduced after 1973 have a significantly lower FTI (with the exception of maprotiline). These findings have

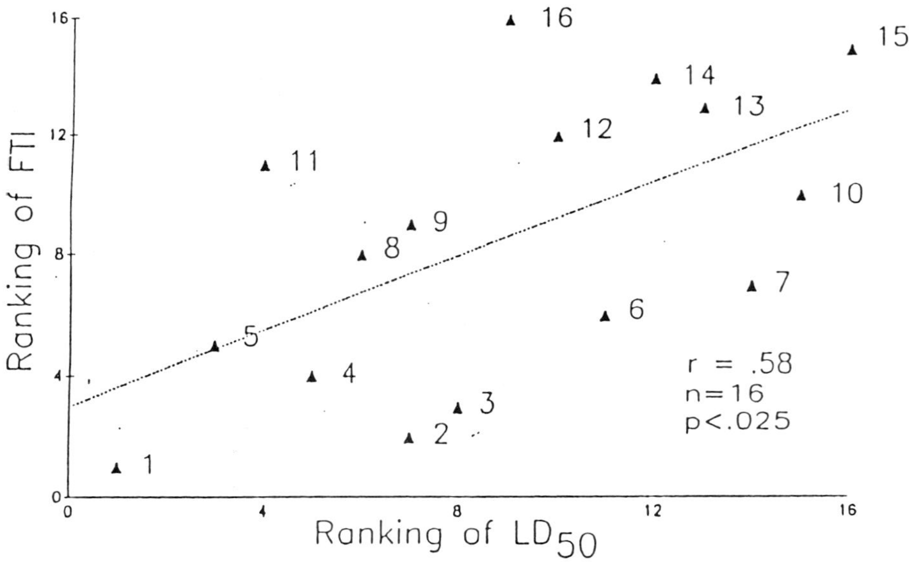

Fig. 1. The correlation between FTI[a] and LD_{50}[b] of antidepressants. [a]FTI values used for ranking taken from [1]; [b]LD_{50} values (in mouse) used for ranking taken from Usdin and Efron, 1972. 1. Lofepramine; 2. Nomifensine; 3. Mianserin; 4. Iprindol; 5. Viloxazine; 6. Protriptyline; 7. Phenelzine; 8. Trimipramine; 9. Imipramine; 10. Doxepin; 11. Maprotiline; 12. Nortriptyline; 13. Amitriptyline; 14 Dothepin; 15. Tranylcyprom; 16. Desipramine.

been relatively consistent over several studies [1,2]. A ranking order of increasing FTI values for these drugs is presented in Fig. 1. A significant positive correlation between LD_{50} ranking of antidepressants in animals and FTI ranking as a measure of toxicity in humans is presented in Fig. 1 ($r = 0.58$, $n = 16$, $P < 0.025$). Thus, it seems that FTI may reflect the inherent toxicity of antidepressants.

The relative toxicity of antidepressants in humans as presented by cases of overdose admitted to hospital seem to support the results obtained by FTI determination. The older antidepressants, maprotiline and amoxapine from the second generation, seem to be associated more frequently with severe cardiac and CNS toxicity and greater mortality. However, newer antidepressants that include mianserine, trazodone, or fluoxetine have been shown to be associated with low mortality and less severe complications even in high doses.

Is suicidal behaviour promoted by antidepressants?

A possible explanation for the incomplete correlation between suicide with antidepressant overdose and the inherent toxicity of these agents may be related to the possibility that some antidepressants induce suicidal behaviour. The emergence of suicidal ideation has been reported in several cases treated with desipramine [3] or fluoxetine [4]. In both reports, it is possible that the appearance of suicidal ideation reflects lack of change or worsening of depression with suicidal ideation being one of its expressions. Obviously, the best way to examine the possible induction of suicidal ideation by antidepressants would be to study prospectively the effect these agents on this behaviour. Studies and reviews that have looked at the effect of fluoxetine, compared with other antidepressants or placebo, on suicidal ideation, in large numbers of patients, have not shown any significant suicidogenic effect of the drug [5]. However, as reviewed by Montgomery et al. [2] and discussed in this volume, another possible explanation for the difference in the frequency with which individual antidepressants are associated with suicide is that certain antidepressants act more effectively to reduce suicidal ideation.

In conclusion, the association between antidepressants and suicide as measured by FTI seems to be related to the inherent toxicity of these agents. The report of cases of patients in which an increase in suicidal thoughts has occurred is not supported by more systematic studies. These anecdotal reports may be related to lack of therapeutic response to the medications and/or worsening of the depressive syndrome with suicidality being one of its several expressions.

References

1. Cassidy J and Henry S (1987) Br. Med. J. 295: 1021–1024.
2. Montgomery AL, Lambert MT and Lynch SP (1988) Int. Clin. Psychopharmacol. 3 (Suppl. 2): 15–24.
3. Damluji NF and Ferguson JM (1988) J. Clin. Psychopharmacol. 8: 342–349.
4. Teicher MH, Gold C and Cole JO (1990) Am. J. Psychiatry 147: 207–210.
5. Muijen M, Roy T, Silverstone T et al. (1988) Acta Psychiatr. Scand. 78: 384–390.

Biological Psychiatry, Volume 1. G. Racagni et al., editors.

Evolution in the concepts of minor depressive disorders and unspecific somatic complaints

Michael Linden
Outpatient Research Group, Department of Psychiatry at the Free University of Berlin, Eschenalee 3, D-1000 Berlin 19, Germany

Since the early days of psychiatry, a distinction has always been made between major and minor disorders. Major psychiatric disorders have been those with a clear-cut prominent symptomatology, which could easily be diagnosed cross-sectionally, where there is usually no doubt that these are abnormal states and which are typically seen as the result of some biological disorder. Minor disorders, in contrast, are much harder to differentiate from normal fluctuations in well-being; they are not so impressive cross-sectionally, which means that they cannot be as easily diagnosed objectively, but their diagnosis is much more dependent on subjective complaints and especially on time-course and duration of complaints. Their aetiology is often seen in psychological factors. This distinction between minor and major disorders has especially been made in the field of depression-like disorders.

For example, in the first monograph on depression, the "Anatomy of Melancholy" published in 1654 by Robert Burton [1] in Oxford, one can find two major sections, one on head, hypochondriac, or windy melancholy and the other on love melancholy. The first is seen as being caused, if not by the devil himself, then by corrupted blood in the brain, overmuch use of hot wines, or default of spleen, belly, bowels or liver and their symptoms being sorrow, restless thoughts, anxiety, or rumbling in the guts, cold sweat, or palpitation and heaviness of the heart. Treatment requires e.g. special diet, herbs, phlebotomy or purging. Love melancholy, in contrast, is caused by provocations of lust and love, opportunity of time and place and natural allurements. Symptoms are paleness, sorrow, anxiety, or neglect of business and the treatment is good counsel or labour.

Minor disorders became really famous in the second half of the 19th century, important publications being the papers and books by the New York physician George M.B. Beard, the first of which was published in 1869 in the Boston Medical and Surgical Journal on "Neurasthenia or nervous exhaustion" [2], or his monograph on "American nervousness, its philosophy and treatment" [3] in 1880. In his handbook of neurasthenia dating from 1893, Franz C. Muller cites more than 800 publications of the time, which are related to the topic of neurasthenic syndromes. The neurologist Beard had basically an organic concept of what neurasthenia means. Living conditions in the societies undergoing the industrial revolution with its high level of environmental pollution were seen as a cause of nervous disorders. The so-called "American nervousness" was therefore seen as a product of the progressive American society, which led to a rapid reaction in Europe, where it was claimed that neurasthenia was also a problem. The first translation of Beard's work on American nervousness into German, for example, had already appeared by 1881.

This primarily biological notion of neurasthenia underwent a major change with the beginning of the 20th century, when Sigmund Freud [4] described neurasthenia as one of the four major classes of neurosis, additional to hysteria, obsessive-compulsive neurosis and anxiety neurosis. The distinction between major disorders, such as organic psychosis, schizophrenia, or endogenous depression on the one hand and minor disorders, such as personality disorders and neuroses on the other hand, delineated in the following decades almost two unrelated areas in psychiatry. The first constituted the topic for psychiatrists with a predominant interest in classification, biological treatment methods and inpatient services and the other was primarily the domain of psychotherapists, who were less interested in classification but in aetiological-functional analyses and preferably with outpatients. Insofar as neurasthenia was concerned, it was now generally accepted that this was a psychodynamic disorder, and the term "pseudo-neurasthenia" was used for neurasthenia-like syndromes with an organic cause [5].

During the last decades, there have been many attempts to come to more operational classifications for minor disorders with predominantly unspecific somatic complaints. In the field of somatic medicine, concepts were introduced such as psychosomatic disorder, vegetative dystonia, or chronic fatigue syndrome [6–9]. The common basis of these concepts is that the feeling of chronic fatigue, exhaustion, dysphoria and multiple unspecific somatic distress is the result of central nervous and vegetative functional regulatory instability, which – according to some authors – has its correlates in an insufficiency of the dynamic regulation of vigilance, which can be seen in the EEC [10]. In spite of this common final pathway, the causes are almost innumerable, ranging from habitual factors to learned, neurotic, or psychological stress reactions and an abundance of organic diseases, including chronic intoxication. There are, for example, many publications on the question of whether the so-called chronic fatigue syndrome may be caused by Epstein-Barr virus infections [8]. In summary, the present state of knowledge on these syndromes of unspecific somatic complaints in the perspective of internal medicine is that they have a high prevalence rate, especially in general medical health care settings [11] that their aetiological specificity is rather low, and that nevertheless, they lead to an impressive demand for medical treatment, albeit only on a symptomatic level [12].

Whereas in general medicine, the trend has been to look for more and more specific causes, which may all lead to a neurasthenic syndrome, in psychiatry a confluence of different categories can be observed. Almost in accordance with E. Kraepelin [13] and K. Schneider [14], in psychiatry these minor unspecific somatic functional disorders have not to such an extent been seen as a somatic problem. Instead, their affective components such as feelings of insufficiency and bad mood have been seen as the predominant features, so that these syndromes have been interpreted as less intense forms of mood disorders or depression. In the newer classification systems, such as RDC and DSM III and DSM III-R, dysthymia has been introduced and neurasthenia – as in DSM III – only listed in the index with reference to dysthymic disorder, and in DSM III-R omitted altogether. The empirical basis for this is that some longitudinal studies have shown that patients with this type of disorder will later show clear depressive episodes in their lives [15,16]. Parallel to this extension of the depression concept, hypochondriasis or somatization disorder, anxiety disorders and hysterical or dissociative disorders have become more narrow in their definitions, for example by introducing the concept of panic disorders as a distinct feature.

What is the conclusion regarding these different developments and what are the perspectives? Neurasthenia is dead, long live neurasthenia! In spite of all the inadequacies in diagnosis of these types of disorder, their prevalence, especially in primary health care settings [17], is reason enough to be sure that concepts like neurasthenia will also be needed in the future. These syndromes will undoubtedly remain a special challenge for a large range of differential diagnoses, but nevertheless there will always be considerable numbers of patients with unknown or known causes of neurasthenia, which will need a specific symptomatic treatment. To return to a neurophysiological functional model of minor unspecific somatic complaints in the sense of neurasthenia – as outlined by Bente [10] – treatments will have to focus on improving and stabilizing regulatory processes of the nervous system. Already there are interesting pharmacological models on how this can be achieved, so it could well be that in the future we will find specific treatments, even for an unspecific syndrome like neurasthenia.

References

1. Burton R (1652) Anatomy of Melancholy. Hen. Grips and Lodo Lloyd, London.
2. Beard GMB (1869) Boston Med. Surg. J. 79: 217–221.
3. Beard GMB (1880) American Nervousness, its Philosophy and Treatment. Virginia M. Mouth, Richmond.
4. Freud S (1895) Uber die Berechtigung, von der Neurasthenie einen bestimmten Symptom-Komplex als "Angst-Neurose" abzutrennen. cit. Freud S (1952) Imago, London.
5. Huber G (1987) Psychiatrie. Schauttauer, Stuttgart.
6. Wiechmann B (1934) Dtsch. Med. Wochenschr. 60: 1500.
7. Lippowski ZJ (1984) Psychosom. Med. 46: 153–171.
8. Nix WA (1990) Nervenarzt 61: 390–396.
9. Linden M (1991) In: Gastpar M (ed.) Psychological Disorders in General Practice. (in press).
10. Bente D (1968) Die Insuffizienz des Vigilanztonus. Med. Habil-Schrift, Erlangen, Nürnberg.
11. Geiselmann B and Linden M (1984) In: Heimann H and Foerster K (eds.) Psychogene Reaktionen und Entwicklungen. Fischer, Stuttgart.
12. Geiselmann B, Linden M, Sachs-Ericsson N (1989) Eur. Arch. Psychiatr. Neurol. Sci. 239: 180–187.
13. Kraepelin E (1906) Psychiatrie. Barth, Leipzig 5. Aufl.
14. Schnieder K (1962) Klinische Psychopathologie. Thieme, Stuttgart 6. Aufl.
15. Akiskal HS (1981) Psychiatr. Clin. North Am. 4: 25–46.

16. Bronisch T (1990) Nervenarzt 61: 133–139.
17. Burvill PW (1990) In: Sartorius N, Goldberg D, De Girolamo G, Costa E, Silva JA, Lecrubier Y and Wittchen HU (eds.) Psychological Disorders in General Medical Settings. Hogrefe, Toronto.
18. Binder H (1960) In: Gruhle HW, Jung R, Mayer-Gross W and Müller M (eds.) Psychiatrie der Gegenwart. Springer, Berlin.

Biological Psychiatry, Volume 1. G. Racagni et al., editors.

A prospective study of diagnostic change in dysthymic disorder

Nicholas Seivewright[1] and Peter Tyrer[2]
[1]University of Manchester Department of Psychiatry, Rawnsley Building, Manchester Royal Infirmary, Oxford Road, Manchester, M13 9WL; and [2]St Charles Hospital, Exmoor Street, London, W10 6DZ, U.K.

Two-hundred and ten psychiatric outpatients diagnosed as generalized anxiety disorder (GAD) (71), panic disorder (PD) (74), or dysthymic disorder (DYS) (65) using a structured interview schedule for DSM III also had their personality status assessed and ratings made on a scale for a mixed anxiety-depressive disorder, the general neurotic syndrome. During a comparison of the effects of drug and psychological treatment diagnostic assessments using the same structured interview schedule were made at weeks 10, 16, 32, 52 and 104 weeks after initial assessment. There were no significant interactions between original diagnosis and treatment and diagnostic status changed fundamentally in over 80% of the patients during the course of the 2 years.

Diagnostic assessments and ratings

All assessments were carried out by psychiatrists. After initial diagnosis and treatment allocation each patient was seen by the same assessor throughout the two years wherever possible so that inter-rater variability was reduced. The assessors were masked with respect to treatment; each patient was instructed by the clinical team involved in treatment that this should not be mentioned to their "research doctor" and any problems discussed only with their therapists. If disclosure of treatment was made a different assessor was allocated. Assessments were usually conducted at patients' homes to avoid inconvenience and improve compliance. All assessors received prior training in the use of each of the schedules until agreement reached acceptable levels [1]. Diagnostic assessments of mental state were made using the 1983 version of the Structured Clinical Interview for DSM III [2] and of personality status using the Personality Assessment Schedule [3].

Diagnostic changes over time

In analysing changes in diagnosis it was appreciated that patients who improved during treatment and subsequently received no psychiatric diagnosis could not be regarded as having changed from one diagnosis to another. However, those who improved from one DSM III diagnosis which also included another diagnosis which was lower in the diagnostic hierarchy (e.g. DYS and GAD) so that the main

Table 1. Changes in DSM III diagnoses in 181 patients seen on 6 occasions over 2 years

Initial diagnosis	n	No change of improvement to no diagnosis	Changes to other diagnoses							
			GAD	DYS	AG	PAG	PD	MDE	MEL	OC
GAD	59	11 (19%)	n/a	34	12	4	10	18	1	4
DYS	56	8 (14%)	15	n/a	8	5	5	32	3	3
PD	66	3 (5%)	16	23	24	18	n/a	30	3	3

χ^2 (MDE differences only) = 8.3, df 2, $P < 0.02$; AG = agoraphobia; MEL = melancholia; OC = obsessive-compulsive disorder.

diagnosis was replaced by the subsidiary one at follow-up, were regarded as having changed their diagnostic status. All changes in status were recorded, so that if for example, a patient with an original diagnosis of DYS who had a diagnosis of PD at weeks 10, 32 and 104, but GAD at weeks 16 and 52, would be recorded as having 5 diagnostic changes over the 2 years.

The results showed that diagnosis changed frequently with an average of 1.5 changes per patient during the 2 years. No fixed pattern of change was shown. In particular, the prediction that PD would progress to agoraphobia with panic (PAG) as postulated by Klein [4] was only partly sustained, with nearly twice as many patients with PD having an episode of major depression (MDE) than developed PAG (Table 1). This is in keeping with other prospective studies which find panic to be an unstable diagnosis with most frequent change to depressive illness [5,6]. DYS changed less than PD and GAD but this is at least partly explained by the differences in diagnostic criteria for the disorders, DYS requiring the presence of depressive symptoms for most of the previous two years whereas GAD and PD require a minimum duration of symptoms of four weeks or less before the diagnoses are satisfied.

The results give some support to the concept of dysthymia as a norm of depression associated with personality disturbance, but the substantial degree of overlap between other diagnoses over time undermines its clinical validity [7] and gives credence to unitary concepts of neurotic disorder such as the general neurotic syndrome [8].

References

1. Landis JR and Koch GG (1977) Biometrics 33: 159–174.
2. Spitzer R and Williams JB (1983) Structured Clinical Interview for DSM III (1983 Version). New York Psychiatric Institute, New York.
3. Tyrer P and Alexander J (1979) Br. J. Psychiatry 135: 163–167.
4. Klein DF (1981) In: Klein DF and Rabkin JG (eds.). Anxiety: New Research and Changing Concepts. Raven Press, New York, pp. 235–263.
5. Thompson AH, Bland RC and Orn HT (1989) J. Nerv. Ment. Dis. 177: 456–463.

6. Angst J and Wicki W (1991) The epidemiology of frequent and less frequent panic attacks. Br. J. Psychiatry (Suppl.) (in press).
7. Kendell RE (1989) Psychol. Med. 19: 45–55.
8. Tyrer P (1985) Lancet i: 685–688.

Biological Psychiatry, Volume 1. G. Racagni et al., editors.

The pharmacological treatment of dysthymia

G.B. Cassano[1], M. Savino[2], G. Perugi[2] and P. Medda[2]
[1]*Institute of Clinical Psychiatry, II Chair of Clinical Psychiatry, University of Pisa; and* [2]*Institute of Clinical Psychiatry, University of Pisa, Italy*

Chronic depression represents a major problem for the clinician, both with regards to diagnostic and therapeutic aspects. Since Kraepelin's [1] observations on the chronic course of some depressive syndromes, an increasing number of studies [2,3] has progressively provided new data, allowing a better definition and a more effective treatment of these conditions [4].

Major chronic depression can be easily recognized because of its typical and severe symptomatology, while some kinds of *minor chronic depressions* are often misdiagnosed. In fact, chronic course, mild depressive symptoms, relative resistance and scarce compliance to medication [5,6], frequent comorbidity phenomena with anxiety states [7] and reactive mood and maladjustment have favoured, in the past, the adoption of diagnoses such as "neurotic depression" and "depressive personality". Recent advances in psychopharmacology have led to a better delimitation of minor chronic depressions from both anxiety states and personality disorders (Table 1). The major dilemma remains whatever minor chronic conditions may be separated from major depressive episodes and not considered as attenuated conditions belonging to the same category.

The term "neurotic depression" [8] was substituted by DSM III [9] dysthymic disorder, this also including the "depressive personality" of previous classifications. This important step in considering these conditions not linked to stable and unmodifiable characterological features, was confirmed and ameliorated by the definition of dysthymia in the revised version of the manual. In fact, DSM III-R [10] provides a sharper delimitation of this condition from sequels of major depressive episode, that has to be ruled out during the first 2 years of the disorder. DSM III-R [10] also considers the diagnosis of chronic major depressive episode – over 2 years of full-blown major depression – thus implying a clear-cut distinction between full-blown prolonged episodes, minor chronic and phasic conditions with prolonged periods of well-being.

Table 1. Personality disorders vs. dysthymia

- Early onset
- Enduring
- Pervasive
- Interpersonal
- Egosyntonic

Table 2. Core clinical manifestations of dysthymia (Akiskal, 1990)

Mood	Vegetative	Cognitive	Psychomotor
Anhedonia	Insomnia	Low self-esteem	Poor concentration
Depression	Hypersomnia	Guilty ruminations	Fatigue
		Hopelessness	Reduced interests
		Suicidal ideation	Social withdrawal

Despite its low-grade symptomatologic expression, dysthymia can produce severe maladjustment in familial, interpersonal and work areas [11]. The patient's insight is often affected and the insidious early onset and the long-lasting course are associated with a worse prognosis than that of chronic major depression, the latter showing higher treatment-induced recovery rates [12]. Moreover, dysthymia is often accompanied by a high risk of substance abuse and dependence, as well as suicidal behaviour [13].

A disabling condition such as dysthymia (Table 2) often requires long-term, high-dose pharmacological treatment. The therapeutic choice will follow an accurate evaluation of symptomatologic features, course and patient's family history.

The effective doses of trycyclic antidepressants (TCAs) – such as imipramine, clomipramine and amitryptiline – are rarely inferior to 150–200 mg daily. Desimipramine and nortryptiline are indicated if side-effects are relevant and affect compliance. On the basis of course of family history and symptomatology, as well as when the response to TCAs is incomplete, lithium salts [14] may be added.

TCA-resistant depressions and comorbidity conditions with panic disorder or with other anxiety disorders may benefit from monoamino-oxidase inhibitors (MAOIs) [15].

In our experience, serotonin re-uptake inhibitors (SRI) are also effective and well-tolerated in long-term treatment: fluoxetine at 20–60 mg daily and fluvox-

Table 3. Ritanserin studies in dysthymia

Study	Patients	mg	Evaluations		
			CGI	HAMA	HAMD
Arriaga et al., 1986	43	10	N.S. (0.05)		N.S. (0.05)
Bersani et al., 1988	29	10	0.01	0.01	0.001
Hoppenbrouwers et al., 1986	53	20	N.S. (0.05)		N.S.
Meco et al., 1989[a]	36	10–20	N.S.	N.S.	N.S.
Murphy and Checkley, 1988	17	10	N.S.	N.S.	N.S (0.05)
Paiva et al., 1987	23	10	N.S.	N.S.	N.S
Reyntjens et al., 1986	93	20	N.S. (0.05)		N.S.

[a] Compared with amitriptyline 25–50 mg daily.

amine at 150–300 mg daily are frequently effective in treating dysthymia without significant side-effects.

Sleep-deprivation [16] may be associated to other treatments.

Nowadays, an increasing number of new compounds – such as bupropion, moclobemide and bufloramine – is widening the range of therapeutic opportunities and a new serotonergic agent, the highly specific 5-HT_2-blocker ritanserin, has recently been proposed for drug therapy of dysthymia [17,18]. Ritanserin has a high in vitro affinity to 5-HT_2 receptors [19] which are exclusively post-synaptic and do not modify 5-HT release. In spite of what usually happens, chronic stimulation of 5-HT_2 receptors with antagonists does not determine receptor supersensitivity but, indeed, it brings about a prolonged subsensitivity [20]. This direct down-regulating action of 5-HT_2 receptor blocking drugs has been hypothesized as the reason for the shorter latency period of their therapeutic effect when compared with other antidepressants [17].

The antidepressant action of 5-HT_2 receptors blocking drugs is based on the hypothesis of a 5-HT_2 receptor up-regulation as a primary condition in the origin of depression [21].

Ritanserin increases slow wave sleep [22], has a negligible sedative potential on CNS [23], has no effects on blood pressure [24] and has shown a better efficacy than placebo in several psychiatric disorders [25,26] showing both anti-anxiety and antidepressive properties. Double-blind placebo-controlled studies involving patients with dysthymia suggested the effectiveness and the safety (Table 3) of ritanserin, in doses ranging from 10–20 mg daily [26].

In this paper we have briefly summarized and discussed preliminary data derived from a multicenter double-blind, placebo-controlled study focused on the treatment of dysthymia (RID – ritanserin in dysthymia) (Cassano GB, Casacchia M, Faravelli C, Sacchetti E and Smeraldi E) with ritanserin. Patients with primary dysthymia (DSM III-R) were recruited from different Italian university clinics; the sample consisted of 45 patients: 15 patients were male (33.3%) and 30 were female (66.7%), while the mean age was 41.9, ranging from 16–62 years. Clinical evaluations were conducted at baseline, 1st, 2nd, 4th, 6th and 8th week utilizing

Table 4. Symptomatological features (HAM-D)

	Ritanserin 5 mg (n = 12)		Ritanserin 10 mg (n = 7)		Placebo (n = 8)	
	Baseline	Week 8	Baseline	Week 8	Baseline	Week 8
Anxiety/somatization	0.8	0.5	0.8	0.5	0.8	0.7
Weight	1.0	0.7	0.7	0.4	0.8	0.6
Cognitive disorders	0.3	0.3	0.4	0.2	0.4	0.2
Diurnal variation	0.4	0.6	0.4	0.2	0.5	0.3
Motor retardation	1.4	0.9	1.1	0.8	1.1	0.7
Sleep disorders	0.7	0.4	0.9	0.2	0.8	0.5

(Cassano GB, Casacchia M, Faravelli C, Sacchetti E and Smeraldi E.)

Table 5. Symptomatological features (HSCL 90)

	Ritanserin 5 mg (n = 12)		Ritanserin 10 mg (n = 7)		Placebo (n = 8)	
	Baseline	Week 8	Baseline	Week 8	Baseline	Week 8
Somatization	1.0	0.5	0.9	0.5	0.9	0.5
Obsession-compulsion	1.4	0.7	1.6	1.0	1.4	0.7
Sensitivity	0.7	0.4	1.4	0.8	1.5	0.7
Depression	1.4	0.8	1.9	1.1	1.7	0.7
Anxiety	0.9	0.6	1.2	0.6	1.0	0.5
Hostility-anger	0.5	0.2	1.0	0.5	1.0	0.4
Phobic anxiety	0.6	0.2	0.7	0.1	0.6	0.1
Paranoidism	0.7	0.4	1.0	0.6	1.1	0.4
Psychoticism	0.7	0.3	0.7	0.4	0.7	0.3

(Cassano GB, Casacchia M, Faravelli C, Sacchetti E and Smeraldi E.)

HAM-D [27], SRS [28], HSCL-90 [29] and other validated rating scales. At baseline patients were assessed by SID [30] and social adjustment was explored by SAS [31] at baseline and at the end of the study.

The sample was treated with ritanserin 5 mg/day (17 patients) and 10 mg/day (14 patients); placebo was given to 14 patients. Two patients refused the treatment after baseline evaluation, 6 were treated only for 1 week, 6 for 2 weeks, 2 reached the 4th week, 2 reached the 6th week and 27 completed the 8 weeks of treatment.

As a consequence of the limited number of patients available for evaluation for each treatment group, it is not possible to draw any firm conclusion from our preliminary results. As far as symptomatological features (Tables 4 and 5), social adjustment (Table 6) and global improvement are concerned, the differences between the two groups treated with ritanserin and the group treated with placebo failed to reach statistical significance. However, the group treated with 5 mg of ritanserin tended to present a lower number of "dropouts" (Fig. 1) and a certain efficacy at a symptomatological level. Concerning social adjustment, the 2-month period appears too short to show any significant improvement.

Table 6. Social adjustment scale

	Ritanserin 5 mg (n = 12)		Ritanserin 10 mg (n = 7)		Placebo (n = 8)	
	Baseline	Week 8	Baseline	Week 8	Baseline	Week 8
Work	4.66	4.50	4.42	4.14	4.37	3.87
Household	3.91	3.97	4.14	4.57	4.12	4.75
External family	5.33	4.33	4.42	4.57	5.12	4.87
Social/leisure	4.83	4.25	4.57	4.57	4.37	4.12
Global adjustment	4.33	3.91	3.38	4.00	4.12	3.85

(Cassano GB, Casacchia M, Faravelli C, Sacchetti E and Smeraldi E.)

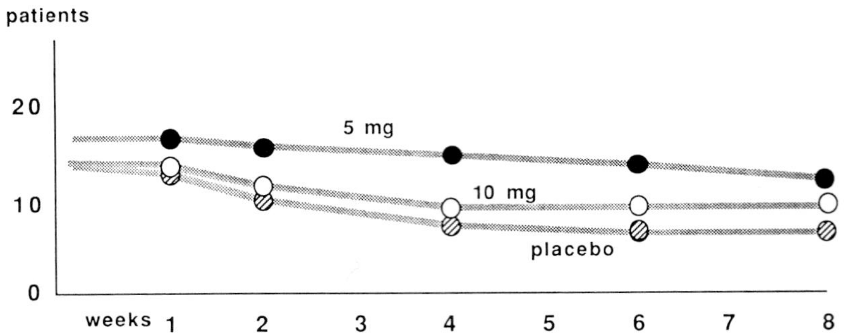

Fig. 1. Attrition in RID (Cassano GB, Casacchia M, Faravelli C, Sacchetti E and Smeraldi E).

Treatment with ritanserin, at dose levels utilized in our sample, was very well tolerated and side-effects appeared clinically negligible. Further studies are required to determine the reported effectiveness of ritanserin in dysthymia.

References

1. Kraepelin E (1913) Lectures on Clinical Psychiatry. Bailliere Tindall and Cox, London.
2. Akiskal KS (1983) Am. J. Psychiatry 140: 11–20.
3. Robins E and Guze S (1969) In: Williams TA, Kats MM and Shield JA (eds.) Recent Advances in the Psychobiology of Depressive Illness. Proceedings of Workshop Sponsored by the Clinical Research Branch Division of Extramural Research Programs NIMH, April 30–May 2, 1969.
4. Akiskal HS (1985) J. Clin. Psychiatry 46: 32–36.
5. Akiskal HS (1982) J. Clin. Psychiatry 43: 266–271.
6. Kerr TA, Roth M, Schapira K and Gurney C (1972) Br. J. Psychiatry 121: 167–174.
7. Weissman MM, Leaf PJ, Bruce ML and Florio L (1988) Am. J. Psychiatry 145: 815–819.
8. American Psychiatric Association (1968) Diagnostic and Statistical Manual of Mental Disorders, 2nd Edn. Am. Psychiatr. Assoc., Washington D.C.
9. American Psychiatric Association (1983) Diagnostic and Statistical Manual of Mental Disorders (DSM III). Am. Psychiatr. Assoc., Washington D.C.
10. American Psychiatric Association (1987) Diagnostic and Statistical Manual of Mental Disorders (DSM III-R), 3rd Edn. Revised. Am. Psychiatr. Assoc., Washington D.C.
11. Cassano GB, Perugi G, Maremmani I and Akiskal HS (1990) Social adjustment in dysthymia. In: Burton and Akiskal (eds.) Dysthymic Disorder. Gaskell, London.
12. Gonzales LR, Lewinsohn PM and Clarke GN (1985) J. Consult. Clin. Psychol. 53: 461–469.
13. Freidman R, Clarkin J, Lorn R, Aronoff M, Hurt S and Murphy M (1982) J. Nerv. Ment. Dis. 170(9): 511–521.
14. Akiskal HS, Rosenthal TL, Haykal RF et al. (1980) Arch. Gen. Psychiatry 37: 777–783.
15. Akiskal HS (1985) J. Clin. Psychiatry 46: 31–36.
16. Rihmer Z (1990) dysthymia: A clinician's perspective. In: Burton and Akiskal (eds.) Dysthymic Disorder. Gaskell, London.
17. Bersani G, Marini S and Grispini A (1988) Psychopharmacology (Suppl.) 96: 244.
18. Murphy D and Checkley SA (1988) Psychopharmacology (Suppl.): 109.
19. Leysen JE, Awouters F and Kennis L (1981) Life Sci. 28: 1115–1122.
20. Leysen JE, Van Gompel P and Gommeren W (1986) Psychopharmacology 88: 434–444.

21. Deakin JFW (1989) In: Archer T et al. (eds.) Behavioural Pharmacology of 5-HT. Lawrence Erlbaum, New York, pp. 179–204.
22. Dugovic C and Wauquier A (1987) Eur. J. Pharmacol. 137: 145–146.
23. Roth G, Gillner A and Siwers B (1986) In: XVth CINP Book of Abstracts, p. 180.
24. Hedner T, Petterson A and Persson B (1987) Acta Med. Scand. 222: 307–310.
25. Reyntjens AJM, Gelders YG, Hoppenbrouwers M and Vanden Bussche G (1986) Drug Dev. Res. 8: 205–211.
26. XVth CINP (1986) Congress, Book of Abstracts.
27. Hamilton M (1960) J. Neurol. Neurosurg. Psychiatry 23: 56–62.
28. Widlocher D (1983) Psychiatr. Clin. North Amer. 6: 27–40.
29. Derogatis LR, Lipman RS and Rickel SK (1973) The Hopkins Symptoms Checklist (HSCL): A measure of primary symptom dimensions in psychological measurement. In: P Pichot (ed.) Modern Problems in Pharmacopsychiatry. Karger, Basel.
30. Cassano GB, Akiskal HS, Musetti L, Perugi G, Soriani A and Mignani V (1989) Psychopathology 22: 278–288.
31. Schooler NR, Hogarty GE and Weissman MM (1979) In: Argreaves et al. (eds.) Resource Material for Community Mental Health Program Evaluators. U.S. Dept. of Health, Education and Welfare, Washington D.C., pp. 290–330.

Biological Psychiatry, Volume 1. G. Racagni et al., editors.

Biochemical correlates of postnatal depression

Vivette Glover, Pat Hannah, Diana Adams, Julia Littlewood and M. Sandler
Department of Chemical Pathology, Queen Charlotte's and Chelsea Hospital Goldhawk Road, London W6 OXG, U.K.

Postnatal mental disturbance is currently classified in three ways: the blues (which occurs in about 50% of women), postnatal depression (10%) and postnatal psychosis (0.2%), which is frequently of the manic depressive type. The risk of psychosis is increased 100-fold in women with a history of bipolar affective disorder [1]. The relationship between these different clinical states is not yet clear, nor is it known the extent to which the depressive episode is biologically triggered. At least half the cases of postnatal depression appear to start in the first 2 weeks after parturition and there is evidence of a significant correlation between depression in the first postpartum week and the persistence of later depression [2]. Illness in this early onset subgroup might plausibly be triggered by the large hormonal changes associated with parturition and probably should be investigated separately from later onset depression.

There are very substantial changes in the circulating concentrations of several hormones at parturition, including β-endorphin, oestrogens and progesterone. Cortisol economy is also disturbed and the dexamethasone suppression test is abnormal in the majority of women at this time [3,4]. High values of plasma cortisol may be associated with the blues [5]. No convincing association, however, has yet been found with circulating levels of either progesterone or oestrogen and postnatal blues or depression [e.g. 6].

In a recent study, we have determined whether the tyramine test [7] is useful for the detection of vulnerability to postnatal depression. This test appears to be a trait marker for endogenous unipolar depression, but not for "neurotic" or bipolar depression, even if endogenous features are present [8]. The test, in fact, was quite negative in the 37 patients in whom it was employed (both early and late onset), including a subgroup with endogenous features. This finding suggests that vulnerability to unipolar endogenous depression does not predispose to postnatal depression; this disorder seems more likely to occur in those vulnerable to the neurotic or bipolar subtypes of depressive illness.

We have also observed another clinical phenomenon, which has not previously been focussed on. About 15% of the 200 postpartum women we have studied showed what we have termed the postnatal "highs" in the first postpartum week, euphoria associated with other features of hypomania. These patients were twice as likely to show later depression (Edinburgh Postnatal Depression Score 10+ at 6 weeks postpartum) than women with no psychopathology at that time ($P < 0.01$).

In some women, these symptoms appeared to coexist with those of depression, and this group was also particularly vulnerable to a persisting depression.

There is some evidence that circulating cyclic AMP is raised in the subgroup of women with elevated mood in the first postpartum week [9]. A possible explanation for the "postnatal highs" is that the profound hormonal changes of parturition disturb membrane and second messenger function. Several models for bipolar disorder are currently focussing on this system [e.g. 10,11]. In many women, this disturbance might lead to the emotionally labile state termed the blues; in a substantial subgroup, it may cause mild euphoria, often followed by depression. In a small predisposed minority, it may trigger postnatal psychosis.

References

1. Kendell RE (1985) J. Psychosom. Res. 29: 3–11.
2. Hannah P, Adams D, Lee A, Glover V and Sandler M (1991) Br. J. Psychiatry (in press).
3. Greenwood J and Parker G (1984) Aust. N.Z. J. Psychiatry 18: 282–284.
4. Singh B, Gilhotra M, Smith R, Brinsmead M, Lewin T and Hall C (1986) J. Affective Disord. 11: 173–177.
5. George A and Sandler M (1988) In: Kumar R and Brockington IF (eds.) Motherhood and Mental Illness 2. Wright, London, pp. 78–112.
6. Nott PN, Franklin M, Armitage C and Gelder MG (1976) Br. J. Psychiatry 128: 379–383.
7. Hale AS, Walker PL, Bridges PK and Sandler M (1986) J. Psychiatr. Res. 20: 251–261.
8. Hale AS, Sandler M, Hannah P, Glover V and Bridges PK (1991) J. Psychiatr. Res. (in press).
9. Ballenger CB, Kay DSG, Naylor GJ and Smith AHW (1982) Psychol. Med. 12: 549–556.
10. Lachman HM and Papolos DF (1989) Life Sci. 45: 1413–1426.
11. Wachtel H (1989) J. Neural Transm. 75: 21–229.

Biological Psychiatry, Volume 1. G. Racagni et al., editors.

Oestradiol in the treatment of postnatal depression

Alain Gregoire[1], Ramesh Kumar[1], Anne Henderson[2] and John Studd[2]
[1]Institute of Psychiatry, DeCrespigny Park, London, SE5; and [2]Dulwich Hospital, East Dulwich Grove, London, SE22, U.K.

During the reproductive years depression is twice as common in women as compared to men. Much research has focussed on the possible hormonal contribution to depression, premenstrually, postnatally and in the climacteric. Results from this research demonstrate a significant therapeutic effect of oestrogens on mood and associated depressive symptoms in the premenstrual syndrome [1] and in the climacteric [2]. A hormonal aetiology for postnatal depression has long been suggested. However, despite much research, no clear association between sex hormone levels or activity and mood postnatally has been found [3,4]. A number of explanations have been given for this failure to demonstrate any clear association. These include:

a) methodological problems in the measurement of plasma hormone levels;
b) the unknown relationship between peripheral and central hormone levels;
c) the difficulties in assessing CNS hormone receptor activity, and the lack of knowledge about the significance of any change which might occur in these receptors.

It is of course possible that there is no relationship between oestrogens and mood changes, but a number of observations in the literature do support such a relationship:

1. Women with premenstrual syndrome have a more frequent history of puerperal depression and have a greater history of depression in the subsequent perimenopausal years [5]. Oestrogens appear to be effective in the treatment of premenstrual depressive symptoms and climacteric depressive symptoms [1,2].
2. Repeated premenstrual relapse of puerperal depressive psychosis has been reported [6].
3. The only double-blind randomised study of oestrogen treatment for antidepressant resistant depression in women found a significant improvement in those women receiving oestrogens compared to placebo [7].
4. Oestrogens have effects on a number of CNS neurotransmitter systems including the noradrenergic and serotonergic systems which are associated with affective disorders [8]. It has been suggested that oestradiol withdrawal postpartum may reverse the antidepressant effect of oestrogen on these systems [9]. One of the main criticisms of this hypothesis concerns the variable and sometimes lengthy symptom-free period which may occur between delivery and the onset of depression. The peak prevalence for postnatal depression of 6 weeks is not consistent with a direct effect of oestrogen withdrawal. However,

it is clear from our knowledge about delayed therapeutic effects of antidepressants that central biochemical changes can have delayed effects on clinical state. Furthermore, experimental work on the effects of oestrogen on the rat CNS has demonstrated changes which may be delayed by eight weeks or more [10]. Thus although our understanding of precise mechanisms of oestrogenic effects is still limited, a valid hypothesis can be made of delayed effects of oestrogen withdrawal on depressive symptoms.

5. Studies examining psychosocial correlates of postnatal depression, of which there have now been many, have produced inconsistent results [11]; even in factors which do emerge with some consistency, such as psychosocial stressful events, the power of the association may not be great, leading some authors to suggest that important organic factors are involved in the genesis of this disorder [12].

We are currently carrying out a double-blind, prospective, randomised, placebo-controlled study of transdermal oestrogen administration over a six-month period for the treatment of postnatal depression. It is hoped that through careful methodology and attention to a number of factors which may affect treatment outcome, we will be able to assess the effectiveness of oestradiol therapy and eventually identify those women who are most likely to respond.

Acknowledgement

We are grateful to Ciba-Geigy for financial support.

References

1. Watson NR, Studd JWW, Savvas M, Garnett T and Baber RJ (1989) Lancet ii: 730–734.
2. Montgomery JC, Brincat M, Tapp A, Appleby L, Versi E, Fenwick PBC and Studd JWW (1987) Lancet i: 297–299.
3. Nott PN, Franklin M, Armitage C and Gelder NG (1976) Br. J. Psychiatry 128: 379–383.
4. Kuevi V, Carson R, Dixson AF et al. (1983) Clin. Endocrinol. 19: 39–46.
5. Studd JWW and Watson NR (1988) Estrogens and depression in women. The Proceedings of the XIIth World Congress of Gynecology and Obstetrics, Rio de Janeiro.
6. Brockington IF, Kelly A, Hall P and Deakin W (1988) J. Affective Disord. 14: 287–292.
7. Klaiber EL, Brauverman DM, Vogel W and Kubariashi Y (1979) Arch. Gen. Psychiatry 36: 550–554.
8. Oppenheim G (1983) Neuropharmacol. Mechanisms Biol. Psychiatry 18; 6: 721–725.
9. Deakin JFW (1988) In: Kumar R and Brockington IF (eds.) Motherhood and Mental Illness 2. Wright, London.
10. Naftolin F, MacLusky NJ, Leranth CZ, Sakamoto HS and Garcia-Segura LM (1988) J. Steroid Biochem. 30: 1–6, 195–207.
11. Kendell RE (1985) J. Psychsom. Res. 29; 1: 3–11.
12. Martin CJ, Brown GW, Goldberg DP and Brockington IS (1989) J. Affective Disord. 16: 283–293.

Biological Psychiatry, Volume 1. G. Racagni et al., editors.

Prophylactic lithium in puerperal psychosis: Three centres' experience*

D.E. Stewart, J.L. Klompenhouwer, R.E. Kendell and A.M. van Hulst
St. Michael's Hospital, 30 Bond Street, Toronto, Ontario M5B 1W8, Canada

Introduction

Women with a history of bipolar affective disorder or previous puerperal psychosis have a greatly increased risk of psychosis following pregnancy. A number of investigators have suggested lithium carbonate prophylaxis following delivery in these high-risk women [2,3] but there has been no consensus. This paper will report the experience of four clinicians at three centres (Universities of Toronto, Rotterdam, and Edinburgh) who agreed to collect and pool data on this problem to systematically obtain a larger sample.

Materials and Methods

Consecutive high-risk women given prophylactic lithium carbonate by one of the investigators to prevent postpartum psychosis were identified in Toronto, Rotterdam and Edinburgh. To qualify, the women must have had one previous postpartum psychosis requiring admission and have agreed to take lithium after delivery or commencing late in pregnancy, to have regular serum lithium determinations performed for six months after delivery, and agree not to breastfeed or become pregnant while on lithium. In Toronto and Rotterdam, lithium was initiated within 24 h of delivery and in Edinburgh it was administered from week 34 of gestation. Women were seen by one of the investigators after delivery and followed regularly as outpatients for 6 months. A standard data form was used to collect information regarding previous non-puerperal, gestational and puerperal disorders using Research Diagnostic Criteria [4]. Frequency and length of hospital admission and diagnoses for all episodes were obtained. Onset after delivery of previous puerperal episodes was recorded, as was a family history of mental illness. Information was collected about the dosage, timing of administration, and serum levels of lithium following delivery.

*Originally published in Br. J. Psychiatry (1991) 158: 393–397.

Results

Twenty-one high-risk postpartum women, mean age 31.2 years, received prophylactic lithium in the three centres. Mean number of previous puerperal illnesses was 1.5 episodes with a mean duration of 21.6 weeks (see Table 1). Sixteen women had a family history of mental illness in first and second-degree relatives, the majority of which were affective illnesses. Nineteen women suffered no puerperal psychosis while on lithium, although three had mild brief psychological symptoms treated as outpatients, while two women suffered a recurrence of puerperal psychosis. The mean dose of lithium after delivery was 900 mg (range 750–1200 mg) a day to achieve a serum level of 0.8 mmol/l by postpartum day 7. There was one full-term stillbirth, cause undetermined, to a woman who received lithium carbonate from 34 weeks' gestation and whose serum lithium during pregnancy ranged from 0.55 to 0.69 mmol/l.

Table 1. Results of lithium prophylaxis in 21 women with previous puerperal psychoses

A	B	C	D	E	F	G
1	2	0	2	5	8	Mild symptoms
2	1	2	1	6	8	–
3	2	1	1	3	8	–
4	1	1	1	3	4	Mild symptoms
5	0	0	2	10	72	–
6	2	0	3	6	43	Mild symptoms
7	1	6	1	3	24	–
8	1	0	2	4	94	–
9	2	0	1	3	27	–
10	0	0	1	3	10	–
11	1	0	1	2	12	–
12	4	4	1	13	26	–
13	1	0	2	5	19	–
14	2	1	2	7	13	–
15	0	1	1	2	11	–
16	1	1	1	5	17	–
17	1	2	3	19	20	–, Stillbirth
18	3	2	2	5	5	Major depression
19	0	12+	1	8	16	Bipolar I
20	0	5	1	90	8	–
21	1	7	2	43	8	Relapse at 3 months after lithium discontinued

A: Patient No.; B: number of family members with history of mental illness; C: number of previous non-puerperal episodes in patient; D: number of previous puerperal episodes in patient; E: mean onset of puerperal psychosis: days after delivery; F: mean duration of puerperal psychosis: weeks; G: recurrence of puerperal illness on lithium carbonate.

Discussion

This report of prophylactic use of lithium carbonate in women at high risk for puerperal psychosis is an attempt to approach the problem from the perspective of an affective disorder precipitated by the many biological and psychological changes of pregnancy and parturition in the postpartum period. The three women who experienced mild confusion, insomnia, tiredness and depression after giving birth are of interest, as these symptoms may represent attenuated forms of puerperal illness. It is also of interest that one of the women with recurrence of puerperal illness (No. 18) had a shorter illness while on lithium carbonate. In view of the strong family history of affective disorders, the high proportion with bipolar disorder and the previous occurrence of puerperal psychosis, these 21 women given prophylactic lithium were at very high risk for a recurrence of puerperal psychosis. Various predictions from 20 to 50% for the risk of recurrence can be found in the literature depending on the specific risk factors surveyed [5–7]. However, predictive figures were not available for the multiple risk factors present in all but one of our patients given prophylactic lithium. The recurrence rate of 10% in our series thus falls well below the most conservative single factor estimates of recurrence risks. Although this finding requires replication in a larger sample in a randomized, double-blind, placebo-controlled study, there now seems to be some grounds for the use of prophylactic lithium immediately after delivery in women who have previously suffered from either puerperal psychosis or bipolar disorder.

References

1. Kendell RE (1985) J. Psychosom. Res. 29: 3–11.
2. Stewart DE (1988) J. Nerv. Ment. Dis. 176: 485–489.
3. Van Hulst AM and Klompenhouwer JL (1989) In: Van Hall EV and Everaerd W (eds.) Proc. of the 9th Int. Congr. of Psychosomatic Obstetrics and Gynaecology. The Parthenon Publishing Group Ltd., Carnforth, Lancs, U.K., pp. 417–423.
4. Spitzer RL, Endicott J and Robins E (1978) Arch. Gen. Psychiatry 35: 773–782.
5. Bratfos O and Haug JO (1966) Acta Psychiatr. Scand. 42: 285–294.
6. Reich T and Winokur G (1970) J. Nerv. Ment. Dis. 151: 60–68.
7. Abou-Saleh MT and Coppen A (1983) Br. J. Psychiatry 142: 539.

Biological Psychiatry, Volume 1. G. Racagni et al., editors.

Dopamine receptor hypersensitivity precedes puerperal affective psychosis: A possible link with perinatal changes in oestrogen production

A. Wieck, A.D. Hirst, M.N. Marks, I.C. Campbell, S.A. Checkley and R. Kumar
Institute of Psychiatry, De Crespigny Park, London SE5 8AF, U.K.

Introduction

Childbirth is a potent precipitator of affective psychosis [1] and it is likely that endocrine factors are involved in the pathogenesis. As oestrogens are known to have pronounced effects on the function of central dopaminergic neurotransmitter systems in laboratory animals [2] it has been proposed that the precipitous fall in oestrogen production after childbirth triggers the onset of affective psychosis by inducing dopaminergic dysfunction in predisposed women [3]. We tested this hypothesis by measuring the growth hormone (GH) response to apomorphine (APO) as an index of hypothalamic D_2 receptor function in postnatal women who had had an affective psychosis in the past. This group of women are particularly vulnerable after childbirth and have a relapse rate of about 50% in the postnatal period [4,5].

Since the interaction of oestrogen with the dopaminergic system has only been demonstrated in laboratory animals we also measured the APO-GH response in the changing hormonal milieu of the menstrual cycle in women without a history of psychiatric disorder.

Some of the results presented here have been described in detail elsewhere [6].

Methods

Fifteen postnatal women with a history of bipolar or schizo-affective illness and fifteen controls with no past psychiatric disorder were included in the study. All subjects had been free of psychotropic medication for at least two months and had no major obstetric complications. The APO-GH was carried out on the fourth day after delivery between 9 and 12 a.m. after overnight fasting according to the procedure of Corn et al. [7]. After a resting period of one hour, venous blood samples for GH estimations in plasma were taken at intervals of 15 min during 30 min before and 90 min after the administration of APO-HCL (0.005 mg/kg s.c.). During the test the mothers were separated from their babies and not permitted to breastfeed. GH concentrations in plasma were measured by immunoradiometric assay using commercial kits (Novo BioLabs, U.K.).

Clinical assessments were made at 36 weeks of pregnancy and 6 months postpartum using the Schedule for Affective Disorders and Schizophrenia and psychiatric illnesses were categorized according to the Research Diagnostic Criteria. The postnatal period was defined as 90 days after childbirth.

Five drug-free and regularly menstruating women with no past psychiatric disorder volunteered for the menstrual cycle study and had an APO-GH test in the early follicular phase when sex steroid plasma levels are low (4–6 days after onset of menstruation), in the midluteal phase when sex steroid plasma levels are at a stable high plateau (7–9 days after ovulation) and the endluteal phase when sex steroid levels are falling (12–13 days after ovulation). The time of ovulation was determined by detection of the midcycle LH surge in urine using a commercial self-test.

Results

Postpartum subjects

None of the women had a psychiatric illness in the 2 months before delivery. Eight "at risk" women relapsed after childbirth (n = 5: mania, n = 1: schizo-affective mania, n = 2: major depressive disorder) and 6 of these became ill within the first week after delivery. None of the control mothers became ill. The relapsed group had significantly higher GH responses to APO than the 15 controls (average peak GH increase and AUC increase after APO, $P < 0.05$) and also higher GH responses than the 7 women who remained well (average peak GH increase, $P < 0.05$). These results were not due to differences in the duration of the neuroleptic-free period, medication administered during labour or breastfeeding before the GH test [6].

Spontaneously cycling subjects

In the non-childbearing women the average GH peak increase was higher in the mid-luteal phase of the menstrual cycle (9.09 ± 2.76 mU/l $\pm$ S.E.M.) than in the early follicular (2.55 ± 2.81, mU/l $\pm$ S.E.M.) and the endluteal phase (3.66 ± 2.19, mU/l $\pm$ S.E.M.) taken together (Mann-Whitney U-test, $P < 0.05$).

Discussion

The data suggest that the onset of puerperal affective psychosis is preceded by an enhanced GH response to apomorphine indicating an increased sensitivity of (probably postsynaptic) D_2 receptors. The function of these receptors has also been shown in this study to be markedly modulated by physiological variations in oestrogen levels in normally cycling women confirming the findings in experimental animals. These results support the hypothesis that perinatal changes in oestrogen production trigger puerperal affective psychosis via effects on central dopaminergic systems. The neurochemical mechanism by which oestrogens alter the sensitivity to dopaminergic stimulation in spontaneously cycling women and induce the abnormal responsiveness in mothers who have recently delivered and who subsequently develop an affective psychosis requires further investigation.

Acknowledgements

The project has been funded by the Medical Research Council (U.K.) and the Health Promotion Research Trust (U.K.).

References

1. Kendell RE, Chalmers JC and Platz C (1987) Br. J. Psychiatry 150: 662–673.
2. Van Hardtesveldt C and Joyce JN (1986) Neurosci. Biobehav. Rev. 10: 1–14.
3. Cookson JC (1982) Lancet ii: 672.
4. Dean C, Williams JR and Brockington IF (1989) Psychol. Med. 20: 637–647.
5. Marks MN, Wieck A, Checkley SA and Kumar R (1990) Br. J. Psychiatry 158 (10): 45–49.
6. Wieck A, Kumar R, Hirst AD, Marks MN, Campbell IC and Checkley SA (1991) Br. Med. J. (in press).
7. Corn T, Hale AS, Thompson C, Bridges PK and Checkley SA (1984) Br. J. Psychiatry 144: 636–639.

Biological Psychiatry, Volume 1. G. Racagni et al., editors.

Physiopathological and pharmacological aspects of the stress response

Bruno Silvestrini
Istituto di Farmacologia e Farmacognosia, Universita' degli Studi 'La Sapienza', P. le Aldo Moro 5, 00185 Rome, Italy

Summary

The stress response is a defence mechanism that in situations of danger either extra-activates or depresses various processes. Its physiological and pathological effects vary from person to person, depending on the individual reaction to stress. Its core medium is a sympathetic discharge controlled by a positive feedback process, that provides a key to the pharmacological control of various pathological conditions, but requires an adjustment according to the individual reaction to stress.

Physiological and pharmacological aspects

Since the pioneering studies of [1], emotional and physical stress is known to induce a mass sympathetic discharge with a fight or flight reaction. This phenomenon is called "sympathetic alarm or stress response", "fight or flight reaction" or, more concisely, "stress response" and is generally viewed as a defensive reaction to danger. The stress response is described as two complementary sets of effects [2]:

a) an extra activation of some processes, i.e., heart rate, blood pressure, blood coagulation, pulmonary ventilation, glucose supply, mydriasis, mental alertness and muscle strength; and
b) a depression of other momentarily useless processes, including hunger and sexuality, with a reduction of blood flow in tissues not involved in the stress response.

In some individuals there is also a state of physical and mental analgesia that permits the performance to be increased over the critical level normally signalled by pain.

The "surrender stress response" is a third type of reaction to danger that was first described in detail in different animal species [3], but is common in man too [4,5]. It is observed in persons that react to danger not by an active fight or flight response, but by submission to the adversary. The decision among these 3 choices – fight, flight or surrender – depends on various factors, i.e. animal species, sex, age, previous experience, education and temperament. The role of the latter will be discussed later in greater detail.

Also the single effects of the stress response present ample variations, that to some extent are independent from the above mentioned behavioural patterns. Some individuals become pale, others flush. Some have a craving for food, an increased sexual drive, a sense of sufferance. The sympathetic discharge produces opposite effects: hyperglycemia, which is a well known signal for suppressing, rather than increasing hunger; a detumescence, rather than a tumescence of erectile genital tissues; analgesia, rather than an increased pain perception. Nevertheless, these paradoxical effects of the stress response should not be considered paradoxical both because they are observed rather commonly and because in the logics of survival they can be as useful as the orthodox responses.

Another interesting feature of the stress response is its physiologic control. Most systems of the body are regulated by a process of negative feedback, in which the response is negative to the initiating stimulus. This does not seem to be the case of the stress-induced sympathetic discharge. In this respect, it should be recalled that a stress that persists sufficiently induces a secretion from the medulla of both cortisol and epinephrine [6]. Cortisol has negative feedback effects on the hypothalamus to decrease the formation of CRF (corticotropin-releasing factor) and ACTH (adrenocorticotropic hormone). On the contrary, the intravenous injection of epinephrine has been shown to produce a subcortical EEG activation in cats [7]. The stimulation of subcortical structures, on the other hand, produces a state of rage and transmits signals downward through the reticular formation to induce the sympathetic discharge [2]. Therefore, it appears that in the sympathetic discharge epinephrine functions at the same time as response and initiating stimulus. This deduction is supported by results of a pharmacological study with trazodone that will be described later. The positive feedback control of the stress response is useful as in a situation of danger, that is potentially life-threatening, it permits an organism to squander all its energies. The limiting factor of the stress response is its exhaustion. This parameter has not yet been investigated in detail, but a study performed on volunteers has shown that a protracted epinephrine infusion triggers an arterial hypertension lasting 18 h [8]. This result provides an indirect indication that the sympathetic discharge produced by a strong stimulus can last several hours.

Obviously this extra activation of the body involves some risks at the pathological level, particularly when it is prolonged, excessive or associated with cofactors. For instance, the increase of blood pressure and coagulation rate can progress to stroke or infarct [9]. The inhibition of appetite can result in severe anorexia [10]. The stress response has also been implicated in psychotic states [11], insomnia, functional impotence in man, frigidity in women and depression [12,13].

It is known that the features of stress-related pathology depend on the basal, physiological reactivity to stress. For instance, the A type behaviour, marked by easily aroused hostility, has been reported to be associated with a more marked increased risk of coronary artery disease than the B type behaviour [14]. A significant correlation was reported between the paradoxical stress-associated hunger and overweight [15]. Likewise, it was speculated that the paradoxical increase of sexual drive associated with stress is related to deviations in which stress is necessary for sexual activity [5]. Likewise, the mental pain hypothesis of depression proposes that this condition develops more easily in individuals that

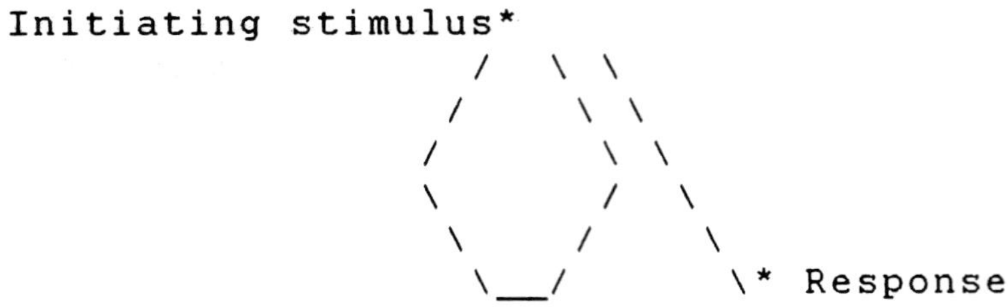

Fig. 1. The pharmacological control (*) of positive feedbacks is exerted both at the level of response and initiating stimulus.

under stress feel a sense of dysphoria and sufferance, rather than of euphoria and analgesia [16].

Pharmacological aspects

The pharmacological control of a positive feedback process raises the interesting problem of drugs that influence the same phenomenon both at the level of its initiating stimulus and response (Fig. 1).

The pharmacological modulation can consist of either inhibition or activation. Trazodone is a typical case of an agent having such an inhibitory action on the sympathetic system. It possesses a peripheral sympatholytic action, which, however, takes place preferentially at the α-adrenoceptors. At the same time, it reduces the sympathetic discharge following electrical stimulation of the reticular formation (unpublished results). Epinephrine, however, which is the main transmitter of the sympathetic discharge stimulates both the α and β-adrenoceptors. Therefore, trazodone possesses either an α or an α and β-blocking activity depending on whether it acts on the peripheral response of the sympathetic discharge or it acts indirectly, by inhibiting the epinephrine release.

To my knowledge, the effects of sympathomimetic drugs on the stress-induced sympathetic discharge have not been investigated, except at the peripheral site of catecholamine release from their stores. It appears reasonable, therefore, to speculate that sympathomimetic drugs have mirror-like effects to those of trazodone on the stress-induced sympathetic discharge.

Thus sympatholytic and sympathomimetic agents provide a tool for the treatment of pathological conditions depending on an exaggeration or failure of the stress response. The pattern and the single effects of the stress response, however, depend on individual reaction to stress or temperament. This latter factor, therefore, must also be taken into consideration at the pharmacological level. Some practical implications of this notion are shown in Table 1.

To simplify matters, it is assumed that there are two different stress-responders: γ, with increased mental alertness, analgesia and decrease of sexuality and appetite; and δ responders, with opposite effects. The same drug produces opposite effects

Table 1. Temperament and stress response pharmacological control. The γ responder reacts to stress with increased mental alertness, analgesia, and decreased sexuality and appetite; the δ with opposite effects

Responder	Drugs	Mental alertness, pain, sexuality, appetite
γ	Sympatholytics	Decrease
	Sympathomimetics	Increase
δ	Sympatholytics	Increase
	Sympathomimetics	Decrease

according to whether a person belongs to one or the other of these two categories of stress responders. The effects of the stress response, however, most probably vary not only as a group, but independently of one another. Thus, before initiating a drug treatment of stress-related disorders the individual reaction to stress should be determined in detail.

A case of special interest is that of antidepressants marked respectively by a sympatholytic and sympathomimetic action. The former is the case of trazodone and its derivatives etoperidone and dapiprazole, the latter of fluoxetine. If the above-mentioned notions are correct, their efficacy on some symptoms commonly associated with depression – such as sexuality and appetite disorders – could be improved by taking into consideration the individual reaction to stress.

Conclusions

To conclude, the stress response has some interesting physiopathological and pharmacological features:

a) it consists of an extra activation of some processes and a depression of others that in conditions of stress are respectively useful and useless;
b) the physiological and pathological effects of the stress response, however, vary from person to person, depending on the individual reaction to stress;
c) the sympathetic discharge controlled by a positive feedback process is central to the stress response;
d) it provides a key to the pharmacological control of various stress-related conditions, but it requires a specific adjustment according to the individual reaction to stress.

There is a progression in this list from traditional to new notions and from them to the working hypothesis that the treatment of stress-related disorders should be guided by the individual reaction to stress, rather than by objective assessment of its symptoms. This latter concept, however, is not new as it dates back to the Hippocratic tradition of "temperament" or "temper" that conditions the response to pathogenetic factors and medical treatment.

I would also like to emphasize that the stress response modulates several mechanisms throughout the body. I have focused on the sympathetic discharge essentially because it is one of the landmarks of my personal research. There are others, however, which are equally and perhaps more important. One of them will be described in the lecture by Professor Samuel Gershon of Pittsburgh University.

References

1. Cannon WB (1915) Bodily Changes in Pain, Hunger, Fear and Rage. Appleton, New York, U.S.A.
2. Guyton AC (1986) In: Dreibelbis D (ed.) Textbook of Medical Physiology, 7th Edition. WB Saunders Co., Philadelphia, PA, U.S.A., p. 695.
3. Lorenz K (1967) L'Anello di Re Salomone. Adelphi, Milan, Italy.
4. Silvestrini B (1989) Clin. Neuropharmacol. 12: S4–S10.
5. Silvestrini B and Silvestrini M (1991) In: Proc. Int. Congr. Stress Rel. Disord., Modena, Italy, November 18–22, 1990. Parthenon Publishing, U.K., Ch. 23.
6. Weiner N (1975) In: Blaschko H, Sayers G and Smith AD (eds.) Adrenal Gland. Vol. 6, Sect. 7. Endocrinology, Handbook of Physiology. American Physiological Society, Washington D.C., U.S.A.
7. Longo VG and Silvestrini B (1957) Proc. Soc. Exp. Biol. Med. 95: 43–47.
8. Blankestijn PJ, Man in't Veld AJ, Julen J, et al. (1988) Lancet ii: 1386–1388.
9. Rozanski A, Bairey CN, Krantz DS et al. (1988) N. Engl. J. Med. 318: 1005–1012.
10. Schachter S, Goldman R and Gordon A (1968) J. Pers. Soc. Psychol. 10: 91–97.
11. Osmond H and Smythies JR (1952) J. Ment. Sci. 98: 309–315.
12. Gold PW, Goodwin FK and Chrousos GP (1988a) N. Engl. J. Med. 319: 348–353.
13. Gold PW, Goodwin FK and Chrousos GP (1988b) N. Engl. J. Med. 319: 413–419.
14. Friedman M (1989) Am. J. Cardiol. 64: 12C–19C.
15. Silvestrini M and Paga C (1991) In: Proc. Int. Congr. Stress Rel. Disord., Modena, Italy, November 18–22, 1990. Parthenon Publishing, U.K., Ch. 12.
16. Silvestrini B (1990) J. Clin. Psychiatry 51(9): 6–8.

Biological Psychiatry, Volume 1. G. Racagni et al., editors.

Altered sleep, depression and antidepressant efficacy

Martin B. Scharf
Center For Research In Sleep Disorders, Inc., 1275 E. Kemper Road, Cincinnati, OH 45246, U.S.A.

The purpose of this study was to systematically evaluate the effectiveness of trazodone on insomniac depressed patients for antidepressant efficacy, polysomnographically determined sleep architecture and sedative effects.

Methods

Subjects. Twelve patients, 5 men (40.8 ± 10.45 years) and 7 females (36.6 ± 15.27 years), between 20 and 58 years of age were enrolled in this 9-week single-blind treatment study. All patients met the diagnostic criteria for major depression and insomnia secondary to psychiatric illnesses defined by the DSM III-R criteria. REM density was evaluated by determining the number of 3-s REM epochs in which at least one eye movement was present divided by the total number of 3-s epochs.

Procedures

Following a 1-week placebo baseline period, patients were entered into the trazodone treatment period. Patients received 150 mg of trazodone for 2 days, which was increased to 200 mg for 2 more days and then to 250 mg for the remaining 3 days of the 1st week. Patients whose therapeutic benefit after 1 week was not considered optimal were given an increased dose up to a maximum of 400 mg over the course of the remaining 4 weeks of treatment. Following the 5 weeks of trazodone administration, patients received placebo for 2 consecutive weeks.

Clinical symptoms were assessed using the Hamilton Anxiety and Hamilton Depression Scales at pretreatment, after the initial placebo period, at the end of 1, 2 and 5 weeks of active therapy and again following the placebo withdrawal period. Patients were evaluated polysomnographically during the initial placebo period, at the end of 1, 2 and 5 weeks of therapy and again during the first and last 3 days of the 2-week placebo-withdrawal period.

Statistical analysis

All variables were analyzed using a one-way repeated measures analysis of variance over the different time periods of the study. The 1st night of each sleep lab period was used as an adaptation night and was not included in the data analysis. Post hoc analyses were considered appropriate when overall $P < 0.05$. The follow-up comparisons were made using Bonferroni adjusted probabilities.

Results

Substantial improvement in both HAM-A and HAM-D scales were observed in all subjects receiving trazodone. Improvement was evident at the end of the 1st treatment week and progressively increased with continued drug administration. There were no noticeable responses to placebo during the placebo period.

With drug administration, the persistent sleep latency dramatically decreased reaching statistical significance by the end of 2 weeks of therapy. The efficacy was maintained throughout the remaining weeks of therapy. Similarly, total sleep time improved considerably and remained improved throughout the remainder of the drug administration period. Trazodone administration improved sleep efficiency in a similar fashion.

No significant changes in sleep stage percentages were noted with administration of trazodone throughout the 5 weeks of drug administration or following withdrawal (Tables 1 and 2) except for an increase of stage 2 sleep during the 1st week of drug therapy. While REM percent remained essentially unchanged, REM latency showed a progressive increase reaching statistical significance at the end of 5 weeks. Slow wave sleep (stages 3 and 4) individually or separately showed little change from baseline throughout the period of drug administration.

Figure 1 shows the effects of trazodone on REM density. Trazodone administration resulted in a progressive and sustained decrease that was followed by a rebound increase following withdrawal.

Table 1. The effect of trazodone on objective sleep parameters in depressed patients

	Baseline	Acute effect	1 week	2 weeks	5 weeks
Persistent sleep latency (min)	52.9±38.79	37.8±32.65	38.1±37.63	29.6±19.54[a]	26.6±16.96[a]
Total sleep time (min)	383.7±43.79	411.2±39.83	419.1±35.0[a]	419.3±51.13[a]	436.0±18.01[b]
Stage I (%)	11.3± 5.04	10.7± 6.42	8.9± 3.07	8.1± 4.54	9.7± 2.69
Stage II (%)	57.7± 8.10	58.6± 7.66	63.5± 8.01[a]	61.5± 8.50	61.1±10.10
Stage III (%)	6.0± 4.18	6.1± 4.60	5.4± 6.00	4.3± 3.74	6.6± 4.91
Stage IV (%)	2.7± 3.62	1.6± 2.91	3.1± 3.23	2.4± 4.01	3.5± 3.83
REM (%)	22.6± 3.10	22.3± 3.73	20.4± 6.73	23.1± 4.47	20.1± 5.27
REM latency (min)	78.1±26.75	85.3±30.18	98.3±24.67	104.8±46.19	121.8±40.87[a]
No. awakenings	4.5± 2.34	5.4± 2.22	3.5± 2.00	3.5± 3.37	3.9± 1.55
Sleep efficiency (%)	79.9± 9.14	84.6±11.19	87.3± 7.29[a]	87.3±10.67[a]	89.6± 5.53[b]

[a]Significantly different from baseline $P \leq 0.05$; [b]Significantly different from baseline $P \leq 0.01$.

Table 2. The effect of trazodone withdrawal on objective sleep parameters in depressed patients

	Baseline	Acute W/D	Long W/D
Persistent sleep latency (min)	52.9 ± 38.79	40.5 ± 25.30	26.8 ± 21.36
Total sleep time (min)	383.7 ± 43.79	398.7 ± 57.75	397.0 ± 53.40
Stage I (%)	11.3 ± 5.04	12.0 ± 6.07	11.7 ± 4.89
Stage II (%)	57.7 ± 8.10	56.3 ± 6.82	61.2 ± 6.76
Stage III (%)	6.0 ± 4.18	5.9 ± 5.14	4.9 ± 5.25
Stage IV (%)	2.7 ± 3.62	2.4 ± 3.80	0.67 ± 1.36
REM (%)	22.6 ± 3.10	23.3 ± 3.91	22.1 ± 5.20
REM latency (min)	78.1 ± 26.75	82.6 ± 21.83	86.8 ± 28.88
No. awakenings	4.5 ± 2.34	4.2 ± 1.36	4.5 ± 1.76
Sleep efficiency (%)	79.9 ± 9.14	83.1 ± 12.05	82.5 ± 11.01

Discussion

Patients in this study showed a simultaneous progressive and consistent decrease in both depression and anxiety during the 5 weeks of trazodone dosing. These clinical improvements occurred in conjunction with improvements in overall sleep duration and sleep difficulty.

No change in REM sleep percentages were noted during drug administration or withdrawal in this study. This is consistent with reports of others, but contrasts with findings reported for most antidepressants. Vogel and coworkers have pro-

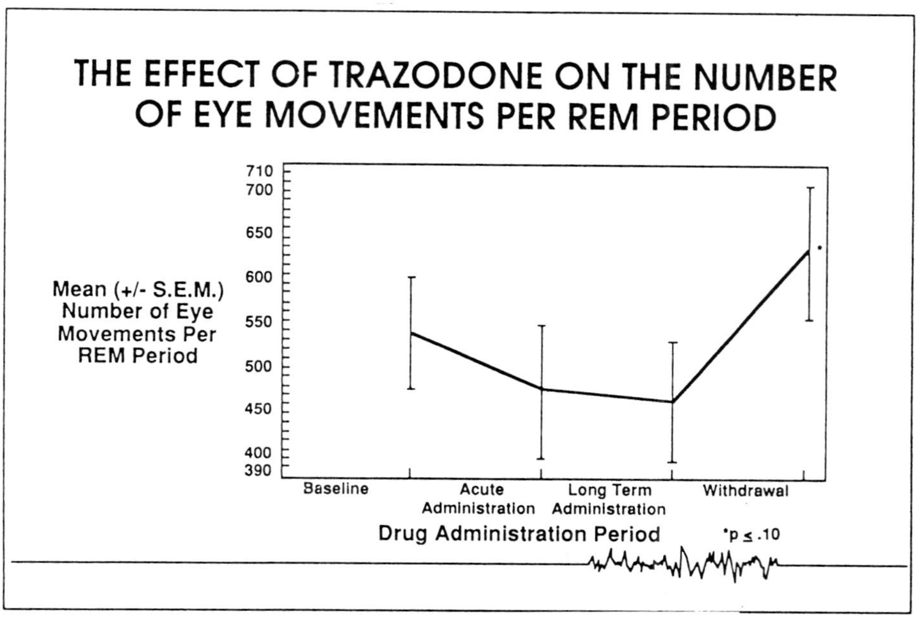

Fig. 1.

posed that REM sleep deprivation actually improves endogenous depression and is a consistent concomitant of most effective treatments for depression. However, trazodone has not been shown to suppress REM sleep or cause a REM rebound following withdrawal.

Most REM suppressant agents suppress both phasic and tonic aspects of REM sleep and their withdrawal results in REM rebound, including an increase in eye movement density. The trazodone-induced decrease in eye movement density with the subsequent rebound, however, suggests that trazodone may exhibit its antidepressant efficacy through REM mechanisms. The progressive delay in REM latency with drug administration suggests a shift in REM distribution, such that there is a decrease in REM sleep in the early part of the night with a rebound in the second part of the night. Thus, both phasic and tonic REM components may be implicated in the clinical mechanism of trazodone efficacy. Trazodone administration results in a consistent normalization of overall sleep patterns, with a reduction in sleep difficulty in conjunction with clinical improvement in depressed insomniac patients.

References

1. Reynolds, FC (1989) In: Kryger MG, Roth T and Dement WC (eds.) Principles and Practice of Sleep Medicine. W.B. Saunders, Philadelphia, U.S.A., pp. 413–415.
2. Montgomery I, Oswald I, Morgan K et al. (1983) Br. J. Clin. Pharmacol. 16: 139–144.
3. Muratoria A, Maggini C, Coccagna G and Guazzilli M (1979) In: Ban TA and Silvestrini B (eds.) Trazodone Mod. Probl. Pharmacopsychiatry. Karger, Basel, pp. 182–189.
4. Vogel GW (1983) Prog. Neuro-Psychopharmacol. Biol. Psychiatry 7: 343–349.

Biological Psychiatry, Volume 1. G. Racagni et al., editors.

Antidepressants and sympatholytic activity: The case of etoperidone, a new triazolone derivative

John P. Feighner and William F. Boyer
The Feighner Research Institute, San Diego, California, U.S.A.

Pharmacology

Etoperidone is a triazolone derivative which is difficult to classify. Although etoperidone has sedative properties, it interacts differently to sedatives with brain neurotransmitters, it lacks anticonvulsant effects, and has different behavioral effects at high doses. Etoperidone differs from the tricyclic antidepressants by not antagonizing reserpine in the rat or potentiating L-dopa's behavioral effects in the mouse. It is not a monoamine oxidase inhibitor [1]. Etoperidone is similar in some aspects to the neuroleptics since it produces analgesic, deconditioning and sedative effects at low doses. However it does not block central dopaminergic receptors. Etoperidone also differs from these drugs in its capacity to selectively inhibit the response of animals to unpleasant stimuli at doses which do not produce other pharmacological effects. In this etoperidone resembles trazodone, to which it is structurally related [2].

Both etoperidone and trazodone produce MCPP, a serotonergic agonist, as a metabolite [3]. Etoperidone has both peripheral and central effects on neurotransmitters. It inhibits the peripheral effects of norepinephrine and serotonin. It also inhibits the head-twitch reaction in mice and rats induced by 5-HT, suggesting central activity on serotonergic function [4]. Etoperidone applied to rat brainstem blocks the excitatory but not the inhibitory neuronal responses to ACh, 5-HT and NA [5]. This property may conceivably be related to its beneficial psychotropic effects.

Open studies in depression

Miano and Ottaviani investigated etoperidone in 20 patients on a general ward with symptoms of anxiety and depression. Etoperidone exhibited satisfactory activity in alleviating anxiety, somatization, hypochondria, and depression. The absence of side-effects and the excellent tolerance made the drug useful in treating both anxious and depressive symptoms [6].

Antonelli administered etoperidone to 24 depressed outpatients in a 27-day trial. Twenty patients completed the study. The result was deemed excellent or good in 15 cases. No side-effects were noted. Etoperidone was particularly helpful in treating somatization due to depression [7].

Alessandrini and colleagues administered etoperidone to 40 geriatric patients with anxious depression. Favorable effects on somatization, sleep disturbances, depression and anxiety were seen. No side-effects or changes in laboratory testing were noted [8].

Controlled studies in depression

Several controlled studies of etoperidone in depression have been published (Table 1). These indicate that etoperidone's antidepressant activity is superior to placebo and comparable to reference antidepressants. Patients tend to report few side-effects. Tolerance is usually described as "excellent". Occasional nausea and drowsiness are reported.

Several 6-week double-blind multicenter studies of etoperidone and reference antidepressants have been conducted (Table 2). These 3 trials show no significant differences in antidepressant activity between etoperidone and the standard antidepressant as measured on the Hamilton Depression Rating Scale. If one considers the numbers of patients who reported no side-effects, which is a very stringent criterion of medication acceptability, etoperidone clearly surpassed the standard antidepressants.

Table 1. Controlled studies in depression

Investigator	Control group	Sample size	Outcome	Side-effects
DePasquale et al. [9]	Placebo	20	Etoperidone significantly superior to placebo	No "relevant side-effects" were observed
Forin and Bruno [10]	Placebo	30	Etoperidone significantly superior to placebo	Tolerance was "excellent"
Lieto et al. [11]	Nomifensine Trazodone	20	Good outcome in: 6/7 etoperidone 4/7 nomifensine 5/6 trazodone	Good tolerance in: 6/7 etoperidone 5/7 nomifensine 5/6 trazodone
Roccatagliata et al. [12]	Trazodone Mianserin	38	Good outcome in: 7/12 etoperidone 9/12 mianserin 12/14 trazodone	Nausea reported by 1 etoperidone patient
Muller et al. [13]	Amitriptyline	30	No significant differences	8/12 etoperidone patients dropped out due to lack of efficacy or side-effects (unclear)

Table 2. Six-week, double-blind multicenter studies of etoperidone in depression

Comparison group	Sample	Maximum dosage	Decrease in HAM-D	Percentage reporting no side-effects
Clomipramine (CLOM)	39 inpatients with various depressive diagnoses	ETO 375 mg/day CLOM 175 mg/day	ETO 67.5% CLOM 79.8%	ETO 43% CLOM 27%
Amitriptyline (AMI)	32 inpatients with DSM III-R major depression	ETO 400 mg/day AMI 200 mg/day	ETO 57.4% AMI 75.5%	ETO 50% AMI 12.5%[a]
Imipramine (IMI)	40 outpatients with DSM III-R major depression	ETO 400 mg/day IMI 200 mg/day	ETO 58.8% IMI 70.1%	ETO 40% IMI 5%[a]

[a]$P < 0.05$.

Dementia

Some data suggest that etoperidone may have beneficial effects in the treatment of the behavioral aspects of organic mental disorders. Lieto and Del-Gaizo reported beneficial effects of etoperidone in patients suffering from vascular organic mental syndromes [14]. Spagnola and colleagues conducted a controlled, double-blind study of etoperidone in elderty subjects with severe dementia. Etoperidone had a significantly beneficial effect on resocialization [15].

Summary

The available evidence indicates that etoperidone is a relatively unique psychotropic agent with significant antidepressant and anxiolytic activity. Its mechanism of action may be related to its adrenolytic activity and/or its effects on serotonergic function. Etoperidone's benign side-effect profile appears especially promising. It may have advantages in the treatment of depression, mixed anxiety-depression, and the behavioral problems accompanying dementia.

References

1. Hyslop DK, Allen LE and Taylor DP (1988) Drug Dev. Res. 12(1): 77–79.
2. Lisciani R, Baldini A, De-Feo G et al. (1978) Arzneim. Forsch. 28(3): 417–423.
3. Fong MH, Garattini S and Caccia S (1982) J. Pharm. Pharmacol. 34(10): 674–675.
4. Przegalinski E and Lewandowska A (1979) J. Neural Transm. 46(4): 303–312.
5. Janiri L, Salera P and Tempesta E (1986) Arzneim. Forsch. 36(12): 1721–1726.
6. Miano G and Ottaviani G (1976) Lav. Neuropsichiatr. 59(3): 101–109.

7. Antonelli F (1977) Med. Psicosom. 22(3): 259–265.
8. Alessandrini A, Tiberi F, Morbidelli C et al. (1976) Acta Gerontol. 26(3): 181–184.
9. De-Pasquale C, Civelli L, Ongaro A et al. (1976) Acta Gerontol. 26(4): 252–259.
10. Forin G and Bruno S (1976) Acta Gerontol. 26(4) 264–273.
11. Lieto L, Sena M, Govetto G et al. (1983) Rass. Stud. Psichiatr. 72(2): 331–340.
12. Roccatagliata G, Albano C, Serati C et al. (1985) Rass. Stud. Psichiatr. 74(2): 1–6.
13. Muller N, Schmauss M, Scherer S et al. (1989) Pharmacopsychiatry 22(5): 208.
14. Lieto L and Del-Gaizo F (1980) Lav. Neuropsichiatr. 66(1–2): 147–155.
15. Spagnolo C, Dallasta D, Iannucelli M et al. (1983) Drugs Exp. Clin. Res. 9(12): 873–880.

Biological Psychiatry, Volume 1. G. Racagni et al., editors.

Stress and aging brain: Markers of adaptation in dementia of the Alzheimer's type

Giuseppe Nappi[1], Emilia Martignoni[1], Alfredo Costa[1], Felice Petraglia[2], Giorgio Bono[1] and Andrea R. Genazzani[2]

[1]*Department of Neurology III, Neurological Institute "C. Mondino", University of Pavia, Pavia; and* [2]*Department of Obstetrics and Gynecology, University of Modena, Italy*

Introduction

Over the past few years, a relationship between the stress-related phenomena and the mechanisms of the aging brain has been claimed, particularly on the basis of experimental evidence in animal studies [1]. The major issues raised by these reports concern: the suitability of animal models to humans; whether human aging is associated with impaired stress response; whether chronic stress can accelerate the aging processes. In this respect, the neuroendocrine approach to aging brain can provide simple tools to investigate the activity of neurotransmitters and neurohormones in the central nervous system. A number of observations point to a derangement of some neuroendocrine axes during aging [2], these changes being even more pronounced in the case of the pathological aging brain [3]. Despite the great number of morphological and biochemical studies on brain tissues, dementia of the Alzheimer type (DAT) has only recently become one of the targets of psychoneuroendocrine research. DAT is associated with defects in several biochemical pathways along with typical structural changes in the cerebral cortex [4,5]. The neuropathological features, however, also involve subcortical sites [6] including the hypothalamus, which controls the secretion of the pituitary hormones. Most of the endocrine studies carried out in DAT focus on the function of the hypothalamus-pituitary-adrenal (HPA) axis, although it has been reported that the secretory patterns of other hormones are also affected [3,7]. It is well known that the HPA axis and the sympathetic nervous system (SNS) play a crucial role in the stress response, in that they counteract stressors and maintain homeostasis. While the activity of the HPA axis in normal aging remains controversial, it has been strongly suggested that an adrenocortical overactivity is a common finding in DAT patients [8–10]. As far as the SNS is concerned, a sympathetic hyperactivity seems to represent a biochemical marker of normal aging in humans [11]. Plasma noradrenaline (NA) is considered as a reliable index of peripheral SNS activity, while cerebrospinal fluid (CSF) NA is believed to derive solely from the central nervous system, thus reflecting central noradrenergic activity [12]. Both plasma and CSF NA levels seem to increase throughout life [11,13]. The heightened noradrenergic tone in the normal elderly has been explained in terms of increased

NA release, a lack of the inhibitory α_2 receptor activity being a possible mechanism of action [13]. Conversely, it has been hypothesized that DAT is characterized by a noradrenergic deficit. Indeed, neurohistologic studies have shown cell loss in the locus caeruleus [6] and reduced NA content has been found in several brain areas of DAT patients [14]. However, previous studies on plasma and CSF NA in DAT have provided conflicting results [15,16], the noradrenergic activity in this neurodegenerative disease remaining a controversial issue.

We further explored the function of the HPA axis and the sympathetic activity in DAT patients by measuring plasma cortisol and cerebrospinal fluid (CSF) corticotropin releasing factor (CRF), as well as plasma and CSF NA levels, respectively.

HPA axis findings

We examined 35 patients (29 males and 6 females, age range 55–75 years) suffering from mild to moderate primary dementia, according to DSM III-R criteria. As controls we considered 21 age-matched subjects, 17 males and 4 females, ranging in age between 57 and 74 years. DAT patients showed morning plasma cortisol levels (176.1 ± 77.2 ng/ml, M ± S.D.) which were significantly higher than those of the controls (115.1 ± 27 ng/ml) ($P < 0.01$) and directly correlated to the Global Deterioration Scale (GDS) score ($y = 3.39 + 5.68x$, $r = 0.51$, $P < 0.01$). In 10 patients, the analysis of the cortisol circadian rhythm (cosinor) showed a greater mean 24-h value (mesor) of cortisol secretion (106.4 ± 28.7 ng/ml M ± SD) and a greater amplitude of the rhythm (52.5 ± 8.8 ng/ml) than the controls (70.8 ± 22 ng/ml and 31.5 + 15.6 ng/ml, respectively, $P < 0.01$). The times of cortisol nadir, maximum and acrophase did not differ between the 2 groups. CSF CRF levels (462 ± 288 pg/ml, M ± S.D.) were significantly higher in 9 of the patients, compared to 11 control subjects (158 ± 122 pg/ml) ($P < 0.01$). Moreover, CRF values proved to be inversely correlated with the severity of the cognitive decline, as assessed by Mini-Mental State (MMS) ($y = 20.41x - 3.73$; $r = -0.53$; $P < 0.05$). Ten of our DAT patients and 11 age-matched controls also underwent DST and CRF tests. Six out of the 10 DAT patients showed an escape from dexamethasone suppression, whereas no major difference in cortisol secretion was observed after CRF systemic administration. In the DAT group, however, we found an inverse correlation between age and the maximum percentage of increase in cortisol plasma levels (Δ% max.) in response to CRF ($r = -0.76$; $P < 0.01$).

Sympathetic activity findings

In 18 out of the DAT patients the plasma NA levels (220.4 ± 119 pg/ml) were not different from those of 23 age-matched controls (260.9 ± 131.3 pg/ml). Significantly decreased HA concentrations were found instead in the CSF from 18 patients (93.3 ± 45 pg/ml, controls (n = 28) 142.5 ± 79.1 pg/ml, $P < 0.05$). No correlation was found between the NA levels and the severity of the cognitive impairment or other clinical variables.

Comments

As a whole, the data on HPA axis confirm that a state of adrenocortical overactivity, possibly originating at hypothalamic level, occurs in degenerative dementia. The increased CSF CRF content found in our DAT patients could directly reflect a hypothalamic CRF hypersecretion, thus supporting the findings by other authors [17]. Moreover, the CSF CRF determination in DAT patients could be of some clinical significance, providing a useful tool to follow the progression of dementia. The finding of a similar acute cortisol response to CRF in patients and controls suggests that in DAT there is, in principle, a normal pituitary responsiveness, which may progressively decrease with age (receptor desensitization?).

As far as the sympathetic activity is concerned, the reduced CSF NA levels observed in our patients seem to be directly related to the loss of cortical and subcortical neurons, thus being consistent with a central noradrenergic impairment in DAT. On the other hand, the peripheral sympathetic tone, as expressed by plasma NA, does not seem to be affected by the disease. Moreover, our observations do not suggest that the cognitive deficits in the DAT subjects are related to a deranged noradrenergic activity. Noradrenergic changes might rather underlie the behavioural aspects of the disease: such neurons, in fact, project from the locus caeruleus and other brainstem structures to the limbic system and neocortex and influence the higher processing of sensory perception and the response to external events, including stressors [18].

In conclusion, our data on the activity of two of the major systems involved in the stress response support the view that their disruption in DAT may lead to a lack of adaptation, and a reduced ability to cope with the environmental changes which in turn, may be relevant to the further evolution of the disease.

References

1. Sapolsky RM, Krey LC and McEwen BS (1986) Endocrinol. Rev. 7(3): 284–301.
2. Everitt AV and Burgess JA (eds.) (1976) Hypothalamus, Pituitary and Aging. Charles C. Thomas, Springfield, Illinois.
3. Christie JE, Brown NS, Dick H, Rosie R and Sanches-Watts G (1985) In: Von Hahn HP (ed.) Interdisciplinary Topics in Gerontology. Karger, Basel, 19, pp. 131–142.
4. Coyle JT, Price DL and DeLong MR (1983) Science 219: 1184–1190.
5. Rossor M and Iversen LL (1986) Br. Med. Bull. 42: 70–74.
6. Bondareff W, Mountjoj CQ and Roth M (1981) Lancet i: 783–784.
7. Cramer H (1988) In: Valenti G (ed.) Psychoneuroendocrinology of Aging: Basic and Clinical Aspects. Springer Verlag, Berlin, pp. 97–111.
8. Greenwald BS, Mathe AA, Mohs RC, Levy MI, Johns CA and Davis KL (1986) Am. J. Psychiatry 143: 442–446.

9. Martignoni E, Petraglia F, Costa A, Bono G, Genazzani AR and Nappi G (1990) Acta Neurol. Scand. 81: 452–456.
10. Oxenkrug GF, Gurevich D, Siegel B, Dumlao MS and Gershon S (1989) Psychiatr. Res. 29: 169–175.
11. Palmer CJ, Ziegler MG and Lake CR (1978) J. Clin. Pharmacol. 19: 458–466.
12. Ziegler MG, Lake CR, Wood JH, Brooks BR and Ebert MH (1977) J. Neurochem. 28: 677–679.
13. Veith RC and Raskind MA (1988) Neurobiol. Aging 9: 101–117.
14. Yates CM, Ritchie IM, Simpson J, Maloney AFJ and Gordon A (1981) Lancet ii: 39–40.
15. Mann JJ, Stanley M, Neophytides A, de Leon MJ, Ferris SH and Gershon S (1981) Neurobiol. Aging 2: 57–60.
16. Raskind MA, Peskind ER, Halter JB and Jimerson DC (1984) Arch. Gen. Psychiatry 41: 343–346.
17. Powers RE, Walker LC, De Souza EB, Vale WW, Struble RG, Whitehouse PJ and Price DL (1987) Synapse 1: 405–410.
18. Cotman CW and McGaugh JL (eds.) (1980) Behavioural Neuroscience. Academic Press, New York.

Biological Psychiatry, Volume 1. G. Racagni et al., editors.

Phosphodiesterase inhibitors as antidepressants

Helmut Wachtel

Department of Neuropsychopharmacology, Schering AG, Müllerstrasse 170–178, W-1000 Berlin 65, Germany

It has previously been proposed that affective disorders arise from the dysbalance of the two major intraneuronal signal amplification systems, i.e. the adenylate cyclase (AC)/cAMP kinase system and the phospholipase C (PLC) system including the Ca^{2+}-calmodulin (CaM) kinases and the protein kinases C (C kinases); according to the second messenger dysbalance hypothesis, depression results from underfunctioning of the AC-cAMP kinase pathway associated with dominance of the PLC-CaM/C kinase system and mania resulting from the converse [1]. This hypothesis harmonizes the classic monoamine (MA) deficiency hypothesis, the cholinergic-adrenergic hypothesis, and the output deficiency hypothesis and explains the therapeutic and prophylactic effect of lithium in bipolar depression [1]. Lithium's antimanic effect would result from dampening the overactive AC system because of its AC inhibitory action [2,3] and its prophylactic effect in depression from preventing overactivity of the PLC system due to attenuation of phosphatidylinositol-4,5-biphosphate (PIP_2) resynthesis by inhibition of inositol-1-phosphatase [4]. The functional cAMP deficiency in depression may result from defects at the level of: a) the presynaptic neuron (impaired MA turnover); b) the postsynaptic MA receptors (decreased or increased density and affinity of MA receptors coupled stimulatory (G_s) or inhibitory (G_i) to AC, respectively); c) the AC (impaired or enhanced coupling between the catalytic subunit and G_s or G_i, respectively); and d) the phosphodiesterase (PDE) inactivating cAMP (increased activity), or it may result from an absolute preponderance of the PLC-CaM/C kinase system. Therefore, conceivable pharmacological manipulations to restitute second messenger balance are: a) selective inhibition of the low-K_m, high-affinity cAMP PDE isoenzyme, e.g. by rolipram (see below); b) deactivation of PLC by preventing PIP_2 resynthesis, e.g. by lithium (see above); c) selective stimulation of the catalytic subunit of AC, e.g. by forskolin [5]; d) selective inhibition of PLC; e) antagonism of CaM [6]; and f) selective inhibition of C kinase isoenzymes.

As catabolism of cAMP by PDEs is the only known enzymatic mechanism for terminating the action of cAMP, PDEs play a crucial role in determining the intensity and duration of the effector cell to the intraneuronal signal. Although the low-K_m, high-affinity cAMP PDE isoenzyme (now termed type IV or rolipram-sensitive PDE [7]) contributes only a small percentage of the total cerebral PDE activity, it represents a functionally important PDE isoenzyme which is primarily responsible for cAMP decay in intact neurons at physiological cAMP levels [8]. According to the second messenger dysbalance hypothesis, the selective inhibition of this cAMP PDE isoenzyme should increase neuronal cAMP availability and exert antidepressant activity. Pursuing this approach, rolipram was predicted to show antidepressant activity at much lower dosages than conventional drugs and to lack anticholinergic side-effects; this prediction has been confirmed in open and controlled clinical trials [1].

Rolipram causes a characteristic behavioral syndrome in rats consisting of head twitches, increased grooming, decreased locomotor activity and hypothermia [9] and reverses hypokinesia and hypothermia in MA-depleted mice [10]; these effects can be mimicked by membrane-penetrating cAMP analogues or the AC activator forskolin [5,11] indicating that they represent behavioral correlates of enhanced cerebral cAMP availability. We tested a variety of PDE inhibitors with different selectivity for distinct isoenzymes and their capability to elicit head twitches and grooming in rats and to reverse the hypokinesia and hypothermia in mice depleted of endogenous brain MAs by pretreatment with reserpine (10 mg/kg i.p.; 4 h) plus α-methyl-p-tyrosine (250 mg/kg i.p.; 3.5 h) and p-chlorophenylalanine (400 mg/kg i.p.; 24 h). Only the compounds shown in Table 1 were effective, whereas selective cGMP PDE inhibitors (zaprinast, MY-5445) or preferential inhibitors of cGMP-inhibited PDE (imazodan, SKF 94120, cilostamide, trequinsin) were inactive in this respect. Inhibitors of CaM-dependent PDE (tiflucarbine) or non-selective PDE inhibitors (papaverine, caffeine, theophylline, enprofylline, verofylline, IBMX) were either inactive or weakly effective at high, subtoxic doses. As the compounds of Table 1 have been shown to be preferential inhibitors of the low-K_m, high-affinity cAMP PDE isoenzyme in biochemical studies [7], our findings illustrate that the quantitative assessment of head twitches and grooming in rats represents a useful and reliable in vivo method for separating compounds with preferential

Table 1. Efficacy in vivo of preferential inhibitors of the rolipram-sensitive cAMP PDE in rats and MA-depleted mice

Compound	Minimal effective dose (mg/kg i.p.)			
	Induction of		Reversal of	
	Head twitches[a] Rats	Grooming[a] Rats	Hypokinesia[b] Mice	Hypothermia[c] Mice
Rolipram	1.56	0.39	0.39	0.39
ICI 63197	1.56	0.39	0.39	0.39
Ro 20-1724	25	6.25	6.25	6.25
Nitraquazone	6.25	1.56	1.56	6.25
Denbufylline	6.25	1.56	1.56	1.56

[a]The number of head twitches and grooming sequences was assessed by observation of the animals during 1 h starting at the 15th min after vehicle or drug administration;
[b]Locomotor activity was recorded immediately after vehicle or drug injection for 1 h;
[c]Rectal temperature was measured 30 min after vehicle or drug administration.

inhibitory action on the type IV cAMP PDE isoenzyme for development as potential antidepressants.

References

1. Wachtel H (1990) Pharmacopsychiatry 23: 27–32.
2. Dousa T and Hechter O (1970) Lancet i: 834–835.
3. Newman M, Klein E, Birmaher B, Feinsod M and Belmaker RH (1983). Brain Res. 278: 380–381.
4. Hallcher LM and Sherman WR (1980) J. Biol. Chem. 225: 10896–10901.
5. Wachtel H and Löschmann PA (1986) Psychopharmacology 90: 430–435.
6. Schmidt BH and Schultz JE (1986) Eur. J. Pharmacol. 130: 27–35.
7. Beavo JA and Reifsnyder DH (1990) Trends Pharmacol. Sci. 11: 150–155.
8. Whalin ME, Garrett RL Jr, Thompson WJ and Strada SJ (1988–1989) Second Messengers Phosphoproteins 12: 311–325.
9. Wachtel H (1982) Psychopharmacology 77: 309–316.
10. Wachtel H and Schneider HH (1986) Neuropharmacology 25: 1119–1126.
11. Wachtel H, Löschmann PA, Schneider HH and Rettig KJ (1987) Neurosci. Lett. 76: 191–196.

Biological Psychiatry, Volume 1. G. Racagni et al., editors.

Effect of lithium on adenylate cyclase in rat brain

Arne Mørk and Arne Geisler
Department of Pharmacology, University of Copenhagen, Juliane Maries Vej 20, 2100 Copenhagen, Denmark

Several studies have shown that lithium (Li^+) in vitro and ex vivo, i.e. after chronic treatment, inhibits the activity of adenylate cyclase. It has been observed repeatedly that Li has no effect on the basal enzyme activity, but modifies its stimulated activities. Lithium decreases the function of cerebral β-adrenergic receptors by interacting with the associated adenylate cyclase. Activation of the enzyme by GTP alone is unaffected by Li^+ ex vivo, but neurotransmitter-induced GTP activation is inhibited. Further, Li^+ in vitro as well as ex vivo impairs the activity of the catalytic subunit of the enzyme when stimulated by calcium-calmodulin or forskolin. The in vitro effects of Li^+ seem to be due to a competition between Li^+ and intracellular magnesium. However, Li^+ seems to have a more complex effect on the adenylate cyclase during chronic treatment. Thus, our studies on rat brain adenylate cyclase suggest that the inhibitory actions of Li in vitro and ex vivo on the enzyme activity differ. The mechanisms by which Li^+ exerts its ex vivo effects are unknown, but Li^+ may modify the fluidity of the cell membrane or influence protein kinases which modulate the adenylate cyclase activity by phosphorylating the proteins of the enzyme.

Studies on cerebral adrenergic receptors have given contradictory results. Presumably, Li^+ has no effect on the number of adrenergic receptors or the binding affinity to these receptors. Further, it has been observed that Li may increase the release of norepinephrine by an interaction with presynaptic α-adrenergic receptors, but other studies have not confirmed this observation. Lithium ex vivo reduces the density of pre- and postsynaptic 5-HT receptors without changing their affinities. In addition, it has been observed that chronic Li^+ treatment enhances 5-HT-stimulated adenylate cyclase activity in rat hippocampus. In accordance, electrophysiological studies have demonstrated that short-term lithium treatment enhances serotonergic activity in the rat brain. This enhancement of serotonergic processes may be involved in the therapeutic action of Li^+, since an enhanced serotonergic function may also modulate the adrenergic receptor activity. In fact, it has been demonstrated that drug-induced down-regulation of β-adrenergic receptors depends upon an intact serotonergic function.

It is not known whether the actions of Li^+ on the cyclic AMP formation mentioned are related to its therapeutic properties.

Biological Psychiatry, Volume 1. G. Racagni et al., editors.

Lithium selective interaction with G proteins in the CNS

Gabriel Schreiber and Sofia Avissar

Beer-Sheva Mental Health Center and Ben Gurion University of the Negev, PO Box 4600, Beer Sheva 84140, Israel

G proteins play a pivotal role in post-receptor information transduction. An important characteristic of G proteins is their increased guanine nucleotide binding following agonist stimulation, which in turn leads to their activation. We have developed a method which enables the measurement of early events in signal transduction beyond receptors, through activated receptor-coupled guanine nucleotide exchange on G proteins. Lithium was recently shown to inhibit the coupling of both muscarinic cholinergic and β-adrenergic receptors to pertussis toxin-sensitive and cholera toxin-sensitive G proteins, respectively, thus suggesting alteration of the function of G protein by lithium, as the single site for both the antimanic and antidepressant effects of this drug. One of the most puzzling aspects of the ability of lithium to ameliorate the manic depressive condition is its relatively selective action upon the central nervous system (CNS). It was previously shown that lithium selectively attenuated the function of G_s proteins in the CNS. In the present study we show that inhibition by lithium of muscarinic receptor-coupled G protein function is also selective to the CNS.

G proteins are distributed in cells throughout the body [1–3]. If these proteins are suggested as the biochemical target sites for the action of lithium, it has yet to be explained how lithium selectively alters the function of G proteins in the CNS, with only few peripheral side-effects. In the present study the effects of lithium on the function of receptor-coupled G proteins were compared between central (cerebral cortex) and peripheral (cardiac ventricles) tissues of the rat. We have previously shown that lithium selectively attenuated the function of G_s proteins in the CNS. Therapeutic concentrations of lithium (1–1.5 mM in vitro) inhibited the function of G_s protein in the cerebral cortex of the rat, while 4- to 6-fold larger concentrations of lithium were required to alter the function of G_s protein equivalently in the cardiac ventricles of the rat. Chronic administration of lithium totally abolished the effect of isoproterenol on the binding of GTP in the CNS, but did not affect the function of peripheral cardiac G_s protein [4]. It remains to be shown that inhibition by lithium of muscarinic receptor-coupled function is also selective to the CNS. Comparison of muscarinic agonist-coupled G protein function between the CNS and peripheral systems as exemplified by cardiac ventricles is, however, more complicated.

In contrast to isoproterenol, carbamylcholine does not induce any detectable increases in GTP binding capacity in rat cardiac ventricles. These differences in the ability of the β-adrenergic and the muscarinic agonists to alter GTP binding characteristics in cardiac membranes may be explained by the findings of Gilman et al. and [5], who reported that at low concentrations of Mg^{2+}, the tendency of G_i to dissociate appears to be greater than that of G_s. This characteristic of G_i is an important feature in the subunit dissociation model of action of this protein as an inhibitory regulator of adenylate cyclase activity [6]. In a previous study, we showed that pertussis toxin-blockable, carbamylcholine-induced increases in GTP binding capacity are mediated by the pharmacologically defined M_1 muscarinic receptors, as M_1-selective antagonists had a 100-fold greater ability than M_2-selective antagonists to block carbamylcholine effects in rat cerebral cortex [7]. Moreover, the carbamylcholine effect was exclusively detected in tissues such as the cerebral cortex and hippocampus, which are predominantly populated by M_1 receptors, whereas cerebellum and cardiac ventricles, which are mostly populated by M_2 receptors, failed to show carbamylcholine effects on GTP binding to G proteins [7]. The underlying biochemical mechanisms of these differences in the carbamylcholine effect are still unknown and may stem from different coupling mechanisms of the various muscarinic receptor subtypes. The fact that carbamylcholine does not induce increases in GTP binding capacity to pertussis toxin-sensitive G proteins in cardiac ventricles [7] is advantageous for exploring the

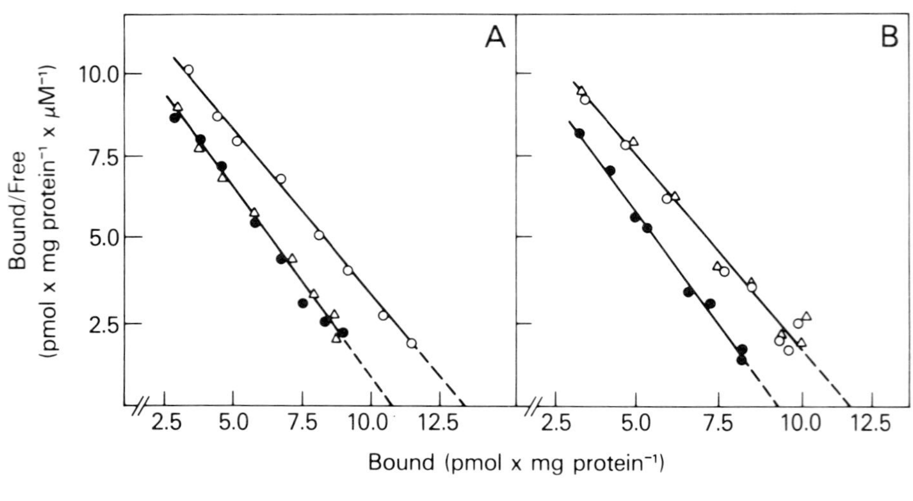

Fig. 1. Pertussis toxin-blockable muscarinic agonist inhibition of β-adrenergic agonist-induced increases in GTP binding capacity. Representative Scatchard plots of basal (●) and isoproterenol-induced [^{3}H]-GTP binding in the absence (○) or presence (Δ) of carbamylcholine to membranes prepared from rat cardiac ventricles. A) Untreated membranes exposed to ribosylation conditions in the absence of pertussis toxin; B) Membranes pretreated with pertussis toxin. Briefly, [^{3}]-GTP binding was carried out as follows: 200 μl of membranes were suspended in 25 mM Tris (pH 7.4), 1 mM ATP, 2 mM $MgCl_2$, 1 mM EGTA, 1 mM DTT were pipetted into microfuge tubes containing varying concentrations of [^{3}H]-GTP (0.05–5 μM). Incubation was carried out at room temperature under equilibrium conditions and the reaction was terminated by the addition of 5 volumes of ice-cold buffer followed by centrifugation at 10,000 g for 2 min. The pellets were rapidly washed 3 times and then re-suspended in 200 μl buffer. Bound radioactivity was measured by liquid scintillation spectrometry. All assays were carried out in triplicate, together with triplicate control samples containing 100 μM unlabeled Gpp(NH)p for determination of non-specific binding.

possibility of a muscarinic receptor-coupled effect through G_i on G_s protein function proximal to adenylate cyclase.

Figure 1A shows that carbamylcholine attenuates isoproterenol-induced increases in GTP binding capacity to G_s. This carbamylcholine effect reflects inhibitory influences exerted by a pertussis toxin-sensitive G_i protein on G_s as the inhibition of carbamylcholine of β-adrenergic-coupled G_s function was totally abolished by pretreatment of the cardiac membranes with pertussis toxin (Fig. 1B). Administration of lithium via rat chow containing lithium carbonate to rats for 3 weeks did not affect the ability of isoproterenol to induce increases in the binding capacity of GTP to G_s protein in rat cardiac membranes. It also did not affect the ability of carbamylcholine to inhibit isoproterenol effects in a pertussis toxin-sensitive manner. Thus, neither the function of peripheral cardiac G_s protein, nor the function of peripheral cardiac non-G_s proteins (i.e., G_i, G_o, G_p) were inhibited by lithium treatment.

The functions of both G_s and non-G_s proteins were previously shown to be sensitive to inhibition by lithium in rat cerebral cortex [7,8]. As subtypes of muscarinic receptors differ in their primary transducing effect (i.e., induction of PI turnover vs. adenylate cyclase inhibition) [9–11], different members of the G protein family (i.e. G_i, G_o, G_p) may be involved in the coupling of the various muscarinic receptor subtypes to their second messenger signalling systems [12]. Lithium selective effects on muscarinic receptor-coupled G protein function on the CNS vs. peripheral cardiac ventricles may stem from its differential interaction with M_1 receptor-coupled G_p in contrast to M_2 receptor-coupled G_i. It should be noted that heterogeneity exists with respect to α_s, α_i and α_o subunits of G proteins, and that differences may exist in their tissue distribution. Differential lithium interactions with the various α subunits may be a potential neurochemical explanation for its selective effects on brain G proteins.

Acknowledgement

This study was supported in part by a grant from the Chief Scientist Office of the Ministry of Health, Israel.

References

1. Gilman AG (1987) Annu. Rev. Biochem. 56: 615–649.
2. Casey PJ and Gilman AG (1988) J. Biol. Chem. 263: 2577–2580.
3. Neer E and Clapham DE (1988) Nature 333: 129–134.
4. Schreiber G, Avissar S, Aulakh CS and Murphy DL (1990) Neuropharmacology 29: 1067–1071.
5. Katada T, Bokoch GM, Northup JK, Ui M and Gilman AG (1984a) J. Biol. Chem 259: 3568–3577.
6. Katada T, Northup JK, Bokoch GM, Ui M and Gilman AG (1984b) J. Biol. Chem. 259: 3578–3585.
7. Avissar S and Schreiber G (1989) Biol. Psychiatry 26: 113–130.
8. Avissar S, Schreiber G, Danon A and Belmaker RH (1988) Nature 331: 440–442.

9. Gil DW and Wolfe BB (1985) Pharmacol. Exp. Ther 232: 608–616.
10. Peralta EG, Ashkenazi A, Winslow JW, Ramachandran J and Capon DJ (1988) Nature 334: 434–437.
11. Barnard EA (1988) Nature 335: 301–302.
12. Cockcroft S (1987) Trends Biochem. Sci. 12: 75–78.

Biological Psychiatry, Volume 1. G. Racagni et al., editors.

Interaction of antidepressants with phosphoinositide turnover in rat brain and human platelets

G.M. Pandey, S.C. Pandey and J.M. Davis
Illinois State Psychiatric Institute, 1601 West Taylor Street, Chicago, IL 60612, U.S.A.

Introduction

There is some evidence to suggest that the phosphoinositide (PI) signalling system may be involved in the mechanism of action of antidepressant drugs. Receptor-mediated activation of phospholipase C (PLC) causes breakdown of inositol phospholipids, leading to the formation of inositol triphosphate (IP_3) and diacyl-glycerol (DG), both of which function as second messengers [1]. The observation that lithium interferes with the PI turnover by inhibiting inositol-1-phosphatase raises the possibility that other psychoactive drugs may also interact with the PI signalling system and this interaction may be related to their mechanism of action [2]. We have therefore studied the in vitro effects of antidepressant drugs on PI turnover and inositol phospholipids in human platelets and rat brain.

Methods and Materials

Determination of PI turnover and inositol phospholipids in human platelets and rat brain

Inositol phosphate formation in human platelets and rat cortical slices was determined according to the method describd by Pandey et al. [3] and Berridge et al. [4], respectively. Inositol phospholipids were determined by a procedure described by Pandey et al. [3]. The platelet or cortical slices were incubated with ^{3}H-myoinositol in the presence or absence of test drugs for 3 h and 1 h respectively at 37°C. Inositol phospholipids were extracted by shaking with a $CHCl_3$, methanol, and HCl mixture. Aqueous and organic phase were separated by centrifugation, and organic phase was used for the determination of various inositol phospholipids by TLC.

Results

Effect of antidepressants and neuroleptics on inositol phosphate formation and inoitol phospholipids

We observed that the tricyclic antidepressants, desipramine (DMI), imipramine

(IMI), and amitriptyline (AMI) as well as the atypical antidepressant iprindole (IP) and the neuroleptics thioridazine (TH) and chlorpromazine caused a significant inhibition of thrombin (4 units/ml) stimulated IP_2 and IP_3 but not IP_1 formation in human platelets. We also observed that other antidepressants, trazodone, mianserine, and phenelzine, as well as the neuroleptic haloperidol did not cause a significant inhibition of inositol phosphate formation (Table 1). These results thus suggested that tricyclic antidepressants and phenothiazines caused inhibition of thrombin stimulated IP_2 and IP_3 formation. We also determined the effect of antidepressant and neuroleptics on various inositol phospholipids in human platelets and, as reported previously by us [3], we observed that DMI, IP, IMI and AMI caused a significant increase in all three phospholipids, that is, PI, PIP and PIP_2. Thioridazine caused a significant increase in the [^{3}H]-PI levels but a slight decrease in the levels of [^{3}H]-PIP and ^{3}H-PIP_2. Haloperidol, which had no significant effects on IP_2 and IP_3 formation, also caused a small but significant increase in the inositol phospholipids [3]. However, phenelzine and mianserine had marginal effects on inositol phospholipids.

In rat brain it is difficult to measure the initial product of PIP_2 hydrolysis, that is, IP_2 and IP_3, and most studies have used the method of Perridge et al. [4], which measures the accumulation of IP_1 in the presence of lithium. We observed that the tricyclic antidepressants DMI and IMI caused significant inhibition of norepinephrine (NE) and serotonin (SHT) stimulated IP_1 formation in rat cortex (Table 1).

We also observed that DMI and IMI caused a significant increase in ^{3}H-PI, ^{3}H-PIP and ^{3}H-PIP_2 inositol phospholipids in rat cortex (Table 2). Our results thus suggested that similar to the platelets tricyclic antidepressants caused an inhibition of agonist-stimulated inositol phosphate formation as well as an increase in the levels of ^{3}H-inositol phospholipids in rat brain.

Table 1. Effect of psychoactive drugs on inositol phosphate formation in human platelets and rat brain

Human platelets				Rat cortex	
Drugs	[^{3}H]IP_1	[^{3}H]IP_2	[^{3}H]IP_3	Drugs	[^{3}H]-IP_1
Thrombin	100 ± 4.6	100 ± 12.1	100 ± 10.5	NE	100 ± 16.6
Thrombin + iprindole	94 ± 3.9	44 ± 7.1	42 ± 8.5	NE + DMI	30 ± 5.7
Desipramine	96 ± 3.6	48 ± 6.8	59 ± 8.8	5-HT	100 ± 8.5
Imipramine	89 ± 7.1	64 ± 6.6	57 ± 10.7	5-HT + DMI	39 ± 1.8
Amitriptyline	98 ± 5.8	65 ± 3.8	72 ± 12.7	NE	100 ± 4.4
Chlorpromazine	95 ± 3.7	43 ± 5.2	40 ± 10.8	NE + IMI	32 ± 5.9
Thioridazine	86 ± 5.0	41 ± 11.5	53 ± 12.5		
Haloperidol	95 ± 2.3	102 ± 24.3	101 ± 9.3		
Trazodone	98 ± 2.0	93 ± 17.8	73 ± 8.0		
Mianserin	105 ± 3.2	101 ± 21.4	108 ± 11.5		
Phenelzine	95 ± 6.2	90 ± 15.4	89 ± 14.7		

Values are mean ± S.E.M. from 3-10 determinations and represented as percent of controls. Concentration of drugs, NE and 5-HT are 10^{-4} M.

Table 2. Effect of antidepressant drugs on the levels of [^{3}H]-PI, [^{3}H]-PIP and [^{3}H]-PIP_2 in rat cortex

	[^{3}H]-PI	[^{3}H]-PIP	[^{3}H]-PIP_2
None (4)	2808 ± 550	365 ± 87	106 ± 15
Desipramine (4)	5853 ± 1935	900 ± 304	214 ± 44
Imipramine (3)	5783 ± 1741	1537 ± 674	247 ± 67

Each value is mean ± S.E.M. and represented as DPM/mg protein. Values within brackets indicate number of determinations.

Several factors may account for the observed decrease in inositol phosphate formation in human platelets by tricyclic antidepressants and thioridazine. These include a decrease in phosphoinositide substrate due to inhibition of PI and PIP kinase, or stimulation of PIP and PIP_2 phosphomonoesterase, or inhibition of the enzyme phospholipase C. Since antidepressants cause an increase in the level of ^{3}H-inositol phospholipids, it is quite likely that this decrease is related to the inhibition of the enzyme PLC rather than increased dephosphorylation or decreased phosphorylation of the inositol phospholipids. This inhibition of PLC may be either due to the blockade of thrombin receptors, the decreased coupling of G protein to the receptors, or the inhibition of the enzyme itself by antidepressants. It is least likely that the decrease in inositol phosphate formation by antidepressants is due to the blockade of thrombin receptors.

We also observed that DMI and IMI caused a significant inhibition of agonist stimulated IP_1 formation in rat cortex and increased the levels of ^{3}H-PI, ^{3}H-PIP and ^{3}H-PIP_2. The effects thus appear to he similar to that observed in platelets. Our results are similar to those of Li et al. [5] who also observed a decrease in NE stimulated inositol phosphate formation by DMI and IMI. The effect of acute and chronic treatment with antidepressants has been studied by several investigators and it has been observed that chronic treatment with antidepressants caused a decrease in 5-HT_2 receptors and 5-HT stimulated inositol phosphate formation in rat brain [6]. Thus, it appears that in vitro effects of antidepressants on PI turnover may differ from chronic effects. Whereas under in vitro conditions, the inhibition of inositol phosphate formation in rat brain may be related to the inhibition of the enzyme phospholipase c, the decrease in PI turnover observed after chronic treatment with antidepressants is related to a decrease in 5-HT_2 and/or α_1-adrenergic receptors. This difference in the effects of antidepressants under in vitro conditions and after chronic treatment should be taken into account in attempts to understand the therapeutic mechanism of action of antidepressant drugs. Further studies are needed to precisely examine the site of interaction of antidepressant drugs with PI turnover.

References

1. Berridge MJ (1987) Ann. Rev. Biochem. 56: 159–193.
2. Allison JH and Stewart MA (1971) Nature New Biol. 233: 267–268.
3. Pandey SC, Davis JM, Schwertz DW and Pandey GM (1991) J. Pharmacol. Exp. Ther. 256: 1010–1018.
4. Berridge MJ, Downes CP and Hanley MR (1982) Biochem. J. 206: 587–595.
5. Li PP, Warsh JL, Sibon D and Chiu A (1988) Neurochem. Res. 13: 1111–1118.
6. Kendall DA and Nahorski SR (1985) J. Pharmacol. Exp. Ther. 233: 473–479.

Biological Psychiatry, Volume 1. G. Racagni et al., editors.

ECS effect on second messengers in rat brain

Jerzy Vetulani

Department of Biochemistry, Institute of Pharmacology, Polish Academy of Sciences, Smetna 12, 31-343 Kraków, Poland

Introduction

Since the discovery that chronic ECS, similarly to other antidepressant treatments, down-regulates β-adrenoceptor responses [1], its neurochemical effects have been thoroughly studied, particularly as the treatment is regarded as one of the most efficient in alleviating depression [2], and studies on its mechanism of action are simplified because of absence of pharmacokinetic complications. The action of ECS on second messenger systems is of particular importance, as changes in this system reflect the functional effects of the treatment more than the alterations of receptor parameters. In this paper the results of our studies on second messenger systems linked with adrenoceptors will be briefly reviewed.

Effect of ECS on phosphatidylinositol system

Immediately after a single or repeated ECS the hydrolysis of membrane polyphosphoinositides is augmented (possibly because of receptor-mediated activation of protein kinase C (PKC) due to enhanced neurotransmitter release) [3], but we observed no effect of chronic ECS on basal inositol phosphate (IP) level 24 h after the last treatment. As several authors, including our group (cf. [4]), reported an increase in α_1-adrenoceptor density in the rat cerebral cortex after prolonged ECS, we investigated whether a functional up-regulation of α_1-adrenoceptor exists, which might be reflected by an increase in the accumulation of IP upon exposure to noradrenaline. However, chronic ECS, and also imipramine, in normal rats tended to depress rather than augment the IP response ([5,6] and unpublished results). In another experiment we confirmed the findings of Newman et al. [7] that carbachol-induced IP accumulation in cortical slices is unaffected by ECS.

Several other authors also reported no effect of ECS on noradrenaline-induced IP accumulation, but Newman et al. [7] have observed an increase in noradrenaline-induced IP accumulation after a single or chronic ECS. A possibility that this was a response characteristic for the Sabra strain of rats used in their work cannot be excluded as ECS may elevate IP accumulation if the animals are particularly sensitive to α_1-adrenergic stimulation. This was demonstrated by our finding that in rats with noradrenergic system made hypersensitive by mild reserpinization not only the ECS-induced increase in the number of α_1-adrenoceptors was further augmented, but also the sensitivity of the IP generating system to noradrenaline was increased, as indicated by a decline in the noradrenaline E_{50} from 7.6 to 2.3 μM without change in the maximum effect [6].

Effect of ECS on cyclic AMP generating system

α-β-Adrenoceptor interaction as a target of ECS action

Responses to noradrenaline, isoproterenol and 6-fluoronoradrenaline. The fact that a mixed β- and α-adrenoceptor agonist noradrenaline is more efficient in stimulation of cyclic AMP accumulation than a pure β-adrenoceptor agonist isoproterenol and that after central chemosympathectomy the response to noradrenaline is much more up-regulated than that to isoproterenol [8] suggested the importance of α-adrenoceptor for cyclic AMP generation. Pilc and Enna [9] postulated that a possible site for antidepressant-induced down-regulation of β-adrenoceptors is the synergistic interaction between the adrenoceptor subclasses. For chronic ECS, it was established that the treatment does not depress the response of the cyclic AMP generating system to isoproterenol, although it reduces the responses produced by noradrenaline or a mixture of isoproterenol and a nonspecific α-adrenoceptor agonist, 6-fluoronoradrenaline [5]. In contrast, our recent results (to be published) indicate that chronic administration of imipramine induces down-regulation of the cyclic AMP response both to noradrenaline and to isoproterenol. This seems to be an important difference in the mode of action of ECS and imipramine. It should be added, however, that the results may also depend on the intensity of treatment and the strain: Pilc and Enna [9] did not find down-regulation of cyclic AMP response to desipramine in Sprague-Dawley rats, and a scrutiny of the results of Pilc et al. [5], carried out on Wistar rats, suggest that ECS may produce a weak down-regulatory response to isoproterenol.

Cyclic AMP responses after α-adrenoceptor destruction with EEDQ. To study the involvement of α-adrenoceptors in more detail we used the compound EEDQ, which in lower doses selectively destroys α-adrenoceptor binding sites [10]. Pretreatment with EEDQ, which by itself caused a depression in the cyclic AMP response to noradrenaline but did not affect β-adrenoceptor density, accelerated β-adrenoceptor down-regulation induced by short-term ECS (3 shocks) measured by the depression of the density of dihydroalprenolol binding sites, but did not produce any further down-regulation in cyclic AMP response [11]. We interpreted these results assuming that the functional down-regulation produced by EEDQ without depression of the density of β-adrenoceptor binding sites was caused by destruction of α-adrenoceptors. On the other hand, the depression by ECS of β-adrenoceptor density without functional down-regulation might be either due to a large β-adrenoceptor reserve or to a compensatory increase in the efficiency of coupling between the β-adrenoceptor and G_s protein.

The role of protein kinase C (PKC). We have proposed that protein kinase C, which is intimately involved in α-β-adrenoceptor coupling, may play an important role in the antidepressant-induced β-down-regulation [12]. Activation of α_1-adrenoceptor leads to formation of IP and diacylglycerol, and the latter activates PKC. PKC phosphorylates, among others, G proteins coupled to α_1- and β-adrenoceptors. As phosphorylation of G_i inhibits its activity, and phosphorylation of G_s increases it, the net result of PKC activation will be an increase in formation of cyclic AMP (cf. [12] for references). A PKC activator, phorbol ester TPA, increased the cyclic AMP response to noradrenaline by 40%, while the response to isoproterenol was augmented by 206% [13]. The down-regulation of the response to noradrenaline or isoproterenol produced by ECS was negligible in the presence of TPA: activation of PKC restored the responsiveness of the cyclic AMP generating system depressed by ECT. In contrast, the down-regulation produced by chronic imipramine was well expressed (particularly for the response to isoproterenol) also in the presence of TPA [13]. In an in vitro experiment it was demonstrated that imipramine directly inhibits PKC [12]. As responses to forskolin, a direct activator of adenylate cyclase were affected neither by antidepressant treatment nor by TPA [13], it could be concluded that β-adrenoceptor down-regulation does not involve processes related to changes in the adenylate cyclase activity, and therefore is restricted to the recognition and transduction units of the β-adrenoceptor complex. PKC may be specifically involved in β-adrenoceptor regulation produced by some antidepressant drugs, but not by ECS. Specifically, the difference between the β-down-regulation produced by ECS and imipramine (and possibly other antidepressants of this class) is that imipramine inhibits PKC activity in a mode that is irreversible by TPA. The lack of inhibition of PKC by ECS may be one of the factors responsible for the high efficiency of ECS in the clinic.

References

1. Vetulani J and Sulser F (1975) Nature 257: 495–496.
2. Fink M (1979) Lancet i: 1303–1304.
3. Vadnal RE and Bazan NG (1987) Neurosci. Lett. 80: 75–79.
4. Green AR (1990) In: Heal DJ and Marsden CA (eds.) The Pharmacology of Noradrenaline in the Central Nervous System. Oxford University Press, Oxford, pp. 316–348.
5. Pilc A, Chalecka-Franaszek E, Nalepa I, Vetulani J and Enna SJ (1988) Eur. J. Pharmacol. 156: 143–147.
6. Pilc A, Nalepa I and Vetulani J (1988) Eur. J. Pharmacol. 157: 231–234.
7. Newman ME, Miskin I and Lerer B (1987) J. Neurochem. 49: 19–23.
8. Vetulani J, Stawarz RJ and Sulser F (1976) J. Neurochem. 27: 661–666.
9. Pilc A and Enna SJ (1985) Life Sci. 31: 1183–1194.
10. Pilc A, Vetulani J, Nomura S and Enna SJ (1989) Brain Res. 493: 8–13.
11. Pilc A and Vetulani J (1990) Neuropharmacology 29: 469–473.
12. Nalepa I and Vetulani J (1991) Neuroscience (in press).
13. Nalepa I and Vetulani J (1991) J. Neurochem. (in press).

Biological Psychiatry, Volume 1. G. Racagni et al., editors.

Second messenger transduction associated with 5-HT in the pathogenesis and treatment of affective disorders

Michael E. Newman, Baruch Shapira, Pesach Lichtenberg and Bernard Lerer
Yaacov Herzog Centre for Brain and Psychiatry Research, Ezrath Nashim Hospital, P.O.B. 140; and Biological Psychiatry Laboratory, Department of Psychiatry, Hadassah University Hospital, P.O.B. 12000, Jerusalem 91120, Israel

There is much evidence for a role of serotonin (5-HT) in the pathogenesis of depression and the mechanism of action of antidepressant drugs. Two possible modes of action have received attention; an effect on the 5-HT uptake site or transporter which binds the antidepressant drug imipramine and an effect on 5-HT_2 receptors. Studies involving repeated treatment of rats with antidepressants have not on the whole shown any alterations of the binding of ^{3}H-imipramine or ^{3}H-paroxetine to membranes of cerebral cortex [1]. Recent findings [2,3] have also cast doubt on the original demonstration [4] of up-regulation of 5-HT_2 receptors in cortical samples from postmortem suicide brains. In addition, the effects of antidepressants to down-regulate 5-HT_2 receptors in rat cortex [5] do not extend to an important non-pharmacological treatment, electroconvulsive shock [6,7] where up-regulation is observed instead. Furthermore, 5-HT_2 receptors show abnormal regulation in that they are not up-regulated after destruction of serotonergic neurons or antagonist administration, and in some cases are even down-regulated. This has led Leysen [8] to propose that these receptors receive little stimulation under normal physiological conditions and may exist in a supersensitive state.

There has recently been increasing evidence for involvement of 5-HT_{1A} receptors in antidepressant action. 5-HT_{1A} agonists are active in several animal models of depression [9–12] and were effective in both open and controlled clinical trials of depressed patients [13–16]. Chronic administration of antidepressants including Li and ECS to animals reduced both the hypothermia and the behavioural syndrome induced by the 5-HT_{1A} agonist 8-OH-DPAT [17], and also reduced the degree of inhibition of forskolin-stimulated adenylate cyclase activity induced by 5-HT in rat hippocampal membranes [18–20]. Changes in this latter parameter have in some cases been shown to accompany changes in binding of ^{3}H-8-OH-DPAT to rat hippocampal membranes. There is also preliminary evidence for a change in the density of 5-HT_{1A} receptors in hippocampus of postmortem suicide brains [21].

Human platelets have been extensively used as models for neurones [22] and many studies of both 5-HT uptake and 5-HT_2 receptor number in platelets from depressed patients have been conducted. It is now considered doubtful whether the density of the 5-HT uptake site in platelets is decreased in affective disorders as first reported [1]. Biegon et al. [23–25], using ^{3}H-ketanserin as ligand, demonstrated increased 5-HT_2 receptor number in platelets from depressed patients and attempted suicides, and a reduction in this parameter after antidepressant treatment, findings which match both the initial findings in postmortem suicide brain [4] and the effects of antidepressants on rat brain 5-HT_2 receptors [5]. Similar findings of elevated 5-HT_2 receptor number in platelets of depressed patients were obtained by Arora and Meltzer [26] and Pandey et al. [27] using either ^{3}H- or ^{125}I-LSD. However, Cowen et al. [28,29] using the same ligands, did not observe a change in platelets from depressed patients, and in addition observed an increase rather than a decrease in binding after antidepressant treatment. The same authors [30] also failed to observe a change in ^{125}I-LSD binding to platelets of depressed patients after Li treatment.

We have recently [31] provided preliminary evidence that in human platelet membranes 5-HT both stimulates adenylate cyclase activity under basal conditions, and inhibits adenylate cyclase activity when the enzyme is stimulated by forskolin. These activities parallel those observed with 5-HT and certain of its analogs at the 5-HT_{1A} receptor in rat or guinea pig hippocampal membranes [32–34]. The possibility thus exists that a receptor similar to the 5-HT_{1A} receptor found in several regions of human and animal brain may also exist in human platelets. This receptor is distinct from the site on human platelets labelled by ^{3}H-8-OH-DPAT, a ligand with high affinity for 5-HT_{1A} receptors, which was concluded by Ieni and Meyerson [35] to represent a component of the 5-HT transporter. In the present work we have examined the effect of 5-HT to inhibit

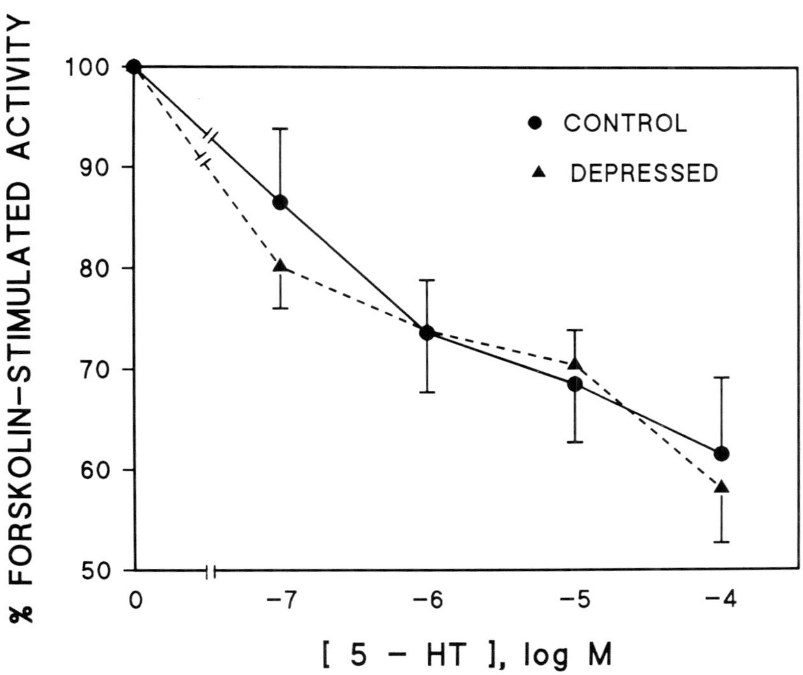

Fig. 1.

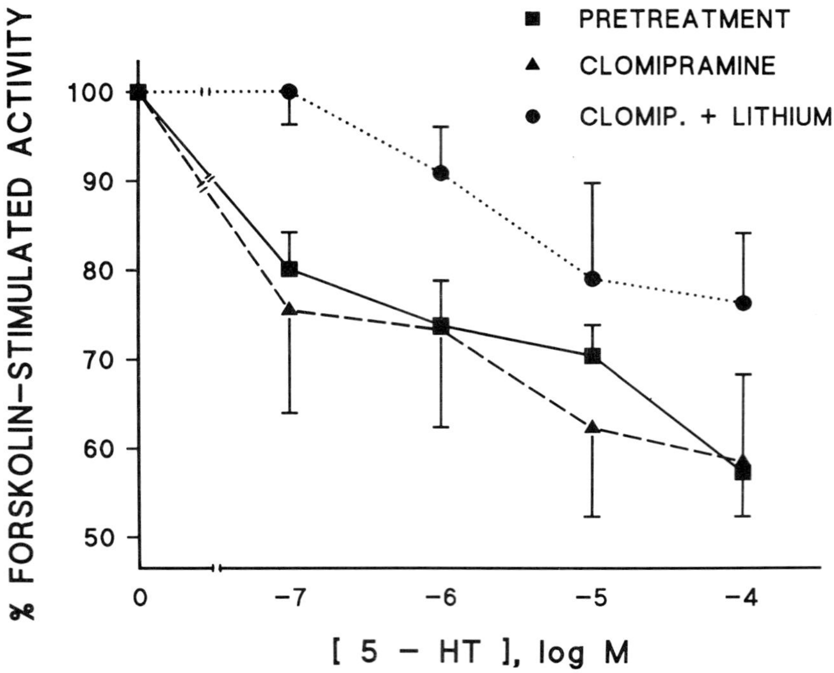

Fig. 2.

forskolin-stimulated adenylate cyclase in platelet membranes derived from control subjects, depressed patients and patients before and after treatment with the tricyclic antidepressant clomipramine with and without Li supplementation. Maximum inhibition in membranes from 10 control subjects was 34.6 ± 2.7% and the EC_{50} for 5-HT 0.19 ± 0.09 μM. There was no difference in the degree of inhibition between membranes from control compared to depressed subjects (Fig. 1), and treatment of the same depressed subjects with 250 mg/day clomipramine for 4 weeks had no effect (Fig. 2). However, addition of Li for a further 3 weeks to the clomipramine regimen resulted in a decrease in the degree of inhibition by 5-HT, an effect similar to that seen in hippocampal membranes from rats which had received a combination of DMI and Li [20]. We conclude that 5-HT inhibition of forskolin-stimulated adenylate cyclase in platelet membranes is capable of showing adaptive changes and may represent a useful peripheral measure of human serotonergic function. The relationship of this activity to the 5-HT_{1A} receptor remains to be determined.

Acknowledgement

This work was supported by Grant No. MH 43873 from the National Institutes of Health, U.S.A.

References

1. Marcusson JO and Ross SB (1990) Psychopharmacology 102: 145–155.
2. Cheetham SC, Crompton MR, Katona CLE and Horton RW (1988) Brain Res. 443: 272–280.
3. Gross-Isseroff R, Salama D, Israeli M and Biegon A (1990) Brain Res. 507: 208–215.
4. Stanley M and Mann JJ (1983) Lancet i: 214–216.
5. Peroutka SJ and Snyder SH (1980) Science 210: 88–90.
6. Kellar EJ, Cascio CS, Butler JA and Kurtze RN (1981) Eur. J. Pharmacol. 69: 515–518.
7. Vetulani J, Lebrecht U and Pilc A (1981) Eur. J. Pharmacol. 76: 81–85.
8. Leysen JE (1990) Clin. Neuropharmacol. 13 (Suppl. 2): 230–231.
9. Cervo L and Samanin R (1987) Eur. J. Pharmacol. 144: 223–229.
10. Kennett GA, Dourish CT and Curzon G (1987) Eur. J. Pharmacol. 134: 265–274.
11. Wieland S and Lucki I (1990) Psychopharmacology 101: 497–504.
12. Martin P, Beninger RJ, Hamon M and Puech AJ (1990) Behav. Brain Res. 38: 135–144.
13. Schweitzer EE, Amsterdam JD, Rickels K, Kaplan M and Droba M (1986) Psychopharmacol. Bull. 22: 183–185.
14. Amsterdam JD, Berwish N, Potter L and Rickels K (1987) Curr. Ther. Res. 41: 185–193.
15. Kurtz NM, Keppel-Hesselink J, Beneke M and Heller AH (1990) Clin. Neurophmacol. 13 (Suppl. 2): 95–96.
16. Robinson DS, Gammans RE, Shrotriya RC, Jenkins SW, Andary JJ, Alms DR and Messina ME (1990) Clin. Neuropharmacol. 13 (Suppl. 2): 228–229.
17. Goodwin GM (1989) Prog. Neuro-Psychopharmacol. Biol. Psychiatry 13: 445–451.
18. Newman ME and Lerer B (1988) Eur. J. Pharmacol. 148: 257–260.
19. Sleight AJ, Marsden CA, Palfreyman AG, Mir AK and Lovenberg W (1988) Eur. J. Pharmacol. 154: 255–261.
20. Newman ME, Drummer D, Lerer B (1990) J. Pharmacol. Exp. Ther. 252: 826–831.
21. Cheetham SC, Crompton MR, Katona CLE and Horton RW (1990) Psychopharmacology 102: 544–548.
22. Pletscher A (1986) Clin. Neuropharmacol. (Suppl. 4): 344–346.
23. Biegon A, Weizman A, Karp L, Ram A, Tiano S and Wolff M (1987) Life Sci. 41: 2485–2492.
24. Biegon A, Grinspoon A, Blumenfeld B, Bleich A, Apter A and Mester R (1990) Psychopharmacology 100: 165–167.
25. Biegon A, Essar N, Israeli M, Elizur A, Bruch S and Bar-Nathan AA (1990) Psychopharmacology 102: 73–75.
26. Arora RC and Meltzer HY (1989) Life Sci. 44: 725–734.
27. Pandey GN, Pandey SC, Janicak PG, Marks RC and Davis JM (1990) Biol. Psychiatry 28: 215–222.
28. Cowen PJ, Geaney DP, Schachter M, Green AR and Elliott JM (1986) Arch. Gen. Psychiatry 43: 61–67.
29. Cowen PJ, Charig EM, Fraser S, Elliott JM (1987) J. Affective Disord. 13: 45–50.
30. Glue PW, Cowen PJ, Nutt DJ, Kolakowska T and Grahame-Smith DG (1986) Psychopharmacology 90: 398–402.
31. Newman ME and Lerer B (1990) Clin. Neuropharmacol. 13 (Suppl.2): 237–238.
32. de Vivo M and Maayani S (1986) J. Pharmacol. Exp. Ther. 238: 248–253.
33. Markstein R, Hoyer D and Engel G (1986) Naunyn-Schmiedebergs Arch. Pharmakol.333: 335–341.
34. Shenker A, Maayani S, Weinstein and Green JP (1987) Mol. Pharmacol. 31: 357–367.
35. Ieni JR and Meyerson LR (1988) Life Sci. 42: 311–320.

Biological Psychiatry, Volume 1. G. Racagni et al., editors.

Effects of antidepressants and electroconvulsive shock on coupling of G protein to adenylate cyclase

Hiroki Ozawa[1], Shinichi Hatta[2], Mark M. Rasenick[3], Naohiko Takahata[1] and Toshikazu Saito[1]

[1]Department of Neuropsychiatry; and [2]Department of Pharmacology, Sapporo Medical College, Sapporo 060, Japan; [3]Department of Physiology and Biophysics, University of Illinois College of Medicine, Chicago, IL 60680, U.S.A.

Introduction

A monoamine theory was proposed in the 1960s, and a β-adrenergic receptor or 5-HT_2 receptor downregulation theory in the late 1970s on the action of antidepressants. However, recently many studies have not been in agreement with the above theories. Antidepressants have effects on multiple loci which contain dopamine, $GABA_B$, acetylchloride and neuropeptides, alone or in combination [1]. Thus, a single neurotransmitter is unlikely to account for the common mechanisms of antidepressant action. Our group first reported that long-term treatment by antidepressants and electroconvulsive shock (ECS) enhance Gpp(NH)p stimulated adenylate cyclase (AC) activity in rat cerebral cortex membranes [2]. This laboratory and others have postulated that G proteins form part of a molecular locus for antidepressant action, but additional data are required to clarify hypothesis. In the search for a single common mechanism for antidepressant and ECS action, the present study examines effects of antidepressants and ECS on β-adrenergic receptor, G protein mediated stimulation (Gs) or inhibition (Gi) of adenylate cyclase in a membrane preparation from rat cerebral cortex.

Methods

Male Sprague-Dawley rats (150–200 g) were injected (intraperitoneally) once daily for 1 day (acute) or 21 days (chronic) with desipramine, amitriptyline, iprindole (10 mg/kg) or saline (as control). ECS treatment was administered with sinusoidal current (80 mA, 60 Hz, 0.2 s) using ear clip electrodes. This treatment caused typical tonic clonic convulsion for 10–30 s. ECS was administered every other day between 1 and 11 times for 22 days. Sham treatment consisted of electrodes applied without current. Animals were sacrificed 24 h after the last treatment and cerebral cortex membranes were prepared and assayed for adenylate cyclase or analyzed by SDS-PAGE.

Results and Discussion

The long-term administration of tricyclic antidepressants or ECS induced a significant decrease in β-adrenergic receptor number and isoproterenol stimulated adenylate cyclase (AC) activity in membrane preparation of brain cortex. In contrast to the above results, Gpp(NH)p, NaF or forskolin stimulated AC activity was increased in rat cerebral cortex membranes. Inhibition of AC was not affected by this treatment. The chemical elimination of Gs functions (low pH treatment) abolished all differences between treated and control groups. Non-neuronal tissues from treated animals showed no differences in AC to those from control animals. The dissociation constant (K_d) and maximal binding (B_{max}) for AAGTP (a hydrolysis-resistant, photoaffinity GTP analog) to synaptic membrane G proteins was unchanged after antidepressants or ECS treatment (Fig. 1). Thus, it is unlikely that there was any change in the quantity or GTP-binding capacity of Gs. However, the transfer of [^{32}P]-AAGTP from Gi/o to Gs was accelerated by this treatment.

Recently, it has been reported that although AC appears to bind calmodulin, the regulation of enzyme activity by that compound is complicated and likely to involve G proteins. When membranes were assayed under conditions in the absence of 1 mM EGTA, chronic treatment with antidepressant increased basal AC

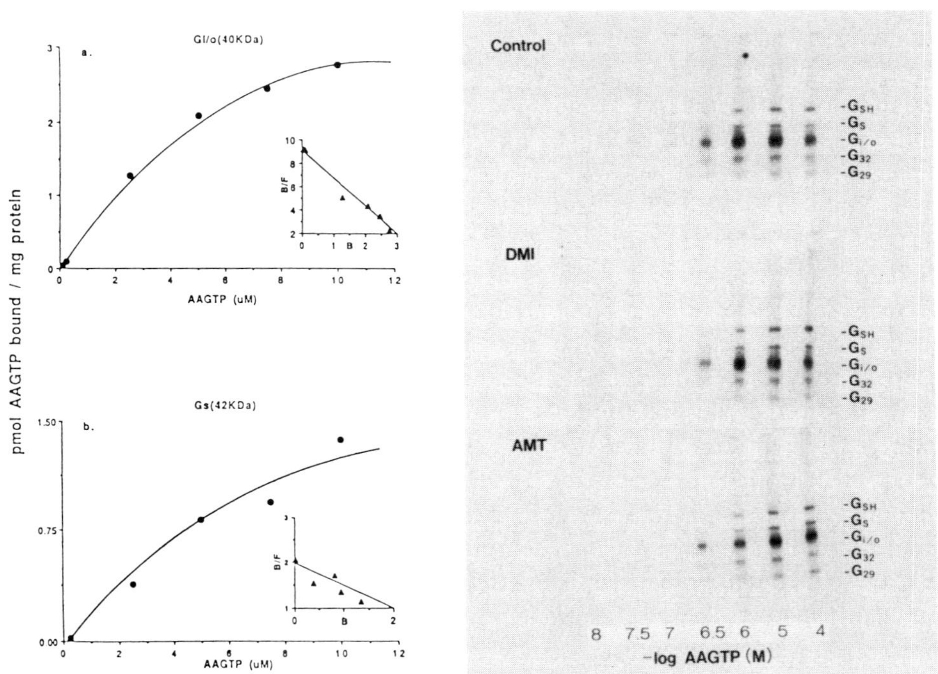

Fig. 1. Kinetics of nucleotide binding to G proteins after chronic antidepressant treatment. Isotherms and Scatchard plots of AAGTP binding (left), a representative autoradiogram of SDS-PAGE of membrane proteins labelled with [^{32}P]-AAGTP (right).

activity but not in the presence of EGTA. Enhancement of GppNHp stimulated AC activity by antidepressants; however, it was not affected by EGTA. Ca^{2+} dependent AC activity was enhanced in membranes from rats chronically treated with antidepressants by the addition of 1 μM calmodulin. In the absence of calmodulin, however, Ca^{2+} dependent AC activity was not altered by chronic antidepressant treatment. Ca^{2+} dependent AC activity stimulated by Gpp(NH)p was increased in membranes from rats treated by chronic antidepressants with or without calmodulin.

These results suggest that enhanced AC after chronic treatment by antidepressants and ECS is due to a change in the nature of Gs or increased coupling between Gs and the catalytic unit of AC, but no direct effects on Gi. Furthermore increased sensitivity of Ca^2/calmodulin by chronic antidepressant treatment on the AC system may be attributed to enhanced coupling between Gs and the catalytic unit of AC. Thus, the molecular locus of action of antidepressant and ECS may reside at the stimulatory GTP-binding protein (Gs).

The β and D_1 receptor appears to be the major Gs-linked receptor types. The observation of downregulation of these receptors or the subsensitivity of the receptor agonist mediated cAMP accumulation seems to contrast with the observation of guanine nucleotide stimulated adenylate cyclase activity. However, recent work from our laboratory has suggested that the receptor coupled to a G protein prevents the G protein (specifically Gs) from interacting with the catalytic subunit of adenylate cyclase and activating that enzyme [3]. Thus, if a G protein is freed from the constraints of receptor coupling, it would be expected to interact more successfully with the appropriate intracellular effector molecule. Thus, downregulation of a Gs-linked receptor might result in increased adenylate cyclase activity within an affected neuron by increasing receptor-independent activation of that enzyme which is the increased coupling between Gs and the adenylate cyclase catalytic moiety. A similar speculation may occur in effects of chronic antidepressant treatment on D_1 receptor-adenylate cyclase system [4].

What is the physiological meaning of the reconciliation of receptor-G protein-effector regulation on the action of antidepressant? The possibility of intracellular (receptor-independent) activation of neuronal adenylate cyclase has been proposed previously by this laboratory. Much of the rationale for such endogenous regulation resides in the fact that, in the mammalian brain, the quantity of neurotransmitter capable of stimulating adenylate cyclase is at least 100-fold lower than amount of neurotransmitter capable of inhibiting that enzyme. The current paradigms involved to explain the dual regulation of adenylate cyclase require inhibition of a stimulated enzyme. Thus, neurotransmitters that act by inhibiting adenylate cyclase might be expected to be ineffective without prior exposure of a cell to a stimulatory agonist. Therefore, intraneuronal regulation of adenylate cyclase could provide the basis for a hypothesis on new treatment and pathogenesis in depression.

GsH or Gs is a cholera toxin substrate which stimulates adenylate cyclase (PAGE M_r 52 kDa, 42 kDa respectively). Gi is a pertussis toxin substrate which inhibits adenylate cyclase (PAGE M_r 40 kDa). Go is a pertussis toxin substrate, slightly smaller than Gi (PAGE M_r 39 kDa) without a clear function in second messenger systems. Gi/o is a mixed band of Gi and Go. These GTP binding proteins were indicated by ADP ribosylation and Western blots with antibodies supplied by S. Mumby and A. Gilman. G_{32} or G_{29} is a major AAGTP binding protein in rat cerebral cortex synaptic membranes; however, it is not clear whether this species functions in signal transduction.

References

1. Heninger GR and Charney DS (1987) Psychopharmacology, The Third Generation of Progress. Raven Press, New York, pp. 535–544.
2. Menkes DB et al. (1983) Science 129: 65–67.
3. Rasenick MM et al. (1988) Brain Res. 488: 105–113.
4. De Montis GM et al. (1990) Eur. J. Pharmacol. 180: 169–174.

Biological Psychiatry, Volume 1. G. Racagni et al., editors.

Mechanisms of lithium in modulation of postreceptor second messenger function in rat brain

Arne Mørk and Pia Hollund
Department of Pharmacology, University of Copenhagen, Juliane Maries Vej 20, DK-2100 Copenhagen, Denmark

It has been demonstrated that lithium in vitro and ex vivo, i.e. after chronic treatment, affects the levels of second messengers generated by adenylate cyclase and phospholipase C in the brain [1]. The neurotransmitter stimulation of adenylate cyclase is analogous to activation of phospholipid hydrolysis insofar as the neurotransmitter-receptor signal is transferred to the second messenger generating enzyme via proteins belonging to the family of G proteins [2]. Thus, stimulatory and inhibitory neurotransmitter signals are transferred to the catalytic unit of adenylate cyclase by G_s and G_i respectively, and signals to phospholipase C are transferred by G_p [2].

Recent studies have suggested that lithium inhibition in vitro of adenylate cyclase activity is competitive with magnesium ions (Mg^{2+}) [3,4], suggesting that lithium in vitro interacts with the Mg^{2+} ion sites on the G proteins and/or the catalytic unit. Furthermore, Mg^{2+} has been reported to reverse lithium inhibition in vitro of β-adrenoceptor- and muscarinic receptor-induced GTP binding in rat cerebral cortex [5]. This lithium-Mg^{2+} interaction may have significant clinical implications. However, studies from our laboratory indicate that the chronic effect of lithium is different from the in vitro effect, since: 1) the inhibitory action of lithium ex vivo on adenylate cyclase activity is not antagonized by Mg^{2+}; 2) the sensitivity of adenylate cyclase activity to lithium in vitro is unaltered after chronic lithium treatment; and 3) the lithium inhibition ex vivo is still persistent after washing the brain tissue [6]. In addition, the action of lithium ex vivo on both guanylyl-5'-imidodiphosphate (Gpp(NH)p)- and β-adrenoceptor-stimulated adenylate cyclase can be observed at both 3 and 10 mM Mg^{2+} [7].

The inhibitory action of chronic lithium treatment on forskolin-, manganese- and calcium-stimulated adenylate cyclase activity in rat cerebral cortex suggests that lithium reduces the activity of the catalytic unit [4,6,8]. However, recent studies on neurotransmitter receptor-mediated processes indicate that lithium ex vivo exerts more than one effect on the second messenger system generating cAMP. Lithium ex vivo inhibits isoprenaline-induced GTP stimulation of adenylate cyclase but does not affect the enzyme activity stimulated by GTP alone [9,10], suggesting that lithium influences the mechanisms by which the β-adrenoceptor enhances GTP-stimulated adenylate cyclase activity via G_s. This assumption is supported by the fact that lithium ex vivo decreases isoprenaline-induced GTP binding in rat brain without affecting the basal GTP binding [11,12]. It has been demonstrated that lithium ex vivo reduces the degree of inhibition of forskolin-stimulated adenylate cyclase by 5-HT in rat hippocampus [13]. We have, furthermore, demonstrated that 5-HT_{1A} receptors are negatively coupled to calcium-stimulated adenylate cyclase in rat hippocampus [14]. Chronic lithium treatment reduces 5-HT inhibition of calcium-stimulated adenylate cyclase and reduces 5-HT-induced GTP inhibition of this parameter [8], suggesting an influence on G_i. Such studies have thus demonstrated that lithium ex vivo decreases GTP-dependent processes mediated by β-adrenergic- [8–11], M_1 muscarinic- [12], 5-HT_{1A} serotonergic- [8,14] and α_1-adrenergic receptors [15].

The receptor-G protein interaction has, furthermore, been studied by investigating the hysteretic activation of adenylate cyclase by Gpp(NH)p in rat cerebral cortex after chronic lithium treatment. Adenylate cyclase responds hysteretically, i.e. with a lag period upon exposure to Gpp(NH)p and this lag period preceding the onset of steady-state activation may reflect the time required to convert G_s from its inactive to active form [16,17]. Both the rate and extent of this activation is regulated by Mg^{2+} [16,17]. The steady-state concentration of active G_s is dictated by the rate of GDP/GTP exchange, which can be catalyzed by β-adrenoceptors in the presence of a receptor agonist. Thus, stimulation of adenylate cyclase in rat cerebral cortex by Gpp(NH)p occurs with an observable lag period, and the addition of isoprenaline in the presence of Gpp(NH)p results in a near abolishment of this lag period [7]. Chronic lithium treatment reduces Gpp(NH)p- and isoprenaline-stimulated adenylate cyclase activities. Lithium treatment does not alter the lag period preceding the onset of the steady-state activation by Gpp(NH)p, indicating that lithium does not affect the rate of activation of G_s but decreases adenylate cyclase activity stimulated by Gpp(NH)p, presumably by an effect on G_s or the catalytic unit. Furthermore, the isoprenaline-induced reduction of the lag period is smaller in membranes from rats treated with lithium than from untreated rats. This decreased β-adrenoceptor-induced shortening of the lag period in lithium-treated animals suggests that the coupling between the receptor and G_s is impaired [7]. However, these lithium effects do not seem to involve a Mg^{2+}-interaction, since all effects were measured both at 3 and 10 mM Mg^{2+} [7]. The molecular mechanisms by which lithium exerts these effects are unclear. Lithium ex vivo may affect some G proteins, rendering them resistant to receptor activation. Another possibility is that lithium influences the receptor-G protein coupling by altering the phosphorylation of some proteins in the membrane. Several studies have demonstrated that protein kinases modulate the activities of second messenger systems [1,18]. Furthermore, chronic lithium treatment causes alterations in protein kinase C and cAMP-dependent protein phosphorylation in the rat brain [19]. While no decisive biochemical alteration can be ascribed to lithium, a distinct profile of the action of lithium on second messenger systems in brain has emerged. The activity of second messenger systems may be exposed to at least two inhibitory effects of lithium during chronic treatment: 1) the lithium-Mg^{2+} interaction [3–5] that can be measured in vitro and which might reflect the in situ effect of lithium; and 2) the chronic effect which, once generated, can be measured ex vivo in the absence or presence of very small concentrations of lithium [6]. The observations that lithium ex vivo reduces neurotransmitter-induced GTP regulation of G proteins [7–12] is intriguing, since the G protein familiy is linked to many neurotransmitter receptors and may explain several observations of lithium upon neurotransmitter functions in the past. These actions of lithium may be involved in the antimanic and antidepressant effects of lithium, since lithium could stabilize abnormal oscillations in neurotransmitter function, which might occur in mania and depression.

References

1. Mørk A (1990) Lithium 1: 131–147.
2. Bimbaumer L, Abramowitz J, Yatani A et al. (1990) Crit. Rev. Biochem. Mol. Biol. 25: 225–244.
3. Mørk A and Geisler A (1987) Pharmacol. Toxicol. 60: 241–248.
4. Newman ME and Belmaker RH (1987) Neuropharmacology 26: 211–217.
5. Avissar S, Murphy DL and Schreiber G (1991) Biochem. Pharmacol. 41: 171–175.
6. Mørk A and Geisler A (1989) Neuropharmacology 28: 307–311.
7. Mørk A and Geisler A (1991) Lithium (in press).
8. Mørk A and Geisler A (1989) Eur. J. Pharmacol. 168: 347–354.
9. Mørk A and Geisler A (1989) Biol. Psychiatry 26: 279–288.
10. Mørk A, Klysner R and Geisler A (1990) Neuropharmacology 29: 261–267.
11. Avissar S, Schreiber G, Danon A and Belmaker RH (1988) Nature 331: 440–442.
12. Avissar S and Schreiber G (1989) Biol. Psychiatry 26: 113–130.
13. Newman ME, Drummer D and Lerer B (1990) J. Pharmacol. Exp. Ther. 252: 826–831.
14. Mørk A and Geisler A (1990) Eur. J. Pharmacol. 175: 237–244.
15. Casebolt TL and Jope RS (1989) Biol. Psychiatry 25: 329–340.
16. Iyengar R and Bimbaumer L (1981) J. Biol. Chem. 256: 11036–11041.
17. Iyengar R (1981) J. Biol. Chem. 256: 11042–11050.
18. Huganir R and Greengard P (1990) Neuron 5: 555–567.
19. Casebolt TL and Jope RS (1991) Biol. Psychiatry 29: 233–243.

Biological Psychiatry, Volume 1. G. Racagni et al., editors.

Oral or ICV injection of compounds that reduce cyclic AMP affect rat behavior

O. Kofman[1] and R.H. Belmaker[2]
[1]*Department of Behavioural Sciences, Beersheva Mental Health Center, P.O. Box 46, Beersheva; and* [2]*Division of Psychiatry, Ben Gurion University, Beersheva, Israel*

Since inhibition of agonist-stimulated cyclic AMP (cAMP) is a major biochemical effect of lithium, it may be useful to evaluate other drugs with similar biochemical properties to see if they have potential for treatment of bipolar affective disorder. Two such drugs are the tetracycline derivatives demethylchlortetracycline (DMC) and minocycline (MIN) [1]. Although these drugs are not noted for their psychoactive properties, it had been noted that tetracyclines, and especially DMC, cause a pronounced diuresis. Examination of the mechanism of this diuresis revealed that it was due to inhibition of ADH-sensitive adenylate cyclase, distal to the ADH receptor similar to the effect of lithium on the kidney. Since it is rare to find pharmacological effects distal to the receptor, we hypothesized that these tetracyclines and lithium may share some common pharmacological effects [2].

The ability of DMC and MIN to attenuate agonist-stimulated increases in cAMP in vitro and ex vivo in male Sabra rats has been previously reported [3]. DMC alone had no effect on accumulation of cAMP in cerebral cortical slices incubated with various concentrations ranging from 0.1 to 100 μM. DMC produced a dose-dependent decrease in the stimulatory response to 50 μM NA, which was significant at concentrations of DMC of 10 μM and above. In the chronic ex vivo experiment, animals that had been fed 0.8% DMC for 2 weeks had increased basal cAMP levels compared to slices from control animals, but a total (100%) reduction in the response to 100 μM NE. MIN produced significant decreases in NE stimulated cAMP at concentrations equal to and above 0.1 μM.

Baseline open field activity and post-amphetamine hyperactivity were tested following an acute injection of DMC (166.8 mg/3 cc/rat) or an equal volume of physiological saline 4 h prior to the test. Immediately before placing them in the open field, half the animals in each group were injected with physiological saline, and half with 0.8 cc of a 1 mg/ml solution of d-amphetamine, i.p. Thus the animals received either saline-saline, saline-amphetamine, DMC-saline or DMC-amphetamine. Amphetamine significantly increased motor activity, as expected ($P < 0.001$) and DMC significantly suppressed motor activity ($P < 0.05$).

Three groups of 15 rats were fed a diet containing various concentrations of powdered DMC: 0%, 0.4% or 0.8% DMC mixed with powdered commercial rat chow during 2 weeks. They were then tested for baseline activity in an open field for 30 min. Then they were fed for one more week with the DMC diet and tested again in an open field following an injection of 0.5 mg/kg d-amphetamine, i.p. Amphetamine increased activity only for the group that was not fed DMC, suggesting that chronic DMC attenuates amphetamine-induced hyperactivity.

MIN is a tetracycline which is more lipophilic than DMC and caused attenuation of agonist-stimulated accumulation of cAMP similar to that of DMC. In order to determine if acute systemic injections of MIN would affect motor activity, 40 rats were divided into 4 groups of 10, receiving either saline-saline, saline-amphetamine, MIN-saline or MIN-amphetamine. The pretreatment (saline or 100 mg/kg minocycline hydrochloride) was injected subcutaneously in a volume of 1 mg/ml 4 h prior to treatment. Immediately before the test, the rats were injected with either physiological saline or amphetamine (1 mg/kg), i.p. Rats were placed in an open field and crossings of peripheral and central squares and number of rears were monitored manually every 5 min for 30 min. Post-hoc Scheffe tests showed that amphetamine increased activity in saline-treated rats ($P < 0.001$), but not in MIN-treated rats. These data suggest that MIN, like lithium, effectively reduces amphetamine-induced hyperactivity more than it reduces baseline motor activity. Neither DMC nor MIN was effective in reducing apomorphine-induced stereotypy [3].

Subcutaneous DMC or MIN could cause pain or other peripheral effects and thereby artifactually affect behavior. Thirty-two rats, divided into 4 groups of 8 were implanted with cannulae (Plastic Products) in the lateral ventricle using standard stereotaxic procedures. After 1 week rats were injected subcutaneously with either isotonic saline or d-amphetamine (1 mg/kg) in a volume of 1 ml/kg, and placed in their home cages for 5 min. Next, they were injected i.c.v. with either 50 μg minocycline hydrochloride (pH 2.4) or isotonic saline brought to pH 2.4 with hydrochloric acid. Amphetamine significantly increased total activity ($F = 48.72$, $P = 0.00001$), ambulatory activity ($F = 35.85$, $P = 0.00002$) and rearing ($F = 20.65$, $P = 0.00024$). MIN had no effect on total activity and ambulatory activity, but significantly reduced rearing behaviour ($F = 4.97$, $P = 0.03$) There was a significant interaction between MIN and amphetamine on rearing behaviour ($F = 4.55$, $P = 0.039$), indicating that MIN was more effective in amphetamine-treated rats. A test of simple main effects showed that amphetamine significantly increased activity for the vehicle injected rats ($F = 22.29$, $P < 0.001$), but not for the rats that received MIN i.c.v. ($F = 2.91$, n.s.) These data demonstrate that MIN acts centrally to reduce baseline rearing and amphetamine-induced increases in rearing.

References

1. Singer I and Rotenberg D (1973) Ann. Intern. Med. 79: 679–683.
2. Belmaker RH (1984) Pharmacopsychiatry 17: 9–15.
3. Kofman O, Klein E, Newman M, Hamburger R, Kimchi O, Nir T, Shimon H and Belmaker RH (1990) Pharmacol. Biochem. Behav. 37: 417–424.

Biological Psychiatry, Volume 1. G. Racagni et al., editors.

Lessons from the withdrawal of lithium prophylaxis

G.M. Goodwin[1], F.G.M. Souza[2] and A.J. Mander[3]
[1]MRC Brain Metabolism Unit, Royal Edinburgh Hospital, Morningside Park, Edinburgh EH10 5HF, U.K.; [2]Universidade Estadual do Ceara, Hospital de Saude Mental de Messejana, Fortaleza, Brazil; and [3]Royal Park Hospital, Melbourne, Australia

The withdrawal of lithium is an everyday clinical event. Studies at the Royal Edinburgh Hospital employing a case register to monitor the impact of lithium withdrawal on the risk of subsequent admission to hospital have helped to define the practical impact of lithium prophylaxis in relation to the course of affective illness; this has then prompted controlled studies to clarify the clinical phenomena.

Bipolar illness

Mander [1] showed that lithium discontinuation was associated with a high risk of readmission with manic illness in bipolar patients. However, the increase in risk of recurrence was largely confined to the 3 months following withdrawal. The validity of withdrawal mania in bipolar patients stopping lithium prophylaxis was confirmed in a small stable sample of 14 patients who underwent double-blind discontinuation under close clinical supervision as outpatients [2]. Eight patients had manic mood changes in the month of lithium withdrawal, with a mean delay of 21 days. The design of this study allowed a variety of clinical and specifically endocrine factors to be examined experimentally. Lithium withdrawal was associated with a rebound rise of thyroxine levels (and a fall in TSH). However, these changes were within normal limits for euthyroid function and no difference in endocrine function was detected in patients who became manic compared with those who did not. Cortisol tended to fall following lithium withdrawal but this similarly failed to account for manic relapse. The lessons for the management of bipolar patients are that withdrawal of lithium is accompanied by a short-term increase in the risk of recurrence, but if no recurrence occurs, the prognosis in the medium-term is as good as for patients not taking lithium. The lithium withdrawal paradigm is potentially useful for subsequent prospective investigation of biological markers in bipolar illness.

Unipolar illness

In unipolar depression, the prophylactic efficacy of lithium has been the subject of considerable debate. A positive effect of lithium in reducing the frequency of recurrence has been found in a number of uncontrolled as well as controlled studies; however, others have failed to find such an effect. The withdrawal of lithium in unipolar patients offers further evidence on this matter [3]. The admissions of unipolar patients satisfying DSM III-R criteria for major depression have been analysed in relation to lithium prophylaxis. Forty patients who discontinued lithium therapy were retrospectively compared with 105 patients who continued the drug and served as a control group. The time to readmission from starting on lithium was compared in a phase while both groups were still on lithium and in a second phase after discontinuation in one group and further continuation in the control group. The progressive increase in the probability of recurrence over a 2-year follow-up interval was greatest after discontinuation of lithium. For the patients who eventually discontinued lithium, the cumulative probability of recurrence in 2 years was 0.08 on lithium and 0.58 after stopping it. The probability of recurrence was unchanged over the duration of the study for patients who continued to take lithium. There was no evidence of a lithium withdrawal syndrome within 3 months of stopping the drug. The results support the view that the everyday clinical use of lithium as prophylaxis confers a significant benefit in unipolar depression.

In view of the contradictions exposed by these studies we have recently completed a meta-analysis of treatment trials for lithium in unipolar depression [4]. This shows indubitably that trials of lithium versus placebo are homogeneous and demonstrate a benefit of lithium prophylaxis. Even the largest of the "negative" studies [5] is not in conflict with the results from other studies when viewed in terms of effect size and confidence interval. It simply shows a positive effect of lithium but with a sample size that does not allow statistical significance. This, in a nutshell, illustrates the difference in emphasis between a statistical analysis based on significance levels compared with one based on effect size. Further, the difference is not a trivial one, because the analyses lead to opposite conclusions: that lithium is ineffective (because it is "not significant") or that it may be effective but that the confidence interval is too great to allow certainty. It appears self-evident which is the most clinically useful.

Inositol and lithium withdrawal

Lithium withdrawal should also be mimicked by any treatment that prevents its action. One way in which this might be achieved is by the addition of inositol to the diet of patients on lithium. The rationale follows from the observation that lithium inhibits the enzyme inositol phosphatase, which converts inositol-1-phosphate to inositol in the cycle of phosphoinositides (PI) observed in a wide variety of tissues [6]. Lithium treatment may thereby deplete the stores of myoinositol in target organs or tissues. Supplementation of the diet with inositol might reverse lithium action. This would be an important indicator that the PI cycle is involved in the action of lithium in man. Secondly, it could provide a way of preventing the side-effects of lithium, particularly in peripheral tissues. Patients and controls were studied in a single-blind design for 12 days. For the first and last 2 days of this period, patients added a sachet of glucose (2 g) to food. Inositol was started at 2 g daily on the third day for 2 days followed by 4 g for 2 days, followed by 6 g for 2 days, followed by 8 g for 2 days. The tenth day of the trial was the last day of inositol administration. The administration of inositol at a dose of 1 g daily increases plasma inositol levels and changes the amplitude of peripheral nerve action potentials in diabetics within 2 weeks [7]. However, our own findings with doses of inositol increasing from 2–8 g over a week were entirely negative. Protection from the effects of lithium for example, in teratogenesis, have been described from the administration of inositol [8]. That it fails to work in man is disappointing, but perhaps not entirely surprising. First, the capacity for inositol to reverse lithium effects may depend crucially upon its access to different physiological compartments. Secondly, actions of lithium other than those on PI function may be more relevant to hormone secretion and the side-effects we could measure.

References

1. Mander AJ (1986) Br. J. Psychiatry 149: 498–501.
2. Mander AJ and Loudon JB (1988) Lancet ii: 15–17.
3. Souza FGM, Mander AJ and Goodwin GM (1990) Br. J. Psychiatry 157: 718–722.
4. Souza FGM and Goodwin GM (1991) Br. J. Psychiatry 158: 666–675.
5. Prien RF, Kupfer DJ, Mansky PA, Small JG, Tuason VR, Voss CB and Johnson WE (1984) Arch. Gen. Psychiatry 41: 1096–1104.
6. Berridge MJ, Downes CP and Hanley MR (1989) Cell 59: 411–419.
7. Salway JG, Finnegan JA, Barnett D, Whitehead L, Karunanayaka A and Payne RB (1978) Lancet ii: 1282–1284.
8. Busa NB and Gimlich R.D. (1989) Dev. Biol. 132: 315–324.

Biological Psychiatry, Volume 1. G. Racagni et al., editors.

The influence of lithium and rubidium on cyclic AMP formation in vitro and ex vivo

Arne Mørk and Arne Geisler
Department of Pharmacology, University of Copenhagen, Juliane Maries Vej 20, 2100 Copenhagen, Denmark

Lithium (Li^+) exerts an antimanic, a prophylactic effect against affective disorders, and possibly, an antidepressive effect. It is unclear how Li^+ exerts these therapeutic actions. In this context it is of interest that another monovalent ion, rubidium (Rb^+), seems to be an antidepressant agent. Further, Rb^+ can prolong the period of mania and increase its severity. This is of experimental interest since it has been reported that Rb^+ exerts "opposite" neurochemical and physiological effects to those of Li^+.

For example, it has been shown that Rb^+ and Li^+ have opposite effects on the circadian rhythm of locomotor activity in the cockroach. Similarly, it has been shown that Li^+ attenuates while Rb^+ increases shock-induced changes in open-field activity of rats. Furthermore, it has been shown that rats consume significantly more alcohol when treated with Rb^+ while Li^+ treatment significantly reduces the intake of alcohol. Also at the molecular level Li^+ and Rb^+ have opposing effects. Thus, we have observed that the two ions have different effects in vitro on norepinephrine-induced cyclic AMP (cAMP) formation in cortical slices from rat brain. In this preparation 2 mM of Rb^+ increased the hormone-induced cAMP formation, while 2 mM Li^+ inhibited cAMP accumulation. Combination of the two ions neutralized these effects. On the other hand, neither Rb^+ nor Li^+ influenced the basal activity of the enzyme. Further, it was observed using dose-response curves that Li^+ inhibited the enzyme in a non-competitive manner, while Rb^+ had a potentiating effect over the whole concentration range of added norepinephrine (10^{-7}–10^{-3} M); even at maximal concentrations of norepinephrine, Rb^+ enhanced the formation of cAMP. In recent experiments we have observed that 2 mM Li^+ inhibits the β-adrenergic agonist isoproterenol stimulation of cAMP formation in cortical slices. In accordance with our previous results it was observed that 2 mM Rb^+ enhanced isoproterenol-stimulated cAMP accumulation. Further, it was shown that 2 mM cesium, which may influence human mood, had a similar effect to that of Rb^+ on the cAMP formation. In contrast, it was observed that adenylate cyclase stimulated by GTP with and without isoproternol was not influenced by Rb^+ in rat brain cortical slices from rat brain.

Chronic influence of Rb^+ on isoproterenol-stimulated cAMP formation in rat brain cortical slices was studied by giving the rats tap water containing RbCl (40 mM) for 14 days. This treatment showed that chronic Rb^+ administration had no effect on the basal activity of the enzyme while the isoproterenol-stimulated cAMP formation was significantly reduced.

Rb^+ in vitro had no effect on adenylate cyclase activity in cell-free systems. Thus, Rb^+ does not seem to interact directly with the adenylate cyclase. In intact tissue, Rb^+ had no effect on the unstimulated activity of the enzyme but enhanced the isoproterenol-stimulated cAMP formation. However, Rb^+ also increased forskolin-stimulated cAMP accumulation in rat brain cortical slices. These results show that Rb^+ potentiation can also be observed even when the enzyme is stimulated beyond the receptor. Thus, the effect of Rb^+ in vitro on the adenylate cyclase seems to require an intact cell and may be exerted by an effect independent of the receptor stimulation. After chronic treatment with Rb^+ a decreased isoproterenol-stimulated cAMP formation was observed. This may be explained by Rb^+-induced release of norepinephrine from presynaptic terminals. However, this conclusion does not correspond with the fact that Rb^+ in vitro has no effect on the unstimulated cAMP formation in rat brain cortical slices, but enhances the enzyme activated with maximal concentrations of norepinephrine. Thus, further studies are necessary to clarify the mechanisms by which Rb^+ modulates cAMP formation in brain.

Biological Psychiatry, Volume 1. G. Racagni et al., editors.

Rapid re-entrainment of the circadian clock in “jet-lag” paradigm: Role for behavioral feedback

Olivier van Reeth, Carmen Wickland and Fred Turek

IRIBHN Universite Libre de Bruxelles, Brussels, Belgium; and Department of Neurobiology and Physiology, Northwestern University, Evanston, Illinois, U.S.A.

Introduction

A large number of environmental or chemical stimuli that can alter the phase and/or the period of the mammalian circadian clock have now been identified [1]. The general shape of the phase response curves (PRCs, i.e. a plot of the phase shifts as a function of the time of presentation of the stimulus) generated to these stimuli in hamsters fall into one of two categories, whereby the stimuli mimic either the effects of a short light pulse or a short dark pulse on the circadian clock [2,3]. An interesting common feature shared by some of the agents inducing a “dark pulse type” PRC (e.g. the short-acting benzodiazepine, triazolam [4], or the presentation of a dark pulse on a background of constant light [5,6]) is that their acute presentation to hamsters induces a short-term increase in locomotor activity that lasts for 3–6 h. These observations, coupled with findings indicating that activity bouts themselves are capable of shifting the circadian clock [7,8], led to the hypothesis that the effects of triazolam or dark pulses on the clock might be mediated through this acute hyperactivity. Indeed, we recently demonstrated that the phase shifting effets of these two stimuli on the free-running activity rhythm of hamsters were completely blocked by immobilizing the animals for 6 h after presentation of the stimulus [9]. In the present paper, we determined whether the ability of triazolam to accelerate the rate of reentrainment of the circadian clock of hamsters subjected to a shift in the LD cycle [10] is also modified by immobilization of the animals after treatment.

Methods

Ten-week old hamsters (n = 20) kept under a 14:10 LD cycle (light intensity 600 lux at cage floor level) were subjected to an 8-h advance in the LD cycle on four consecutive occasions separated by 23–42 days. On the day of the shift in the LD cycle, the animals received an i.p. injection of the vehicle DMSO (V and V_r) or 2.5 mg triazolam (T and T_r) 6–7 h prior to the expected onset of locomotor activity on that day [10], and were then either left undisturbed in their cage (V, T) or immobilized in a restraining device for 6 h (V_r, T_r). The time taken for reentrainment to the new LD cycle (i.e. the transient period, defined as the number of days needed for the animal to eventually begin locomotor activity within 30 min of lights-off of the new LD cycle) was assessed and compared in the various groups of animals by using unpaired Student's *t*-tests modified by Bonferroni.

Results

Following the 8-h advance in the LD cycle, the animals began their activity earlier each day until eventually the onset of activity once again occurred near the time of lights-off (Fig. 1). The mean transient period in the group of undisturbed vehicle-treated animals (V) averaged 13 ± 0.9 days. As expected from results of a previous study [10], triazolam significantly reduced the transient period in undisturbed animals (T, mean transient period 6 ± 0.8 days, $P < 0.001$ compared to V). Immobilisation had no effect on the rate of reentrainment of vehicle-treated animals (V_r, mean transient period 12 ± 0.5 days; $P = 0.2$ compared to V), but completely blocked the accelerating effects of triazolam on the resynchronization to the new LD cycle (T_r, mean transient period = 14 ± 0.8 days; $P = 0.6$ compared to V.

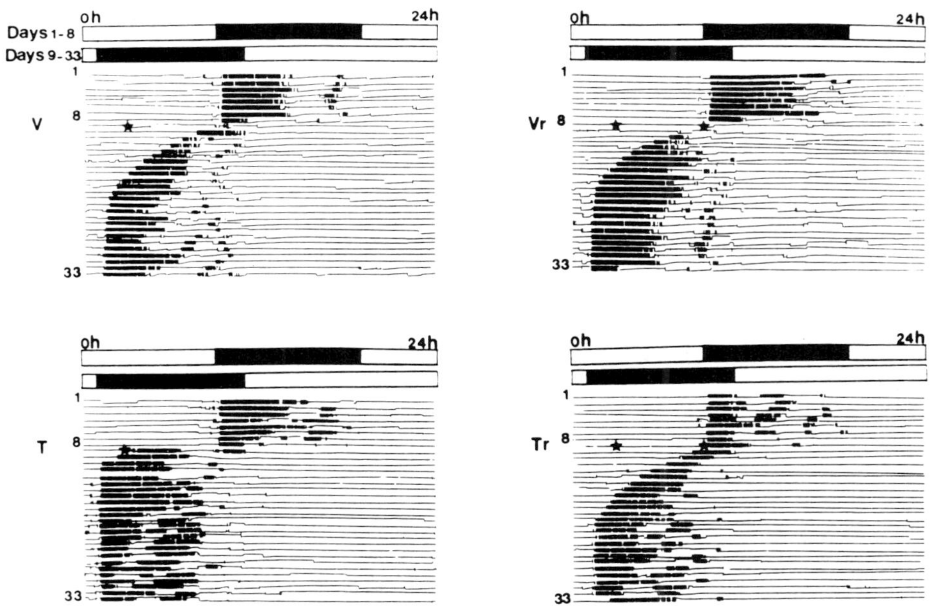

Fig. 1. Representative sections of the activity records from four hamsters subjected to an 8-h advance in the LD cycle on day 8. The LD cycles before and after the shift are shown above each record. On the day of the shift in the LD cycle, the animals received a single injection of either vehicle (V and V_r) or 2.5 mg of triazolam (T and T_r) 6–7 h prior to the expected onset of activity and the animals were then either left undisturbed (V and T) or restrained for 6 h (V_r and T_r). The precise time of the infection for each animal is denoted by a star.

Discussion

These results confirm our findings that the phase shifting effects of triazolam on the hamster clock are mediated through changes in the level of locomotor activity [9]. Previous studies demonstrated that immobilisation during the highly active part of the activity cycle induces phase delays in the activity rhythm of hamsters [3]. Thus, a number of experiments have demonstrated that stimulation of activity during the normal rest period or prevention of activity during the normal active period can induce phase shifts in the circadian clock. Taken together, these findings support the hypothesis that feedback signals during both the rest and active phases of the activity-rest cycle influence the circadian clock.

For many years the possibility that alterations in behavioral states might modify the performance of circadian pacemakers was ignored by most investigators because of the prevailing hypothesis that the insensitivity of circadian systems to feed-back effects originating in the overt rhythms driven by the pacemaker (i.e. locomotor activity, sleep) was essential for the optimal functioning of the pacemaker as a circadian clock. We have now provided extensive experimental evidence that this hypothesis is incorrect and that circadian pacemakers are in fact very responsive to various signals originating in the internal as well as the external milieu. In addition to providing new insights into neurochemical and/or molecular events underlying circadian rhythmicity, experiments using diverse powerful pharmacological or environmental probes might prove to be useful in identifying drugs or behavioral techniques which can be utilized in the treatment of various physical and mental illnesses (i.e. jet lag, shift work, dysomnias, SAD) that have been associated with disorders in circadian time-keeping.

Acknowledgements

Work supported by a Grant from the Ministère Belge de la Politique Scientifique, MN Research Grant ND-09885 and NIMN Research Grant MH-41211. O.V.R. is senior research assistant of the Belgian F.N.R.S. and recipient of a NATO Fellowship for Scientific Research.

References

1. Turek FW (1987) Trends Pharmacol. Sci. 8: 212–217.
2. Smith RD, Inouye SIT and Turek FW (1989) J. Comp. Physiol. 164: 805–814.
3. Van Reeth O, Hinch D, Tecco JM and Turek FW (1991) Brain Res. 545: 208–214.
4. Turek FW and Losee-Olson S (1986) Nature 321: 167–168.
5. Boulos Z and Rusak B (1982) J. Comp. Physiol. A 146: 411–417.
6. Ellis GB, McKlveen RE and Turek F W. (1982) Am. J. Physiol. 242, R44–R50.
7. Reebs S and Mrosovsky N (1989) J. Biol. Rhythms 4: 39–48.

8. Wickland C and Turek FW (1991) Am. J. Physiol. (in press).
9. Van Reeth O and Turek FW (1989) Nature 339: 49–51.
10. Van Reeth O and Turek FW (1987) Am. J. Physiol. 253: R204–R207.

Biological Psychiatry, Volume 1. G. Racagni et al., editors.

Energy and metabolism in depression: A circadian link between synapse and symptom

J.L. Anderson

Laboratory for Circadian and Sleep Disorders Medicine, Brigham and Women's Hospital and Harvard Medical School, 221 Longwood Ave., Boston, MA 02115, U.S.A.

Since the advent of the recent biological psychiatry movement, the collection of data on the physiology of affective disorders has been shaped by available technologies and by influential hypotheses. The latter include the catecholamine hypothesis of affective disorders and other amine hypotheses [1], hypotheses concerning separation and loss of reward [2], learned helplessness [3], up-regulated β-adrenergic receptors [4], sensitization and kindling [5] and the dysregulation hypothesis [6].

Under these influences a great deal of data has been collected and the treatment of affective disorders has developed. However, a considerable gap remains in our understanding of the physiology of affective disorders. A wide range of biological anomalies and abnormalities have been observed in patients and in many cases quantified. Although many of the abnormalities have been related to situational precipitants such as separation and loss [2] and stress [3,7], the relationship between the biological abnormalities and the symptom of affective disorders is not well understood. Moreover, our knowledge of the physiological relationships among these variables is incomplete [8,9]. Hypotheses are needed that meaningfully integrate these observations. Therefore, it may be fruitful to ask of the various approaches to affective disorders research, "how might this approach help us to conceptualize the links among the synaptic, cellular and hormonal abnormalities that frequently accompany affective disorder and the actual symptoms and complaints of our patients?"

The study of circadian rhythms in affective disorders may be uniquely positioned, at this point in history, to advance the process of hypothesis development. Chronobiological investigation may offer both a) an emphasis on the importance of timing in understanding neuroendocrine events, and b) a *physiological* schema in which to conceptually integrate observations from intracellular, synaptic and neurotransmitter system levels. Chronobiology moves us beyond gross analysis of levels of substances, to highlight the temporal pattern of availability of each and to analyse the impact of the temporal sequence of neuroendocrine events on receptive tissues [10]. Studies of the internal regulation of timing and the role of the endogenous circadian pacemaker in particular, also have provided an entrée into the investigation of a functional physiological system, integrated in the hypothalamus, whose crucial survival function is to fuel the body's chemical reactions and remove heat energy that is generated as a by-product. This physiological system utilizes a neuroendocrine network that includes the circadian pacemaker. Examination of circadian rhythms of body-core temperature, used as a marker for the output of the circadian pacemaker, has yielded evidence of reversible thermoregulatory abnormalities in depressed patients. Moreover, the multiply-regulated system of energy metabolism and thermoregulation incorporates many of the variables shown to function abnormally in individuals who are depressed, including biogenic amines, other synaptically-active compounds, receptor proteins and second-messengers, as well as neuropeptides and hormones such as cortisol, TSH, vasopressin and prolactin. This raises the possibility that our understanding of affective disorders may be advanced by attempting to understand how observed abnormalities in these variables [e.g. 1,4–9,11,12] impact physiological processes of energy metabolism and thermoregulation.

The idea that **energy metabolism** may be faulty in depression has been raised over the years by several authors [13–15]. The potential connection to many symptoms of depression is quite straightforward. Among recognized symptoms of depression are *fatigue or loss of energy* and *psychomotor retardation* [16]. Energy can be understood not only phenomenologically, but also at the level of organs, cells and molecules: biochemical reactions transfer chemical energy from food to vital cellular activities [17].

Mood disorders involve more than fatigue. Seasonal change in weight is one symptom of seasonal mood disorders, and *weight loss or gain* plus *changes in appetite* are symptoms of depressive syndromes in general. These symptoms also have a clear relationship to physiologic systems regulating energy metabolism and body temperature, as do the of symptoms insomnia or hypersomnia. *Depressed mood, decreased active engagement, psychomotor agitation* and *mental slowing* can also be related to these systems. It is the symptoms of *guilt/worthlessness* and *suicidality*, most explicitly involving cognitive processes, that require considerable invocation of mediating processes in order to be related to physiologic systems for energy metabolism.

Ironically, a connection between physiological systems of energy metabolism and many symptoms of depression is easy to entertain, but there is a paucity of relevant data [18]. On the other hand, the connection between **thermoregulatory** mechanisms and affective disorders is more difficult to conceptualize, but a bit more empirical evidence has been collected which supports such an association. Reports of elevated nighttime body-core temperatures in depressed patients include that of Avery et al. nearly 10 years ago [13]. Since that time Wehr [19,20] has led the systematic investigation of thermoregulatory processes in affective disorders, linked to exploration of the effects of sleep and sleep deprivation on these disorders. Wehr [19] has proposed that the process of sleep is physiologically akin to heat exposure, with thermolytic neuroendocrine changes increasing at sleep onset (including inhibited secretion of TSH and increased secretion of prolactin) while resting metabolic rate and thermogenic processes decrease. Conversely, sleep deprivation (which has marked antidepressant effects in a large proportion of patients) is proposed to have effects similar to cooling, including increased secretion of TSH and inhibited secretion of prolactin. The observation by Wehr's group that the antidepressant effects of sleep deprivation are blocked if it is conducted in an overheated room indicates that these processes may have an etiological significance [20].

Multiple rhythms are involved in the neuroendocrine network of energy metabolism and thermoregulation. A key component in the relationship between rhythms is the amount of time that elapses between a given event in one rhythm and a specific event in the other rhythm. Fine-tuning of metabolic regulation is possible in part due to the number of neurochemicals with different temporal patterns that can each affect a given cellular process. The chronobiologic approach suggests that greater attention be focussed on temporal neuroendocrine abnormalities. Disturbances in the temporal relationships among rhythms might produce reversible dysfunctions in energy level, appetite and related processes, as well as potentially accounting for their diurnal, catamenial and seasonal patterns of recurrence. Chronobiologic investigations of affective disorders using the physiological schema of energy metabolism and thermoregulation may facilitate the development of integrative hypotheses that can bridge the existing conceptual gap between intracellular, synaptic and symptomatic events.

Acknowledgement

Supported by the Swiss National Science Foundation (83NI-028030).

References

1. Potter WZ, Rudorfer MV and Goodwin FK (1987) In: Hales RE and Frances AJ (eds.) American Psychiatric Association Annual Review, Vol. 6. American Psychiatric Press, Washington DC, pp. 32–60.
2. Akiskal HS and McKinney WT Jr. (1975) Arch. Gen. Psychiatry 32: 285–305.
3. Garber J and Seligman MEP (1980) Human Helplessness: Theory and Applications. Academic Press, New York.
4. Sulser F (1983) Psychopharmacol. Bull. 19: 300–304.
5. Post RM (1990) Pharmacopsychiatria 23: 3–17.
6. Siever LJ and Davis KL (1985) Am. J. Psychiatry 142: 1017–1031
7. Gold PW, Goodwin FK and Chrousos GP (1989) N. Engl. J. Med. 319: 413–420.
8. Jarrett DB, Pollock B, Miewald JM and Kupfer DJ (1991) Biol. Psychiatry 29: 3–14.
9. Rudorfer MV, Risby ED, Osman OT, Gold PW and Potter WZ (1991) Biol. Psychiatry 29: 253–264.
10. Hastings MH (1991) Neuroendocr. Rhythms (in press).
11. Bauer MS and Whybrow PC (1988) Integr. Psychiatry 6: 75–85.
12. Post RM and Ballenger JC (eds.) (1984) Neurobiology of Mood Disorders. Williams and Wilkins, Baltimore.
13. Avery DH, Wildschiødtz G and Rafaelsen OJ (1982) J. Affective Disord. 4: 61–71.
14. Rosenthal NE (1986) Arch. Gen. Psychiatry 43: 188–189.

15. Avery DH (1987) In: Halaris AS (ed.) Chronobiology and Psychiatric Disorders. Elsevier, New York, pp. 75–101.
16. APA (1987) Diagnostic and Statistical Manual of Mental Disorders (3rd Edn., Rev.). American Psychiatric Association, Washington DC.
17. Miller A Jr (1968) Energy Metabolism. Physiology Series. FA Davis Co., Philadelphia.
18. Zach J and Ackerman SH (1988) Psychosomat. Med. 50: 454–468
19. Wehr TA (1990) In: Montplaisir J and Godbout R (eds.) Sleep and Biological Rhythms. Oxford Press, London, pp. 42–86.
20. Wehr TA, Joseph-Vanderpool JR and Kasper S (1989) Sleep Res. 18: 381.

Biological Psychiatry, Volume 1. G. Racagni et al., editors.

The role of HPA hormones in the neuroregulation of sleep in affective disorders

Axel Steiger, Ulrich von Bardeleben, Jürgen Guldner, Christoph Lauer, Barbara Rothe and Florian Holsboer
Max-Planck-Institute of Psychiatry, Kraepelinstrasse 2–10, 8000 Munich 40, Germany

Introduction

Among the most robust findings of psychiatric research during the last 25 years there are changes of sleep structure and of endocrine activity in depressed patients. Abnormalities of sleep-EEG, i.e. a shortened REM-latency, an enhanced REM-activity, reduced slow wave sleep (SWS) and a disturbed sleep continuity [1] and aberrancies of hormonal secretion, particularly an overactivity of the hypothalamic-pituitary-adrenocortical (HPA) axis [2] are well documented. During sleep the cyclic occurrence of periods of REM- and non-REM-sleep is recorded by sleep-EEG and also characteristic patterns of the secretion of several hormones – like the growth hormone (GH) peak near to sleep onset and the cortisol rise in the early morning – are detectable [3]. Synchronous registration of sleep-EEG and nocturnal hormonal secretion is an attractive approach to elucidate the interaction between sleep-EEG and sleep-associated hormonal secretion.

We entered a series of studies in patients with major depression and in normal controls to investigate the role of HPA hormones in the neuroregulation of sleep in affective disorders. We performed a longitudinal study to compare sleep structure and nocturnal hormonal secretion in depressed patients during acute illness and after recovery; in control subjects we examined sleep-endocrine effects of cortisol, of desoxycorticosterone (DOC), a neurosteroid, which binds predominantly to mineralocorticoid receptors and of repetitive infusion of the neuropeptide corticotropin-releasing hormone (CRH) and of the synthetical ACTH(4-9) analog ebiratide (HOE 427).

Methods

All studies were performed in the sleep laboratory applying a "through-the-wall-technique", which has been described in detail elsewhere [4]. During investigation nights, which were preceded by 1 or 2 adaptation nights, sleep-EEG was recorded between 11 p.m. and 7 a.m. Blood for later analysis of the plasma concentrations of cortisol and GH was sampled every 20 min between 8 p.m. and 7 a.m. In the sample of patients with depression additionally prolactin and – every hour – testosterone were collected.

Twelve male patients with an acute episode of major endogenous depression (mean age 46.4 ± 11.3 years) were investigated during acute illness (HAMD score 27.7 ± 6.8 points) and after recovery.

In male healthy paid volunteers (20–35 years old) the effect of the following substances (n = 8 to 11 subjects) was examined according to randomized schedules:

1. pulsatile application of cortisol according to a total dose of 1 mg/kg body weight, a loading dose of 20% of the total dosage at 5 p.m., further continued with an oral dosage of 6% or placebo (PL);
2. oral application of 2 mg DOC or PL at 10 p.m.;
3. infusions of 4 × 50 μg CRH or PL at 10 p.m., 11 p.m., 12 p.m., 1 a.m.;
4. infusions of 4 × 120 μg HOE 427 or PL at same time points as in study 3.

Results

In the depressed patients sleep-EEG variables did not differ between acute depression and recovery except for a significant decrease of sleep stage 4. Also the relatively low GH concentration remained unchanged after recovery. In contrast, cortisol concentration decreased significantly and cortisol rise appeared at a later clocktime. Testosterone concentration showed a significant increase after remission. No differences in prolactin secretion were found between both time points. Prolactin variables were in a similar range as found in a sample of younger normal controls.

Under cortisol a significant increase of SWS and GH concentration and a suppression of stage REM were found.

No sleep-EEG changes were detectable after 2 mg DOC.

Repetitive infusion of CRH prompted an elevation of cortisol concentration and a blunted GH peak during the first half of the night. SWS decreased significantly during the second half of the night, while stage REM was reduced during the total night.

Under pulsatile application of HOE 427 a decrease in sleep efficiency, a prolonged sleep latency, an increase of time spent awake and a decrease in SWS during the first third of the night occurred. Cortisol and GH variables remained unaffected by the substance.

Discussion

Our data show that an elevated cortisol concentration, an advanced occurrence of the cortisol rise and a blunted testosterone concentration are state markers of acute depression. Sleep structure and GH concentration do not normalize after clinical remission; the persistence of the abnormality of these variables may represent long-lasting “scars” mirroring the metabolic aberrancies during acute illness. It is also evident that cortisol normalizes independently from sleep structure. Therefore, it is unlikely that shallow sleep contributes to the changes of cortisol secretion during acute depression. It is demonstrated that prolactin secretion is not affected by depression.

Artificial enhancement of the cortisol concentration by infusion of cortisol did not prompt sleep endocrine changes similar to those during elevated cortisol release in depression. In contrast, in the controls who received cortisol, SWS and GH increased. This effect of a glucocorticoid differs from that of DOC, which is predominantly a mineralocorticoid receptor ligand. DOC did not induce sleep-EEG changes. These findings suggest that different steroids exert specific effects on sleep.

In contrary to cortisol CRH induced some of the changes, which are characteristic of acute depression – decrease of SWS and GH and enhancement of cortisol. This finding corroborates the view that overactivity of CRH in depression does not only play a key role in the regulation of the HPA axis, but also contributes to a wide range of behavioral changes during affective disorders [2].

Our finding of shallow sleep under the ACTH(4-9) fragment ebiratide (HOE 427) – which is different from the effects of CRH – gives further evidence that neuropeptides of the HPA axis exert specific effects on sleep-EEG. Since GH and cortisol secretion remain unchanged under this substance, it is demonstrated that peripheral application of neuropeptides allows challenge of changes in CNS activity which are not mediated by modulation of peripheral endocrine secretion.

Acknowledgement

Research supported by a grant from the Deutsche Forschungsgemeinschaft (Ste 486/1-1).

References

1. Reynolds CF and Kupfer DJ (1987) Sleep 10: 199.
2. Holsboer F (1989) Eur. Arch. Psychiatr. Neurol. Sci. 238: 302.
3. Steiger A, Herth T and Holsboer F (1987) Acta Endocrinol. (Copenhagen) 116: 36.
4. Holsboer F, von Bardeleben U and Steiger A (1988) Neuroendocrinology 48: 62.

Biological Psychiatry, Volume 1. G. Racagni et al., editors.

Pituitary changes in depression

K. Ranga Rama Krishnan[1], P. Murali Doraiswamy[1], David A. Axelson[1], Scott N. Lurie[1], Gary S. Figiel[1], Mustafa M. Husain[1], Linda Patterson[1], Orest B. Boyko[2], Everett H. Ellinwood Jr.[1,3] and Charles B. Nemeroff[1,3]

[1]Department of Psychiatry; [2]Department of Radiology; and [3]Department of Pharmacology, Duke University Medical Center, Durham, NC 27710, U.S.A.

Hypothalamo-pituitary-adrenal axis (HPA) hyperactivity is a frequent neuroendocrine abnormality in depression [1,2] and may play a role in the pathophysiology of depression. It is characterized by sustained hypercortisolemia and non-suppression of serum cortisol after administration of dexamethasone [1,2]. Central overdrive by corticotropin releasing factor (CRF) of the pituitary corticotroph has been suggested by several studies to be present in patients with depression [3,4]. In addition, Von Bardeleben et al. [5] and Lisansky et al. [6] have shown that the corticotropin (ACTH) response to CRF after metyrapone administration is increased in depressed patients compared to controls. Animal studies have shown that administration of CRF can lead to a marked increase in the number and volume of corticotroph cells (and therefore pituitary volume) [7,8]. This led us to hypothesize that patients with depression may have pituitary enlargement due to hypersecretion of "trophic" releasing factors.

In a preliminary study, we measured pituitary gland size on magnetic resonance images (MRI) centered at the pituitary stalk, in a group of 19 patients with depression in comparison with 19 age and sex-matched controls [9].

We also examined the signal intensity of the posterior and anterior pituitary. The posterior pituitary has a higher signal intensity area called the bright spot. The significance of the bright spot is unclear, although it is believed to be related to vasopressin. In patients with syndrome of inappropriate antidiuretic hormone (SIADH) secretion, the bright spot is usually not seen. Since vasopressin has been implicated in the pathogenesis of hypercortisolemia in depressed patients, assessment of the intensity of the posterior bright spot is of interest.

In an additional phase of the study, we used a stereological method of calculating pituitary volume and evaluated the relationship between pituitary volume and plasma cortisol concentrations from the dexamethasone suppression test (DST).

Nineteen consecutive patients (14 female, 5 male) who satisfied DSM III-R criteria for major depression and met selection criteria and 39 normal volunteers participated in a standardized brain MRI protocol. The selection criteria included screening for medications known to elevate HPA axis activity in patients with affective disorders as well as significant endocrine, hepatic, renal disease or previous neurosurgery [1,9]. Of the 19 patients, 16 had unipolar, 3 had bipolar depression and 14 patients were diagnosed as having recurrent major depression. The control group of 19 was matched from a group of 39 normal community volunteers.

All brain MRI studies were performed on a General Electric 1.5 Tesla Signa System. The MRI acquisition parameters for the T_1-weighted sagittal and coronal images were performed as previously described [9]. Four controls and 1 patient did not complete the protocol beyond the sagittal images, and coronal images were not available in these subjects for measuring pituitary width or estimating pituitary volume. A board-certified neuroradiologist (O.B.B.) evaluated all the scans. Two controls (and none of the 19 patients) had scans suggestive of a partially empty sella, but were included in the analyses since it is a common finding in normals [10]. The midsagittal T_1 image centered at the pituitary stalk was used to measure the central height, maximum length and cross-sectional area of the pituitary gland [11,12]. The coronal T_1 image through the pituitary stalk was used to measure the maximum gland width. Pituitary gland volume was estimated using the formula area × width in the 15 controls and 18 depressed patients for whom width measurements were available. Although pituitary volume estimated by this formula may slightly overestimate actual volume, this method may be adequate for purposes of group comparisons. All measurements were obtained independently by 2 experienced physicians (P.M.D. and S.N.L.), blinded to the clinical diagnosis, on an offline console with the GE CLIPS software program. Anterior and posterior pituitary signal intensity was also measured. Interrater reliability (evaluated with Pearsons correlation coefficient) between the 2 raters was excellent: pituitary area $r = 0.96$, height $r = 0.96$, length $r = 0.83$ and width $r = 0.86$; $P = 0.0001$ for all of the above.

Depressed patients had significantly larger pituitary gland area ($t = -3.62$, $df = 36$, $P = 0.0009$), volume ($t = 2.85$, $df = 31$, $P = 0.007$), and length ($t = 2.05$, $df = 36$, $P = 0.04$) when compared to age and sex-matched controls [9]. Pituitary height and width also tended to be larger in depressed patients. Age was strongly negatively correlated with pituitary area ($r = -0.64$, $P = 0.002$), height ($r = -0.49$, $P = 0.03$), and volume ($r = -0.57$, $P = 0.02$) in controls [9]. Consistent with these correlations, elderly (>50 yrs, $n = 11$) depressed patients had significantly larger pituitary gland areas ($t = -5.15$, $P = 0.0001$), volume ($t = -3.2$, $P = 0.005$), and length ($t = -3.1$, $df = 19$, $P = 0.005$) than elderly controls [9].

The effect of previous lithium treatment on pituitary size was also addressed. Lithium treatment is known to produce hypothyroidism in some patients, which could potentially lead to enlargement of the pituitary gland. Patients in this study had recently been exposed to lithium; they were dropped and the data was reanalyzed using the general linear models procedure on PC-SAS. Diagnosis was significantly related to pituitary area ($F = 9.31$, $P < 0.005$) and pituitary volume ($F = 7.94$, $P < 0.009$) after covarying for age. This suggests that lithium treatment should not affect pituitary size in the absence of hypothyroidism. It will be interesting to study patients on lithium longitudinally to see if there is a change in pituitary size concomitant to changes in plasma thyrotropin stimulating hormone concentrations.

There was no difference in anterior pituitary signal intensity between patients and controls. Posterior pituitary signal intensity was greater in patients as compared to controls ($P < 0.03$). The ratio of posterior to anterior pituitary signal intensity was also higher in patients as compared to controls ($P < 0.04$). This data is preliminary in nature and needs to be further investigated.

In a subsequent study, we evaluated depressed patients with thin (3 mm with no interslice gap) section, sagittal T_1-weighted MR images and the DST. Pituitary volume was related to 10:00 p.m. post-dexamethasone plasma cortisol concentration after covarying for the effect of age and sex ($P < 0.03$). Pituitary volume assessed using a stereological method, in a group of patients who were DST suppressors, was compared to pituitary volume in age-matched controls and was found to be essentially similar.

Discussion

The finding that depressed patients had larger pituitaries than controls may indicate functional as well as structural alterations in the neuroendocrine axis in depression. These findings probably reflect differences in anterior rather than the posterior pituitary size because: a) the posterior pituitary is of neural origin and there are no known conditions (other than non-endocrine tumors) associated with posterior pituitary enlargement; and b) the posterior pituitary comprises less than 20% of the total volume and has to increase several-fold to account for the increase seen in the depressed patients. These studies suggest that pituitary enlargement in depression is related to corticotroph hypertrophy and/or hyperplasia.

There are some limitations in interpreting the findings of this study. We studied a heterogenous group of depressed patients which included first episode depression, recurrent depression and bipolar disorder. Future studies of larger numbers of subjects will allow for these and other clinical variables to be controlled, though the expense of the MRI is a limitation. This study also does not address the causal nature of the link between depression and pituitary size; all the patients had major depression at the time they were studied, and none had a baseline MRI for comparison. Therefore we cannot say whether the pituitary glands of the patients enlarged as a result of their depression or were larger than controls prior to the onset of illness. The higher signal intensity in the posterior pituitary in depressed patients needs to be further investigated. Additional questions which need to be addressed are: whether pituitary size increases in conditions other than depression; whether size increases with depression and changes after treatment; and whether pituitary size reflects the neuroendocrine milieu in depression.

References

1. Carroll BJ, Feinberg M, Greden JF et al. (1981) Arch. Gen. Psychiatry 15–22.
2. Krishnan KRR, Nemeroff CB and Carroll BJ (1989) In: Rose CF (ed.) International Universities Press Inc., Madison 29: 419–435.
3. Nemeroff CB, Widerlov E, Bissette G et al. (1984) Science 226: 1342–1344.
4. Gold PW, Chrousos G, Kellner C et al. (1984) Am. J. Psychiatry 141: 619–627.
5. Van Bardeleben U, Stalla GK, Muller OA and Holsboer F (1988) Biol. Psychiatry 24: 782–785.
6. Lisansky J, Peake GT, Strassman J et al. (1989) Arch. Gen. Psychiatry 46: 641–643.
7. Westlund KN, Aguilera G and Childs GV (1985) Endocrinology 116: 439–445.
8. Gertz BJ, Contreras LN, McComb DJ et al. (1987) Endocrinology 120: 381–388.
9. Krishnan KRR, Doraiswamy PM, Lurie SN et al. (1991) J. Clin. Endocrinol. Metab. 72: 256–259.
10. Chakeres DW, Curtin A and Ford G (1989) Radiol. Clin. North Am. 27: 265–281.
11. Lemort M, Haesendonck P, Louryan S et al. (1988) In: Gouaze A and Salamon G (eds.) Brain Anatomy and Magnetic Resonance Imaging. Springer-Verlag, pp. 158–163.
12. Hayakawa K, Konishi Y, Matsuda T et al. (1989) Radiology 172: 171–177.

Biological Psychiatry, Volume 1. G. Racagni et al., editors.

Aging and the canine hypothalamic-pituitary-adrenocortical (HPA) axis

Johannes M.H.M. Reul[1], Jan Rothuizen[2] and E. Ronald de Kloet[3]
[1]Max Planck Institute for Psychiatry, Clinical Institute, Kraepelinstr. 2, 8000 Munich 40, Germany; [2]Department of Clinical Sciences of Companion Animals, Utrecht; and [3]CBPS, Sylvius Laboratory, Leiden, The Netherlands

Introduction

The aging process of organisms may be regarded as a progressive fall in bodily functions associated with a diminishing ability to maintain homeostasis [1]. Corticosteroids are critical factors in the maintenance of homeostasis and do so via the interaction with two corticosteroid receptor systems in the brain; the mineralocorticoid (MR) and the glucocorticoid receptor (GR) [2,3]. Studies in rats directed at defining the role of MR and GR in control of homeostasis have forwarded the notion that these receptors operate in a coordinate and antagonistic manner [4,5]. Corticosterone exerts via limbic MR a tonic action on brain function. Limbic MR-mediated effects are involved in basal control and set the threshold of responsiveness of the HPA axis [6]. Hypothalamic and hypophyseal GR seem to be involved in the suppression of stress-evoked HPA activity. GR in pyramidal neurons of the hippocampus is involved in suppression of cellular excitability, which is transiently raised by excitatory stimuli [7].

In rats, at senescence, there are considerable individual and strain differences in corticosteroid receptors and HPA dynamics. Rat hippocampal MR level has been found to be reduced [8]. Some studies report a reduced GR number [8], others a decline in the post-adrenalectomy (ADX) rise in GR capacity [9], while GR in old Brown Norway rat is not changed [10]. A progressive deterioration in the control of HPA activity has been found in the aging rat, which may result in increased basal and stress-induced ACTH levels [10], corticosterone levels or both [11,12]. Typically, a prolonged stress-induced adrenocortical secretion has also been observed in some rat strains [13]. In this study, we report age-related changes in neuroendocrine regulation and central corticosteroid receptors in the dog.

Materials and Methods

Animals

Twelve young dogs (9 males, 3 females; age 18–24 months) and 10 aged dogs (6 males, 4 females; age over 11 years (mean 13 years)) were used.

Neuroendocrine challenge tests

Blood samples were drawn by jugular vein puncture and collected in ice-chilled EDTA-coated tubes. The following challenge tests were performed:

1. CRH-test: ovine CRF (o-CRF; 1 μg/kg body weight (b.w.)) was administered intravenously (i.v.);
2. electric footshock stress: the dogs were placed in left lateral recumbency and mild electric shocks (1 mAmps, alternatively on/off for 2 s) were given for 1 min via 2 subcutaneous needles placed 2 cm apart in the dorsal carpal region of one forelimb with an earth connection at the other forelimb;
3. immobilisation stress: dogs were immobilized in dorsal recumbency by fixation of their extremities for 45 min.

Blood samples were drawn 30, 15 min and immediately before the start of each challenge test and with 10 min intervals for 3 h thereafter for measurement of ACt and cortisol. The tests were performed with intervals of 7–10 days. This protocol was approved by the Institutional Committee on Animal Care and Use of the Veterinary Faculty, State University of Utrecht, The Netherlands.

Adrenalectomy and tissue dissection

In order to perform corticosteroid receptor assays, the animals were bilaterally adrenalectomized in order to deplete the body of endogenous corticosteroids. Following ADX the dogs were given 0.9% NaCl (100 ml/kg b.w./24 h) via a jugular vein catheter. The dogs were sacrificed 1 day after ADX with pentobarbital. After sacrifice, the brain and pituitary were rapidly dissected and the dissected tissues were immediately frozen on dry ice and stored at –70 °C until cytosol receptor assay. The methodology of the steroid receptor assay is described elsewhere [13].

Results

Neuroendocrine challenge tests

Figure 1 shows plasma cortisol levels at 4 different time points: pre-challenge basal levels and peak concentrations following o-CRF injection and the two stress tests. From this figure, it is evident that aged dogs displayed higher basal levels of cortisol than young animals (Student's t-test, $P < 0.05$). Basal ACTH levels were also increased (not shown). Moreover, upon administration of o-CRF or application of stress, the aged animals showed a significantly larger responsiveness in cortisol (Student's t-test, $P < 0.05$; Fig. 1) and ACTH (not shown). However, the time span of stress-induced cortisol and ACTH secretion was similar in young and aged animals. No sex differences were apparent in any of the tests.

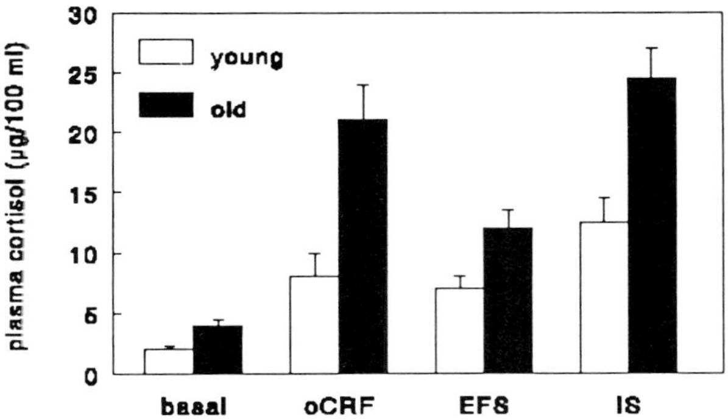

Fig. 1. Basal and peak values (mean ± S.E.M.) of plasma cortisol following o-CRF challenge test, electric footshock stress (EFS) and immobilization stress (IS).

Age-related corticosteroid receptor changes

Figure 2 shows the corticosteroid receptor levels in brain and pituitary of aged dogs, expressed as the percentage of the concentrations found in young animals. The MR concentration was markedly decreased in all examined tissues (minus 50–75%; Student's *t*-test, $P < 0.05$) with highest decrements in the extrahypothalamic limbic brain regions, septum and hippocampus (minus 65–75%). In contrast, GR levels were not changed in the aged canine brain, while GR levels in the anterior pituitary were increased by 70% (Student's *t*-test, $P < 0.05$).

Discussion

In this study, aged dogs displayed hypercortisolemia not only under basal con-

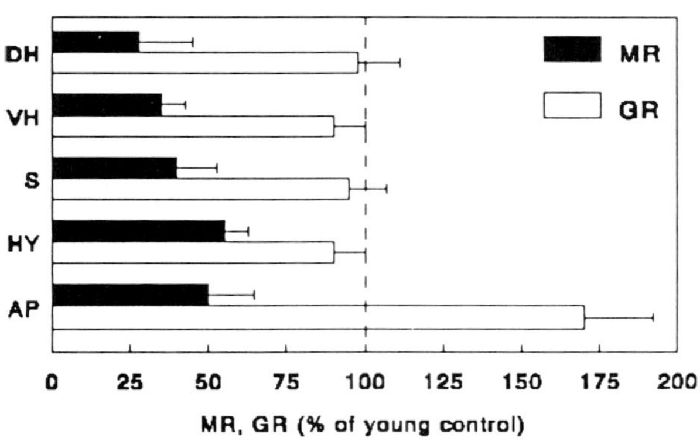

Fig. 2. Age-induced changes in MR and GR capacity in dog brain and pituitary. Abbreviations: DH: dorsal hippocampus; VH: ventral hippocampus; S: septum; HY: hypothalamus; AP: anterior pituitary.

ditions but also as a result of stress or hormonal challenges. In the aged rat, some authors have found elevated basal and stress-induced corticosterone levels [11,12], whereas others have found no such changes [14,15]. The use of different rat strains as well as differences in type and severity of the challenges may underlie the variability in the outcome of the various studies. In addition, a marked sex difference in plasma corticosterone level has been reported in rats [16]. In this study, no sex difference was observed in either young or aged dogs.

Recently, in young and aged male Brown Norway rats, the stress responsiveness of the HPA axis was studied in relation to the properties of the brain and hypophyseal corticosteroid receptors [10]. These aged rats displayed increased stress-responsiveness of the pituitary ACTH release, while plasma corticosterone levels were not different between young and old rats under resting conditions or after stress [10]. In the present study, the pattern of neuroendocrine responses in cortisol in the young and aged dogs largely parallelled the changes in ACTH.

The present study shows for the first time that, in the aged dog, brain and hypophyseal MR are largely decreased, while GR in brain is not affected and is even upregulated in the AP. In aging studies using the rat as an experimental model, the situation is more complex: depending on the rat strain used and the brain tissue under study, some studies report a decrement in both MR and GR [8], while others show a rather specific decrement in MR with no change in the levels of GR [10,17].

It has been hypothesized that corticosterone and cortisol exert a dual control on the activity of the HPA system, being a tonic influence via the limbic MR and a feedback action (post-stress) via GR [2,4,5]. Since MR and GR presumably are colocalized in the pyramidal neurons of the hippocampus and other neurons in limbic structures, it is thought that the balance of MR and GR functioning may be important for the homeostasis of the HPA axis. Recent studies have shown that it is the limbic MR, which is mostly involved in the regulation of basal ACTH secretion [6]. The present study shows that limbic MR levels are diminished in the aged dog brain, which may explain the elevated basal concentrations of plasma ACTH and cortisol and the increased stress responsiveness of these animals. The stress-induced elevations of cortisol and ACTH were not prolonged, which suggests that GR-mediated negative feedback action of glucocorticoids is not altered. This observation is in line with the unchanged brain GR, as reported in this study. In this context the significance of the increased GR capacity in the AP is at present unknown.

Acknowledgement

This study was supported by the Dutch Organization of Advanced Research MEDIGON (Grant No. 900-543-077).

References

1. Everitt A and Meites J (1985) J. Gerontol. 44: B139–B147.
2. Reul JMHM and De Kloet ER (1985) Endocrinology 117: 2505–2511.
3. Reul JMHM, De Kloet ER, Van Sluijs FJ, Rijnberk A and Rothuizen J (1990) Endocrinology 127: 907–915.
4. De Kloet ER and Reul JMHM (1987) Psychoneuroendocrinology 12: 83–105.
5. De Kloet ER (1991) Front. Neuroendocrinol. 12: 95–165.
6. Ratka A, Sutanto W, Bloemers M and De Kloet ER (1989) Neuroendocrinology 50: 117–123.
7. Joels M and De Kloet ER (1989) Science 245: 1502–1505.
8. Reul JMHM, Tonnaer JADM and De Kloet ER (1988) Neurobiol. Aging 9: 253–260.
9. Eldridge JC, Brodish A, Kute TE and Landfield PW (1989) J. Neurosci. 9: 3237–3242.
10. Van Eekelen JAM, Rots NY, Sutanto W and De Kloet ER (1991) (submitted).
11. Dekosky ST, Scheff SW and Cotman CW (1984) Neuroendocrinology 38: 33–38.
12. Landfield PW, Baskin RK and Pitler TA (1981) Science 214: 581–584.
13. Sapolsky RM, Krey LC and McEwen BS (1984) Proc. Natl. Acad. Sci. U.S.A. 81: 6174–6177.
14. Lorens OH, Hata N, Handa RJ, Van De Kar LD, Guschwan M, Goral J, Lee JM, Hamilton ME, Bethea CL and Clancy J Jr (1990) Neurobiol. Aging 11: 139–150.
15. Sonntag WE, Golis AG, Brodish A and Eldridge JC (1987) Endocrinology 120: 2308–2315.
16. Brett LP, Levine R and Levine S (1986) Neurobiol. Aging 7: 153–159.
17. Eldridge JC, Brodish A, Kute TE and Landfield PW (1989) J. Neurosci. 9: 3237–3242.

Biological Psychiatry, Volume 1. G. Racagni et al., editors.

Glucocorticoid receptors in psychiatry: Clinical, functional and molecular aspects

Rainer Rupprecht, Johannes Kornhuber, Norbert Wodarz, Peter Riederer, Dietmar Spengler, Klaus Damm and Florian Holsboer

Max-Planck-Institute for Psychiatry, Kraepelinst. 10, W-8000 Munich 40; and Department of Psychiatry, University Würzburg, Füchsleinstr. 15, W-8700 Würzburg, Germany

Introduction

Abnormalities of the hypothalamic-pituitary-adrenal (HPA) system linked to depression include 24-hour hypersecretion of cortisol during depressive episodes, inadequate suppressibility of cortisol by dexamethasone and hyperresponsiveness of the adrenal cortex to exogenous corticotropin [1]. An escape of plasma ACTH and β-endorphin from dexamethasone suppression in endogenously depressed patients provided evidence for a subtle derangement of the feedback regulation of the HPA system during depression [1]. As hypercortisolemia in depression represents a major confounding factor in accurate assessments of the HPA system and its feedback mechanism, we tried to determine the effects of in vivo and in vitro administered dexamethasone (DEX) in relation to DEX plasma concentrations and glucocorticoid receptor (GR) autoregulation by avoiding the potential effects of hypercortisolemia by metyrapone (MET) induced blockade cortisol synthesis.

Material and Methods

Subjects

Eighteen patients with unipolar major depressive disorder or bipolar depression and 15 healthy controls were studied.

Study design

For determination of leukocyte GR binding characteristics, leukocyte proliferation tests and hormone data baseline values were obtained on day 1. On day 2 the subjects were pretreated with 1.5 g metyrapone (MET) at 9 a.m. 1 mg dexamethasone (DEX) was given orally at 11 p.m. On day 3 administration of 1.5 g MET was performed again.

Assays

The GR binding assay, leukocyte proliferation tests, hormone assays and transfection experiments are described in detail elsewhere [1,2].

Results

Administration of MET resulted in a drastic increase in ACTH in patients and controls. There was a slightly attenuated suppresibility of ACTH by DEX in depressed patients in the face of unchanged DEX plasma concentrations under MET pretreated conditions. Administration of MET induced an upregulation of GR sites per cell in the control group but not in the depressives. While MET and DEX administration did not affect Con A or PHA induced T-cell proliferation, there was a decrease in PWM induced B-cell blastogenesis and an increase in the inhibition of spontaneous leucocyte proliferation by in vitro added DEX following MET administration in the control group. Depressed patients did not change lymphocyte proliferation characteristics following changes of HPA system activity in vivo.

To investigate the hypothesis of whether antidepressants might restore HPA axis function via a direct influence on GR expression, various cell lines were transfected with the glucocorticoid responsive mouse mammary tumor virus (MMTV) promoter fused to the luciferase gene (MMTV-LUC). Incubation of cells with amitryptiline or desmethylimipramine (DMI) did not change the glucocorticoid-induced induction of the MMTV promoter either via endogenous or via co-transfected GRs.

Discussion

Our data suggest that the deranged response to glucocorticoids during depression is not directly related to hypercortisolemia since it persists after depletion of endogenous cortisol by MET. The observation of the inertness of the lymphoproliferative system to major changes of HPA system activity supports the concept of a subtle steroid resistance also at the cellular level during major depressive episodes. The decreased autoregulatory potency of the GR in the depressed patients suggests a diminished functional plasticity of GR regulation as has also been shown in the hippocampus of aged rats. In view of recent findings that antidepressants might upregulate GR mRNA in rat primary neuronal cultures [3] we investigated the influence of antidepressants on GR function at the molecular level. We could not detect a direct influence of antidepressants on the induction of a highly GR responsive promoter. These data suggest that potential influences of antidepressants on GR expression might be tissue-specific and not a general principle of antidepressant action.

References

1. Rupprecht R, Kornhuber J, Wodarz N et al. (1991) Biol. Psychiatry (in press).
2. Arriza JL, Simerly RB, Swanson LW and Evans RM (1988) Neuron 1: 887–900.
3. Pepin MC, Beaulieu S and Barden N (1989) Mol. Brain Res. 6: 77–83.

Biological Psychiatry, Volume 1. G. Racagni et al., editors.

Repression and differential regulation of the hCRH gene promoter through glucocorticoid receptors

D. Spengler, R. Rupprecht, K. Damm and F. Holsboer
Max-Planck-Institute of Psychiatry, Clinical Institute, Department of Neuroendocrinology, Kraepelinstr. 10, 8000 Munich 40, Germany

Introduction

A number of studies on depressed patients indicate that exaggerated activity of corticotrophic and adrenocortical cells is related to central alteration of corticotropin releasing hormone (CRH) regulation.

Expression of the CRH gene in the nucleus paraventricularis of the hypothalamus is implicated in the coordination of HPA-axis activity and feedback inhibition by glucocorticoid receptors. Despite considerable synthesis of CRH in the brainstem, the central nucleus of the amygdala, the bed nucleus of the stria terminalis and frontal cortex CRH function outside the hypothalamus remains unresolved. Repression of CRH gene transcription by glucocorticoids is restricted to the hypothalamus irrespective of highly expressed functional glucocorticoid receptors in other brain areas. Glucocorticoids repress CRH mRNA levels in parvicellular neurons, and conversely increase them in paraventricular neurons with descending projections and in certain magnocellular neurons. Thus in different types of neurons, glucocorticoids may increase, decrease, or have no influence on CRH mRNA levels [1].

Materials and Methods

Plasmid construction

To construct plasmid pBLCRHCAT3, a 760 bp PstI fragment containing the entire hCRH gene promoter and part of the first exon of the hCRH gene was fused to the CAT gene by insertion into the PstI site of pBLCAT3 [2].

Cell culture and DNA transfections

AtT20 and SK-N-MC cells were grown in DMEM supplemented with 10% FCS. JAR-cells were propagated in RPMI. Transfections were performed by calcium phosphate precipitates resp. electroporation [2].

CAT assay

Unmodified chloramphenicol and its acetylated derivatives were separated on TLC plates and quantified after autoradiography by scintillation counting [2].

Results

We transfected the human CRH gene promoter into different cell lines to investigate cis-acting elements involved in repression and differential regulation by glucocorticoids. We studied the regulation of expression of the human CRH gene in a mouse anterior pituitary cell line (AtT20) after transient transfection with a chimeric gene containing the hCRH gene promoter fused to the CAT gene. Expression of the chimeric hCRH CAT gene in AtT20 cells was enhanced by the cAMP analogue (8 Br-cAMP) about 5-fold but not by phorbol 12-myristate-acetate (TPA). The cAMP phosphodiesterase inhibitor isobutylxanthine (IMX) also strongly stimulated 15-fold the expression of the hCRH CAT gene. Coincubation of cAMP analogue and IMX resulted in a moderate 2-fold synergistic enhancement of CAT activity. A core sequence for a cAMP responsive element 5'TGACGTCA-3' at −221 bp relative to the cap site was demonstrated to confer cAMP inducibility on an otherwise unresponsive promoter. Interestingly treatment with 0.5 μM dexamethasone reduced CAT activity about 2-fold in cAMP-stimulated cells. This result suggests that cAMP and glucocorticoids coordinately control hCRH gene expression. Analysis of several neuroendocrine cell lines revealed high expression of the CRH-gene in the human choriocarcinoma cell line (JAR). Promoter activity was enhanced by inducers of the cAMP pathway, though coincubation of cAMP and IMX was neither synergistic nor additive. In contrast to repression of CRH promoter activity in AtT20 cells, we observed an enhancement (about 100%) of cAMP-dependent promotor activity after cotransfection of the GR cDNA.

Further cotransfection experiments into the human neuroblastoma cell line SK-N-MC revealed that basal promoter activity is not regulated by the glucocorticoid receptor. Though the promoter was efficiently stimulated by inducers of cAMP, we observed no modulation of promoter activity by cotransfection of the GR.

Discussion

In summary, our results suggest that differential regulation and repression of the hCRH gene promoter by glucocorticoids can be mimicked in vitro by transfection of the promoter into different cell lines. In future studies we shall attempt to isolate the cis-DNA elements involved in repression and differential regulation.

References

1. Swanson LW and Simmons DM (1989) J. Comp. Neurol. 285: 413–435.
2. Phi Van L, Spengler DH and Holsboer F (1990) Endocrinology 127: 1412–1418.

Biological Psychiatry, Volume 1. G. Racagni et al., editors.

Does depression cause pain or pain cause depression?

Harold Merskey
Research Department, London Psychiatric Hospital, 850 Highbury Avenue, P.O. Box 2532, London, Ontario N6A 4H1, Canada

Pain has repeatedly been found to be associated with psychological illness [1]. This is the case both with psychiatric patients and with patients in other settings. Chaturvedi et al. [2] showed that, among patients with chronic pain and no significant physical lesion, only 14% lacked a psychiatric diagnosis. Where there was physical illness, a psychiatric diagnosis could not be made in 42%. Romano and Turner [3] noted that the frequency of depression in different samples with chronic pain varied greatly according to the source of the samples. In twenty studies of chronic pain, depression occurred in from 10% to 100% of the whole sample, depending upon the source of the sample and the criteria for recording or demonstrating depression. One of the lowest frequencies with standardized tests was found in a population with headache [4], which is traditionally much associated with psychiatric illness. In this population with chronic headache and no major organic lesion, only 7% had troublesome depression, as diagnosed by the Levine-Pilowsky Depression Questionnaire. More had some form of psychiatric illness, including depression, when measured by the General Hospital Questionnaire, the figures for psychiatric disturbance being 52%. Nevertheless, since psychiatric illness may affect 20% to 30% of patients in general practice and in most medical settings [5], the frequency of potential psychiatric illness, including depression, in patients with chronic pain is not particularly high. In consequence, it is essential to recognise the importance of selection in biasing the occurrence of depression and the estimates of other psychological phenomena in different samples of patients with chronic pain.

Crook et al. [6] demonstrated that, in a representative sample of individuals served by a health maintenance organization, 11% of the adult population had persistent pain, defined as pain which often troubled the person and was present during the last 2 weeks. Another 5% had pain which was not persistent, but had been apparent in the same period. The Nuprin study [7] showed that 9% of an adult population, interviewed systematically by telephone, had chronic low back pain. Sternbach noted that 12% of the population in this study had chronic pain defined as pain present for more than 100 days in the last 12 months. Von Korff et al. [8] in a community study found that persistent or recurrent pain affected as many as 45% of the general population, but only 2.7% had severe and persistent pain, which limited activity for seven or more days [8]. The definition of persistent pain, used by Von Korff et al. [8] was “pain that had lasted a whole day or more or that had occurred several times in a year in the back, head, abdomen, face, or chest”. This definition differs from that used by Crook and Tunks [9] and resulted in a much higher frequency of back pain, namely 41% in the general population. Brattberg et al. [10] who also used a much broader definition than Crook and Tunks [9], likewise obtained figures of 40% of the adult population having obvious pain or stiffness, lasting over a period of more than 6 months. Although these studies seem to show wide variations, they also are in reasonable agreement, if one appreciates that each study adopted different definitions of persistence and chronicity.

Crook et al. [9] demonstrated the further importance of sampling technique. Two groups of individuals were examined who reported persistent pain. One came from the original survey above and the other from a specialist pain clinic. Despite being similar on many socioeconomic and demographic variables, the specialist pain clinic group was distinctly different from the family practice pain group on a two-year follow-up with respect to many other variables connected with pain behaviour and emotion. Thirteen percent of those from the pain clinic group, who had had persistent pain, were no longer in pain while 36% of those in the family practice group no longer reported pain as a problem.

In both groups, pain became more intermittent in those who still had pain and the emotional state improved and the use of health services decreased. Persistent pain does not necessarily continue for ever and persistent pain sufferers in the general population have a better prognosis than those referred to a specialist pain clinic. Dworkin et al. [11] further found a relationship between persistent pain and what they considered to be somatization.

Dworkin et al. [11], assessed subjects in an epidemiological survey of pain and evaluated the association of affective disturbance, somatization, and psychological distress from scores on the Symptom Checklist 1990 Revised [12]. They drew measures of somatization from this checklist and a measure of depression, which they translated into an equivalent of a major affective disorder by means of an algorithm. There was a highly significant association between the number of pain conditions reported and elevated levels of somatization. Also, individuals with two or more pain conditions were at increased risk for a diagnosis of major depression, unlike those with only one pain. The number of pains reported was a better predictor of major depression with these measures than were severity or persistence of pain. The authors concluded that pain in several parts of the body had a significant association with somatization. The concept of somatization is a complex one with several subdivisions which cannot be fully discussed here. It is logical to anticipate a relationship between depression and chronic pain, if the latter is severe enough to cause disability. Some evidence to this effect was given in the paper by Dworkin et al. [11] although the authors did not feel it to be important.

The most difficult question, in relation to depression and chronic pain, is the extent to which depression causes pain or pain causes depression. The data which Magni will report in this session indicate that at least 14.4% of a representative adult population suffered from pain in the musculoskeletal system on most days for at least 1 month in the 12 months preceding the interview. Among these patients who definitely had pain, there was more than twice as much evidence of depression as among that portion of the population who definitely did not have chronic pain. It will require longitudinal studies to determine whether specific individuals with chronic pain develop depression more frequently than by chance. Likewise, it would be essential to know if individuals with depression, at one point in time, develop chronic pain subsequently. Only by such a study can a good quantitative comparison be achieved of the relative importance of each phenomenon in causing the other.

References

1. Merskey H and Spear FG (1967) Pain: Psychological and Psychiatric Aspects. Bailliere Tindall, London.
2. Chaturvedi SK, Varma VK and Malhotra A (1984) Pain 19: 87–94.
3. Romano JM and Turner JA (1985) Psychol. Bull. 97: 18–34.
4. Merskey H, Brown A, Brown J et al. (1985) Pain (23) 1: 35–47.
5. Shepherd M, Cooper B, Brown A et al. (1966) Psychiatric Illness in General Practice. Oxford University Press, London.
6. Crook J, Rideout E and Brown G (1984) Pain 18: 299–314.
7. Sternbach RA (1986) Clin. J. Pain 2: 49–53.
8. VonKorff M, Dworkin SF and LeResche L (1990) Pain 40: 279–291.
9. Crook J, Weir R and Tunks E (1989) Pain 36: 49–61.
10. Brattberg G, Thorslund M and Wikman A (1989) Pain 37: 215–222.
11. Dworkin S, VonKorff M and LeResche L (1990) Arch. Gen. Psychiatry 47: 239–244.
12. Derogatis RL, Lipman RS and Covi L (1973) Psycholopharmacol. Bull. 9: 13–28.

Biological Psychiatry, Volume 1. G. Racagni et al., editors.

Chronic abdominal pain and depressive symptoms: An epidemiologic evaluation of the hispanic population in the United States

G. Magni[1], H. Merskey[2], M.R. Rossi[3] and S. Rigatti-Luchini[3]

[1]Wyeth-Ayerst European Clinical Research and Development, Paris, France; [2]Department of Psychiatry, University of Western Ontario, London, Canada; and [3]Department of Statistics, Padua, Italy

Chronic pain and depression frequently coexist; however, it is now evident that the majority of the data on this relationship have been collected in selected populations made up of patients referred to hospitals or psychiatric centers and that patients so channelled more frequently present psychological problems.

Abdominal pain is reported as a frequent complaint in patients seen in general practice [1]. However, very little information is to date available on the epidemiology of chronic abdominal pain in the general population.

We have examined the prevalence rates of depressive symptoms in subjects with chronic abdominal pain who participated to the Hispanic Health and Nutrition Examination Survey (HHANES). This survey was conducted by the National Center of Health Statistics (NCHS) from 1982–1984 to evaluate the physical and mental health of the 3 largest Hispanic groups in the United States: Mexican-Americans, Cuban-Americans and Puerto-Ricans.

The survey was not designed to be a national Hispanic survey; however, it actually sampled about 76% of the population of Hispanic origin in the United States in 1980. A detailed description of the plan and operations of the HHANES is available [2]. Our sample was made up of 5498 subjects, 20–74 years of age (2323 males and 3175 females), who had analyzable data on the relevant variables considered in this report.

The Center for Epidemiologic Studies Depression Scale (CES-D) was used as a measure of depressive symptomatology. Chronic abdominal pain "cases" were subjects who indicated in their response to one question that abdominal pain or lower chest pain had been present for at least 30 days in the 12 months preceding the interview.

The point prevalence rates of chronic abdominal pain were 4.6% in Mexican-Americans and 5.8% in Cuban Americans in a total of 4175 subjects. The rate was 8.3% among 1323 Puerto-Rican Americans. About 1/4 of the sample used drugs for the pain and were hospitalized because of it.

For Mexican and Cuban Americans jointly considered, there were significantly more females ($P < 0.01$) and people with a lower income in the pain group ($P < 0.01$). For Puerto-Ricans the pain group had more females ($P < 0.05$). The mean depression scores in the chronic pain groups were significantly higher than those of the respective samples with no abdominal pain and more subjects with pain scored above the pre-defined CES-D cut-off points (Mexican and Cuban Americans: cut-off $\geq$ 16; 26.7% vs. 12.4% $\chi^2 = 20.8$; df = 1, $P < 0.001$; cut-off $\geq$ 20; 18.7% vs. 8% $\chi^2 = 15.4$; df = 1, $P < 0.001$; Puerto-Ricans: cut-off $\geq$ 16; 47.3% vs. 25.8% $\chi^2 =$ 19.5, $P < 0.001$; cut-off $\geq$ 20; 4.8% vs. 19, 1% $\chi^2 = 20.2$; df = 1, $P < 0.001$). An important difference emerged between the Mexican and Cuban Americans and the Puerto-Ricans in the sense that depressive symptoms were definitely much higher in the Puerto-Ricans, with or without pain.

Logistic regression analyses with backward selection of variables were used to assess the likelihood of becoming depressed, adjusted for possible confounding variables.

As independent variables we considered at starting: sex (male-female), civil status (not married – including widowed, separated, etc. – married), education (low-high), income (expressed as the poverty index, which is a ratio between total annual family income and the updated poverty threshold, where <1 is below the poverty threshold), age (<45 years and ≥45 years) and the presence or absence of chronic abdominal pain.

The variables significantly linked to depressive symptoms with a cut-off of 16 in the Mexican-Cuban Americans sample were: female sex, not being married, low education, low income and presence of chronic abdominal pain. The corresponding figures for a cut-off of 20 were: female sex, not being married, low income and presence of chronic abdominal pain.

The results obtained in the Puerto-Rican sample were very similar to those just mentioned with a notable exception, that female sex did not appear to be a direct risk factor for depression.

This study represents one of the first assessments of the epidemiology of chronic abdominal pain and of its relationship with depressive symptoms in Hispanic Americans. It is evident from the data that subjects with pain present more depressive symptoms than that portion of the population classified as having no pain.

The results of the logistic regression analyses on the probability of becoming depressed are also quite interesting: they show a contribution to depression among Hispanic Americans by some well-recognized socio-demographic variables like female sex, low education, low income and the civil status of not being married, which have long been identified among non-Hispanic whites and blacks. It appears, however, that there are some important differences between Mexican and Cuban Americans and Puerto Ricans in this respect, particularly with regard to female sex which does not seem to be a risk factor in the latter group.

The presence of chronic abdominal pain remains an important risk factor for depressive symptoms in all the analyses considered, both in the Mexican and Cuban Americans and in the Puerto-Rican samples.

We consider that these results clearly show the existence of a close relationship between chronic abdominal pain and depressive symptoms in the Hispanic populations under study, substantially confirming previous results which we analyzed in a sample of 3023 subjects representative of the U.S. population in which musculoskeletal pain was evaluated [3].

References

1. Frolund F and Frolund C (1986) Scand. J. Prim. Health Care 4: 97–100.
2. National Center for Health Statistics (1985) Plan and Operation of the Hispanic Health and Nutrition Examination Survey 1982–1984. Vital and Health Statistics Series 1, No. 19, DHHS Publication No. (PHS) 85–1321, U.S. Government Printing Office, Washington, D.C.
3. Magni G, Calderion C, Rigatti-Luchini S and Merskey H (1990) Pain 43: 299–307.

Biological Psychiatry, Volume 1. G. Racagni et al., editors.

Platelet [^{3}H]paroxetine binding in chronic pain patients

Erling T. Mellerup, Niels-Henrik Jensen, Lise Lauritzen, Marianne Lunde and Per Plenge

Institute of Neuropsychiatry, University of Copenhagen, Rigshospitalet, Blegdamsvej 9, DK-2100, Denmark

Introduction

Binding sites, located on the serotonin transporter, have previously been studied in platelets from depressed patients and in pain patients using the ligand [^{3}H]imipramine. Most studies found decreased binding compared with control persons [1]. In the present study [^{3}H]paroxetine has been used instead of [^{3}H]imipramine.

Methods

Forty-eight ambulatory, non-cancer, pain patients and 29 control persons were included in the study. The pain condition was classified as nociceptive pain, neurogenic pain, or psychogenic pain. Actual pain was measured by a visual analog scale. The affective condition was classified as endogenous depression, non-endogenous or mixed depression by the use of the Diagnostic Melancholia Scale [2]. The severity of depression was quantified by the use of the Hamilton Depression Scale in combination with the Melancholic Scale (10). The severity of anxiety was quantified by the use of the Hamilton Anxiety Scale. Blood sampling, isolation of platelets, preparation of membranes, binding assay and calculations were all as previously described [3].

Results and Discussion

Twelve of the 29 control persons showed actual pain, measured by the visual analog scale. All the chronic pain patients showed actual pain with a mean rating thrice as high as the mean for the 12 controls. One of the 29 control persons showed high ratings for anxiety and depression as well as for pain; the results from this person were excluded from the calculations. Only 4 of the pain patients were below the scores for clinical anxiety and only 14 showed no sign of clinical depression. Of the 34 pain patients, who were clinically depressed, only 3 showed endogenous depression, whereas 31 showed non-endogenous or mixed depression. No connection was found between the pain classification and the type of depression.

Table 1 shows the results of the binding analysis. The whole group of pain

Table 1. Paroxetine binding sites in human platelets

	B_{max} (fmol/mg protein)	*P*
Control persons (28)	1190 ± 170	–
Pain patients (48)	1360 ± 240	<0.01
Without depression (14)	1270 ± 200	n.s.
Endogenous depression (3)	1360 ± 250	n.s.
Mixed depression (12)	1380 ± 260	<0.05
Non-endogenous depression (19)	1400 ± 310	<0.01
Nociceptive pain (17)	1390 ± 260	<0.01
Neurogenic pain (18)	1310 ± 210	<0.05
Psychogenic pain (13)	1370 ± 250	<0.05

patients had significantly higher platelet paroxetine binding than the controls. When the patients were divided according to pain classification, no difference between the nociceptive, neurogenic or psychogenic pain patients was observed and all three groups remained significantly higher than the controls.

When the patients were divided according to type of depression no statistically significant difference was found between the different groups, but the non-endogenous and the mixed depression groups were higher than the control persons.

Almost all patients received multiple medication and 13 received, among other drugs, tricyclic antidepressants. However, no difference in B_{max} or K_d was found between those who received antidepressants, those who received other drugs or those who were drug-free. The only exception was that whereas mean K_d was 0.025 nM, range 0.01–0.04 nM, K_d in 2 patients who received chlorimipramine was 0.05 and 0.09 nM, respectively.

No correlations were found between age, sex, pain intensity and any of the binding parameters. However, a significant correlation was found between pain intensity in the patients and score for endogenous features in the Diagnostic Melancholia Scale.

The main result of the present study was that the pain patients, who also were depressed, had higher platelet paroxetine binding than the control persons; a result which is opposite to previous studies of pain patients. One explanation for this lack of consistency may be the use of [^{3}H]paroxetine instead of [^{3}H]imipramine. If this explanation is true, wholly or partly, it may imply that many other studies using [^{3}H]imipramine should be repeated with [^{3}H]paroxetine as marker of the serotonin transporter; and only such studies, on the other hand, can answer the question. Another explanation could be that the present patient population is different from previous populations regarding pain classification and pain intensity. A third explanation could be that higher platelet binding is characteristic of non-endogenous depression, as such a result has been obtained in a study of depressed patients [4].

References

1. Mellerup ET and Plenge P (1988) Acta Psychiatr. Scand. 78 (Suppl. 345): 61–68.
2. Bech P, Kastrup M and Rafaelsen OJ (1986) Acta Psychiatr. Scand. 73 (Suppl. 326): 1–37.
3. Plenge P and Mellerup ET (1991) J. Neurochem. 56: 248–252.
4. Mellerup ET, Langer SZ et al. (1990) Pharmacopsychiatry 23: 113–117.

Biological Psychiatry, Volume 1. G. Racagni et al., editors.

Common pathogenetic mechanisms in chronic pain syndromes and in depressive disorders

Lars von Knorring
Department of Psychiatry, University Hospital, S-751 85 Uppsala, Sweden

Introduction

For several decades, it has been noted that a subgroup of chronic pain patients exists in which no organic pathology can be found to account for the pain. The syndrome has been discussed under many different names. Today it is named the idiopathic pain syndrome or in DSM III-R, the somatoform pain syndrome. It has long been noted that there are clinical similarities between the chronic pain syndromes and depressive disorders. Thus, it has been suggested that the two syndromes at least share a common pathogenetic mechanism [1].

Clinical and family studies

It has been known for a long time that depressive symptoms and depressive syndromes are very common in idiopathic pain syndromes [2]. However, only about 25% of the patients [3] fulfill the DSM III criteria for major depressive disorders. Katon et al. [4] could demonstrate that more than 50% of their patients with chronic pain syndromes had had episodes of major depression and/or alcohol abuse before the onset of the pain syndrome. Sixty percent had first degree relatives with chronic pain syndromes, 38% with alcoholism and 30% with affective disorders. In a later study, Eberhard et al. [2] reported affective disorders in 31% of the first-degree relatives of their patients with idiopathic pain syndromes.

Personality traits

There are certain personality traits that are regarded as important in patients with depressive disorders, including somatic and psychic anxiety, muscular tension, and inhibition of aggression as determined by means of the Karolinska Scales of Personality (KSP). By means of these personality traits, 81.3% of the subjects could be correctly classified as earlier depressed or healthy when a discriminant analysis was made [5]. In patients with idiopathic pain syndromes, many of the same personality traits exist [6] and at least 50% of the patients have the same discriminant function that is typical of patients who have had depressive episodes.

Biological markers

In an early study, Blumer et al. [7] demonstrated that 40% of the patients with idiopathic pain syndromes had shortened REM latency in sleep EEG, 50% had borderline values while only 10% had normal REM latencies. Hypercortisolemia and pathological DST are also common in patients with idiopathic pain syndromes [7,8].

In patients with idiopathic pain syndromes, low concentration of 5-HIAA in CSF have been demonstrated [9]. A significant positive correlation ($r = 0.31$) was found between the concentrations of 5-HIAA in the CSF and the duration of the chronic pain syndrome [10] and thus it is possible that the low 5-HIAA concentrations already existed before the onset of the pain syndrome. Low concentrations of MAO in platelets have also been demonstrated in patients with idiopathic pain syndromes [11]. As platelet MAO activity is stable over time and seems to be almost entirely dependent upon genetic factors with a negligible influence of environment, at least the low platelet MAO activity ought to have existed before the onset of the chronic pain syndrome. As a significant positive correlation existed between 5-HIAA in CSF and platelet MAO activity, both ought to have been present for a long time. In patients with idiopathic pain syndromes, low levels of substance P in CSF have been demonstrated [12]. As substance P and serotonin may coexist in some neurons, the results may indicate low serotonergic turnover.

Another model for the study of central serotonergic function is the high-affinity binding of ^{3}H-imipramine to platelet membranes. ^{3}H-imipramine binding has been demonstrated to be low in patients with idiopathic pain syndromes [13]. In a fenfluramine test, patients with idiopathic pain syndromes had significantly stronger cortisol and prolactin responses [14], probably indicating an increased postsynaptic receptor sensitivity in the serotonergic systems. Patients with idiopathic pain syndromes have also been demonstrated to have low concentrations of melatonin in serum and urine [15]. This finding provides a further support for the hypothesis that the depressive syndromes and the idiopathic pain syndromes at least share a common pathogenetic mechanism.

Response to treatment

ECT and antidepressants have been used for a long time in patients with idiopathic pain syndromes. Today, there are at least 40 double-blind, placebo-controlled studies in which tricyclic antidepressants have been found to be significantly more effective than placebo [16]. The mean percentage of improved patients is about 65%, which is about the same improvement rate as that found when antidepressants are used for the treatment of patients with depressive disorders. In most of the studies, amitriptyline, imipramine or clomipramine have been used. All three drugs are strong serotonin reuptake inhibitors. As there are a series of results indicating a role for serotonin in the pathogenesis of chronic pain syndromes, it is of interest that chronic pain syndromes can be relieved by means of treatment with the serotonin precursor tryptophan, by means of tricyclic antidepressants with a strong effect as serotonin reuptake inhibitors such as amitriptyline and imipramine [16] or by means of selective serotonin reuptake inhibitors such as zimelidine, fluoxethine, fluvoxamine or clomipramine. Furthermore, there are results indicating that the serotonin reuptake inhibitors are more effective than the noradrenaline reuptake inhibitors in the treatment of idiopathic pain syndromes [17].

Acknowledgement

Supported by Grants from the Swedish Medical Research Council B91-21X-09523-01A.

References

1. von Knorring L (1975) Umeå University Medical Dissertations, New Series, No. 2, Umeå University, Umeå.
2. Eberhard G, von Knorring L, Nilsson HL, Sundequist U and Wåhlander L (1989) Nord. J. Psychiatry (Suppl. 11) 43: 114–120.
3. Pilowski I (1988) In: Dubner R, Gebhart GF and Bond MR (eds.) Proc. Vth World Congress on Pain. Elsevier, Amsterdam, pp. 263–275.
4. Katon W, Egan K and Miller D (1985) Am. J. Psychiatry 142: 1156–1160.
5. von Knorring L, Perris C, Eisemann M and Perris H (1987) Arch. Psychiatr. Neurol. Sci. 234: 202–205.
6. von Knorring L, Almay BGL and Johansson F (1987) Acta Psychiatr. Scand. 76: 490–498.
7. Blumer D, Zorick F, Heilbronn M and Roth T (1982) J. Nerv. Ment. Dis. 170: 425–428.
8. Almay BGL (1987) Umeå University Medical Dissertations, New Series, No. 191, Umeå University, Umeå.
9. Almay BGL, Häggendal J, von Knorring L and Oreland L (1987) Biol. Psychiatry 22: 403–412.
10. von Knorring L (1988) In: Dubner R, Gebhart GF and Bond MR (eds.) Proc. Vth World Congress on Pain. Elsevier, Amsterdam, pp. 276–285.
11. Almay BGL, von Knorring L and Oreland L (1987) J. Neural Transm. 69: 243–253.
12. Almay BGL, Johansson F, von Knorring L, Le Grevés P and Terenius L (1988) Pain 33: 3–9.
13. Eberhard G, von Knorring L, Mellerup ET, Nilsson HL, Plenge P and Sundequist U (1989) Pain 38: 261–267.
14. von Knorring and Almay BGL (1989) Nord. J. Psychiatr. (Suppl. 20) 43: 61–65.
15. Almay BGL, von Knorring L and Wetterberg L (1987) Psychiatr. Res. 22: 179–191.
16. Eschalier A (1990) In: Besson J-M (ed.) Serotonin and Pain. Excerpta Medica Int. Congr. Series 897, Amsterdam, pp. 305–326.
17. Eberhard G, von Knorring L, Nilsson HL, Sundequist U, Björling G, Linder A, Svärd KO and Tysk L (1988) Neuropsychobiology 19: 25–34.

Biological Psychiatry, Volume 1. G. Racagni et al., editors.

Serotonergic agents in tricyclic non-responsive depressions

Steven P. Roose

College of Physicians and Surgeons, Columbia University, 722 West 168th Street, New York, NY 10032, U.S.A.

The recent availability of specific serotonin reuptake blockers raises a number of questions as to the efficacy of these drugs in depressed patients that are treatment-refractory, specifically:

1. are these drugs more effective than the standard tricyclics?
2. are these drugs effective where tricyclics have not worked, specifically is a serotonin reuptake blocker effective when a noradrenergic reuptake blocker has failed?

The availability of serotonin reuptake blockers has revived interest in a hypothesis that was prominent in the early 1970s, namely that there are two distinct biological subtypes of affective disorder: a) a neuroadrenergic depression which is characterized by deficient norepinephrine which is reflected by a low MHPG and which would respond preferentially to a drug that blocks the reuptake of norepinephrine; and b) a serotonin-deficient depression which is reflected by a low spinal fluid 5-HIAA and which would respond to a drug that blocks the reuptake of serotonin. Early studies which tried to demonstrate that patients who failed to respond to a neuroadrenergic tricyclic such as desmethylimipramine would then respond to a serotonergic agent such as amitriptyline were not able to demonstrate preferential drug response. Part of the problem in the 1970s was that there really were no specific serotonin reuptake blockers available, and in the dosages that were used clinically, all tricyclics block both reuptake of serotonin and norepinephrine. Furthermore, the blockade of reuptake is not the direct antidepressant mechanism of action of the tricyclics.

The availability of specific serotonin reuptake blockers has revived interest in the biological subtypes of depression. However, though these new agents specifically block the reuptake of serotonin, do they exclusively affect the serotonin system? Data from Potter et al. [1] have demonstrated that after 3 weeks of treatment, both the serotonin reuptake inhibitor zimelidine and the noradrenergic reuptake inhibitor desmethylimipramine reduce MHPG and 5-HIAA; Potter concluded "that there is an increasing body of data showing neuroanatomical and functional links between the neuroadrenergic and serotonergic systems in the central nervous system such that drugs affecting one are likely to affect the other." Though it would appear that no available drug has exclusive effects on the serotonergic vs. adrenergic system, that does not mean that all drugs are the same. As Fuller [2] noted, "a change in the metabolism of some neurotransmitter other than serotonin (e.g. norepinephrine) is not in itself evidence for non-specificity for action of a serotonergic agent. Such metabolic changes may be a result of increasing serotonergic input to these neurons as a consequence of inhibiting serotonin reuptake."

Is there evidence that serotonergic agents are as effective or more effective than standard tricyclic antidepressants? In considering the multiple studies addressing this issue one has to maintain a critical perspective for a number of reasons. First, most of these studies are funded by the drug company testing a new drug so there is an a priori desire to find that the new drug is equal to or better than the standard tricyclic. This will lead companies to use sub-optimal tricyclic treatment for comparison to their new agent. Moreover, one must ask not only are these studies comparing comparable doses of the drug, but also for how long is the drug given and what is the measure of outcome, e.g. are the studies using reduction in Hamilton score or a categorical recovered vs. not recovered outcome? The available data provide no evidence that any of the serotonergic agents are more effective than tricyclic antidepressants in patients with major depressive disorder, and there is at this point some suggestion that they may not be as effective for patients with melancholia.

But what about the effectiveness of the specific serotonergic agents where standard tricyclics have not worked? These studies generally follow the idea of comparing the specific serotonin reuptake blockers to neuroadrenergic tricyclics. Nystrom and Hallstrom [3] looked at the response of maprotiline vs. zimelidine and reported that in 7 maprotiline non-responders 6 of the 7 responded to zimelidine whereas in 7 zimelidine non-responders 6 of the 7 responded to maprotiline. Aberg-Wistedt [4] reported that in 5 zimelidine non-responders 3 of 5 responded to desipramine whereas in 11 desipramine non-responders treated with zimelidine, 8 of 11 responded. In a methodologically excellent study Delgado et al. [5] reported a 20% response rate in 28 patients who had not responded to 4 weeks of a therapeutic plasma level of tricyclics or a minimum of 300 mg of imipramine or its equivalent who were subsequently treated with 300 mg of fluvoxamine. In the largest study to date addressing this issue, Nolen et al. [6] studied 68 patients who had not responded to a minimum of 150 mg of imipramine or its equivalent for 4 weeks with a minimum post-treatment Hamilton score greater than 18, in a crossover design using oxaprotiline vs. fluvoxamine. In the first phase, 27% (9 out of 33) of patients treated with oxaprotiline responded, and of the 35 patients treated with fluvoxamine none responded. In the crossover phase of the 21 oxaprotiline non-responders treated with fluvoxamine 10% responded, and in the 31 fluvoxamine non-responders treated with oxaprotiline 38% responded.

The studies to date report a consistent, but not robust, effect of serotonergic agents when a neuroadrenergic agent has failed. Furthermore, in a new study by Beasley et al. [7] reporting on fluoxetine treatment in patients who have failed to respond to tricyclics, a 50% reduction of Hamilton score was achieved in 50% of tricyclic non-responders. However, if one looks at the categorical response of recovered vs. not recovered, then only 17% of the fluoxetine-treated patients responded. Thus, the evidence that serotonergic agents are an effective treatment when a standard tricyclic, noradrenergic or otherwise, has been ineffective is limited. However, there do seem to be some promising results when a serotonergic agent is combined with a tricyclic antidepressant. Weilburg et al. [8], in an open study of fluoxetine augmentation in 28 patients who had been unresponsive to tricyclic antidepressants, reported that 24 out of 28 (88%) had a robust response to this augmentation strategy. This needs to be replicated in a double-blind, placebo-controlled design. Of further interest is a recent report by Nelson et al. [9] combining desmethylimipramine with fluoxetine (20 mg per day administered between day 2 and 14 of the tricyclic treatment). Patients on the combined treatment had a faster response and at endpoint were significantly better than the patients on desmethylimipramine alone. Again, this was an open study that needs double-blind placebo replication. However, both the Weilburg and Nelson studies raise the question of whether increased specificity of antidepressant agents works against, rather than for, treatment response.

In summary, there has been revision of the original hypothesis that there are noradrenergic vs. serotonergic depressions, such that it may be that both systems are disrupted in affective disorder. It is known that an intact serotonin system is necessary to down-regulate β-receptors, which is presumed to be a mechanism of action of antidepressant medications. It may be that drugs, or combinations of drugs, which affect both receptor systems directly are more robust in the treatment of depression, particularly in cases labeled treatment-refractory.

References

1. Potter WZ, Calil HM, Extein I et al. (1981) Acta Psychiatr. Scand. (Suppl.) 290: 152–170.
2. Fuller RW (1987) J. Clin. Psychiatry 48 (Suppl. 3): 5–11.
3. Nystrom C and Hallstrom T (1987) Acta Psychiatr. Scand. 75: 377–382.
4. Aberg-Wistedt A (1982) Acta Psychiatr. Scand. 66: 129–138.
5. Delgado PL, Price LH, Charney DS et al. (1988) J. Affective Disord. 15: 55–60.
6. Nolen WA, van de Putte JJ, Dijken WA et al. (1988) Acta Psychiatr. Scand. 78: 668–675.
7. Beasley CM Jr, Sayler ME, Cunningham GE, Weiss AM and Masica DN (1990) J. Affective Disord. 20: 193–200.
8. Weilburg JB, Rosenbaum JF, Biederman J et al. (1989) J. Clin. Psychiatry 50: 447–449.
9. Nelson JC, Mazure CM, Bowers MB Jr and Jatlow PI (1991) Arch Gen. Psychiatry 48: 303–307.

Biological Psychiatry, Volume 1. G. Racagni et al., editors.

Lithium addition in treatment-resistant depression: Evidence for the involvement of the serotonin system

Claude de Montigny
Neurobiological Psychiatry Unit, Department of Psychiatry, McGill University, 1033 Pine Avenue West, Montreal, Quebec, Canada H3A 1A1

The notion of a possible synergism of lithium and antidepressant drugs in major depression emerged in the 1970s [1–3]. However, the first prospective clinical trial on the effectiveness of lithium addition in tricyclic antidepressant-resistant depression was carried out in 1981 [4]. The study was devised to put to the test the hypothesis that tricyclic antidepressant treatment induces in humans a sensitization of postsynaptic neurons to serotonin. It was predicted that, by enhancing serotonin neuron function, lithium would unveil the sensitization of postsynaptic neurons induced by the prior unsuccessful tricyclic antidepressant treatment. The development of this therapeutic strategy was based on several observations of the neurobiological effects of tricyclic antidepressant drugs and of lithium on the serotonin system. First, long-term tricyclic antidepressant treatment induces a selective increase of the responsiveness to serotonin in the rat dorsal hippocampus [5], which has been recently shown to be mediated by 5-HT_{1A} receptors [6], consistent with the increased density of 5-HT_{1A} binding sites detected in this region of the limbic system following such a treatment [7]. Second, several behavioral, biochemical and electrophysiological studies have demonstrated the enhancement of serotonin neuron function by lithium [8–10]. It is of major importance that the long-term administration of several types of antidepressant treatments, such as tricyclic antidepressant drugs, monoamine oxidase inhibitors, serotonin reuptake blockers and electroconvulsive shocks, has been shown in humans, using neuroendocrinological paradigms, to enhance hormonal responses to the serotonin precursor L-tryptophan or to the serotonin releaser fenfluramine [11–15], in keeping with animal studies which have shown that these treatments increase serotonin neurotransmission [16]. Furthermore, other neuroendocrinological studies have shown that, as in animals, in humans lithium augments the function of the serotoninergic system [17–20].

Since the initial report on the effectiveness of the lithium augmentation strategy in tricyclic antidepressant-resistant depression [4], more than 55 clinical reports have not only confirmed its efficacy, but, strikingly, extended its usefulness in depressions resistant to a wide variety of antidepressant treatments (for a recent review see [17]). In the first studies, it was reported that in most patients responsive to lithium addition, a marked alteration of depressive symptoms occurred within 24 to 48 h. However, subsequent reports have well documented that many patients require a longer period of treatment for lithium addition to produce a clinically significant improvement. Since low plasma levels of lithium are generally sufficient to achieve a robust antidepressant effect, remarkably few side-effects were reported when lithium was added at doses of 900 to 1200 mg per day to diverse types of antidepressant drugs. It is now clear that lithium addition is effective in both unipolar and bipolar treatment-resistant depression. The remarkable potency of this pharmacological strategy is indicated by its effectiveness in treatment-resistant psychotic depression [18–20] and in patients unresponsive to electroconvulsive therapy [21]. There are several case reports of "switch" into mania of treatment-resistant depressed patients shortly after addition of lithium [22–25]. Interestingly, the lithium addition strategy has also been found to be as efficacious in treatment-resistant depression in adolescents [26] and in the elderly [27,28]. Furthermore, some reports suggest that it might also be effective in some other psychiatric disorders not responding satisfactorily to an antidepressant treatment such as panic disorder and obsessive-compulsive disorder [29–35], although it would appear that the degree of improvement as well as the rate of response to lithium addition are greater in the former than in the latter disorder [36].

Several lines of evidence suggest that the potentiation of antidepressant treatments by lithium might be mediated by an enhancement of serotonin neurotransmission. In particular, it is striking that the effectiveness of lithium addition in treatment-resistant depression constitutes the exact mirror image of the reversal of the therapeutic effect of antidepressant treatment obtained by decreasing serotonin synthesis [37–39]. Taken together, these observations provide strong evidence for the pivotal role of the serotonin system in mediating the antidepressant response.

References

1. Zall H (1971) Am. J. Psychiatry 127: 1400–1403.
2. Himmelhoch JM, Detre T, Kupfer DJ, Swartzburg and Byck R (1972) J. Nerv. Ment. Dis. 155: 216–220.
3. Lingjaerde O, Edlund AH, Gormsen CA, Gottfries CG, Haugstad A, Hermann IL, Hollnage P, Makimattila A, Rasmussen KE, Remvig J and Robak OH (1974) Acta Psychiatr. Scand. 56: 233–242.
4. de Montigny C, Grunberg F, Mayer A and Deschesnes JP (1981) Br. J. Psychiatry 138: 252–256.
5. de Montigny C and Aghajanian GK (1978) Science 202: 1303–1306.
6. Chaput Y, de Montigny C and Blier P (1991) Neuropsychopharmacology (in press).
7. Welner S, de Montigny C, Desroches J, Desjardins P and Suranyi-Cadotte BE (1989) Synapse 4: 347–352.
8. Grahame-Smith DG and Green AR (1974) Br. J. Pharmacol. 52: 19–26.
9. Broderick P and Lynch V (1962) Neuropharmacology 21: 671–679.
10. Blier P and de Montigny C (1985) Eur. J. Pharmacol. 113: 69–77.
11. Charney DS, Heninger GR and Steinberg DE (1984) Arch. Gen. Psychiatry 41: 359–365.
12. Price LH, Charney DS and Heninger GR (1985) Life Sci. 37: 809–818.
13. Cowen PJ, Geaney DP and Schachter M (1986) Arch. Gen. Psychiatry 43: 61–67.
14. Price LH, Charney DS, Delgado PL, Anderson GM and Heninger GR (1980) Arch. Gen. Psychiatry 46: 625–631.
15. Shapira B, Gropp C and Lerer B (1989) Biol. Psychiatry 25 (7A): 110A.

16. Blier P, de Montigny C and Chaput Y (1990) J. Clin. Psychiatry 51 (Suppl. 4): 14–20.
17. Nierenberg AA and White K (1990) Psychopharmacol. Bull. 26: 429–460.
18. Price LH, Conwell Y and Nelson JC (1983) Am. J. Psychiatry 140: 318–322.
19. Weaver KEC (1983) Am. J. Psychiatry 140: 962–963
20. Nelson JC and Mazure CM (1986) Am. J. Psychiatry 143: 363–366.
21. Shapira B, Kindler S and Lerer B (1988) Convulsive Ther. 4: 192–198.
22. Louie AK and Meltzer HY (1984) J. Clin. Psychopharmacol. 4: 316–321.
23. Price LH, Charney DS and Heninger GR (1984) J. Clin. Psychopharmacol. 4: 361–362.
24. Delisle JD (1986) Am. J. Psychiatry 143: 1326–1327.
25. Yuvarajan R and Yousufzai NM (1988) Br. J. Psychiatry 153: 828–830.
26. Ryan ND, Meyer V, Dachille S, Mazzie D and Puig-Antich J (1988) J. Am. Acad. Child Adolesc. Psychiatry 27: 371–376.
27. Kushnir SL (1986) Am. J. Psychiatry 143: 378–379.
28. Finch EJL and Katona CLE (1989) Int. J. Geriatr. Psychiatry 4: 41–46.
29. Rasmussen SA (1984) Am. J. Psychiatry 141: 1283–1285.
30. Cournoyer J (1986) Can. J. Psychiatry 31: 335–338.
31. Pope HG Jr (1988) Am. J. Psychiatry 145: 1292–1294.
32. Feder R (1988) J. Clin. Psychiatry 49: 458.
33. Camara EG (1990) J. Clin. Psychopharmacol. 10: 225–226.
34. Feder R (1990) Am. J. Psychiatry 147: 1091–1092.
35. Jones BD (1991) Can. J. Psychiatry 36: 154–155.
36. McDougall C, Price LH, Goodman WK, Charney DS and Heninger GR (1990) Am. Psychiatr. Assoc., New Res., p. 163.
37. Shopsin B, Gershon S, Goldstein M, Friedman E and Wilk S (1975) Psychopharmacol. Commun. 1: 239–249.
38. Shopsin B, Friedman E and Gershon S (1976) Arch. Gen. Psychiatry 33: 811–819.
39. Delgado PL, Charney DS, Price LH, Aghajanian GK, Landis H and Heninger GR (1990) Arch. Gen. Psychiatry 47: 411–418.

Biological Psychiatry, Volume 1. G. Racagni et al., editors.

Monoamine oxidase inhibitors in resistant major depression

Willem A. Nolen, Paul F. Bouvy and P.M. Judith Haffmans
Department of Biological Psychiatry, Psychiatric Centre Bloemendaal, Monsterseweg 93, 2553 RJ, The Hague, The Netherlands

Introduction

Since 1959 when West and Dally [1] found that the monoamine oxidase inhibitors (MAOIs) are especially effective in patients with "atypical depression" and 1965 when the Medical Research Council [2] in a study in depressed patients with some melancholic features found phenelzine to be less effective than imipramine and electroconvulsive therapy (ECT), the use of MAOIs in major depression has been very restricted.

Nevertheless, besides lithium-addition and ECT, MAOIs are also advocated for those 20–30% of the patients with major depression who do not respond to treatment with (tri-)cyclic antidepressants (TCAs). Several case-reports and open studies have been published, as well as one double-blind controlled study (Table 1) [3–10].

From these studies it can be concluded that MAO-inhibitors are an effective alternative for patients not responding to TCAs. Although most studies have not specifically described the characteristics of the patients who responded to MAOIs, it has become clear that patients with major depression with melancholic and/or psychotic features do respond [3,8,9].

Classical non-selective MAOIs vs. selective MAO-A inhibitors

In the studies presented in Table 1 only classical MAOIs were used. These MAOIs are characterized by their irreversible binding to both the MAO-A and MAO-B form of the enzyme. Their use is sometimes accompanied by severe adverse effects (orthostatic hypotension, dizziness, sleep disturbances) and the risk of interactions with tyramine and several other drugs.

The new reversible and selective MAOIs (moclobemide and brofaromine) have been found to cause lesser adverse effects, while they also can safely be combined with tyramine, which is substrate for both MAO-A and MAO-B. Until now moclobemide has not systematically been studied in patients with major depression resistant to TCAs.

Table 1. Studies of MAOIs in resistant depression

Author(s)	Patients	Design	Treatment(s)	Results
Lieb and Collins (1978)	4 psychotic depressed	Cases	Tranylcypr.	Response 4/4
Larsen et al. (1980)	17 resistant to TCAs	Cases	Isocarboxazide	Effective in follow-up
Georgotas (1983)	20 elderly resist. to TCAs	Open	Phenelzine 15–75 mg	13/20 marked response
Nolen et al. (1985)	26 resist. to –oxaprotiline –fluvoxamine –sleep depr.	Open rand. cross-over	Tranylcypr. max. 100 mg L-5-HTP max. 250 mg	Response (incl. cr. over) tran.: 16/26 L-5-HTP: 0/17
Thase and Kupfer (1985)	19 resist. to imipramine and IPT	Open	Phenelzine 5, 60–75 mg tranylcypr. 14, 20–60 mg	Response 11/19
Roose et al. (1986)	14 melanch. non-psychotic resist. to TCAs	Open	Phenelzine tranylcypr. ECT	Response MAOI: 5/5 ECT: 9/10
Nolen et al. (1988)	21 resist. to –oxaprotilne –fluvoxamine	Double-blind cross-over	Tranylcypr. max. 100 mg nomifensine max. 250 mg	Response (incl. cr. over) tran.: 10/19 nomif.: 1/15
Amsterdam and Berwish (1989)	14 resist. to ±5 TCAs	Cases	Tranylcypr. mean 113 mg	Good response good tolerance

Brofaromine vs. tranylcypromine in resistant depression

In a recently completed double-blind study, we compared brofaromine (BROF, n = 22, max. 250 mg) with tranylcypromine (TRAN, n = 17, max. 100 mg) in hospitalized patients with major depression who had not responded to treatment with maprotiline or nortriptyline, both given for four weeks and during which plasma levels were within the therapeutic ranges for the last three weeks.

Measured on the Hamilton Rating Scale for Depression (response ≥ 50% decrease) 10/22 of the patients responded to BROF and 5/12 to TRAN. Measured on the Hamilton Depression Subscale [11] (6 items, without a.o. sleep items) another 2 patients responded to TRAN.

Adverse effects were less with BROF. Orthostatic hypotension (drop in blood pressure >30 mm after standing) occurred in both groups (BROF 36.4%, TRAN 30.8%), but both lying and standing blood pressure decreased significantly more with TRAN than with BROF. Also dizziness developed significantly more with TRAN (60%) than with BROF (9.5%).

Sleep disturbances were observed both with BROF and TRAN: reduction of REM with BROF, the practical disappearance of REM with TRAN, increase of stage II with both, increased awakenings with BROF, reduction of shifts with TRAN.

It can be concluded that BROF appears to be as effective as TRAN in resistant major depression, and is better tolerated.

References

1. West ED and Dally PJ (1959) Br. Med. J. i: 1491–1494.
2. Medical Research Council (1965) Br. Med. J. ii: 881–886.
3. Lieb J and Collins L (1978) J. Nerv. Ment. Dis. 166: 805–808.
4. Larsen JK and Rafaelsen OJ (1980) Acta Psychiatr. Scand. 60: 456–463.
5. Georgotas A, Friedman E, McCarthy M et al. (1983) Biol. Psychiatry 18: 195–205.
6. Nolen WA, Van de Putte JJ, Dijken WA et al. (1985) Br. J. Psychiatry 147: 16–22.
7. Thase ME and Kupfer DJ (1985) Abstract, IVth World Congress Biological Psychiatry 271.
8. Roose SP, Glassman AH, Walsh BT et al. (1986) Am. J. Psychiatry 143: 345–348.
9. Nolen WA, Van de Putte JJ, Dijken WA et al. (1988) Acta Psychiatr. Scand. 78: 676–683.
10. Amsterdam JD and Berwish NJ (1989) Pharmacopsychiatry 22: 21–25.
11. Bech P, Allerup P, Gram LF et al. (1981) Acta Psychiatr. Scand. 63: 290–299.

Biological Psychiatry, Volume 1. G. Racagni et al., editors.

ECT in the treatment of medication-resistant depression

Harold A. Sackeim

Department of Biological Psychiatry, New York State Psychiatric Institute and the Department of Psychiatry, College of Physicians and Surgeons, Columbia University, 722 West 168th Street, New York, NY 10032, U.S.A.

Introduction

It has long been assumed that the prior treatment history of depressed patients has no bearing on their response to ECT. In general, it is believed that approximately 70–80% of depressed patients will respond to ECT regardless of their treatment history [1]. In addition to its practical implications, this view has important ramifications in considering the mechanisms of action of antidepressant treatments. If, indeed, history of failure to respond to prior adequate antidepressant medication trials has no predictive relation with ECT response, then it would appear that distinct biological processes subserve the therapeutic effects of antidepressant medications and ECT. However, until recently, there had been no attempts to examine empirically the relations between medication resistance and ECT response.

A conceptually related issue concerns the pharmacological prevention of relapse following response to ECT. Tricyclic antidepressant (TCA) medication is the standard continuation therapy in unipolar depression following ECT response [2]. Use of TCAs to prevent relapse in ECT responders is based primarily on the findings of three clinical trials conducted in England during the 1960s [3–5]. These trials were characterized by a number of methodological shortcomings, which are reviewed elsewhere [6]. The most critical limitation in this work was limited applicability to the types of patients that presently receive ECT. At the time of these trials, ECT was often used as a treatment of first choice and in none of this work was the prior treatment history of patients documented. Failure to respond to adequate antidepressant trials (medication resistance) has now become the leading indication for the use of ECT [7]. Consequently, it is common to administer as continuation therapy following ECT the very same class of medications that patients failed during treatment of the acute episode. Were this practice effective, it would also have implications for theories of mechanisms. It would suggest either that ECT has altered the neurobiological substrate so that antidepressant medications now produce an action that was absent (or weak) during the acute episode; or that what needs to be accomplished neurobiologically to prevent relapse differs from what is needed to treat the acute stage of illness. However, the efficacy of the common practice of using TCAs to prevent relapse in patients who failed acute phase TCA treatment has never been substantiated empirically.

Medication resistance and short-term ECT outcome

To address the relations between prior treatment history and short-term ECT response, we examined clinical outcome in 53 patients who received bilateral ECT [8]. Patients met the RDC for major depressive disorder on the basis of SADS interviews and, with the exception of low doses of lorazepam, were medication-free throughout the ECT course. Prior treatment during the current episode was evaluated by two psychiatrists, using rating scales that have been published [9]. Separate criteria were used for psychotic and non-psychotic patients. In dichotomous classification, non-psychotic patients met criteria for medication resistance if they had been administered at least 200–299 mg/day (imipramine equivalents) of a TCA for at least 4 weeks. Medication-resistant psychotic patients had to meet the same criteria and concurrently receive an antipsychotic medication at a dose ≥400 mg/day (chlorpromazine equivalents) for at least three weeks. Medication-resistance was also evaluated with more quantitative ratings. Each medication trial during the index episode was rated on a 0–5 scale for its relative strength [9]. A score for the strongest trial was determined, as well as the total score across all trials. The two independent raters showed excellent reliability, and means across the two raters were used.

The major findings were consistent across the three methods of evaluating medication resistance and different methods of evaluating ECT outcome. Patients who had not received an adequate medication trial during the index episode (due to severity of symptomatology, limiting side-effects, etc.) had superior ECT outcome. Using our standard criteria for ECT response, 50% of the medication-resistant patients and 86% of those who had not failed an adequate antidepressant trial were classified as ECT responders. This effect also held when examining the subgroup of patients who had previously never received ECT. The other major finding pertained to the issue of psychosis. Psychotic patients were over-represented in the group that came to ECT without having failed an adequate medication trial. When medication-resistance and psychosis were examined conjointly in prediction of ECT outcome, only medication resistance had significant relations. The subgroups of non-psychotic and psychotic patients who had not failed adequate medication trials had a strong ECT response. Non-psychotic and psychotic patients who were medication-resistant both showed a less impressive clinical outcome.

These findings suggest that history of non-response to adequate antidepressant medication trials is predictive of ECT outcome. Furthermore, the findings of other investigators suggesting that delusional or psychotic depression may have a preferential rate of ECT response may have been due to confounds with medication resistance. Patients with psychotic depression are particularly likely to come to ECT without having failed adequate combination treatment.

Medication resistance and pharmacotherapy following ECT

In another study, we followed the clinical course of 58 patients who had responded to ECT [9]. Patients were interviewed every two weeks for the first three months following clinical response, followed by monthly interviews until relapse or for one year. Post-ECT pharmacotherapy was uncontrolled, as patients were treated by their original referring physicians. Using survival analysis techniques, we examined the relations of pre-ECT pharmacotherapy and post-ECT pharmacotherapy to the rate and timing of relapse.

The major findings in this study were that when relapse occurs it is rapid. Approximately 80% of the patients who relapsed during the first year did so within 16 weeks of ECT termination. This suggests that the period immediately following ECT is the most critical in preventing relapse. Medication resistance during the index acute episode was a potent predictor of relapse, regardless of the methods used to evaluate medication resistance. Of the patients who failed at least one adequate antidepressant trial during the acute episode, 64% relapsed by the end of the first year. In contrast, in patients who had come to ECT without having failed an adequate medication trial, only 32% relapsed. The adequacy of post-ECT pharmacotherapy was at best only marginally related to relapse. The subgroup that appeared to have benefited from adequate post-ECT pharmacotherapy were those patients which did not have established medication resistance. All other subgroups had high relapse rates. Specific analyses indicated that "adequate" post-ECT TCA continuation therapy was associated with high rates of relapse in patients who had failed an adequate TCA trial during the acute episode.

Conclusions

There is now preliminary evidence that prior history of clinical response to antidepressant medications has predictive relations to both short-term outcome with ECT and to the efficacy of post-ECT continuation therapy. The medication-resistant patient may have a higher probability of both failing to respond to ECT and, given response, to manifest early relapse. At the clinical level, these findings should be tempered by the realization that even a 50% response rate with ECT in patients with established medication resistance is likely to compare favorably with alternative treatments. However, the high rate of early relapse is particularly worrisome. Prospective, randomized, placebo-controlled trials are needed to examine the efficacy of established and new continuation therapies in ECT responders. At this point it is recommended that when considering continuation pharmacotherapy following ECT, the clinician review the classes of medications (and medication combinations) the patient had failed prior to ECT and to consider use of a different class or combination (e.g., TCA-lithium combination, MAOIs, etc.). Alternatively, ECT is the only biological treatment in psychiatry that is typically stopped once it exerts efficacy. Investigation of the therapeutic properties of continuation ECT is particularly needed.

Acknowledgement

The research summarized here was supported in part by Grant MH35636 from the National Institute of Mental Health.

References

1. Fink M (1990) Neuropsychopharmacology 3: 77.
2. Abou-Saleh M and Coppen A (1988) Convulsive Ther. 4: 263.
3. Imlah NW, Ryan E and Harrington JA (1965) Neuropsychopharmacology 4: 438.
4. Kay DWK, Kahy T and Garside RF (1970) Br. J. Psychiatry 117: 667.
5. Seager CR and Bird RL (1962) J. Ment. Sci. 108: 704.
6. Sackeim HA, Prudic J and Devanand DP (1990) In: A Tasman, SM Goldfinger and CA Kaufmann (eds.) Annual Review of Psychiatry, Vol. 9. American Psychiatric Press, Washington, D.C.
7. Weiner RD, Fink M, Hammersley D, Moench L, Sackeim HA and Small I (1990) The Practice of ECT: Recommendations for Treatment, Training and Privileging – Report of the APA Task Force on ECT. American Psychiatric Press, Washington, D.C.
8. Prudic J, Sackeim H and Devanand D (1990) Psychiatr. Res. 31: 287.
9. Sackeim HA, Prudic J, Devanand DP, Decina P, Kerr B and Malitz S (1990) J. Clin. Psychopharmacol. 10: 96.

Biological Psychiatry, Volume 1. G. Racagni et al., editors.

Psychotherapy of treatment-resistant depression

Ellen Frank, David J. Kupfer and Sheri Johnson

Although much has been written about treatment-resistant and treatment-refractory depression, little attention has been paid to the possible value of psychotherapy as a treatment for this population. It seems clear, however, that psychotherapy, particularly of the depression-specific variety, might have a particularly important role to play in the treatment of those patients who do not respond satisfactorily to aggressive pharmacotherapy.

As Guscott and Grof [1] have recently indicated, there is a problem of definition which must be addressed before any question can be examined with respect to treatment-resistant or refractory depressions. While these terms have often been used interchangeably, each sometimes with very "strict" or very "loose" criteria attached to them, in the context of the present report we will refer to a treatment-refractory depression as an episode which is unresponsive to treatment despite treatment efforts which are of both sufficient intensity and duration to be expected to bring about a good response. Treatment-resistant depression will refer to an episode of depression which requires either more intensive treatment efforts and/or efforts of longer duration, but which ultimately responds with a full and sustained remission of symptoms.

The basis of the present report is the Pittsburgh Study of Maintenance Therapies in Recurrent Depression [2]. In this investigation we were primarily interested in testing the relative efficacy of 5 strategies for prophylaxis in patients with a clear history of recurrent depressive episodes. Patients who met RDC criteria for a current major depressive episode and who were rated as having a score of at least 15 on the Hamilton Rating Scale for Depression and a score of at least 7 on the Raskin Depression Rating Scale; whose most recent previous episode had occurred within the last 2.5 years; had at least one other lifetime episode; had at least a 10-week remission between the index episode and the most recent previous episode and who had no other current Axis I disorder, were entered into an acute treatment regimen consisting of imipramine (generally in the range of 150–300 mg, although higher doses were permitted in unresponsive patients) and interpersonal psychotherapy [3]. Patients were seen weekly for the first 12 weeks, then every other week for 8 and finally, monthly until they had sustained an HRSD of $\leq$ 7 and a Raskin of $\leq$ 5 for a period of 3 weeks. Patients were then entered into a 17-week continuation treatment phase during which imipramine was continued and IPT was stepped down to monthly visits if that had not already occurred. At the end of this acute and continuation treatment period, during which Hamilton and Raskin scores were required to remain in the remitted range, patients were randomly assigned to 1 of 5 maintenance treatment conditions: IPT alone, IPT with active imipramine, IPT with placebo tablet, medication clinic visits with active imipramine, or medication clinic visits with placebo tablet. The results of this maintenance treatment investigation indicated a highly significant prophylactic effect for active medication ($P < 0.0001$) and a modest prophylactic effect for psychotherapy ($P < 0.05$) and are described in detail in Frank et al. [2].

The focus of the present report is on the response of patients in the acute treatment phase. In a number of earlier papers [e.g. 4,5], we have described the extent of variability in acute treatment response in this population. For the purposes of the present report, we selected the 15 patients who required the longest time period (all ≥50 weeks) to complete the acute and continuation treatment phases but, nonetheless, were able to achieve a sustained remission and enter the maintenance phase of the study. These 15 patients were matched with 15 "normal responders", patients who required ≤28 weeks to complete the acute and continuation treatment. The 2 groups of patients were matched on number of previous episodes and duration of index episode.

A review of demographic, psychiatric history and clinical characteristics of these 2 groups of patients reveals a number of interesting differences, as well as some surprising similarities. The 2 groups did not differ on age at the time they were screened for entry into the study, sex, marital status, or education. Differences were observed, however, in baseline severity of depression, with the treatment-resistant patients being more severely depressed than the normal responders ($P < 0.04$). Not surprisingly, the treatment-resistant patients were receiving significantly higher doses of imipramine (190 vs. 260 mg, $P < 0.003$) at the time of assignment to maintenance. Interestingly, however, the combined IMI/DMI plasma level at the point of entry into maintenance did not differ between the 2 groups (259 ng/ml vs. 312 ng/ml, $P = 0.24$). The 2 groups also did not differ in terms of the probability of meeting the criteria for endogenous subtype according to RDC. We had hypothesized that the treatment-resistant patients might be characterized by more personality pathology. However, when we examined the total Personality Assessment Form score for the 2 groups, no significant differences were observed. Finally, there was no difference between the 2 groups in terms of the likelihood of having experienced a severely threatening life event in the 12 weeks prior to entry into the study.

In terms of psychiatric history characteristics, there were no significant differences between the 2 groups in terms of age at onset of first episode of depression, with the modal patient in both groups experiencing onset in the mid- to late-20s. The 2 groups did not differ in terms of the probability of having met criteria for bipolar II disorder.

In order to examine whether the normal responders differed from the treatment-resistant in terms of what may be considered psychosocial vulnerability factors or aspects of their psychotherapeutic treatment, we carried out a blind chart review of the 30 patient charts. We hypothesized that the treatment-resistant patients might be more likely to have had a history of childhood victimization, to be currently involved in a discordant or violent marriage, to be experiencing severe financial problems, or to lack sources of social support. As anticipated, there were trends for the treatment-resistant patients to be experiencing more marital problems and to be more likely to report a history of childhood victimization. There were no differences between the groups in the probability of a notation of marital violence, severe financial problems, or lack of social support. The 2 groups did differ, however, in the total number of these vulnerability factors, with the treatment-resistant patients having a larger number of psychosocial vulnerability factors.

Interpersonal psychotherapy requires that the therapist and patient agree on 1 of 4 problem areas as the focus of the acute psychotherapeutic work. The problem areas designated by Klerman and colleagues [3] as being characteristic of the treatment of major depression are grief, role transitions, interpersonal disputes and interpersonal deficits. We thought it likely that the treatment-resistant patients would differ from the normal responders in terms of the nature of the IPT problem area identified and, perhaps, in the number of IPT problem areas which required attention. Although differences did not reach conventional levels of statistical significance, it appeared that the treatment of the normal responders was more likely to focus on role transitions, while the therapy of the treatment-resistant patients was more likely to focus on role disputes. There was no difference between the 2 groups in terms of the number IPT problem areas identified. A quite striking finding to emerge from the chart review was the frequency with which the therapist noted a difficulty "engaging" those patients subsequently identified by us as treatment-resistant. While such a notation was found for 8 of the 15 treatment-resistant patients, it appeared in the chart of only 1 of the 15 normal responders. Thus, it appears that these patients were treatment-resistant both with respect to pharmacotherapy and with respect to psychotherapy. In the chart it was not unusual to find comments such as "highly intellectualized defensive style", "dissatisfaction expressed through vague complaints", "the patient's missionary-like quality has, at the same time, served to make it more difficult for her to accept any help when she is herself depressed", "engaging this patient has been a formidable task", "minimally motivated for treatment; mostly noncommunicative in sessions" and "IPT sessions, initially, have really been cognitive battles". Comments like these were strikingly absent from the charts of the patients characterized by a more normal and rapid response to combined pharmacotherapy and IPT.

Thus, it appears that the treatment-resistant patient may differ from the patient who has a more normal response to a combination of pharmacotherapy and psychotherapy in terms of at least two psychosocial vulnerability factors (childhood victimization and current marital problems), in terms of being more likely to have problems which are ongoing and chronic rather than those which may be more of a short term-nature and, most clearly, in terms of capacity to engage in the psychotherapeutic process. What the present report cannot address, because of the nature of the study design, is the extent to which the addition of interpersonal psychotherapy may have helped to convert these 15 patients from treatment-refractory to treatment-resistant. If nothing else, it seems likely that although these patients were difficult to engage in psychotherapy, the presence of the psychotherapeutic relationship, however tenuous, may have served to sustain them during their long road to recovery.

References

1. Guscott R and Grof P (1991) Am. J. Psychiatry 148(6): 695–704.
2. Frank E, Kupfer DJ, Perel JM, Cornes C, Jarrett DB, Mallinger AM, Thase M, McEachran AB and Grochocinski VJ (1990) Arch. Gen. Psychiatry 47: 1093–1099.
3. Klerman GL, Weissman MM, Rounsaville BJ and Chevron ES (1984) Interpersonal Psychotherapy of Depression. Basic Books Inc., New York.
4. Frank E, Jarrett DB, Kupfer DJ and Grochcinski VJ (1984) Psychiatr. Res. 13: 315–324.
5. Frank E, Kupfer DJ, Jacob M and Jarrett D (1987) J. Pers. Disord. 1: 14–26.

Biological Psychiatry, Volume 1. G. Racagni et al., editors.

Schedule of ECT administration: Implications for antidepressant efficacy and adverse effects

B. Shapira[1,2], J. Hadjez[1], A. Calev[1] and B. Lerer[2]

[1]Depression Treatment Unit, Herzog Hospital; and [2]Department of Psychiatry, Hebrew University Medical School, Jerusalem, Israel

Introduction

Optimization of ECT administration implies the achievement of maximal therapeutic effects in the context of minimal impairment of cognitive function. The major treatment parameters which need to be defined to attain this objective are stimulus waveform, electrode placement, stimulus intensity and schedule of administration. In order to define an optimum treatment schedule, the most appropriate rate of ECT administration (i.e. number ECTs per week) and total number of ECTs in the series must be established. Previous work has shown that increased frequency of ECT administration and a greater total number of treatments are associated with more severe cognitive impairment [1]. It is, however, still not clear to what extent these parameters can be reduced without impairing therapeutic efficacy or significantly slowing the rate of response.

Previous studies

Surveys of clinical practice indicate that 3 times weekly ECT (with a total of ≈9 treatments) is the predominant schedule in the U.S.A. while in the U.K., twice weekly ECT with a median total of 6.5 treatments is applied in about 80% of cases [2,3]. That ECT administered twice weekly is clinically effective has been demonstrated in a series of controlled studies comparing real and simulated ECT (anesthesia and muscle relaxant) (e.g. [4,5]). Two studies directly comparing different schedules of administration have yielded differing results. Both employed unilateral ECT. Stromgren [6] reported that 4 times weekly ECT led to a shortening of the treatment period. Even though more ECT's were administered than to patients treated twice weekly, the more frequent schedule did not increase memory impairment or subjective complaints. McAllister et al. [7] found no difference in the therapeutic response of depressed patients administered twice or 3 times weekly ECT. Both groups improved significantly; however, cognitive impairment was greater in the patients administered the more frequent schedule (who received a larger total number of treatments). Neither of these studies was double-blind in design.

Double-blind evaluation of ECT schedules

In order to directly address these issues, patients with major depression: endogenous subtype (RDC) were randomly assigned to twice (2×) and 3 times (3×) weekly ECT administration. Double-blind conditions were achieved by the administration of 1 simulated ECT per week to the 2× weekly group. Both schedules were administered over 4 weeks giving a total of up to 12 real ECTs in the 3× weekly group and up to 8 in the 2× weekly group. Patients did not receive any adjunctive medication other than chloral hydrate for nocturnal sedation.

An interim evaluation of the results in 40 patients has been performed. Nineteen were randomly assigned to the 2× group and 21 to the 3× group. In terms of overall outcome, there was no difference between the 2× and 3× weekly schedules (comparing Hamilton Depression Rating Scale – HDRS – scores pretreatment and 1 week following the termination of the series). As defined by the schedules, the 3× group received significantly more real ECTs. Rate of response was compared by analyzing HDRS scores the day after each treatment (real or simulated) and showed a significant advantage for the 3× weekly schedule ($P < 0.001$). This was due to the greater frequency of real ECT administration since rate of improvement emerged as identical when real treatments administered to each group were juxtaposed and HDRS scores the day after each treatment compared. However, comparison of memory function on an extensive battery of tests evaluating both verbal and visual components (anterograde and retrograde) showed a clear trend towards greater impairment in those patients who were administered 3× weekly real ECT.

Conclusions

Available evidence suggests that 2× weekly ECT is a clinically effective schedule for treating depressive illness. Use of more frequent administration would be justified if it were shown that this accelerates antidepressant response or improves final therapeutic outcome. Two published studies [6,7] as well as the presently discussed interim findings of a double-blind controlled trial suggest that more frequently-administered ECT does not lead to better therapeutic results at the end of the series. However, administration of a greater number of ECTs within a shorter time period would seem to accelerate antidepressant effects and lead to earlier improvement. This is achieved (in our experience) at the cost of greater memory impairment. If so, the therapeutic advantage of earlier improvement would need to be balanced against the increased cognitive morbidity with which it is associated.

A possible avenue for reducing cognitive morbidity could be a lower total number of treatments in the series. Presently available data do not allow the relative impact of frequency and number of treatments on cognitive function to be teased apart. It is also not yet clear how the end-point of an ECT series should be defined and at what stage treatment should be terminated once a plateau of clinical improvement has been achieved. These questions need to be addressed in order to clearly establish an optimum schedule of ECT administration and thus further rationalize the clinical application of the treatment.

Acknowledgement

Supported in part by NIMH Grant No. 40734.

References

1. Squire LR (1982) In: Abrams R and Essman WB (eds.) Electroconvulsive Therapy: Biological Foundations and Clinical Applications. Spectrum Publications, New York, pp. 169–186.
2. American Psychiatric Association (1978) Electroconvulsive Therapy: Task Force Report #14. American Psychiatric Association, Washington, D.C.
3. Pippard J and Ellam L (1981) In: Electroconvulsive Treatment in Great Britain 1980. Gaskell, London.
4. Brandon S, Cowley P, McDonald D, Neville P, Palmer R and Wellstood-Eason S (1984) Br. Med. J. 226: 22–25.
5. Gregory S, Shawcross CR and Gill D (1985) Br. J. Psychiatry 146: 520–524.
6. Stromgren LS (1975) Acta Psychiatr. Scand. 52: 246–255.
7. McAllister DA, Perri MG, Jordan RC, Rauscher FP and Sattin A (1987) Psychiatr. Res. 21: 63–69.

Biological Psychiatry, Volume 1. G. Racagni et al., editors.

Effects of stimulus electrode placement on therapeutic outcome

Richard D. Weiner[1] and C. Edward Coffee[2]
[1]Department of Psychiatry, Duke University Medical Center, Durham, NC 27705; and [2]Department of Psychiatry, Allegheny Campus, Medical College of Pennsylvania, Pittsburgh, PA 15212, U.S.A.

Introduction

The precise placement of stimulus electrodes with electroconvulsive therapy (ECT) has and continues to be controversial [1]. While there is considerable agreement that non-dominant unilateral electrode placement (UL) produces significantly less severe and persistent cognitive impairment than bilateral (BL) placement [2], data concerning the relative efficacy of these two types of ECT modifications remain mixed [3]. The present studies were designed to compare the efficacy of UL and BL ECT.

Material and Methods

Study 1

Fifty-three right-handed subjects referred for ECT treatment of major depression were randomly assigned to receive either right UL (d'Elia placement [4]) or BL ECT. All subjects were free of pre-existing cerebral disease. Stimulus dosing was moderately suprathreshold. Therapeutic outcome measures included the Hamilton Depression Rating Scale, the Brief Psychiatric Rating Scale (including global ratings), the Zung Self-Rating Depression Scale and a global improvement rating based on the subject's clinical discharge summary. Memory measures, selected to be sensitive to ECT-induced changes, included delayed verbal paired-associate recall, delayed reproduction of complex figures, recall of famous events from the past several years, recall of mainly recent autobiographic memory events and various self-ratings. Assessment was carried out, blind to subject group assignment, prior to ECT and both 2–3 days and 6 months following completion of the ECT course.

Study 2

This investigation was designed to serve as a replication and extension of Study 1. Its design followed basically the same format as Study 1, except for a variety of minor modifications designed to augment sensitivity, and an inclusion of a

1-month post-ECT test session to assess sub-acute effects. A total of 43 subjects were entered.

Study 3

This study is an ongoing investigation in subjects aged 60 years or older who were referred for a course of pulse right UL ECT (administered as described above) for treatment of major depression. As opposed to Studies 1 and 2, subjects with pre-existing cerebral disease were not excluded. In this case, UL ECT non-responders following the sixth treatment were randomly assigned in a double-blind fashion to either continue on UL ECT or be switched to BL ECT (response is defined as at least a 50% drop from pre-ECT levels in Montgomery Asberg Depression Rating Scale (MADRS) scores). Therapeutic and memory outcome measures are similar to those used above. Subjects are assessed prior to ECT and both 2–3 days and 1 month following completion of the ECT course. Out of 53 subjects who have so far begun the index ECT course, 29 (55%) were non-responders following the sixth treatment, of which 25 either eventually met responder status or continued for at least 4 more treatments.

Results

Study 1

Therapeutic outcome
There were no intergroup differences for any of the therapeutic outcome measures at baseline or with respect to either acute or long-term effects.

Memory effects
At 2–3 days post-ECT, BL subjects showed greater decrease than UL subjects in recall/reproduction scores for all memory measures ($P < 0.01/0.0001$ by ANOVA), except for complex figure reproduction (mediated via the non-dominant hemisphere) and self-ratings. At 6 months post-ECT, all subjects demonstrated considerable recovery of memory function, though those receiving BL ECT continued to show diminished recall in autobiographic memory with respect to UL subjects ($P < 0.005$).

Study 2

Therapeutic outcome
Once more, no acute or long-term differences in therapeutic outcome measures were observed.

Memory effects

A repeated measures ANOVA, controlling for pre-ECT scores again demonstrated that BL subjects had greater memory dysfunction at 2–3 days post-ECT than UL subjects, except for self-ratings. In this study, however, differences were present not only for memory functions believed to be primarily subserved by the dominant hemisphere ($P < 0.0001$), but also, to a lesser degree, for complex figure reproduction as well ($P < 0.05$). The persistence of electrode placement differences was also corroborated, with BL subjects performing more poorly than UL subjects on complex figure reproduction, famous events and autobiographic memory tests at one month post-ECT ($P < 0.05$) and more poorly 6 months post-ECT on both of the latter measures ($P < 0.05$).

Study 3

Therapeutic outcome

Due to the ongoing nature of this study, only descriptive statistics are reported. There was no difference in the number of additional (post-six) ECT treatments administered to the 13 elderly subjects switched to BL ECT as compared to the 12 subjects who continued on UL ECT (4.4 vs. 4.3). However, 69% of BL subjects met responder criteria at the end of the ECT course, as compared to 50% for UL subjects. This trend was more dramatic at one month post-ECT, where 69% of BL subjects remained responders, vs. only 20% for UL subjects.

Memory effects

A slight trend favoring subjects continuing on UL ECT was observed.

Discussion

The data presented above indicate that, for a mixed age population, UL ECT may be as effective as BL ECT, and is certainly associated with less objectively demonstrable memory impairment. Study 3, however, suggests that for an elderly population including a substantial fraction with pre-existing cerebral disease, BL ECT may in fact be more effective in sustaining a remission, though the number of subjects is so far too small to allow any conclusion. The differences among these findings could be consistent with a relative difficulty in eliciting fully generalized seizures in elderly, brain-impaired individuals.

Acknowledgements

The authors wish to acknowledge NIMH Grants 30723 and 40159, as well as the Department of Veterans Affairs Medical Research Service.

References

1. American Psychiatric Association (1990) The Practice of ECT: Recommendations for Treatment, Training, and Privileging. American Psychiatric Press Inc., Washington, D.C.
2. Weiner RD, Rogers NJ, Davidson JR and Squire LR (1986) Ann. N.Y. Acad. Sci. 462: 315–325.
3. Abrams R (1986) Ann. N.Y. Acad. Sci. 462: 50–55.
4. D'Elia G (1970) Acta Psychiatr. Scand. (Suppl.) 215: 1–98.

Biological Psychiatry, Volume 1. G. Racagni et al., editors.

Stimulus intensity and the efficacy of ECT

Harold A. Sackeim

Department of Biological Psychiatry, New York State Psychiatric Institute and the Department of Psychiatry, College of Physicians and Surgeons, Columbia University, 722 West 168th Street, New York, NY 10032, U.S.A.

Introduction

In the last decade considerable progress has been made in optimizing ECT technique and challenging fundamental notions about mechanisms of action. Since the classic work of Ottosson [1], it has been widely believed that the production of a generalized seizure of adequate duration provides both the necessary and sufficient conditions for ECT efficacy. Electrical intensity above that which is necessary to produce an adequate generalized seizure does not contribute to efficacy, but aggravates cognitive side-effects. Recent research suggests that this view was wrong. Stimulus intensity may contribute to both the efficacy and side-effects of ECT. Indeed, new data suggest that the degree to which the electrical intensity of the ECT stimulus exceeds the patient's seizure threshold may be a critical factor in determining the likelihood of response, the speed of response, and the magnitude of adverse cognitive effects [2].

Seizure threshold

It has been standard practice in many facilities to administer a set stimulus dose to virtually all patients at all treatments. Based on the original premise that stimulus intensity contributed little to efficacy and greatly to side-effects, this practice could be justified if it were the case that the variability among psychiatric patients in seizure threshold was narrow and that the set dosage was marginally in excess of threshold. However, we had little information on seizure threshold variability. In the early 1980s, my group devised an empirical titration method to quantify seizure threshold in man. This involved delivering a stimulus intensity that was sufficiently modest so that a generalized seizure would be produced in relatively few patients. Under the same anesthesia, the intensity of stimulation was increased in fixed steps until the threshold for an adequate seizure was identified [3]. Various versions of this "empirical titration" method have been adopted by a variety of institutions.

In over 150 medication-free research patients meeting the RDC for major depressive disorder, we have observed a 25-fold range in seizure threshold. This range was extensive despite using an efficient form of electrical stimulation (bidirectional, brief pulse, constant current). In clinical practice, we find that the variability is greater, on the order of 40-fold. This means that when a single set dose is used for all patients, it must be relatively high in order to elicit adequate seizures in patients with elevated seizure thresholds. Consequently, patients with low thresholds may be receiving at each and every treatment doses that are 20, 30, or 40 times that which is minimally necessary. It is likely that much of the toxicity associated with ECT is a result of this practice [2].

The variability in seizure threshold is not random. With brief pulse, constant current stimulation, males have a higher threshold than females [3]. This effect is robust, with the gender difference averaging ~70% over the treatment course. Using the d'Elia placement for right unilateral ECT, the threshold for seizures is considerably lower than with the standard bifrontotemporal (bilateral) placement. This difference is on the order of ~80% [3,4]. Aging also shows a significant relation to seizure threshold, although this effect is less consequential than the gender and electrode placement effects. Indeed, the procedure used by some to adjust stimulus dose only on the basis of patient age may often be too aggressive, resulting in substantially excessive stimulus dose in the oldest age groups. The relations between seizure threshold and gender, electrode placement, and age have recently been replicated in an independent sample [2]. Given the wide variability in seizure threshold, the recent American Psychiatric Association Task Force report [5] on ECT recommends that stimulus dose be adjusted to the needs of each patient. This may be accomplished by either by use of empirical titration (identifying the seizure threshold by trial and error) or by an informed estimate, using knowledge of the predictors of individual differences.

Efficacy

In one random assignment, double-blind study, we contrasted the efficacy and safety of right unilateral and bilateral ECT, when all 52 patients were treated with a minimal electrical dose, just above their individual thresholds [6]. Titrated, low dose bilateral ECT was a powerful antidepressant. Unfortunately, titrated, low dose right unilateral ECT had surprisingly poor efficacy. The two groups did not differ in baseline demographic or psychiatric features, in seizure duration or in the acute cardiovascular effects of seizures [6,7]. Low dose bilateral and right unilateral ECT had response rates of 70% and 28%, respectively.

We hypothesized that the remarkably poor efficacy of titrated, low dose right unilateral ECT was due to the electrical intensity [6]. Specifically we suggested that there was an interaction between electrode placement and electrical dose in determining the efficacy of ECT. At low electrical dose, right unilateral ECT loses therapeutic properties, while bilateral ECT remains an effective treatment. In addition, at the time this trial was conducted, Robin and deTissera [8] reported findings that suggested that higher stimulus intensity may speed clinical response with bilateral ECT. At the outset of our second study we also hypothesized that stimulus intensity has a main effect of the efficiency of ECT. Regardless of electrode placement, patients would achieve clinical remission sooner when treated at higher stimulus dose.

To test these hypotheses, we recently completed a second random assignment, double-blind trial. Patients (n = 96) were assigned to right unilateral or bilateral ECT, with each administered at a stimulus intensity either just above threshold (low dose) or 2.5 times (150% above) the seizure threshold established in the first treatment (high dose). The findings from this trial have supported both hypotheses. Final response rates were 17% for low dose right unilateral ECT, 43% for high dose right unilateral ECT, 65% for low dose bilateral ECT and 63% for high dose bilateral ECT. At all the time points examined, high dose right unilateral ECT was a more effective treatment than low dose right unilateral ECT. Indeed, the differences in efficacy were marked. Nonetheless, high dose right unilateral ECT did not achieve a response rate that was comparable to either of the bilateral conditions. In designing this trial, the choice of stimulus dose for the high intensity conditions was arbitrary, given an absence of prior data on dose/response relations in ECT. At this point, we suspect that we had underestimated the extent to which electrical dose must exceed seizure threshold for right unilateral ECT to achieve comparability with more moderately dosed bilateral ECT. If in fact grossly suprathreshold (450% above threshold) stimulation is required for right unilateral ECT to achieve comparable response rates to bilateral ECT, the issue of whether right unilateral ECT retains advantages with respect to acute and subacute cognitive side-effects will be critical.

Other findings from this trial indicated that speed of clinical response was sensitive to electrical dose, regardless of electrode placement. At times, an increase in stimulus intensity may be a useful strategy to accelerate clinical response. In addition, we observed that the degree to which electrical dose exceeded threshold, and not the absolute electrical dose administered, was related to both the efficacy and side-effect findings. Because there is such wide variability in seizure threshold, a patient treated with a dose of 300 mQ (charge) may be treated just above threshold, while a patient treated with a dose of 150 mQ may be receiving stimulation that greatly exceeds threshold. Our findings indicate that if right unilateral ECT is being administered, the latter patient is considerably more likely to respond, and regardless of electrode placement the latter patient is more likely to have a more rapid response and to display more severe acute cognitive side-effects. In short, these findings suggest that the seizure threshold may act a filter for many of the neurobiological effects of ECT and that electrical dose relative to threshold may serve as the "plasma level" for these effects.

Conclusions

Stimulus intensity can have a substantial effect on the efficacy of ECT. Indeed, it has been established in two independent investigations that generalized seizures of adequate duration can be reliably produced that lack therapeutic properties. Titrated, low dose right unilateral ECT was associated with a 28% response rate in one study and a 17% response rate in a replication, indicating that this form of treatment, regardless of its advantages with respect to cognition, should not be used in clinical contexts. This demonstration indicates that the fundamental belief that the generalized seizure provides both the necessary and sufficient conditions for efficacy was wrong. The generalized seizure of "adequate" duration may be necessary, but is clearly insufficient to guarantee efficacy. There is also new evidence that the degree to which electrical dose exceeds seizure threshold is a critical measure in determining both therapeutic and adverse effects. At the practical level, this underscores the utility of determining the seizure thresholds of individual patients. At the theoretical level, this offers a new opportunity in the investigation of mechanisms. Particularly at issue are the neurobiological events that distinguish therapeutic seizures from non-therapeutic seizures. Investigation of dose/response relations may be useful in addressing this problem.

Acknowledgement

The research summarized here was supported in part by Grant No. MH35636 from the National Institute of Mental Health.

References

1. Ottosson J-O (1960) Acta Psychiatr. Scand. (Suppl.) 145:1.
2. Sackeim HA, Devanand DP and Prudic J (1991) In: Kellner C (ed.) Electroconvulsive Therapy: Psychiatric Clinics of North America (in press).
3. Sackeim HA, Decina P, Prohovnik I and Malitz S (1987) Arch. Gen. Psychiatry 44: 355.
4. Sackeim HA, Decina P, Portnoy S, Neeley P and Malitz S (1987) Biol. Psychiatry 22: 249.
5. Weiner RD, Fink M, Hammersley D, Moench L, Sackeim HA and Small I (American Psychiatric Association) (1990) The Practice of ECT: Recommendations for Treatment, Training and Privileging – Report of the APA Task Force on ECT. American Psychiatric Press, Washington, D.C.
6. Sackeim HA, Decina P, Kanzler M, Kerr B and Malitz S (1987) Am. J. Psychiatry 144: 1449.
7. Prudic J, Sackeim HA, Decina P, Hopkins N, Ross FR and Malitz S (1987) Acta Psychiatr. Scand. 75: 344.
8. Robin A and deTissera S (1982) Br. J. Psychiatry 141: 357.

Biological Psychiatry, Volume 1. G. Racagni et al., editors.

New insights into the neurobiology of ECT: Regionally selective alterations in noradrenaline release revealed by microdialysis

R. Bruce Holman, D. Nigel Thomas and David J. Nutt
Reckitt and Colman Psychopharmacology Unit, School of Medical Science, University Walk, Bristol BS8 1TD, U.K.

Introduction

The acceptance that ECT is the most efficacious treatment for severe depression has given new impetus to the search for the underlying biological mechanisms. Animal experiments have provided a means of directly assessing the effects of electroconvulsive shock (ECS) on brain function. The validity of this approach is supported by evidence that treatment regimes that mimic the human situation produce effects that are congruent with established theories, whereas other forms of ECS administration do not [1]. Animal studies have evolved their focus from assessment of brain concentrations of neurotransmitters, particularly the monoamines, to examination of receptor and second messenger systems and, more recently, of gene products [2,3].

One problem in interpreting these findings is the lack of data relating to the availability of transmitter in the synaptic cleft. For instance, it is not known whether the well-established downregulation of β-receptors is a direct action of the seizure or is due to an increased release of noradrenaline and the subsequent downregulation of receptors. The new technique of brain microdialysis allows in vivo sampling of extracellular concentrations of transmitters and metabolites and thus a means to resolve such questions. We have previously reported that acute ECS elicits regionally different changes in the release of dopamine and noradrenaline. Repeated ECS also caused significant elevations of the basal release of noradrenaline in frontal cortex and of dopamine in the striatum [4]. The present data extend this research into the actions of ECS on noradrenaline function.

Materials and Methods

Male Wistar rats (280–350 g) were anaesthetised with chloral hydrate (400 mg/kg, i.p.) and supplemented (90 mg/kg) as required to abate corneal reflex. Rats were placed into the stereotaxic frame and concentric dialysis probes implanted into either the frontal cortex or hippocampus [5]. Dialysis samples were collected every 15 min and analysed for noradrenaline content using high performance liquid chromatography with electrochemical detection. Sampling for basal noradrenaline release did not begin until at least 1 h after cannula placement and samples were collected until 3 consecutive samples did not differ significantly. At this time, to determine the effects of acute ECS, rats were administered either a single ECS (100 mA, 5 s) or sham (ear clip, 5 s) treatment and dialysis sampling continued for a further 75 min. Animals treated chronically with ECS received once-daily shocks (100 mA; 1 s) for 7 days. On day 8 they were anaesthetised and dialysed for the effect of a further ECS treatment as described above. A subsequent group of animals was treated chronically with ECS for 7 days and dialysed on day 8 to determine the effect on noradrenaline release of a challenge with the α_2-adrenoreceptor antagonist idazoxan (10 mg, s.c.).

Results and Discussion

Acute effects of ECS

In both frontal cortex and HI there was an immediate increase in the release of noradrenaline following the seizure. Table 1 shows the maximum increase in release which occurred during the first sample following ECS. A more detailed time resolution (dialysis sampling every 5 min) revealed that peak noradrenaline release occurred in the first 5-min period. Thus the noradrenaline releasing actions of acute ECS appear to be immediate and short-lived in both brain regions. The regions did, however, differ in terms of the magnitude of response; the hippocampus showed a greater response than frontal cortex. This difference exists even when the data are normalised as percentage response and could simply reflect the difference in tissue content of noradrenaline in the two areas. However, if the release of noradrenaline is a direct result of the convulsion, this could reflect the greater predisposition of the hippocampus to seizure activity. Recent electrophysiological studies have revealed an important role of noradrenaline in potentiating the activity of glutamate in the hippocampus [6] and its release could be predicted to increase seizure activity.

In rats given chronic ECS the magnitude of noradrenaline release evoked by ECS on day 8 was similar to that found after one treatment on day 1. Thus there appears to be no attenuation of this response with repeated seizures, despite other studies (e.g. Sakheim, this symposium) which have found an increase in seizure threshold during a clinical course of ECT. Interestingly, the decrease in frontal cortex presynaptic α_2-adrenoceptor response that we report below does not seem to affect the immediate noradrenaline response to the seizure, perhaps suggesting that the release of noradrenaline following a single ECS is more a reflection of the passage of current than of receptor-regulated noradrenaline release. It would be of interest to attempt to assess whether similar changes occur in human CNS, since ECT increases peripheral noradrenaline concentrations [7].

Table 1. Effects of acute and chronic electroconvulsive shock on noradrenaline release (pg/sample) in the rat frontal cortex and hippocampus

	Frontal cortex		Hippocampus	
	ECS	Controls	ECS	Controls
Acute				
Basal	4.1 ± 0.3	4.6 ± 0.2	4.5 ± 0.3	4.9 ± 0.3
Peak	11.6 ± 1.2	4.1 ± 0.3	21.2 ± 1.3	5.4 ± 0.9
% increase	282	89	475	110
Chronic				
Basal	6.9 ± 0.9	4.3 ± 0.3	4.6 ± 0.4	4.3 ± 0.5
Peak	12.6 ± 2.0	4.2 ± 0.3	20.4 ± 3.8	4.2 ± 0.5
% increase	182	97	443	97
Idazoxan				
% increase	134	231	186	193

Effects of chronic ECS on basal noradrenaline and the response to idazoxan

Chronic administration of ECS caused a significant stable increase in basal release of noradrenaline in the frontal cortex 24 h after the last seizure (Table 1). The increase release occurred only in the frontal cortex and not in the hippocampus. The simplest explanation for this increase in release would be a decrease in the function or downregulation of the presynaptic α_2 autoreceptors. In animals treated chronically with ECS, the response to idazoxan which increases noradrenaline release by blocking the presynaptic α_2 receptors [5], was significantly reduced in the frontal cortex as compared with controls, but was normal in the hippocampus (Table 1). These results support the suggestion that there is a downregulation of the presynaptic α_2 autoreceptors in the frontal cortex. The lack of change in basal noradrenaline release and in the response to idazoxan in the hippocampus suggests that α_2 autoreceptor function is unaltered in this brain region.

It is possible that the transient elevations of noradrenaline seen following each ECS in both frontal cortex and hippocampus lead to the specific increase in basal noradrenaline release in the frontal cortex. But acute ECS increases noradrenaline release in hippocampus and frontal cortex, so why are the responses to idazoxan only decreased in the frontal cortex and not the hippocampus after chronic ECS? We have recently shown that extracellular concentrations of noradrenaline are regulated differently in the frontal cortex as compared with the hippocampus [8]. Although uptake and autoreceptor mechanisms are present in both brain regions, the primary control in the frontal cortex is through activation of autoreceptors and in the hippocampus by uptake of the transmitter. Thus uptake of the transmitter in hippocampus may be so efficient as to prevent the noradrenaline released by ECS from altering autoreceptor sensitivity. Finally, it is tempting to speculate that the regionally specific increase in noradrenaline availability in the frontal cortex may contribute to the therapeutic effects of ECT. In line with this suggestion, we have also shown that several different antidepressants result in a similar increase in frontal cortex noradrenaline release.

References

1. Costain DW et al. (1979) Psychopharmacology 61: 167–170.
2. Nutt DJ et al. (1989) Convulsive Ther. 5: 250–260.
3. Gleiter CH and Nutt DJ (1989) Life Sci. 44: 985–1006.
4. Glue P et al. (1990) Psychopharmacology 100: 60–65.
5. Thomas DN and Holman RB (1991) J. Neurochem. 56: 1741–1746.
6. Nicol RA et al. (1987) In: Meltzer HY (ed.) Psychopharmacology: A Third Generation of Progress. Raven Press, New York, pp. 105–112.
7. Thiagarajan AB et al. (1989) Psychopharmacology 97: 548–552.
8. Thomas DN and Holman RB (1991) Br. J. Pharmacol. 102: 5P.

Biological Psychiatry, Volume 1. G. Racagni et al., editors.

Neurobiological mechanisms of ECT: Clinical studies

J. John Mann and Shitij Kapur
Western Psychiatric Institute and Clinic, 3811 O'Hara Street, Pittsburgh, PA 15213, U.S.A.

Introduction

The effect of antidepressant treatments on the monoamine system has been studied extensively since the promulgation of the monoamine hypothesis of depression. We review the evidence regarding the effect of ECT on dopamine, serotonin and norepinephrine systems.

ECT and the dopamine system

Spontaneous locomotor activity and stereotypic behaviors in rats are augmented by dopaminergic agents [1]. Repeated, not single electroconvulsive shock (ECS) potentiates the dopaminergic enhancement of these behaviors [2]. In humans, the dopamine-mediated neuroendocrine parameters such as prolactin and growth hormone release in response to apomorphine have been studied. Of the growth hormone studies only one out of three found evidence of enhanced dopaminergic function [3]. No studies of prolactin release found increased dopaminergic transmission after antidepressant treatment [4,5].

Studies of dopamine synthesis and turnover show no change in animals or humans [6]. Others suggest that the increased dopamine effect is related to the disruption of the blood-brain barrier, permitting an increased dopamine access to the CNS sites [2]. Decreased autoreceptor sensitivity has been suggested [7]; however, others have been unable to confirm this effect [8]. No increase in the number and affinity of [^{3}H]-spiroperidol binding to D_2 receptor had been found [9]. In contrast, studies using selective ligands for the D_1 receptor found an increase in receptor number, second messenger response and mediated functions [10]. Direct application of the second messenger, dibutyryl cyclic AMP, to the nucleus accumbens in animals treated with chronic ECS resulted in enhanced dopaminergic behaviors suggesting that there may be alterations distal to the postsynaptic receptors that may explain increased dopaminergic behavioral response [11]. Thus, although the enhancement of dopaminergic function by ECS seems well established, its relevance to the antidepressant effect remains uncertain.

ECT and the serotonin system

Direct and indirect acting serotonin agonists produce a behavioral syndrome characterized by a resting tremor, head twitch and hind limb abduction. Chronic ECS when administered in a manner that resembles ECT i.e., multiple spaced convulsive treatments, increases serotonin-mediated behaviors [12]. This effect is not due to non-specific stress. Studies in animals report no change in the serotonin synthesis and turnover after a chronic course of ECS [13]. Human studies of the effect of ECT on the serotonin turnover as measured by CSF 5-HIAA show inconsistent results [14]. Endocrine studies which measure growth hormone and prolactin release in response to serotoninomimetic agents also report conflicting results [15].

In animal studies, chronic ECS results in no change in either the number or the affinity of 5-HT_1 receptors. Studies of 5-HT_2 receptors show a consistent increase in the B_{max} [16]. This finding is interesting, as many pharmacological antidepressants decrease 5-HT_2 receptor number and this may be responsible for the differential efficacy of the two treatments. [^{3}H]-IMI binds to a serotonin transporter site on human platelets. Studies have observed lower [^{3}H]-IMI binding in depressed patients and a normalization after a course of ECT [17]. Studies at the second messenger level reveal no change in the 5-HT_1 receptor number despite diminished 5-HT_1 inhibition of cyclic AMP. In contrast, 5-HT_2 receptors show an increase in number after chronic ECS without a change in the 5-HT_2 stimulation of phosphoinositide hydrolysis [11]. In summary, ECS increases serotonin-mediated behaviors and increases the 5-HT_2 receptor number. Human ECT studies of serotonin responsivity yield conflicting results.

ECT and the norepinephrine system

The studies of the effect of ECS on the turnover of norepinephrine have found an increase in turnover [18]. Studies of ECS in animals show an increase in the brain α_1-receptor number while studies of the α_1-mediated second messenger response as measured by phosphoinositol hydrolysis report conflicting results [19]. The most consistently replicable finding of ECS in animals is the decrease in the β-receptor number after a course of ECS [20]. Consistent with the above, the second messenger system response as measured by the β-agonist stimulated cyclic AMP generation is attenuated [21]. In humans, norepinephrine turnover as measured by urinary, plasma or CSF metabolites reveals no significant change after a course of ECT [22].

Studies of depressed patients find β-adrenergic subsensitivity as shown by a decrease in leukocyte agonist-generated cyclic AMP [23]. A recent study of this marker was conducted by our group in drug-free patients with a diagnosis of depression with melancholia who were given a course of ECT. Patients were severely depressed (average HAMD score = 37) prior to treatment (10.3 ECT sessions, total seizure time 500 s) and had a significant recovery with ECT (average HAMD score = 12). The pre-treatment adrenergic responsivity as measured by isoproterenol-generated cyclic AMP was significantly lower than controls before ECT ($P < 0.001$) and improved significantly ($P < 0.001$) after a course of ECT such that it was not different from control values [23]. This normalization suggests that ECT has corrected a state-dependent abnormality and provides a potential endpoint for clinicians.

Elucidating the mechanism of action of ECT may allow development of new and more potent antidepressant drugs.

Acknowledgement

This work was supported by Grant No. MH40695.

References

1. Willner P (1983) Brain Res. Rev. 6: 211.
2. Gulati A et al. (1987) Neuropharmacology 16: 1733.
3. Costain DW et al. (1982) Lancet ii: 400.
4. Christie JE et al. (1982) Br. J. Psychiatry 140: 268.
5. Baldwin J et al. (1982) Psychopharmacology 76: 371.
6. Linnoila M et al. (1983) Arch. Gen. Psychiatry 40: 1015.
7. Chiodo LA and Antelman SM (1980) Science 210: 799.
8. MacNeil D and Gower M (1982) Nature 298: 302.
9. Atterwill PH (1980) J. Neurochemistry 35: 729.
10. Newman ME and Lerer B (1989) Prog. Neuropsychopharmacol. Biol. Psychiatry 13: 30.
11. Heal DJ and Green AR (1978) Neuropharmacology 17: 1085.
12. Costain DW (1979) Psychopharmacology 61: 167.
13. Lebrecht U and Nowak JZ (1980) Neuropharmacology 19: 1049.
14. Hoffman G et al. (1985) Psychiatr. Res. 16: 199.
15. Balldin J et al. (1980) Psychoneuroendocrinology 5: 329.
16. Kellar KJ (1984) In: Lerer B et al. (eds.) ECT: Basic Mechanisms. American Psychiatric Press, Washington, pp. 46–56.
17. Maj M et al. (1988) Biol. Psychiatry 24: 469.
18. Modigh K (1976) Psychopharmacology 49: 179.
19. Dubeau F and Sherwin AL (1989) Exp. Neurol. 105: 206.
20. Gleiter CH and Nutt DJ (1989) Life Sci. 44: 985.
21. Kellar KJ and Stockmeir CA (1986) Ann. N.Y. Acad. Sci. 426: 76.
22. Cooper SJ et al. (1988) Br. J. Psychiatry 152: 59.
23. Mann JJ et al. (1990) Arch. Gen. Psychiatry 47: 461.

Biological Psychiatry, Volume 1. G. Racagni et al., editors.

Serotonin uptake inhibitors in depression and other indications

Rasmus Fog
St. Hans Psychiatric Hospital, Department P, DK-4000 Roskilde, Denmark

The development in psychopharmacological treatment of various psychiatric disorders has placed serotonin as a very important neurotransmitter in the brain. The 5-HT reuptake inhibitors in particular seem to be effective in a whole range of very different syndromes such as melancholia, major depression, atypical depression, dysphoria, recurrent brief depression, panic disorder, obsessive-compulsive disorder, kleptomania, dementia, pain and alcoholism.

It has therefore been suggested that the 5-HT reuptake inhibitors should be called emotional stabilizers rather than antidepressants. Does serotonin play a specific role in these syndromes, or do the drugs just affect a common pathway?

If we look upon a parallel phenomenon, similarities are obvious. All neuroleptic drugs have antidopaminergic properties. These drugs are effective in treating many very different neuro-psychiatric disorders such as schizophrenia, mania, amphetamine-induced exitation, Huntington's chorea, tardive dyskinesia, Tourette syndrome and pain. Thus it is possible to establish a "dopamine hypothesis" for each of these disorders. The dopamine receptor blocking effect of different neuroleptic drugs is, however, not correlated to the clinical effect in any simple manner.

Just the same could be stated of the drugs affecting serotonin in the brain. We are, therefore, perhaps still not very close to any central pathogenetic mechanism. This does not make the 5-HT reuptake inhibitors less interesting. The important issue is, of course, that they are clinically effective so that the beneficial effect for the patients is obvious. The effects upon neurotransmitters may be far from the etiological factors, but more research in this area may eventually lead us to a better understanding of the biology underlying these syndromes.

Biological Psychiatry, Volume 1. G. Racagni et al., editors.

Psychiatric use of the selective serotonin reuptake inhibitors for indications other than depression

William F. Boyer
Feighner Research Institute, San Diego, California, U.S.A.

The efficacy of the selective serotonin reuptake inhibitors (SSRIs) in depression is reasonably well established [1]. These compounds where they are being employed in an ever-expanding range of conditions. This review will briefly note some of these promising areas.

Obsessive-compulsive disorder (OCD)

A number of double-blind studies of SSRIs in obsessive-compulsive disorder have been reported. With the exception of one small study [2] these have shown clinically and statistically significant effects in OCD [3–8]. Fluoxetine has also been studied in a number of open trials with similarly encouraging results. One study found fluvoxamine to be significantly superior to desipramine in OCD [9].

Panic disorder

Humble and colleagues treated 20 panic disorder patients with citalopram, up to 60 mg per day, in an 8-week open study. Citalopram was effective and well-tolerated [10]. Similar positive results were noted in 2 open trial of fluoxetine [11,12]. One study compared fluvoxamine with maprotiline, a specific noradrenaline uptake inhibitor, in panic disorder. Fluvoxamine was significantly effective, but maprotiline was not [13].

Premenstrual tension

Two double-blind placebo-controlled studies have shown fluoxetine to significantly decrease the affective symptoms accompanying PMS [14,15]. A study with fluvoxamine failed to show significant differences from placebo [16]. This may have been due to the strong placebo effect in this study. It may also suggest that not all of the SSRIs are equally effective for this indication.

Substance abuse

Naranjo and colleagues tested citalopram in 39 non-depressed males who were early problem drinkers. Citalopram, 20 mg/day, did not show an effect but 40 mg/day decreased the number of drinks consumed and increased the number of abstinent days [17]. These same investigators found similar results with other serotonin reuptake blockers [18].

Pollack and Rosenbaum gave fluoxetine to 11 cocaine-abusing heroin addicts in a methadone maintenance program. Of the 8 patients who completed the trial, 5 were successfully treated for cocaine abuse. They concluded that fluoxetine may be a useful addition in the treatment of cocaine abuse [19].

Eating disorders

Enas and colleagues compared 2 doses of fluoxetine in 382 outpatient bulimic women. At 60 mg/day fluoxetine was significantly superior to placebo. Fluoxetine 20 mg/day had an intermediate effect [20].

Gwirtsman and associates reported that 6 patients with chronic anorexia nervosa showed improvement in depression and weight gain with fluoxetine [21]. Ferguson reported successful use of fluoxetine in another patient with anorexia nervosa [22].

Other potential indications

Kafka reported that 9/10 men with DSM III-R nonparaphilic sexual addictions or paraphilias noted improvement in sexual behaviours while treated fluoxetine, imipramine or lithium [23]. Another case report notes the successful use of fluoxetine in treatment of a fetish [24]. Two open studies of fluoxetine have shown significant improvement in patients with severe borderline personality disorder [25,26]. The addition of fluoxetine to neuroleptic medication has also been reported to be helpful in some patients with schizophrenia [27,28].

Conclusions

One or more of the SSRIs has been successfully used in a broad range of psychiatric disorders. These possible indications deserve further study. There are implications not only in the treatment of these conditions but also the nosology, etiology, and interrelationship of these disorders.

References

1. Feighner JP and Boyer WF (1991) Selective Serotonin Reuptake Inhibitors. John Wiley and Sons, Chichester.
2. Jenike MA, Baer L, Summergrad P et al. (1990) Am. J. Psychiatry 147(7): 923–928.
3. Bick PA and Hackett E (1989) In: Stefanis CN, Soldatos CR and Rabavilas AD (eds.) Psychiatry Today: VIII World Congress of Psychiatry Abstracts. Elsevier, New York, p. 152.
4. Chouinard G, Goodman W, Greist J et al. (1990) Psychopharmacol. Bull. 26(3): 279–284.
5. Jenike MA, Hyman S, Baer L et al. (1990) Am. J. Psychiatry 147(9): 1209–1215.
6. Perse TL, Greist JH, Jefferson JW et al. (1987) Am. J. Psychiatry 144(12): 1543–1548.
7. Goodman WK, Price LH, Rasmussen SA et al. (1989) Arch. Gen. Psychiatry 46(1): 36–44.
8. Pigott TA, Pato MT, Bernstein SE et al. (1990) Arch. Gen. Psychiatry 47(10): 926–932.
9. Goodman WK, Price LH, Delgado PL et al. (1990) Am. J. Psychiatry 47(6): 577–585.
10. Humble M, Koczkas C and Wistedt B (1989) In: Stefanis CH, Soldatos CR, Rabavilas AD (eds.) Psychiatry Today: VIII World Congress of Psychiatry Abstracts. Elsevier, New York, p. 151.
11. Schneier FR, Liebowitz MR, Davies SO et al. (1990) J. Clin. Psychopharmacol. 10(2): 119–121.
12. Gorman JM, Liebowitz MR, Fyer AJ et al. (1987) J. Clin. Psychopharmacol. 7(5): 329–332.
13. Den-Boer JA and Westenberg HG (1988) Int. Clin. Psychopharmacol. 3(1): 59–74.
14. Rickels K, Freeman EW, Sondheimer S et al. (1990) Curr. Ther. Res. Clin. Exp. 48(1): 161–166.
15. Stone AB, Pearlstein TB and Brown WA (1990) Psychopharmacol. Bull. 26(3): 331–335.
16. Veeninga AT, Westenberg HG and Wesuten JT (1990) Psychopharmacology 102(3): 414–416.
17. Naranjo CA, Sellers EM, Sullivan JT et al. (1987) Clin. Pharmacol. Ther. 41(3): 266–274.
18. Naranjo CA and Sellers EM (1989) Recent Dev. Alcohol 7: 255–266.
19. Pollack MH and Rosenbaum JF (1991) J. Clin. Psychiatry 52(1): 31–33.
20. Enas GG, Pope HG and Vevine LR (1989) New Research Program and Abstracts. American Psychiatric Association 142nd Annual Meeting, p. 204.
21. Gwirtsman HE, Guze BH, Yager J et al. (1990) J. Clin. Psychiatry 51(9): 378–382.
22. Ferguson JM (1987) Am. J. Psychiatry 144(9): 1239.
23. Kafka MP (1991) J. Clin. Psychiatry 52(2): 60–65.
24. Lorefice LS (1991) J. Clin. Psychiatry 52(1): 41.
25. Cornelius JR, Soloff PH, Perel JM et al. (1990) Psychopharmacol. Bull. 26(1): 151–154.
26. Deitito JA and Stam M (1989) Compr. Psychiatry 30(6): 498–504.
27. Goff DC, Brotman AW, Waites M et al. (1990) Am. J. Psychiatry 147(4): 492–494.
28. Lindenmayer JP, Vakharia M and Kanofsky D (1990) J. Clin. Psychopharmacol. 10(1): 76.

Biological Psychiatry, Volume 1. G. Racagni et al., editors.

Pharmacokinetics of antidepressants: Clinical relevance for citalopram and other 5-HT uptake inhibitors

P. Baumann
Unité de Biochimie et Psychopharmacologie Clinique, Département Universitaire de Psychiatrie Adulte, CH-1008 Prilly-Lausanne, Switzerland

Introduction

The pharmacokinetics and clinical properties of clomipramine, the classic 5-HT reuptake inhibiting antidepressant, are well known. Within the last few years, several more specific and more selective serotonin uptake inhibitors have been introduced into clinical practice. These include citalopram, femoxetine, fluoxetine, fluvoxamine, paroxetine, sertraline and trazodone. As they differ widely in their chemical structure, important differences can be expected with respect to their metabolism and kinetics in man [1].

Biotransformation and kinetics

Role and fate of stereoisomers

Some of these drugs have at least one asymmetrical carbon atom and therefore some enantiomers exist which may differ in their pharmacological and pharmacokinetic properties [2]. Citalopram and fluoxetine are only available as racemates, but the (+)-enantiomers are known to be more selective 5-HT reuptake inhibitors than the corresponding (–)-enantiomers. Unfortunately, nothing is known about a possible enantioselectivity in the kinetics and the metabolism of these drugs. This could have some clinical consequences, as has been seen with another serotonergic agent, fenfluramine, whose (+)- and (–)-enantiomers differ in both the above-mentioned points. In contrast, (+)-femoxetine and (–)-paroxetine are clinically used, as these enantiomers have been shown to be the more selective 5-HT uptake inhibitors. Fluvoxamine, clomipramine and trazodone are devoid of an asymmetrical carbon atom.

Biotransformation and kinetics

Clomipramine, fluoxetine, sertraline, femoxetine and citalopram all have in common the fact that they are N-demethylated to a large extent. However, in the case of clomipramine, its metabolite N-desmethylclomipramine is a very specific and selective norepinephrine uptake inhibitor, in contrast to desmethylcitalopram and didesmethylcitalopram which retain serotonergic properties [3]. Paroxetine and fluvoxamine are metabolized by other oxidizing mechanisms to mostly inactive metabolites, while trazodone yields m-Cl-phenylpiperazine whose pharmacological properties are at least partially antagonistic to those of its parent compound. Most of these drugs have an elimination half-life between 7–33 h, with some exceptions. Figures of 65 h have also been reported for paroxetine. Fluoxetine differs from the other antidepressants in that its plasma half-life ranges from 1–3 days. The plasma half-life of desmethylfluoxetine, a less potent 5-HT uptake inhibitor than its parent compound, reaches 7–15 days [1].

Pharmacogenetics of metabolism

Most tricyclic antidepressants are subjected to a genetic polymorphism of metabolism as a consequence of a genetic deficiency of cytochrome P-45011D6 in part of a population (e.g. 5–10% of the Caucasian population) [4]. However, the question of whether the 5-HT uptake inhibitors are candidates for this genetic polymorphism of metabolism (also called polymorphism of the debrisoquine-sparteine-dextromethorphan type) has not yet been examined. Preliminary results of a study including dextromethorphan-phenotyped depressive patients and treated with citalopram show that in 2 poor metabolisers of dextromethorphane, i.e. presenting a genetic deficiency of the above-mentioned enzyme, citalopram plasma levels are within the range of those observed in extensive metabolisers (Baumann et al., unpublished observations). On the other hand, the metabolic ratio of dextromethorphan is higher in patients phenotyped while in treatment with 40 mg/day citalopram for 4 weeks than that measured before treatment (Baumann et al., unpublished observations). Therefore, it seems that citalopram is an inhibitor of this cytochrome P-450, but probably not a substrate.

Pharmacokinetic interactions

The question of a metabolic interaction between antidepressive 5-HT uptake inhibitors and tricyclic antidepressants has been examined by several authors ([5,6] and S. Vandel et al., this volume). Fluoxetine increases the plasma concentrations of imipramine, desipramine, nortriptyline and also of trazodone: fluvoxamine has been shown to increase those of clomipramine, desmethylclomipramine, amitriptyline and nortriptyline. This increase may lead, at least in some patients, to a potentiation of the antidepressive effect. This is in contrast to a combined treatment of desipramine + fenfluramine, where only an increase of desipramine levels but no additional antidepressant activity has been observed. A single case study shows that a treatment with 40 mg/day of citalopram added to a previously commenced amitriptyline medication (75 mg/day) has no influence on plasma amitriptyline and nortriptyline (Baettig et al., unpublished observations). The exact mechanisms of the above-mentioned metabolic interaction remain to be elucidated, as probably enzymes other than cytochrome P-450IID6 are also inhibited by some of these serotonergic drugs.

Plasma level clinical effectiveness relationship

A clear-cut plasma level-clinical effectiveness relationship has not been clearly shown for any of these recent 5-HT uptake inhibiting antidepressants. In the relative absence of anticholinergic side-effects, we suggest that future studies be centered on defining the upper limit of a "therapeutic window", taking into account the side-effects observed in the presence of a serotonergic syndrome.

References

1. Feighner JP and Boyer WF (eds.) (1991) Perspectives in Psychiatry Vol. 1. John Wiley, Chichester, p. 168.
2. Coutts RT and Baker GB (1989) Chirality 1: 99–120.
3. Milne RJ and Goa KL (1991) Drugs 41(31): 450–477.
4. Brøsen K and Gram LF (1989) 36: 537–547.
5. Bertschy G, Vandel S, Vandel B, Allers G and Volmat R (1991) Eur. J. Clin. Pharmacol. 40: 119–120.
6. Aranow RB, Hudson JI, Pope HG, Grady TA, Laage TA, Bell IR and Cole JO (1989) Am. J. Psychiatry 146: 911–913.

Biological Psychiatry, Volume 1. G. Racagni et al., editors.

Citalopram in panic disorder: Short-term and long-term efficacy. Testing a 5-HT – panic hypothesis

Mats Humble, Charlotte Koczkas, Birgitta Norberg and Börje Wistedt
Department of Psychiatry, Karolinska Institute, Danderyd Hospital, S-182 88 Danderyd, Sweden

Introduction

Panic disorder (PD) is a common, genetically predisposed, multifactorial disorder, often complicated by agoraphobia [1]. The best documented pharmacologic treatments are imipramine, phenelzine and alprazolam. They each have drawbacks; e.g. anticholinergic side-effects, diet restrictions and risk of tolerance. With classical antidepressants, a common problem in chronic treatment is weight gain [2]. Thus, alternative treatments are needed. Many symptoms of PD seem to be related to an increased noradrenergic activity. Hence, noradrenergic regulation and noradrenolytic mechanisms of antipanic drugs have been investigated. This focus on norepinephrine has not enabled prediction of clinically useful antipanic medications, however. Thus, β-blockers, clonidine and maprotiline should be effective, according to noradrenergic hypotheses. Although these drugs are reported to be successful in case reports or short-term trials, none of them has proved useful in clinical praxis, where long-term treatment is often necessary.

Antidepressants also affect serotonergic neurotransmission. Thus, serotonin may be implicated in PD. Symptoms of PD and pharmacological response seem to reflect a deficit of serotonin [2]. In a meta-analysis of different re-uptake inhibitors in open treatment of PD, mean clinical dosage and serotonin re-uptake inhibition of the drugs correlated significantly, i.e. the stronger the serotonergic effect, the lower the sufficient dose. No other biochemical property correlated to dosage [2]. Also, selective serotonin reuptake inhibitors (SSRIs) have been effective in a number of studies [3–6]. In two of these [4,5], the SSRI was superior to imipramine and maprotiline, respectively. Among the SSRIs, citalopram is by far the most selective, and it is not reported to down-regulate β-receptors or 5-HT_2-receptors [7]. Hence, based on a rationale to minimize noradrenergic contribution, citalopram was chosen as an ideal tool for elucidating antipanic mechanisms of antidepressant drugs in an open pilot study.

Material and Methods

Patients

Patients had to fulfill PD criteria according to DSM III-R, have a Clinical Anxiety

Scale (CAS) score of at least 11, indicating moderate to severe anxiety [8], give informed consent and be free of psychotropic drugs for the previous 2 weeks. However, low doses of benzodiazepines were allowed and kept constant or reduced. Twenty patients were included in the study and treated with citalopram. Of the 17 8-week-completers, 13 had PD with agoraphobia and 4 uncomplicated PD, 14 were female and 3 male, the mean age was 33 years; and the mean duration of PD was 10 years.

Treatment

The first phase of this open study lasted for 8 weeks. Citalopram was begun with the low dose 5 mg/day in order to counteract initial jitteriness syndrome (a common problem with tricyclics and SSRIs [2]). The dosage was increased to 20 mg, weeks 2–4, and, if necessary, further to a maximum of 60 mg/day, weeks 6–8. The second phase was flexible dose maintenance treatment for 13 additional months; thus the study lasted for 15 months in total. Mean citalopram dose was: after 8 weeks 41 mg/day, after 15 months 38 mg/day. Compliance was verified by determination of plasma citalopram concentration. No psychotherapy was given.

Assessments

The CAS [9] was chosen as the main efficacy parameter due to its anxiety specificity. Ratings also included MADRS [10] and Clinical Global Impression (CGI). The patients completed a panic inventory and diary, SCL-90, Agoraphobia Scale [11] and other self-rating scales. During the maintenance phase only CGI and side-effects were recorded.

Results

A summary of the patients included in the study and their outcome appears in Table 1.

Dropouts during the 8 weeks were due to nausea, unplanned pregnancy and a dissociative reaction (independent of citalopram treatment), respectively. During the maintenance phase 2 non-responders became late responders, 2 patients (1 non-responder) dropped out due to sexual side-effects, and 3 responders discontinued without implicating side-effects.

Table 1. Patients included in the two study phases

Study phase	Included	Completers	Dropouts	Responders	Non-responders
8 weeks	20	17	3	13	4
15 months	16	11	5	15	1

Psychometric assessments

On the CAS, total score was significantly decreased already after 2 weeks' [1] treatment. After 8 weeks, 13 of 17 patients had at least 50% reduction on the CAS. Eight patients were almost free of symptoms without other measures. Improvement continued far beyond the 8th week. In 7 patients, however, an aggravation, especially of cardiac and respiratory panic symptoms, was noted during the first week of treatment. This represents the jitteriness syndrome that apparently occurred in spite of the very low initial doses.

In spite of not receiving behaviour therapy, our agoraphobic patients improved substantially during the first 8 weeks, as judged by a thoroughly validated agoraphobia scale [11]. The size of the improvement was similar to that obtained with behaviour therapy. In several patients we had the impression that agoraphobia decreased early, while panic attacks responded later. Thus, we cannot exclude the possibility that citalopram exerts a primary antiagoraphobic effect.

Other symptoms that decreased in a clinically and statistically significant way were: somatization, obsessions-compulsions, interpersonal sensitivity and hostility from the SCL-90; depression from MADRS; and derealization and depersonalization from the panic inventory.

During the maintenance phase, improvement continued for the first 6 months from start. No evidence of tolerance was seen, and the gains were maintained during the 15 months.

Side-effects

As expected with a SSRI, side-effects were mild. Initial transient nausea was reported by 8 patients and was the reason for 1 dropout. One responder developed severe asthenia. Two of 3 males reported delayed ejaculation or anorgasmia. During the maintenance phase 10 patients had no side-effects. Mean body weight was constant during the 15 months, although some patients gained weight and others lost. Weight gain was connected to low tryptophan levels.

Discussion

These results (if replicated in a controlled study) and the unique selectivity of citalopram support the hypothesis that facilitation of serotonin may be of pivotal importance in the treatment of PD. Thus, the antipanic effect (and other antianxiety effects) is most likely related to the serotonin reuptake inhibition per se. This may also apply to the initial paradoxical increase of anxiety, the jitteriness syndrome. Whether this anxiety is secondary to undue stimulation of anxiogenic postsynaptic receptors, or to activation of autoreceptors, thereby decreasing serotonin turnover, remains an open question [2]. We may conclude that citalopram is useful as an antipanic drug, but also independently improves other components of anxiety syndromes. The effect seems comparable to, or better than, that of tricyclics. Side-effects are mild and similar to those of other SSRIs. Thus, citalopram is a useful tool in pharmacological dissection.

References

1. Humble M (1987) Acta Psychiatr. Scand. 76 (Suppl. 335): 15–30.
2. Eriksson E and Humble M (1990) In: Pohl R and Gershon S (eds.) Prog. Basic Clin. Pharmacol. Vol. 3. Karger, Basel, pp. 66–119.
3. Koczkas S (1983) Zimelidine Treatment in Phobias. Poster presented at the VII World Congress of Psychiatry, Vienna.
4. Evans L, Kenardy J, Schneider P and Hoey H (1986) Acta Psychiatr. Scand. 73: 49–53.
5. Den Boer JA and Westenberg HGM (1988) Int. Clin. Psychopharmacol. 3: 59–74.
6. Schneier FR, Liebowitz MR et al. (1990) J. Clin. Psychopharmacol. 10: 119–121.
7. Hyttel J, Fredricson Overø K and Arnt J (1984) Psychopharmacology 83: 20–27.
8. Snaith RP, Harrop FM, Newby DA and Teale C (1986) Br. J. Psychiatry 148: 599–601.
9. Snaith RP, Baugh SJ, Clayden AD et al. (1982) Br. J. Psychiatry 141: 518–523.
10. Montgomery SA and Åsberg M (1979) Br. J. Psychiatry 134: 382–389.
11. Öst LG (1990) Behav. Res. Ther. 28: 323–329.

Biological Psychiatry, Volume 1. G. Racagni et al., editors.

New aspects in the treatment of depression

Trevor Silverstone
Department of Psychological Medicine, Medical College of St. Bartholomew's Hospital, London, U.K.

There have been important recent advances in the management of depressive illness. These include development of new selective antidepressant drugs, improvement in the treatment of "resistant" depression and the recognition that depressive illness is frequently recurrent and can benefit from longer-term treatment.

New antidepressant drugs

Standard tricyclic antidepressant compounds have a number of disadvantages:
1. they only work in about 60–70% of patients;
2. they take up to 6 weeks before becoming fully effective;
3. they have a number of unwanted effects, particularly anticholinergic;
4. most are cardiotoxic and can be fatal in overdose.

Newer antidepressants have been introduced in the hope of promoting greater efficacy, faster onset of action, fewer side-effects and increased safety.

Drugs have been developed which selectively inhibit the reuptake of serotonin, thereby promoting neurotransmission in serotoninergic pathways (selective serotonin reuptake inhibitors, SSRI). There are also newer monoamine oxidase inhibitors (MAOI) which are reversible and can be readily displaced from the receptor by tyramine, thereby rendering a cheese reaction less likely.

The SSRI introduced for the treatment of depressive illness are citalopram, fluoxetine, fluvoxamine, paroxetine and sertraline. SSRI do not have anticholinergic properties and they are not cardiotoxic. They are less likely to cause side-effects, or be so dangerous in overdose. However, they are no more effective than standard antidepressants and do not act more quickly.

The pharmacological management of "resistant" depression

Over 20% of patients remain depressed after 2 years despite appropriate treatment with tricyclic antidepressant drugs.

When confronted with a case of resistant depression: a) review the adequacy of previous treatment and reconsider the diagnosis; b) try another type of antidepressant such as a SSRI or MAOI; and c) add lithium. The addition of lithium to standard antidepressant treatment enhances its efficacy; approximately 50% of resistant patients improve, often within a week. Lithium may be acting by promoting serotoninergic neurotransmission.

Another strategy is the addition of L-tryptophan to a MAOI. For psychotic depression, the addition of a neuroleptic to a tricyclic antidepressant is recommended.

Longer-term treatment of depression

Continuation treatment (to prevent relapse of index episode)

If treatment with an antidepressant drug is terminated prematurely (that is within 16 weeks of starting treatment) over 40% of patients are likely to relapse. The World Health Organization in a recent consensus statement recommended that continuation treatment of depression should continue for at least 6 months after recovery.

Prophylactic treatment (to prevent further episodes)

When cohorts of patients admitted for depressive illness have been followed up over a number of years, it has become clear that a large proportion relapse at least once, many several times. To reduce the risk of relapse, long-term treatment extending over years can reduce this risk; for unipolar depression use a TCA or a SSRI, for bipolar depression, lithium or carbamazepine. Greater emphasis needs to be placed on long-term use of antidepressants for high risk patients.

Conclusion

Newer antidepressants, particularly the SSRI, have definite advantages over TCA in terms of side-effects and safety. SSRI may prove effective in patients resistant to treatment with TCA. Patients with recurrent attacks of depressive illness are likely to benefit from long-term prophylactic treatment. While there is still much to be done in improving our treatment of depressive illness, we have made some real advances in recent years.

References

1. Feighner JP and Boyer WF (1991) Selective Serotonin Reuptake Inhibitors. Wiley, Chichester.
2. Leonard B and Spencer P (1990) Antidepressants: Thirty Years On. CNS Publications, London.

Biological Psychiatry, Volume 1. G. Racagni et al., editors.

Citalopram in depression: Meta-analysis of intended and unintended effects

P. Bech and P. Cialdella

Frederiksborg General Hospital, Hillerød, Denmark and Institute of Pharmacology, University of Lyon, France

Introduction

Meta-analysis of clinical trials is a formal, statistical, method of pooling data from several independent studies. This method has been shown to have importance in phase 3 trials where the hypothesis under testing is very clear: the demonstration of small but clinically relevant differences between drugs.

The clinical trials on the antidepressive effect of serotonin reuptake inhibitors have followed the "multiple independent trials approach", where the single center study uses the design for multicenter study in an attempt to make a prospective meta-analysis. By using meta-analysis in this field it was shown [1] that citalopram and fluvoxamine have antidepressive effect. This first meta-analytic study has, however, rightly been criticized for insufficiencies, e.g. lack of testing for homogeneity across trials and for using efficacy data rather than the pure intention to treat approach.

To overcome these insufficiencies a new meta-analysis of citalopram has been performed. The results reported here concern all citalopram trials (published as well as unpublished) where the Hamilton Depression Scale has been used as outcome measures. In the previous study [1] it was shown that a 50% reduction (or more) of the Hamilton baseline scores equals a global clinical improvement score of moderate to excellent degrees. The mean total score of the Hamilton Scale has also been considered. This meta-analysis of the intended effect of citalopram has focussed on subgroup analyses: citalopram vs. placebo, citalopram vs. tricyclics, and citalopram vs. amitriptyline.

Citalopram vs. placebo

Five controlled studies including 399 depressed patients randomized to either citalopram or placebo have been carried out. The analysis showed that they were homogenous. The intention to treat analysis (4 weeks) showed that citalopram was significantly superior to placebo; however, the US trials were more powerful in this respect than the European trials by analogy with the fluvoxamine placebo trials [2]. The efficacy data showed that the difference between response was 18% (confidence limits 9 and 28%) in favour of citalopram.

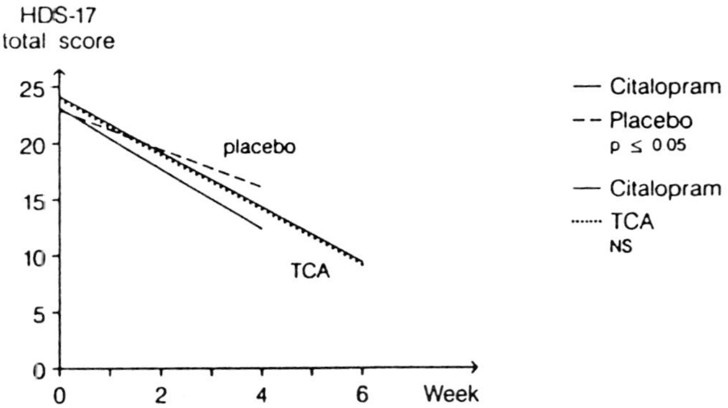

Fig. 1. Citalopram – placebo – TCA. Efficacy patients. End-point score.

Citalopram vs. tricyclics

Five controlled studies including 301 patients randomized to either citalopram or tricyclics (imipramine, clomipramine, nortriptyline or amitriptyline) have been carried out. These trials were found to be homogenous. Both intention to treat and efficacy data showed that there was no statistically significant difference between citalopram and tricyclics. The efficacy data showed a median difference of 1% in favour of tricyclics with confidence limits of 12% and −10%. The largest subgroup of patients received amitriptyline (n = 132) and no difference between citalopram and this drug was seen. However, in another subgroup (clomipramine) the tricyclic drug was found to be superior to citalopram after 5 weeks' of treatment. In this trial a fixed citalopram dose was used; in the other trials a flexible dose was used.

The results of the antidepressive efficacy of citalopram has been summarized in Fig. 1 using mean scores of the Hamilton Depression Scale. The results are very comparable with other antidepressive trials in that placebo after 4 weeks still gives a Hamilton mean score of around 15, whereas active drugs after 6 weeks give scores around 10.

Unintended effects

The meta-analytic method is not particularly suited for measuring unintended effects of drugs, because there are in this area many outcome variables (in contrast to depression, where the Hamilton Scale is the international standard). In this part of the analysis, therefore, only few adverse effects have been considered and only the amitriptyline data have been analysed. After 6 weeks of treatment (Table 1) amitriptyline showed significantly more patients having side-effects (tremor and

Table 1. Adverse effects at week 6. "Intention to treat" patients

Adverse effects	Citalopram % (n = 70)	Amitriptyline % (n = 68)
Tremor	0.0	12.5[a]
Nausea	5.3	4.2
Headache	10.5	12.5
Sweating	19.3	27.1
Dry mouth	3.5	27.1[a]
Global assessment score 2 or 3	3	10

Not corrected for baseline symptoms; [a]$P < 0.05$ (between-group differences).

dry mouth), while no difference between the two drugs was observed concerning nausea, headache and sweating.

Conclusion

This meta-analytic study has shown that citalopram is an antidepressant with few side-effects. The use of meta-analysis has recently been discussed by Souza and Goodwin [3] who emphasized: "Two decades ago, it was possible to write that 'the results obtained with lithium in depressive illness are almost uniformly bad' [4]". In phase 3 trials the judgement of drug effects should be a statistical problem while in phase 2 trials the narrative expert should be consulted.

References

1. Bech P (1989) In: Dahl SG and Gram LF (eds.) Clinical Pharmacology in Psychiatry. Springer-Verlag, Berlin, pp. 81–93.
2. Wagner W, Cimander K, Schnitker G and Koch HF (1986) In: Matussek N and Hippius H (eds.) Differential Therapy and Depression: Possibilities and Limitations. Karger, Basel, pp. 34–56.
3. Souza FGM and Goodwin GM (1991) Br. J. Psychiatry 158: 666–675.
4. Blackwell B and Shepherd M (1968) Lancet i: 968–971.

Biological Psychiatry, Volume 1. G. Racagni et al., editors.

Treatment of depression in elderly patients with and without dementia disorders

C.-G. Gottfries and A.L. Nyth
University of Göteborg, Department of Psychiatry and Neurochemistry, St. Jörgen Hospital, S-422 03 Hisings Backa, Sweden

Introduction

The etiologies of dementia of the Alzheimer type (AD/SDAT) and depression are unknown. It is well known, however, there are serious disturbances of the serotonergic (5-HT) metabolism in the brains of patients with AD/SDAT [1]. It is believed that reduced activity in the noradrenaline and serotonin systems in the brain is related to clinical states of depression. These findings indicate similarities between the biological correlates of AD/SDAT and depression. Thus it may be anticipated that drugs inhibiting the neuronal 5-HT re-uptake might have a beneficial effect both on depressed patients and on patients with AD/SDAT, with or without concomitant depression. Citalopram has been shown to block the entrance of 5-HT into serotonergic neurons, to have no effect on the uptake of noradrenaline or dopamine and to be an effective antidepressant in patients up to 65 years of age [2,3].

Material and Methods

Data from 2 studies investigating the clinical efficacy of citalopram in the treatment of elderly patients are presented. The first study was carried out at 6 centers in Norway, Finland and Sweden and comprised 98 patients with moderate AD/SDAT or VD. The patients, ranging in age from 56–94 years (mean 77.2 years) were studied in a combined placebo-controlled double-blind and open design. The trial consisted of 3 periods of treatment and was carried out over 16 weeks. In a one-week pre-period all patients received placebo. The patients were then randomly assigned to double-blind treatment with either citalopram or placebo during 4 weeks. Then followed 8 weeks treatment with citalopram as a known substance. Finally, the patients were assigned once more to double-blind treatment during 4 weeks with either citalopram or placebo. Assessments were carried out at week −1, 0, 2, 4, 8, 12 and 16 using the Clinical Global Impression Scale (CGI), Montgomery and Åsberg Depression Rating Scale (MADRS) and the Gottfries-Bråne-Steen Dementia Scale (GBS). Safety was assessed by means of the UKU side-effect scale, pulse, blood pressure, ECGs and laboratory tests. Blood samples were drawn for citalopram concentration determination. Treatment dose varied between 10 and 30 mg citalopram or placebo.

The second study comprised 149 patients with a diagnosed depression and a mean age of 77 years. The study was a 6-week double-blind controlled trial carried out at 7 centers in Denmark, Norway and Sweden. In a 1-week pre-period all patients received placebo. In the double-blind phase, the patients started on 10 mg citalopram or placebo. The dose was then increased to 20 mg. The dose could be decreased to 10 or increased to 30 mg. Assessments were carried out at week −1, 0, 2, 4 and 6 using the Hamilton Depression Scale (HDS), CGI, MADRS and GBS. Safety was assessed by means of the UKU side-effect scale, pulse, blood pressure, ECGs and laboratory tests. Blood samples were drawn for citalopram concentration determination.

In both studies patients who suffered from serious somatic illnesses (such as cardiac decompensation and malignant arrhythmias, renal insufficiency, liver dysfunction, general gastrointestinal malabsorption, or disease of the hematopoietic system), those with a history of schizophrenia, epilepsy, alcoholism or drug dependence and those who had recently been treated with monoamine oxidase inhibitors were excluded. Patients with severe dementia were also excluded. No antidepressants other than the test drug were allowed, but patients in stabilized treatment with a neuroleptic or benzodiazepine were not excluded.

Results

The first study

Eighty-nine patients were included in the efficacy analysis. The GBS ratings at baseline indicated moderate cognitive disturbances. In addition, many patients also had depressed mood, reduced motivation, anxiety or confusion. After 4 weeks double-blind treatment, significant improvements were found in the GBS items emotional bluntness ($P \leq 0.05$), confusion ($P \leq 0.01$), irritability ($P \leq 0.01$), anxiety ($P \leq 0.05$), fear-panic ($P \leq 0.05$), depressed mood ($P \leq 0.01$) and restlessness ($P \leq 0.01$) in patients treated with citalopram. No significant improvements were recorded in the placebo-treated patients. Neither motor performance nor intellectual functions were influenced by the treatment. No significant changes were recorded in the VD group during treatment with either citalopram or placebo during the first double-blind phase. For further details see Nyth et al. 1990 [4].

The second study

One hundred and thirty-three patients were included in the efficacy analysis. The CGI severity of illness mean score at baseline was 3.2 in the citalopram group and 3.1 in the placebo group. At week 6 the mean scores were 1.9 and 2.6, respectively. The differences in score and improvement were significant ($P \leq 0.02$ and $P \leq 0.005$).

According to the CGI global improvement scores at week 6, 60% in the citalopram group had improved much or very much versus 24% in the placebo group ($P \leq 0.001$). At week 6 the differences in HDS mean total scores and improvement were statistically significant ($P \leq 0.03$ and $P \leq 0.02$). For a number of single HDS items, the mean scores in the citalopram group improved significantly more than in the placebo group. This was true for depressed mood ($P \leq 0.03$), self-depreciation and guilt feelings ($P \leq 0.03$), suicidal impulses ($P \leq 0.01$), agitation ($P \leq 0.002$) and somatic symptoms ($P \leq 0.04$). The only item with significantly greater improvement in the placebo group was insomnia ($P \leq 0.01$).

Safety

Single side-effects were more frequent in the citalopram group than in the placebo group. Bradycardia was observed in some patients with initially low heart rate. No other clinically significant cardiovascular reactions or blood pressure changes were recorded.

Conclusion

The results of the first double-blind study indicate that emotional disturbances in patients with AD/SDAT diminish when these patients are treated with citalopram, but not with placebo. Since emotional disturbances, which are common in AD/SDAT, are very troublesome for the demented patients themselves and their relatives, citalopram may be valuable in the treatment of elderly demented patients with AD/SDAT and emotional disturbances.

In the second study citalopram showed an antidepressant effect on elderly depressed patients both with and without dementia. Especially the core symptoms of depression were diminished.

Side-effects were few and mostly mild. Thus, citalopram appears to be a good and safe alternative to the classical antidepressants in the treatment of elderly emotionally disturbed patients with or without concurrent dementia.

References

1. Cowburn FR et al. (1989) In: Davies DC (ed.) Alzheimer's disease: Towards an Understanding of the Etiology and Pathogenesis. John Libbey, London/Paris, pp. 9–32.
2. Hyttel J (1982) Progr. Neuro-Psychopharmacol. Biol. Psychiatry 6: 277–295.
3. Shaw DM et al. (1986) Br. J. Psychiatry 149: 515–517.
4. Nyth and Gottifries C-G (1990) Br. J. Psychiatry 157: 894–901.

Biological Psychiatry, Volume 1. G. Racagni et al., editors.

Antidepressant drugs acting on the serotonin transporter

S.Z. Langer, H. Esnaud and D. Graham
Synthélabo Recherche (LERS), 58 rue de la Glacière, 75013 Paris, France

Introduction

The re-uptake of serotonin into presynaptic serotonergic terminals by the sodium-ion coupled serotonin transporter subserves the role of terminating neurotransmission and maintaining low levels of this transmitter in the synaptic cleft. With the hypothesis that serotonergic deficits might be implicated in certain forms of depressive disorders, the sodium-ion coupled serotonin transport system became an important target for antidepressant drug design. This approach has led to the development of a number of selective serotonin uptake inhibitors including fluoxetine, sertraline, citaloprarn, paroxetine and litoxetine [1]. In clinical studies, these selective serotonin uptake inhibitors have proven to be as effective as the antidepressant imipramine, yet devoid of many of the unwanted side-effects displayed by this tricyclic agent.

Studies with radiolabelled selective serotonin uptake inhibitors have indicated that these ligands are highly specific probes of the sodium-ion coupled serotonin transporter. Recently, we have utilized ^{3}H-paroxetine as a tool to delineate details of ligand binding domains on the neuronal sodium-ion coupled serotonin transporter [2]. This work indicated that the tricyclic imipramine and a variety of nontricyclic selective serotonin uptake inhibitors bind to overlapping domains which are sterically mutually-exclusive with the substrate recognition site. Nonetheless, detailed knowledge at the molecular level on the structure and functioning of this transporter will require elucidation of the primary and secondary structure of this protein. For this reason, we have carried out a programme aimed at purifying and eventually cloning the transporter.

Materials and Methods

Membrane preparation

Crude rat cerebral cortical membranes were prepared as described previously [3].

^{3}H-Paroxetine binding assays

^{3}H-Paroxetine binding to either membrane or solubilized forms of the sodium-ion coupled serotonin transporter was performed as described previously [3,4].

Transporter solubilization and purification

Membranes were solubilized using 1% (w/v) digitonin in the presence of a cocktail of protease inhibitors for 1 h at 0°C and then centrifuged at 125,000 × g for 1 h at 4°C.

The supernatant was passed slowly through an agarose support to which an amino derivative of citalopram had been covalently coupled. The affinity-chromatographic support was washed at 4°C and an elution with 1 mM litoxetine performed. The litoxetine eluate was then subjected to wheat-germ agglutinin – sepharose chromatography.

Results and Discussion

Incubation of rat cerebral cortical membranes with 1% (w/v) digitonin resulted in the solubilization of between 40–50% of the total specific ^{3}H-paroxetine binding sites present in the membrane preparation. The pharmacological profile of the solubilized ^{3}H-paroxetine binding sites was similar to that of the parent membrane preparation, indicating that a successful solubilization of the neuronal sodium-ion coupled serotonin transporter had been attained.

For purification of the solubilized serotonin transporter, an affinity-chromatography procedure using a citalopram-based agarose support was chosen. Between 65–80% of the ^{3}H-paroxetine binding sites present in the detergent extracts bound to the chromatographic support. The support was extensively washed and the serotonin transporter eluted using the selective serotonin uptake inhibitor, litoxetine. Equilibrium saturation analysis of ^{3}H-paroxetine binding to aliquots of affinity-purified material subjected to steric-exclusion chromatography revealed the presence of a single class of high-affinity binding sites (K_d = 0.15 nM) and a B_{max} of greater than 1.67 nmol/mg protein. Given that the B_{max} of ^{3}H-paroxetine binding to the rat cerebral cortical membrane preparation was ≈0.5 pmol/mg protein, this affinity chromatography step produced a greater than 3,000-fold purification of ^{3}H-paroxetine binding activity. Citalopram, litoxetine, imipramine and serotonin inhibited ^{3}H-paroxetine binding to the affinity-purified preparation with K_i values of 7 nM, 8 nM, 64 nM and 2.5 μM, respectively. This pharmacological profile thus confirmed that this affinity-purified ^{3}H-paroxetine binding activity was indeed associated with the neuronal sodium-ion coupled serotonin transporter (Table 1).

The affinity-purified transporter preparation was in addition subjected to wheat-germ agglutinin-sepharose chromatography and then an elution with N-acetylglucosamine performed. Analysis of this N-acetylglucosamine eluate by SDS-polyacrylamide gel electrophoresis under reducing conditions permitted identification of the transporter as a polypeptide of 73 kDa. This relative molecular mass corresponds closely to those of the protein sequences predicted from the open reading frames of the cloned cDNAs of the noradrenaline [5] and GABA [6] transporters (M_r of 69,000 and 67,000, respectively).

Table 1. Profile of ^3H-paroxetine binding to the sodium-ion coupled serotonin transporter. Equilibrium saturation and competitive equilibrium inhibition assays of ^3H-paroxetine binding to the membrane and affinity-purified preparations were performed as described previously [4]

Agent	K_i (nM)	
	Membrane-bound	Affinity-purified
Citalopram	1	7
Lixoxetine	3	8
Imipramine	41	64
Serotonin	700	2500

It is hoped that the purification protocol outlined will now permit purification of the sodium-ion coupled serotonin transporter in sufficient quantities for partial protein sequencing.

References

1. Scatton B, Claustre Y, Graham D, Dennis T, Serrano A, Arbilla S, Pimoule C, Schoemaker H, Bigg D and Langer SZ (1988) Drug Dev. Res. 12: 29–40.
2. Graham D, Esnaud H, Habert E and Langer SZ (1989) Biochem. Pharmacol. 21: 3819–3826.
3. Habert E, Graham D, Tahraoui L, Claustre Y and Langer SZ (1985) Eur. J. Pharmacol. 118: 107–114.
4. Habert E, Graham D and Langer SZ (1986) Eur. J. Pharmacol. 122: 197–204.
5. Pacholczyk T, Blakely RD and Amara SG (1991) Nature 350: 350–354.
6. Guastella J, Nelson N, Nelson H, Czyzyk L, Keynan S, Miedel MC, Davidson N, Lester HA and Kanner BI (1990) Science 249: 1303–1306.

Biological Psychiatry, Volume 1. G. Racagni et al., editors.

Adaptation of central 5-HT$_{1A}$ receptors after chronic antidepressant treatment in rats

Michel Hamon, Laurence Lanfumey, Samir Haj-Dahmane, Thierry Jolas, Emma Kidd, Francisco Bolaños and Henri Gozlan

INSERM U.288, Neurobiologie Cellulaire et Fonctionnelle, CHU Pitié-Salpêtrière, 75634 Paris Cedex 13, France

Introduction

Adaptation of central neurotransmitter receptors, notably the β-adrenergic and serotonin 5-HT$_2$ receptors which down-regulate in the cerebral cortex [1], has been reported in rats treated chronically with antidepressant drugs. However, not all antidepressants produce these changes, which raises some doubt with regard to their possible relevance to the neurobiological mechanisms associated with antidepressant therapy. This is the case notably for selective 5-HT uptake inhibitors which are potent antidepressants in man, but are unable to alter the characteristics of cortical β-adrenergic and 5-HT$_2$ receptors either acutely or chronically in rats [2]. Recently a new class of antidepressant drugs, the pyrimidylpiperazine derivatives in the ipsapirone series, have provided new insights into the neurobiological mechanisms associated with antidepressant therapy as these drugs are direct agonists of 5-HT$_{1A}$ receptors [3]. The antidepressant action of ipsapirone develops progressively during chronic treatment, so that adaptation of their molecular target, e.g. the 5-HT$_{1A}$ receptor, might account – at least in part – for the therapeutic effect of this drug. In order to test this hypothesis, we have investigated the binding characteristics and functional properties of 5-HT$_{1A}$ receptors in rats treated for 2 weeks with either ipsapirone or cericlamine, a potent antidepressant with selective 5-HT uptake inhibitory properties [2]. Two main targets were considered: the somato-dentritic 5-HT$_{1A}$ autoreceptors on 5-HT neurones within the dorsal raphe nucleus (DRN) and the postsynaptic 5-HT$_{1A}$ receptors in forebrain areas.

Materials and Methods

Adult male Sprague-Dawley rats (~250 g body weight) were treated twice daily (at 9.00 a.m. and 6.00 p.m.) with saline (controls), ipsapirone (Troponwerke, 1,5 or 10 mg/kg, i.p.) or cericlamine (Jouveinal, 16 mg/kg, i.p.) for 14 days and decapitated 24 h after the last injection. The characteristics of 5-HT$_{1A}$ binding sites were determined using membrane binding assays and quantitative autoradiography with [^{3}H]8-OH-DPAT (100 Ci/mmol, CEA, France) as the radioligand [3]. Measurements of forskolin-stimulated adenylate cyclase activity in hippocampal homogenates were performed with or without various concentrations of the 5-HT_{1A} agonists 8-OH-DPAT and ipsapirone, as previously described [3]. The electrical activity of DRN 5-HT neurones was recorded in vitro, in brain stem slices prepared immediately after the sacrifice. Briefly, 1 corona slice was dissected from each rat, and continuously superfused with artificial CSF while a glass micropipette (15 MΩ) filled with 2 M NaCl was implanted into the DRN area for recording 5-HT neuronal activity.

Results

Binding studies indicated that neither the K_d nor the B_{max} or [^{3}H]8-OH-DPAT specific binding sites in membranes from the hippocampus, cerebral cortex and septum (where 5-HT_{1A} receptors are located postsynaptically) were significantly altered in rats treated with ipsapirone or cericlamine as compared to controls. Quantitative autoradiography confirmed that the binding characteristics of [^{3}H]8-OH-DPAT were similar in the 3 groups of rats at any level of the brain: hippocampus, cerebral cortex, septum and also the DRN, amygdala, interpeduncular nucleus, etc.

As expected from the negative coupling of postsynaptic 5-HT_{1A} receptors with adenylate cyclase [3], 8-OH-DPAT ($IC_{50} = 7.5$ nM) and ipsapirone ($IC_{50} = 43$ nM) inhibited ($I_{max} = -20\%$) forskolin-activated production of (^{32}P) cyclic AMP from [^{32}P]α-ATP by hippocampal homogenates from control rats. The characteristics of the enzyme inhibition by both drugs were unaltered after a 2-week treatment with ipsapirone (5 mg/kg, twice daily).

The stimulation of somato-dendritic 5-HT_{1A} receptors by 8-OH-DPAT or ipsapirone triggered a concentration-dependent inhibition of the 5-HT neuronal discharge in the DRN from control rats (Fig. 1), which could be reversed by 5-HT_{1A} antagonists such as (–)propranolol, (–)pindolol and (–)tertatolol [4]. Both agonists also inhibited the electrical activity of DRN 5-HT neurones in ipsapirone- or cericlamine-treated rats, but their potency was significantly less than in controls (Fig. 1). Thus the IC_{50} of 8-OH-DPAT and ipsapirone were 2.5–3.5 times higher after a two-week treatment with either antidepressant than in controls.

Discussion

The chronic stimulation of 5-HT_{1A} receptors by ipsapirone did not alter the number and affinity of corresponding binding sites in any area in the rat brain. In addition, the functional properties of postsynaptic 5-HT_{1A} receptors were also unaffected by this treatment as the efficiency of the negative coupling between these receptors and adenylate cyclase activity was not significantly different in the hippocampus from ipsapirone- or saline-treated rats. In contrast, a functional desensitization of

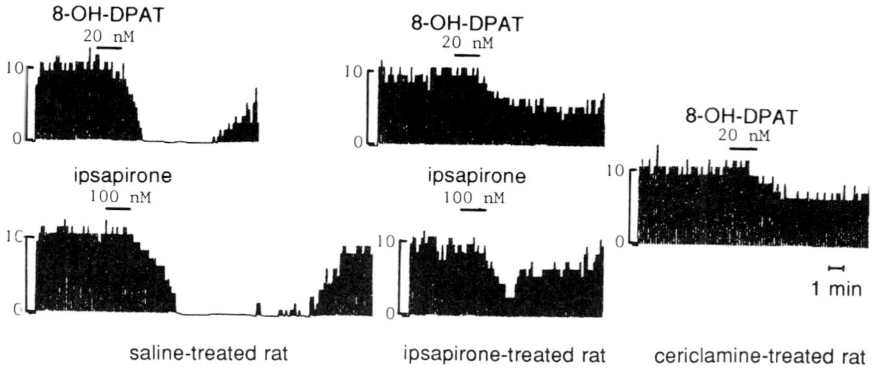

Fig. 1. Inhibitory effects of 8-OH-DPAT and ipsapirone on the firing of DRN 5-HT neurones in brain stem slices from rats treated with saline, ipsapirone (5 mg/kg i.p., twice daily) or cericlamine (16 mg/kg i.p., twice daily) for 14 days. A marked reduction in the potency of both 5-HT_{1A} agonists to reduce the neuronal discharge was observed in rats treated with either ipsapirone or cericlamine as compared to (saline-treated) controls.

somato-dendritic 5-HT_{1A} autoreceptors did occur as a result of their chronic stimulation by ipsapirone. Interestingly, the same adaptive modulation could be induced by the chronic administration of the potent 5-HT uptake inhibitor cericlamine [2], suggesting that a prolonged increase in the extracellular concentration of endogenous 5-HT also led to a functional desensitization of somato-dendritic 5-HT_{1A} autoreceptors in the DRN.

The decreased efficacy of 5-HT_{1A} autoreceptor stimulation to reduce DRN 5-HT neuronal discharge associated with unchanged postsynaptic 5-HT_{1A} receptor function should lead to an enhanced 5-HT neurotransmission during long-term treatment with ipsapirone or cericlamine. Blier and De Montigny [5] have also provided evidence for similar functional alterations of somato-dendritic 5-HT_{1A} autoreceptors in rats chronically treated with other antidepressants. Whether these changes (rather than the down-regulation of cortical β_1-adrenergic and 5-HT_2 receptors [1]) are regularly associated with antidepressant therapy is currently under investigation in our laboratory.

Acknowledgements

This research has been supported by grants from INSERM, Bayer-Pharma and Jouveinal Laboratories.

References

1. Hamon M (1981) Encéphale VII: 381–396.

2. Gouret CJ, Porsolt R, Wettstein JG, Puech A, Soulard C, Pascaud X and Junien JL (1990) Arzneim-Forsch. Drug Res. 40: 633–640.
3. Hamon M, Fattaccini CM, Adrien J, Gallissot MG, Martin P and Gozlan H (1988) J. Pharmacol. Exp. Ther. 246: 745–752.
4. Adrien J, Lanfumey L, Gozlan H, Fattaccini CM and Hamon M (1989) J. Pharmacol. Exp. Ther. 248: 1222–1230.
5. Blier P and de Montigny C (1987) Synapse 1: 470–480.

Biological Psychiatry, Volume 1. G. Racagni et al., editors.

Enhancement of 5-HT synaptic efficacy by antidepressant treatments: A tenable unitary theory?

Claude de Montigny and Pierre Blier

Neurobiological Psychiatry Unit, Department of Psychiatry, McGill University, 1033 Pine Avenue West, Montreal, Quebec, Canada H3A 1A1

Introduction

The serotoninergic (5-HT) system has long been thought to be involved in mediating the therapeutic effect of antidepressant treatments in major affective disorders. Many consider that the 1975–1976 studies of Shopsin et al. [1,2], showing that the therapeutic effects of both imipramine and tranylcypromine could be reversed by blocking 5-HT synthesis with p-chlorophenylalanine, constituted the first compelling clinical evidence for the pivotal role of the 5-HT system in the response to antidepressant drugs. These seminal observations were recently confirmed by the elegant study of Delgado et al. [3] showing that an acute lowering of plasma tryptophan, the precursor of 5-HT, resulted in a reappearance of depressive symptoms in patients treated successfully with different types of antidepressant treatments. In an attempt to characterize the effect of antidepressant treatments on 5-HT neurotransmission, we have carried out in the last several years electrophysiological studies in the rat brain to assess their effects on 5-HT neuron properties as well as on those of postsynaptic neurons.

Tricyclic antidepressant drugs and electroconvulsive therapy

The repeated administration of tricyclic antidepressant (TCA) drugs or electroconvulsive shocks (ECS) were found to increase the responsiveness of dorsal hippocampus pyramidal neurons to 5-HT [4,5] without altering the firing activity of dorsal raphe 5-HT neurons and the sensitivity of their somatodendritic autoreceptors [6,7]. As a result of the sensitization of postsynaptic neurons, the efficacy of the stimulation of the ascending 5-HT pathway in suppressing the firing activity of dorsal hippocampus pyramidal neurons is enhanced following long-term treatment with either a TCA drug or ECS [8].

5-HT reuptake blockers

The therapeutic efficacy of 5-HT reuptake blockers in major depression has been confirmed by numerous clinical studies with several chemically different 5-HT reuptake blockers. In the rat, their repeated administration induces an initial decrease of the firing activity of dorsal raphe 5-HT neurons followed by a progressive and complete recovery. This latter phenomenon has been shown to be due to desensitization of somatodendritic 5-HT autoreceptors [9]. The enhanced effectiveness of the stimulation of the 5-HT pathway, despite an unchanged sensitivity of postsynaptic neurons to 5-HT, has been shown to be due to desensitization of terminal 5-HT autoreceptors following a long-term treatment with a 5-HT reuptake blocker [10].

Monoamine oxidase inhibitors

Long-term treatment with monoamine oxidase inhibitors (MAOI) also results in desensitization of somatodendritic 5-HT autoreceptors [11], without however altering the function of terminal 5-HT autoreceptors [12]. The sensitivity of postsynaptic dorsal hippocampus pyramidal neurons to 5-HT was either unchanged or decreased. However, even in the presence of a desensitization of postsynaptic neurons, the efficacy of the stimulation of the ascending 5-HT pathway was enhanced, presumably due to the increased availability of releasable 5-HT [13].

5-HT$_{1A}$ agonists

Several 5-HT$_{1A}$ receptor agonists have been shown to be effective in the treatment of major depression. As is the case with 5-HT reuptake blockers and MAOI's, their repeated administration induces an initial reduction of the firing activity of dorsal raphe 5-HT neurons followed by a complete recovery, attributable to the desensitization of somatodendritic autoreceptors, which have been shown to be of the 5-HT$_{1A}$ subtype. However, despite being also of the 5-HT$_{1A}$ subtype, the postsynaptic 5-HT receptors of dorsal hippocampus pyramidal neurons are not desensitized by a long-term treatment with a 5-HT$_{1A}$ agonist [14]. In an attempt to provide an explanation for this differential effect, using the 5-HT$_{1A}$ agonist gepirone, we have shown that it acts as a *partial* agonist at postsynaptic 5-HT$_{1A}$ receptors, but as *a full* agonist at somatodendritic 5-HT$_{1A}$ autoreceptors [15]. Hence, it is concluded that the long-term administration of 5-HT$_{1A}$ agonists should lead to an increased activation of normosensitive postsynaptic 5-HT$_{1A}$ receptors, resulting from the concomitant actions of endogenous 5-HT and of the exogenous 5-HT$_{1A}$ agonist.

Clinical studies

In keeping with the enhanced 5-HT neurotransmission observed in the rat following long-term administration of TCA and 5-HT reuptake blockers, these treatments have been shown to increase the prolactin response to intravenous L-tryptophan injection in humans [16–19]. Furthermore, Shapira et al. [20] have observed a similar enhancement of the prolactin response to fenfluramine in depressed patients successfully treated with ECS or imipramine.

The first prospective systematic trial of lithium augmentation in TCA-resistant depression was devised to put to test the hypothesis of an involvement of the 5-HT system [21]. Lithium has indeed been shown to enhance 5-HT neurotransmission in biochemical, behavioral and electrophysiological paradigms [22–25] as well as in humans [26–29]. In the last decade, more than 50 reports have confirmed the efficacy of the lithium augmentation strategy, not only in TCA-resistant depression, but also in depression resistant to a wide variety of antidepressant treatments [30]. Hence, the potentiation of antidepressant treatments by lithium, as the mirror image of the reduction of the therapeutic effect of these drugs by p-chlorophenylalanine or lowering plasma tryptophan, constitutes further evidence that the 5-HT system might be a nodal point in the neurobiological modifications underlying the antidepressant response.

References

1. Shopsin B, Gershon S, Goldstein M, Friedman E and Wilk S (1975) Psychopharmacol. Commun. 1: 239–249.
2. Shopsin B, Friedman E and Gershon S (1976) Arch. Gen. Psychiatry 33: 811–819.
3. Delgado PL, Charney DS, Price LH, Aghajanian GK, Landis H and Heninger GR (1990) Arch. Gen. Psychiatry 47: 411–418.
4. de Montigny C and Aghajanian GK (1978) Science 202: 1303–1306.
5. de Montigny C (1984) J. Pharmacol. Exp. Ther. 228: 230–234.
6. Blier P and de Montigny C (1980) Naunyn-Schmiedeberg's Arch. Pharmacol. 314: 123–128.
7. Blier P and Bouchard C (1991) Third IBRO World Congress of Neuroscience (in press).
8. Chaput Y, de Montigny C and Blier P (1991) Neuropsychopharmacology (in press).
9. Blier P, de Montigny C and Tardif D (1984) Psychopharmacology 84: 242–249.
10. Chaput Y, de Montigny C and Blier P (1986) Naunyn-Schmiedeberg's Arch. Pharmacol. 33: 342–349.
11. Blier P and de Montigny C (1985) Neuroscience 16: 949–955.
12. Blier P, Chaput Y and de Montigny C (1988) Naunyn-Schmiedeberg's Arch. Pharmacol. 337: 246–254.
13. Blier P, de Montigny C and Azzaro AJ (1986) J. Pharmacol. Exp. Ther. 227: 987–994.
14. Blier P and de Montigny C (1987) Synapse 1: 470–480.
15. Blier P and de Montigny C (1990) J. Clin. Psychopharmacol. 10 (Suppl. 3): 13S–20S.
16. Charney DS, Heninger GR and Sternberg DE (1984) Arch. Gen. Psychiatry 41: 359–365.
17. Price LH, Charney DS and Heninger GR (1985) Life Sci. 37: 809–818.
18. Cowen PJ, Geaney DP and Schachter M (1986) Arch. Gen. Psychiatry 43: 61–67.
19. Price LH, Charney DS, Delgado PL, Anderson GM and Heninger GR (1989) Arch. Gen. Psychiatry 46: 625–631.
20. Shapira B, Gropp C and Lerer B (1989) Biol. Psychiatry 25 (7A): 110A.
21. de Montigny C, Grunberg F, Mayer A and Deschenes JP (1981) Br. J. Psychiatry 138: 252–256.
22. Grahame-Smith DG and Green AR (1974) Br. J. Pharmacol. 52: 19–26.
23. Sangdee C and Franz DN (1980) Biol. Psychiatry 15: 59–75.
24. Broderick P and Lynch V (1982) Neuropharmacology 21: 671–679.

25. Blier P and de Montigny C (1985) Eur. J. Pharmacol. 113: 69–77.
26. Glue PW, Cowen PJ, Nutt DJ, Kolakowska T and Grahame-Smith DG (1986) Psychopharmacology 90: 398–402.
27. Cowen PJ, McCance SL, Cohen PR and Julier DL (1989) Psychopharmacology 99: 230–232.
28. McCance SL, Cohen PR and Cowen PJ (1989) Psychopharmacology 99: 276–281.
29. Price LH, Charney DS, Delgado PL and Heninger GR (1989) Arch. Gen. Psychiatry 46: 13–19.
30. Nierenberg AA and White K (1990) Psychopharmacol. Bull. 26: 429–460.

Biological Psychiatry, Volume 1. G. Racagni et al., editors.

Distinct roles of 5-HT subsystems in panic, anxiety and depression

J.F.W. Deakin
University Department of Psychiatry, Rawnsley Building, Manchester Royal Infirmary, Manchester M13 9WL, U.K.

It is an old idea that 5-HT mediates the effects of punishment on behaviour but little psychological analysis has been given to the varied effects of aversive stimuli and how different 5-HT pathways and receptors are involved. A consideration of the normal psychological functions of the different 5-HT subsystems may clarify the contemporary confusion concerning the role of 5-HT in anxiety and depression [1].

Brain mechanisms of acute aversion

Pain and asphyxia are unconditioned proximal aversive stimuli which evoke the defence reflex: autonomic activation, analgesia, and fight/flight behaviour. The reflex is probably mediated by a neuronal system running from amygdala to hypothalamus to periaqueductal grey (PAG) [2]. Stimulation of these structures evokes the complete reflex in animals and vivid panic-like experiences in humans. Panic disorder may be due to spontaneous activation of escape reflexes in the absence of an unconditioned aversive event.

Stimuli which predict aversion (e.g. sight, sound, smell of predators; conditioned fear stimuli) elicit components of the defence reaction including autonomic activation and analgesia. Such high-order stimuli are thought to be processed in anterior temporal lobe and to acquire their emotional significance through the prominent projections to amygdala – the rostral ganglion of the defence system. However, instead of escape behaviour, behavioural inhibition occurs and allowing learned avoidance strategies to extricate the organism from danger. I have proposed that fear inhibits escape. While the clinical corollorary is paradoxical – anticipatory anxiety inhibits panic, it may account for the ability of relaxation exercises to aggravate or precipitate panic attacks in panic patients [3]. This predicts that anxiolytics which selectively block anticipatory anxiety may aggravate panic.

Modulation of acute aversion by dorsal raphe 5-HT projections

The dorsal raphe nucleus forebrain tract (DRNFBT) innervates $5\text{-}HT_2$, 1C and $5\text{-}HT_3$ receptors in amygdala and other forebrain structures. Animal behavioural evidence suggest that this system facilitates or mediates the central motive state of fear (anticipatory anxiety) which has the adaptive function of guiding the organism from danger cues [1]. In a test of this hypothesis in humans we showed that the 5-HT_2/1C antagonist ritanserin blocked the expression of aversively conditioned skin conductance responses in normal volunteers without affecting orienting responses prior to conditioning [4]. To test the idea that dysfunctional activation of the DRNFBT may underlie phobic and generalised anxiety, we investigated the effect of blocking 5-HT_2/1C receptors with ritanserin in 57 anxious neurotic outpatients. We reported that ritanserin had small but significant anxiolytic effects.

The dorsal raphe periventricular tract (DRNPVT) innervates the PAG. This may mediate inhibition of the flight reflex during anticipation of threat. Certainly 5-HT restrains stimulation-induced aversion with PAG electrodes in experimental animals [5]. The clinical implication is that fear restrains panic through a 5-HT mechanism. 5-HT antagonism should therefore aggravate panic and we have unpublished evidence this may be so. Furthermore, we revealed an inhibitory influence of 5-HT on unconditioned anxiety in normal subjects. In a simulated public speaking task, normal volunteers (15 per group) rated themselves (Speilberger, VARs) as more anxious after treatment with ritanserin (5 or 10 mg, p.o.) than on placebo.

These results suggest that DRN 5-HT projections facilitate anticipatory anxiety but restrain unconditioned flight. Clinically, this conceptualisation could explain why ritanserin may ameliorate generalised anxiety and conditioned autonomic responses but aggravate panic and unconditioned anxiety in the public speaking test. It is predicted that some 5-HT agonists may enhance anxiety but ameliorate panic.

Modulation of chronic aversion by median raphe projections

The median raphe nucleus (MRN) innervates complementary structures to those innervated by the DRN, most prominently the hippocampus and its high concentration of 5-HT_{1A} receptors. It is suggested this system mediates tolerance to unavoidable, persistent aversive stimuli so that acute defensive responses become attenuated with repetition [1,6]. When this system fails learned helplessness and depression would result.

There is indeed neuroendocrine evidence that 5-HT_{1A} function is impaired in depression (blunted hormone responses to tryptophan [7], fenfluramine and ipsapirone). Impaired 5-HT_{1A} function may cause depression – the neuroendocrine disturbance recovers with clinical recovery [8] all effective antidepressants enhance 5-HT_{1A} function [9] and intact 5-HT function is necessary for antidepressants to work [10].

Known causal mechanisms in humans include chronic psychosocial stress and social isolation. In our neuroendocrine studies [7] chronic stress was associated with hypercortisolaemia and this predicted blunted PRL responses to tryptophan. Thus chronic stress may predispose to depression by undermining 5-HT_{1A} neurotransmission via steroid-5-HT interactions. Experiments in animals suggest that social stimuli have major influences on 5-HT function. It can be seen that the social origins of depression may be transduced by MRN-5-HT_{1A} mechanisms.

References

1. Deakin JFW (1989) In: Bevan P, Cools AR and Archer T (eds.) Behavioural Pharmacology of 5-HT. Lawrence Erlbaum Associates, Hillsdale, New Jersey, pp. 179–204.
2. Graeff FG (1989) In: Bevan P, Cools AR and Archer T (eds.) Behavioural Pharmacology of 5-HT. Erlbaum, New Jersey, pp. 425–443.
3. Adler CA et al. (1987) Integr. Psychiatry 2: 94–112.
4. Hensman R, Guimaraes FS, Wang M and Deakin JFW (1991) Psychopharmacology (in press).
5. Audi EA, de Aguiar JC and Graeff FG (1988) Psychopharmacology 2: 26–32.
6. Kennett GA, Dickinson S and Curzon G (1985) Brain Res. 330: 253–263.
7. Deakin JFW, Pennell I, Upadhyaya AK and Lofthouse R (1990) Psychopharmacology 101: 85–92.
8. Upadhyaya AK, Pennell I, Cowen PJ and Deakin JFW (1991) J. Affective Disord. 21: 213–218.
9. Blier P, de Montigny C and Chaput Y (1987) J. Clin. Psychopharmacol. 7(6): 24S–35S.
10. Delgado PL, Charney DS, Price LH, Aghajanian GK, Landis H and Heninger GR (1990) Arch. Gen. Psychiatry 47: 411–418.

Biological Psychiatry, Volume 1. G. Racagni et al., editors.

Pilot studies in major depression of litoxetine: A selective 5-HT uptake inhibitor

M. Garreau, M. Bourgeois, M. Escande, J. Mendlewicz, M.F. Poirier and P. Legris
Synthelabo Recherche (LERS) 58, Rue de la Glacière, F-75013, Paris, France

Introduction

Litoxetine is a novel, non-tricyclic competitive inhibitor of neuronal serotonin uptake. It possesses an antidepressant activity in numerous animal models [1].

The selectivity of litoxetine for the inhibition of neuronal 5-HT uptake in comparison with the inhibition of noradrenaline and dopamine uptake is higher than for imipramine or fluoxetine [1].

The in vivo administration of litoxetine resulted in a significant dose-dependent inhibition of ex-vivo serotonin uptake in human platelets: 51% on 5 mg b.i.d., 62% on 10 mg b.i.d. and 87% on 25 mg b.i.d. These inhibitory effects remained constant after 7 days of treatment [1].

Preliminary pharmacokinetic data show that the maximum plasma concentrations of litoxetine are reached within 4 h, with a terminal elimination half-life of about 9 h. The kinetics appear to be linear, the C_{max} and AUG increasing proportionally with the dose. The initial pharmacodynamic studies in humans detected a potentially stimulant effect, with a decreased reaction time after 25 and 50 mg b.i.d. and an increased number of symbols substituted after 25 mg b.i.d. No deleterious effect on memory was observed on 50 mg b.i.d., and an increase in the recall time was noted after 25 mg b.i.d.

The safety profile showed minor adverse drug reactions nausea and gastric discomfort on 50 mg b.i.d. No effect on hemodynamic parameters or blood pressure were seen.

Methods

In order to assess the efficacy and safety of litoxetine in depressed patients, an open pilot study was performed in 4 psychiatric centers in France and Belgium.

The present paper discusses the preliminary results on the 40 patients included, who were suffering from major affective disorders according to DSM III-R [2]: bipolar disorder depressed, major depression recurrent or single episode. They also fulfilled the Feighner criteria for primary depression with a severity of illness defined by a total score of more than 25 on the Montgomery Asberg Depression Rating Scale (MADRS).

All patients who had received antidepressants prior to the study or ECT on the preceding 3 months had to be excluded. In case of necessity, a concomitant treatment with benzodiazepines was allowed. Litoxetine was administered orally for a period of 28 days the initial daily dose was 25 mg twice a day, with an increase up to a maximum of 50 mg twice daily from day 14, depending on the patient's clinical condition. Patients were assessed for efficacy and safety before entering the trial period (day 0), after 4 and 7 days of treatment and at weekly intervals thereafter.

Depression was assessed using the MADRS [3], the Hamilton Depression Rating Scale (HDRS) [4] and a Visual Analogue Scale (VAS). The overall clinical response was assessed by the investigators according to a Clinical Global Impression (CGI) four-point scale (very good, good, moderate, unchanged) [5]. Safety was assessed at the same time intervals on the basis of adverse event reports, vital sign measurements, EKG and laboratory tests for renal, liver and hemopoietic functions.

Results

Forty patients, 16 males and 24 females, entered the study. Their age ranged from 22 to 61 years with a mean age of 44.6 years. According to the severity of the disease, as described in the CGI, the majority of the 40 patients were at least severely ill. The mean total scores of the population were 32.4 for the MADRS and 27.9 for the HDRS. Twenty-seven of the 40 patients had had a previous antidepressant treatment.

Thirty-four patients completed the study period, 6 patients were withdrawn because of inefficacy, 4 patients after day 14 and 2 after day 21. Twenty-one patients responded favourably to treatment and had a good to very good response to treatment, according to the CGI.

The total MADRS score decreased from 32.4 on day 0 to 14.9 on day 28. Parallel results have been found with the total HDRS score, decreasing from 27.9 on day 0 to 12.5 on day 28.

The profile of non-responders seems to correspond to severely ill patients, with an initial MADRS total score exceeding 40, their disease lasting for more than 5 years and the majority of them being resistant to other antidepressant drugs. No patient dropped out because of adverse events. Twenty-one patients developed transient adverse events. The principal events were nausea for 4 patients in the first week of treatment, dizziness for 3 patients, headache for 3 patients and dryness of the mouth for 3 patients.

No abnormalities were detected with regards to vital signs, EKG and laboratory tests. The onset of action seems to be rapid, the first patients having responded within 4 days of treatment.

The effective daily dose in this study was 25 mg, twice daily. The dose increase did not appear to increase the number of responders.

Conclusion

These results on the efficacy and the good safety of the drug in 40 patients suffering from a major affective disorder substantiate the possible interest of litoxetine in depression and need to be confirmed in a larger population of patients in double-blind studies comparing litoxetine with placebo and reference drugs.

References

1. Scatton B, Claustre Y, Graham D et al. (1988) Drug Dev. Res. 12: 29–40.
2. American Psychiatric Association (1987) Diagnostic and Statistical Manual of Mental Disorders, Third Edition Revised (DSM III-R). Washington D.C.
3. Montgomery SA and Asberg M (1979) Br. J. Psychiatry 134: 382–385.
4. Hamilton M (1967) Br. J. Psychiatry 6: 278–296.
5. Guy W (1976) Ecdeu Manual for Psychopharmacology. National Institute of Mental Health, Rockville.

Biological Psychiatry, Volume 1. G. Racagni et al., editors.

New antidepressants: Chemical diversity but unity of action?

B.E. Leonard
Pharmacology Department, University College, Galway, Ireland

Introduction

The accidental discovery of the first tricyclic and monoamine oxidase antidepressants some 30 years ago, and the subsequent finding that these drugs caused cages in the availability of availability in the rat brain, has focused research onto noradrenaline and serotonin as a possible basis for the mode of action of antidepressants. In the last 20 years, antidepressants have been developed that show a high degree of selectivity for the monoaminergic systems, while others appear to show selectivity for the dopaminergic and GABAergic systems. While there is no evidence that the newer antidepressants are therapeutically more effective than the older tricyclic antidepressants, they are safer and better tolerated because of their fewer side-effects. This raises the question of whether or not they have a common mode of action irrespective of their chemical structure and presumed specificity of action on one or more transmitter systems in the CNS. Table 1 classifies some of the antidepressants that have become available in the last 2 decades.

Changes in transmitter receptors in rat brain following chronic antidepressant treatment

While there is considerable controversy regarding the nature of a common pathway

Table 1. Some second-generation antidepressants that combine specificity of action on central neurotransmitters with therapeutic efficacy

1.	MAO-A inhibitors	Brofaromine, cimoxatone, moclobemide
2.	α_2 adrenoceptor antagonists	Mianserin, mepirzapine, idazoxan
3.	Serotonin re-uptake inhibitors	Fluoxetine, fluvoxamine, citalopram, sertraline, paroxetine
4.	Noradrenaline re-uptake inhibitors	Nomifensin[a], oxaprotiline levoprotiline[b]
5.	Serotonin re-uptake enhancers	Tianeptine
6.	5-HT_{1A} partial agonists	Ipsapirone[b], gepirone[b]
7.	Benzodiazepine analogues	Alprazolam[b], adinazolam[b], zometapine[b]
8.	Drugs modulating dopamine function	Buproprion
9.	GABAmimetics	Fengabine[b], progabide[b]
10.	Novel tricyclics	Lofepramine

[a]Withdrawn because of serious adverse side-effects; [b]clinical efficacy uncertain.

Table 2. Changes in central neurotransmitter receptors function following chronic antidepressant treatment in the rodent brain

1.	Cortical β-adrenoceptors	Decreased functional activity and density
2.	Cortical α_1-adrenoceptors	Increased density
3.	Limbic 5-HT_{1A} receptors	Increased density, decreased functional activity
4.	Limbic 5-HT_{1A} receptors	Decreased functional activity
5.	Cortical GABA-B receptors	Decreased density
6.	Dopamine autoreceptors	Decreased functional activity
7.	α_2 autoreceptors	Decreased functional activity

Data summarized in this table obtained from Charney et al. [1], Heal et al. [2], Blier et al. [3], Serra et al. [4] and Butler and Leonard [5].

through which the antidepressants act, the changes in central adrenoceptors, serotonin and GABA-B receptors do appear to correlate with the time of onset of the therapeutic effects in depressed patients (Table 2).

In addition to the changes shown in Table 2, recent unpublished evidence by Barley et al. [6] suggests that the decrease in cortical muscarinic receptors, which are reduced in density in both the suicide brain and in some animal models of depression, return to control values following chronic treatment with both typical and atypical antidepressants.

From such studies, it may be speculated that antidepressants correct an imbalance in several neurotransmitter systems that may be derranged in depression. Such a restoration of these systems appears to parallel the time of onset of the therapeutic response and forms the basis of the receptor sensitivity hypothesis of depression and the mode of action of antidepressants.

Neurotransmitter changes in depressed patients

What is the evidence implicating changes in central transmitter function in the depressed patient? Studies in patients have necessarily been restricted to monitoring changes in the peripheral nervous system and in blood cells that contain biogenic amine receptors and, in the case of the platelet, serotonin uptake processes. Results from such studies suggest that there is a reduction in the 5-HT uptake and 5-HT_2 receptor function [7]. The finding that the number of 5-HT_2 receptors on the platelet membrane increases even though their functional activity decreases, suggests that there may be a failure of signal action between the receptor and the second messenger (PI system). Such a defect is corrected by effective antidepressant treatment. With regard to the noradrenergic system, there is evidence that the density of β-adrenoceptors is increased, and their activity decreased, on the lymphocyte membrane while the α_2 receptors on the platelet membrane in general appear to be unchanged. The β-receptor density normalises following effective treatment [8].

Endogenous endocoids and depression

Is it possible that the changes in serotonergic function in depressed patients are attributable to the presence of an endogenous factor that initiates the pathological changes? Brussov and colleagues [9] found evidence that a plasma factor in depressed patients that impeded platelet aggregation to serotonin. One possible candidate for this factor is α_1 acid glycoprotein [10]. This protein has been shown to reduce the binding of ^{3}H-imipramine to the serotonin uptake site and may modulate serotonergic transmission by such a mechanism. We have recently shown in our laboratory that a plasma factor is present in depressed patients that not only reduces platelet 5-HT-induced aggregation, but also impedes 5-HT uptake; this factor(s) is absent when the patients recover [11]. Tang et al. [12] have also found evidence that endocoid(s) occur in brain and platelet extracts that inhibit 5-HT uptake and ^{3}H-impramine binding. These endogenous substances have been shown to be similar in function to anti-impramine antibodies, thereby raising the possibility that the endocoids may possess a partial structure of the imipramine molecule.

Post-synaptic events: The final common pathway?

What is the evidence at the cellular level that antidepressants have a common mechanism of action? The observation that all clinically effective antidepressants decrease the functional activity of β-adrenoceptors in rat cortex suggests that these drugs have a common action on post-synaptic receptors. Menkes et al. [13] showed that chronic antidepressant treatment augmented the activation of adenylate cyclase by GTP by promoting the interaction of the regulatory and catalytic sub-units of the cyclase. More recently, Perez et al. [14] have shown that the cAMP binding protein associated with the crude microtubule fraction of the rat cortex could be the site of action of antidepressants. The increased incorporation of cAMP into the microtubule protein only occurred following the chronic administration of the antidepressants. Whether such intracellular events are connected with the modulation of calcium channel flux that is also caused by antidepressants [15] is unknown.

Conclusion

It would appear that the chemically and pharmacologically diverse group of drugs that comprise the antidepressants have 2 things in common. Firstly, they are all of approximately equal clinical efficacy. Secondly, there is increasing evidence that they have a common site of action in modulating post-synaptic receptor activity. Whether such changes are restricted to the serotonergic and/or noradrenergic systems in the depressed patient will be the subject of future research.

References

1. Charney DS, Southwick SM, Delgado PL and Krystal JH (1990) In: Amsterdam JD (ed.) Pharmacotherapy of Depression. Marcel Dekker, New York, pp. 13–34.
2. Heal DJ, Hurst EM, Prow MR and Buckett WR (1990) Psychopharmacology 101: 100–106.
3. Blier P, De Montigny C and Chaput Y (1988) Clin. Neuropharmacol. (Suppl. 2) 11: S1–S10.
4. Serra G, Argiolas V, Fadda F and Gessa GL (1979) Pharmacol. Res. Commun. 12: 619–624.
5. Butler J and Leonard RE (1988) Int. Clin. Psychopharmacol. 3: 343–347.
6. Earley B, Glennon M, Lally M, Leonard BE, Junien JL and Wettstein (1990) Autoradiographic Distribution of Cholinergic Muscarinic Receptors in Olfactory Bulbectomized (OB) Rats after Chronic Treatment with Mianserin and Desipramine. Soc. Neurosci. Abstr. Book.
7. Healy P, 0'Halloran A, Carney PA and Leonard BE (1985) J. Affective Disord. 9: 285–296.
8. Leonard BE (1991) Effect of antidepressants on neurotransmission: a common mechanism of action (in press).
9. Brussov OS, Beliaev BS, Katasonov AB, Zlobina GP, Factor MI and Lideman RR (1989) Biol. Psychiatry 25: 375–381.
10. Nemeroff CB, Krishnan KRR, Knight DL, Benjamin D and Meyerson LR (1990) Arch. Gen. Psychiatry 47: 337–340.
11. McAdams C, Colohan F, Brophy J and Leonard BE (1991) Alteration by a plasma factor of platelet aggregation and 5-HT uptake in depression (in press).
12. Tang SW, Cheung S, Strijewski A, Chidzik J and Helmeste D (1990) Psychiatr. Res. 34: 205–212.
13. Menkes DB, Rasenick MM, Whecher MA and Bitensky MW (1983) Science 219: 65–67.
14. Perez J, Tinelli D, Bianchi E, Brunnello N and Racagni IG (1991) Neuropsychopharmacology 4: 57–64.
15. Lavoie PA, Beauchamp G and Elie R (1990) Can. J. Physiol. Biochem. 68: 1414–1418.

Biological Psychiatry, Volume 1. G. Racagni et al., editors.

Subtypes of depression and serotonin function

Johan A. den Boer, Harold J.G.M. van Megen and Herman G.M. Westenberg
Department of Biological Psychiatry, P.O. Box 85500, 3508 GA Utrecht, The Netherlands

Introduction

Identifying subtypes among depressed patients has theoretical and practical importance. There has been consensus that endogenous depression is a relatively distinct subtype characterized by a high likelihood of responding to tricyclic antidepressants. Also, in several studies it has been suggested that atypical depression is especially responsive to treatment with monoamine-oxidase inhibitors (MAOIs). Along the lines of pharmacological dissection these studies have been used to validate the concept of endogenous depression and atypical depression as distinct diagnostic entities. It is questionable whether such reasoning is valid since pharmacological effects cannot be reliably used as a criterion of classification. More recent studies have suggested that concomitant panic attacks, anxiety or phobic features render depressives particularly responsive to MAOI. Moreover, a variety of anxiety disorders appear to respond to treatment with MAOIs [1]. Thus, based upon treatment studies, attempts to validate diagnostic subtypes have been disappointing.

Postmortem findings

Both the levels of 5-HT and 5-HIAA were consistently found to be reduced in the brain stem of suicide victims, but not in the cerebral cortex [2]. Interestingly, these postmortem reduced 5-HT and 5-HIAA levels were found to cut across diagnostic boundaries, suggesting a correlation with suicidal behavior (ideation and/or attempts) irrespective of a specific psychiatric diagnosis.

Similarly, the number of 5-HT_2 binding sites were reported to be increased in prefrontal cortical areas of suicide victims [3].

In a recent study evidence was found for a regionally increased 5-HT_2 receptor binding in the prefrontal cortex of suicide victims [4]. Also, in blood platelets an increased number of 5-HT_2 binding sites was reported, although irrespective of a previous history of affective disorder, but highly correlated to a recent history of suicide attempts or suicidal ideation [5]. The specificity of this serotonergic "defect" is unclear, since positive correlations were also found between reduced 5-HT function, impulsivity and threshold for violence [6]. Thus, psychopathological correlates of depression that relate to a diminished 5-HT function may be impulsivity, reduced threshold for violence and suicidal behavior and do not appear to be confined to one subtype within the spectrum of affective disorders.

Cerebrospinal fluid studies

In a pilot study comprising 17 patients with major depressive disorder (DSM III-R) we found evidence for a bimodal distribution of CSF 5-HIAA (Fig. 1), whereas the majority of patients showed a reduced CSF level of 5-HIAA (median 15.0; range 9.0–33.0). Interestingly, in patients who showed signs of severe regressive behavior (n = 8), who also fulfilled criteria for major depression or atypical depression, we found CSF 5-HIAA levels within normal limits (median 26.0; range 17.0–44.0; figure not shown).

Decreased baseline CSF concentrations of 5-HIAA have been repeatedly found in unipolar depressed patients, schizophrenia and borderline personality disorder [7–9]. Although most evidence points toward a relationship between 5-HT dysfunction and unipolar depression, melancholic type, the data: 1) are by no means

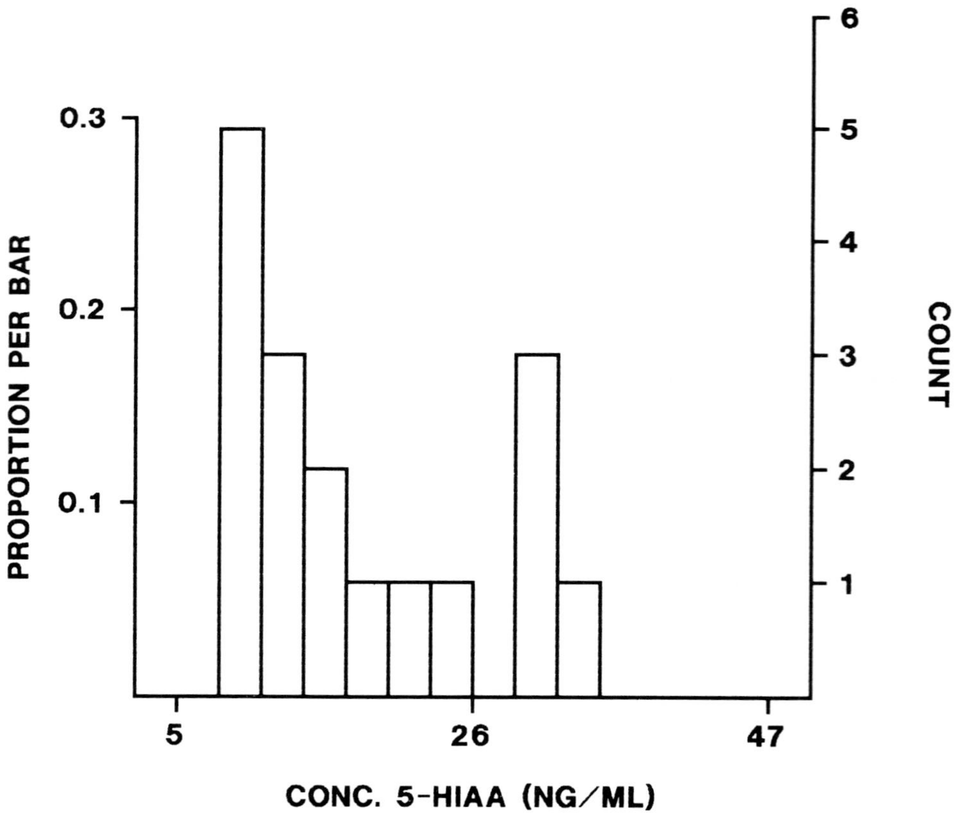

Fig. 1. CSF 5–HIAA in depression.

conclusive with respect to other subtypes of depression; and 2) suggest that this 5-HT dysfunction is not restricted to one psychiatric syndrome.

The effect of treatment with 5-HT uptake inhibitors

So far there is good evidence that selective 5-HT uptake inhibitors are effective antidepressants, but they are also effective in anxiety disorders [10,11], anorexia nervosa and bulimia. These findings suggest that improvement of mood may not be the only treatment effect of antidepressants, but that other symptom dimensions which may be shared by these different disorders respond to treatment with selective 5-HT uptake inhibitors.

Conclusion

Within the realm of DSM III-R subtypes of depression there is little evidence supporting a circumscribed role of 5-HT for specific subtypes like atypical depression, unipolar or bipolar depression. Cutting across the borders of classification systems, there appears to be more convincing evidence for a specific 5-HT-ergic link and behavioral dimensions.

References

1. Vliet IM van, Westenberg HGM and Den Boer JA (1991) Psychopharmacology of social phobia; behavioral and biochemical effects of brofaromine, a selective MAO-A inhibitor (submitted).
2. Owen F, Cross AJ, Crow TJ, Deakin JFW, Ferrier IN, Lofthouse R and Poulter M (1968) Lancet ii: 1256.
3. Mann JJ, Stanley McBride PA and McEwen BS (1986) Arch. Gen. Psychiatry 43: 954–959.
4. Arango V, Ernsberger P, Marzuk PM, Chen JS, Tierny H, Stanley M, Reis DJ and Mann J (1990) Arch. Gen. Psychiatry 47: 1038–1043.
5. Pandey GN, Pandey SC, Janicak PG, Marks RC and Davis JM (1990) Biol. Psychiatry 28: 215–222.
6. Linnoila M (1988) Acta Psychiatr. Scand. 78: 529–535.
7. Traskman L, Asberg M, Bertiilsson L and Sjostrand L (1981) Arch. Gen. Psychiatry 38: 631–636.
8. Van Praag HM (1983) Lancet ii: 977–978.
9. Brown GL, Ebert MH, Goyer PF, Jimmerson DC, Klein WJ, Bunney WE and Goodwin FK (1982) Am. J. Psychiatry 139: 741–746.
10. Den Boer JA and Westenberg HGM (1988) Int. Clin. Psychopharmacol. 3: 59–74.
11. Perse TL, Greist JH and Jefferson JW (1987) Am. J. Psychiatry 144: 1543–1548.

Biological Psychiatry, Volume 1. G. Racagni et al., editors.

Benzodiazepines in the treatment of depressive disorders: An updated review

Alan F. Schatzberg and Joel A. Posener
Massachusetts Mental Health Center, 74 Fenwood Road, Boston, MA 02115, U.S.A.

The antidepressant efficacy of benzodiazepines has been a subject of controversy over the past two decades. Some early literature had suggested that these compounds had therapeutic effects against depression, and 13 years ago we reviewed all double-blind studies comparing benzodiazepines with known antidepressants [1]. We concluded that benzodiazepines have potent anxiolytic and sedative effects but not specific antidepressant activity. Since that time, a new class of benzodiazepines, the triazolobenzodiazepines, has become a focus of clinical and investigational interest. Preclinical studies have found that in contrast to classical benzodiazepines, the triazolobenzodiazepines alprazolam and adinazolam do exert effects on catecholamine and/or indoleamine systems and have some activity in traditional animal models used for testing potential antidepressant properties. Moreover, clincial studies also point to this class of compounds as having antidepressant properties. On the basis of these findings, we re-examined the literature on the clinical antidepressant efficacy of benzodiazepines.

Method

Using a Medline search program, we identified all English language studies published from 1977 through August 1990 in which a benzodiazepine was compared against a known antidepressant or placebo in the treatment of depressive disorders and which employed a double-blind, random assignment paradigm. In this review we examine: the antidepressant efficacy of three different classes of benzodiazepines (i.e. 2-keto-, 3-hydroxy and triazolo-); differentiation between their possible antidepressant and anxiolytic effects; and relationships between possible efficacy and clinical subtypes of depressive disorders.

Results

Classical benzodiazepines

Our search disclosed eight studies that involved non-triazolobenzodiazepines. Of these, three compared the benzodiazepine with placebo and seven involved a comparison with a reference antidepressant. Of the three placebo-controlled studies, two failed to find a difference in antidepressant efficacy between the benzodiazepine and placebo, and one reported a difference (in favor of the benzodiazepine) only for a subgroup of patients with high scores on the Zung Depression Scale. Of these three studies, only one employed DSM III criteria for major depression and this study failed to find a difference between the benzodiazepine and placebo. Of the seven studies comparing a benzodiazepine with a known antidepressant, none found the benzodiazepine to be superior; three found the reference drug to be superior; and four failed to find a significant difference between the two. Only two of these studies employed DSM III or IDC 9 criteria for depressive disorders, and both of these studies found the benzodiazepines to be less effective than the reference antidepressant. On the basis of these findings, our review provides further evidence that classical benzodiazepines do not have antidepressant activity.

Alprazolam

We identified twenty-one studies in which alprazolam was compared with placebo or a known antidepressant. One study reported an aggregate of data that were apparently reported separately in three other publications and our comments will focus on the larger study; for the remainder of this discussion, we will address a total of eighteen papers. Two of these were comparisons with placebo alone; five additional studies that employed a placebo control also compared alprazolam with another active compound. Seven studies compared alprazolam with amitriptyline; six with imipramine; and two each with desipramine and doxepin. Fifteen studies required subjects to have a diagnosis of major depression according to DSM III, Research Diagnostic Criteria (RDC) or Feighner Criteria. The remaining three studies did not employ standard operational criteria for a diagnosis of depression. Only two studies involved a significant proportion of inpatients. Mean final tricyclic doses ranged from 63.8 mg/day to 243 mg/day with seven studies employing comparison tricyclic doses of 150 mg/day or greater.

Of the seven studies comparing alprazolam with placebo, six found the drug was significantly superior and only one failed to find a significant difference from placebo. When the two studies which did not employ a standard, operational diagnosis are excluded, four of the remaining five studies found alprazolam to be superior and one found no difference. It is noteworthy that in the one study which did not find a significant difference between alprazolam and placebo, baseline scores on the Hamilton Rating Scale for Depression (HAMD) prior to treatment were significantly higher in the group receiving alprazolam than in the group receiving placebo. Four of the studies reported results separately for subscales on the HAMD. A review of these data does not support the hypothesis that the superiority of alprazolam to placebo is due solely to effects on anxiety symptoms.

Of the sixteen studies comparing alprazolam to a tricyclic antidepressant, none found alprazolam to be superior, three found the tricyclic to be significantly superior and thirteen found no overall statistically significant difference between alprazolam and the tricyclic. To provide a more rigorous test of the comparative efficacy of these two drug treatments, we eliminated those studies which did not require a standard, operationally defined diagnosis of major depression and those studies which did not report a mean final tricyclic antidepressant dose of at least 150 mg/day. Of the remaining seven studies, five found no statistically significant difference between alprazolam and the tricyclic, and two found the tricyclic to be superior. One of the latter two employed imipramine as the reference drug; the other, amitriptyline. Particularly striking was the observation that the two studies which found a tricyclic antidepressant to be significantly superior to alprazolam were also the only studies that employed a significant proportion of inpatients.

Subscales of the HAMD were examined, whenever reported, to determine whether the overall tabulation of results might obscure more specific differences between the effects of alprazolam and tricyclics on different classes of symptoms. Of the 16 studies making comparisons between alprazolam and a reference drug, 11 reported results for various subscales of the HAMD. While there was some evidence that alprazolam may be more effective for anxiety and sleep disturbance, there was no evidence that alprazolam and tricyclics had differential efficacy on core depressive symptoms.

Adinazolam

Our search identified five studies employing adinazolam. Three of these were comparisons against placebo alone; two were comparisons against a reference antidepressant, one of which also employed a placebo cell. All five studies required patients to meet DSM III and/or RDC criteria for major depression. Imipramine at a mean maximum dose of 173 mg/day was the comparison drug in one study and amitriptyline, at a mean maximum dose of 236 mg/day was the comparison drug in the other. Three of the studies included outpatients only and two studied samples were composed only of inpatients. Of the four studies that compared adinazolam with placebo, three found the drug to be significantly superior. Of the two studies that compared adinazolam with a reference antidepressant drug, one found no significant difference between adinazolam and imipramine and one found amitriptyline to be superior to adinazolam. One of the studies involving inpatients found adinazolam to be superior to placebo. However, the only study that found adinazolam was both inferior to a reference tricyclic and not significantly different from placebo included only inpatients. Three studies, all comparisons between adinazolam and placebo, reported results for subscales of the HAMD. All of these found adinazolam to be superior to placebo in reducing core depressive symptoms.

Conclusion

We reviewed 34 randomized clinical trials comparing benzodiazepines with placebo or known antidepressants in order to present an update of our 1978 review, in which we concluded that the evidence did not support specific antidepressant efficacy for benzodiazepines. With regard to classical benzodiazepines (i.e. non-triazolobenzodiazepines), the studies reviewed here do not lead us to modify that conclusion. However, our earlier statement must be adjusted in the case of triazolobenzodiazepines. The studies reviewed here provide evidence that alprazolam is superior to placebo in the treatment of depressive symptoms in major depression. Alprazolam also appears to be roughly equivalent in antidepressant efficacy to tricyclics for outpatient populations. Similarly, we conclude that in the treatment of outpatient depression, adinazolam is superior to placebo and may be equivalent in efficacy to tricyclic antidepressants. Further studies on inpatients with major depression are required. Data to date suggest that alprazolam is less effective than tricyclic antidepressants in this population. Limited data to date on adinazolam in inpatients are equivocal. Further research can elucidate the clinical and biological characteristics that may predict antidepressant response to triazolobenzodiazepines.

Acknowledgements

This work was supported in part by grants from the National Institute of Mental Health (MH16259) and the Poitras Charitable Foundation. Ms. Linda Messier prepared this manuscript.

Reference

1. Schatzberg and Cole (1978) Arch. Gen. Psychiatry 75: 1359–1365.

Biological Psychiatry, Volume 1. G. Racagni et al., editors.

α_2-Adrenoceptor antagonists as antidepressants: New developments

Roger M. Pinder
Scientific Development Group, Organon International B.V., P.O. Box 20, 5340 BH Oss, The Netherlands

Inhibitors of monoamine oxidase or reuptake are presumed to act as antidepressants in part by rapidly elevating synaptic levels of noradrenaline (NA) and serotonin (5-HT). Synaptic levels of NA, however, are not controlled entirely by reuptake and metabolic processes, but are under the additional influence of a negative feedback inhibition mediated by an agonist action of NA itself upon α_2-adrenoceptors located presynaptically on the noradrenergic nerve terminal [1,2]. Antagonism of these so-called autoreceptors leads to enhancement of the release of NA from its storage sites in the nerve terminal and thereby to a situation akin to that following uptake inhibition. α_2-Autoreceptors have been demonstrated to exist at almost all noradrenergic axons where postsynaptic α_2-adrenoceptors are known to occur and they are widely distributed in the brain particularly in the cortex. They also occur on 5-HT terminals as heteroceptors where they play a role in controlling the release of 5-HT.

The first indication that antidepressant drugs might block α_2-autoreceptors was provided by mianserin, which not only potentiated NA release from rat brain slices but also reversed the inhibiting effect of the α_2-agonist clonidine [3]. The possibility that α_2-autoreceptor antagonism might lead to antidepressant properties stimulated the development of a number of putative therapeutic agents which vary widely in their potency and selectivity [1–5]. Such compounds also provide tools to investigate α_2-adrenoceptor function, which may be abnormally sensitive in depression. However, while more potent and selective agents have given better tools, their therapeutic efficacy is still largely unproven. Indeed, convincing evidence of antidepressant efficacy exists only for the three tetracyclic α_2-antagonists mianserin, setiptiline and mirtazapine. A fourth and more potent tetracyclic α_2-antagonist, aptazapine, failed to reach clinical trials [5]. Thus mianserin and setiptiline were introduced in 1974 and 1989 respectively, while placebo controlled studies have demonstrated the efficacy of mirtazapine prior to introduction [6,7]. None of these drugs is a selective α_2-antagonist and all block histamine and 5-HT receptors to a greater degree [5]. Their minimal inhibitory effects in vitro upon NA reuptake, which are largely absent in vitro, are unlikely to play a role in their antidepressant activity, but it is possible that antagonism at 5-HT_1, 5-HT_2 and 5-HT_3 receptors influences their antidepressant and anxiolytic properties. Histamine-1 receptor antagonism appears to be significant only for the sedative action of the tetracyclics.

The search for α-antagonists with greater selectivity for α_2-adrenoceptors and higher potency than mianserin and its analogues has focussed upon structural modifications of the classical α_2-antagonist yohimbine, an agent with a variety of other receptor interactions, and of the non-selective α-antagonists phentolamine and piperoxan [1–5]. The strategy has been to eliminate affinity for α_1-adrenergic and other types of receptors as well as any effect upon NA reuptake. While presynaptic α_2-selectivity is a priori desirable for an NA-releasing effect, available evidence suggests that pre- and post-synaptic α_2-adrenoceptors are identical [8]. Nevertheless, presynaptic selectivity has been reported for yohimbine [9] and (+)-idazoxan [10], and α_2-adrenoceptor heterogeneity provides further opportunities for selective drug design [11]. Of the several candidate substances – piperoxan/phentolamine analogues (idazoxan, imiloxan, fluparoxan), yohimbine derivatives (CH-38083, L-654,284, L-657,743, Wy 26703), imidazoles (atipemazole, midaglizole, idazoxan, imiloxan) and azepines (BHT-958, SKF 86466) – clinical data have been published only on imiloxan, atipemazole and idazoxan. Both imiloxan [12] and atipemazole [13] showed effects in healthy volunteers typical for α_2-adrenoceptor antagonists, but imiloxan has not been evaluated in depressed patients and the poor oral bioavailability of atipemazole makes unlikely its routine use in depression. Yohimbine also suffers from often poor and highly variable oral bioavailability [14] which may partly explain its inability to augment desipramine treatment of depressed patients with a history of non-response to standard antidepressant drugs [15]. Published data are available in depression only for idazoxan although studies are in progress with fluparoxan.

Montgomery [16] compared idazoxan 20 mg or 40 mg three times daily with amitriptyline 50 mg 3 times daily in patients with major depression. Response to idazoxan at the lower dose was significantly worse than that to amitriptyline in the first part of the study which saw 97 patients completing 3 weeks and 88 completing 4 weeks of treatment. This advantage for amitriptyline was more apparent in the more severely depressed patients. When idazoxan was given at the higher dose there was no apparent difference in efficacy between it and amitriptyline in 65 patients. Furthermore, a transient advantage for idazoxan in moderately depressed patients was observed, supporting theoretical predictions from animal studies of a faster onset of action with α_2-antagonists. In a placebo-controlled double-blind longitudinal study in two refractory bipolar depressed patients, idazoxan 60–120 mg/day was effective in ameliorating the current depressive episode and maintaining the response when given with lithium for 9 to 10 months [17]. MA levels in plasma were rapidly raised and maintained by short-term idazoxan treatment while CSF levels were significantly increased only after 4–6 weeks of treatment.

Large placebo-controlled studies are needed to test the antidepressant properties of selective α_2-adrenoceptor antagonists like idazoxan and fluparoxan. It is currently not possible to decide whether they are effective antidepressants. Such studies would also assist in assessing whether the α_2-adrenoceptor antagonism of the non-selective tetracyclic antidepressants contributes substantially to their undoubted efficacy in depression.

References

1. Pinder RM (1985) Drugs Future 10: 841–857.
2. Clark RD, Michel AD and Whiting RL (1986) Prog. Med. Chem. 23: 1–39.
3. Baumann PA and Maitre L (1977) Arch. Pharmacol. 300: 31–37.
4. Pinder RM and Sitsen JMA (1987) In: Dahl SG, Gram LF, Paul SM and Potter WZ (eds.) Clinical Pharmacology in Psychiatry. Springer-Verlag, Berlin, pp. 107–112.
5. Pinder RM (1990) In: Leonard BE and Spencer PSJ (eds.) Antidepressants: Thirty Years On. CMS Publishers, London, pp. 334–348.
6. Claghorn JL, Johnstone EE, Studebaker RM and Ajeman SA (1987). Psychopharmacol. Bull. 23: 160–161.
7. Smith WT, Glaudin V, Panagides J and Gilvary E (1990) Psychopharmacol. Bull. 26: 191–196.
8. Connaughton S and Docherty JR (1990) Br. J. Pharmacol. 99: 97–102.
9. Starke K, Borowski E and Endo T (1975) Eur. J. Pharmacol. 34: 385–388.
10. Martire M, Pistritto G and Peziori P (1988) Neurosci. Lett. 86: 328–333.
11. Bylund DB (1988) Trends Pharmacol. Sci. 9: 356–361.
12. Dow RJ and Whiting RL (1985) Br. J. Pharmacol. 18: 288P–289P.
13. Karhuvarra S, Kallio A, Scheinin M, Anttila M, Salonen JS and Scheinin H (1990) Br. J. Clin. Pharmacol. 30: 97–106.
14. Guthrie SK, Hariharan M and Grunhaus LJ (1990) Eur. J. Clin. Pharmacol. 39: 409–411.
15. Charney DS, Price LH and Heninger GR (1986) Arch. Gen. Psychiatry 43: 1155–1161.
16. Montgomery SA (1989) In Dahl SG and Gram IF (eds.) Clinical Pharmacology in Psychiatry. Springer-Verlag, Berlin, pp. 105–108.
17. Osman OT, Rudorfer MV and Potter WZ (1989) Arch. Gen. Psychiatry 46: 958–959.

Biological Psychiatry, Volume 1. G. Racagni et al., editors.

GABAergic drugs as putative antidepressants: A review of available data

Paolo Lucio Morselli and Marine Garreau
Clinical Research Department, Synthelabo Recherche (LERS), 75622 Paris, France

Several data in the recent literature suggest that GABAergic drugs may have an antidepressant action and that the GABA system may play an important role in the pathogenesis of depressive disorders.

At an experimental level, in animal behavioral models of depression the action of GABAergic drugs is comparable or superior to that observed with tricyclic antidepressants (TCAs) [1–3]. Such an effect is antagonized for both TCA and GABAergic drugs by GABA receptor antagonists such as bicuculline and picrotoxine [3]. A repeated (but not acute) administration of TCAs leads to an upregulation of cerebral $GABA_B$ receptors [4] and downregulation of β-adrenoceptors; the same effects have been observed with GABA mimetic agents [3–5].

While no effects on monamine uptake or monoamine oxidase activity have been noted with GABA mimetic drugs, an activation of noradrenaline neuron activity has been observed following administration of progabide and fengabine [5,6]. Taken together, the available data at experimental level suggest a direct or an indirect involvement of GABA function in the therapeutic effect of classical antidepressants and a possible antidepressant action of GABAergic drugs.

Furthermore, low CSF GABA levels have been reported in depressed patients with an apparent relationship between GABA-CSF concentrations and clinical status [7,8].

The data available at clinical level refer mostly to two GABA mimetic agents which have been extensively tested in human depression [9–13].

A first series of observations conducted with progabide, the first GABAergic drug extensively studied in depression, indicated a clear therapeutic effect in depressive syndromes, both in open pilot studies [9] and in controlled double-blind trials vs. imipramine and nortriptyline [10,11]. The therapeutic action was evident in major depressive disorders, dysthymic disorders or adjustment disorders with depressive mood.

However, none of the above-mentioned studies was run against placebo, and the data indicating an antidepressant effect in about 65–70% of the patients should be considered as suggestive of a potential antidepressant action. The development of progabide as an antidepressant has been abandoned because of its hepatotoxic potential.

Further data have been collected with fengabine, another GABAergic agent chemically related to progabide [11].

In a first series of pilot observations a good response was recorded in 65% of the cases [10,11]. A second series of 6 controlled randomized double-blind studies with parallel group design included more than 400 patients treated over a 4-week period with either fengabine or TCAs (IMI, AMI, CLOMI) [10–13].

An overall analysis of these 6 studies [12] indicated that a clear antidepressant effect was present in all studies for both treatment groups, without significant differences between treatments. Responders were between 70 and 78% for fengabine and between 72 and 80% for TCAs.

TCAs appeared to be slightly better in major depressions, while the contrary was evident for other type of depressive disorders. The therapeutic index ratio was significantly better with fengabine.

However, no data for progabide against placebo are available in the literature and the paper by E.S. Paykel (personal communication) indicates no differences between placebo and fengabine. The development of fengabine has been halted during Phase III studies because of adverse effects on cholesterol plasma levels during long-term trials.

On the whole, the clinical data available for progabide and fengabine are consistent with experimental behavioral and biochemical data. Even if the lack of data against placebo does not permit a conclusive assessment, they are strongly suggestive for a therapeutic action of GABAergic drugs in human depression. The experimental and clinical findings support the GABAergic hypothesis of depression [3,9,14,15] as well as its interest at both euristic and pragmatic levels.

A confirmation of such a hypothesis is linked to the future availability of better tolerated GABAergic drugs.

References

1. Lloyd KG, Morselli PL, Depoortere H et al. (1983) Pharmacol. Biochem. Behav. 18: 957–966.
2. Lloyd KG, Zivkovic B, Sanger DJ et al. (1987) J. Pharmacol. Exp. Ther. 241: 245–250.
3. Lloyd KG and Morselli PL (1987) In: Meltzer HY (ed.) Psychopharmacology: The Third Generation of Progress. Raven Press, New York, pp. 183–195.
4. Pilc A and Lloyd KG (1984) Life Sci. 35: 2149–2154.
5. Scatton B, Lloyd KG, Zivkovic B et al. (1987) J. Pharmacol. Exp. Ther. 241: 251–257.
6. Scatton B, Zivkovic B, Dedek J et al. (1982) J. Pharmacol Exp. Ther. 220: 678–687.
7. Gerner RH and Fairbanks L (1986) In: Shagass C et al. (eds.) Biological Psychiatry 1985. Elsevier, New York, pp. 853–855.
8. Joffer J, Post RM, Rubinov DR et al. (1986) In: Shagass C et al. (eds.) Biological Psychiatry 1985. Elsevier, New York, pp. 1553–1558.
9. Morselli PL, Bossi L, Henry JF et al. (1980) Brain Res. Bull. 5: 411–414.
10. Morselli PL, Priore P, Loeb C et al. (1988) In: Lerer B and Gershon S (eds.) New Directions in Affective Disorders. Springer Verlag, New York, pp. 660–664.
11. Bartholini G, Lloyd KG and Morselli PL (1986) GABA and Mood Disorders: Experimental and Clinical Research. Raven Press, New York.
12. Magni G, Garreau M, Orofiamma B et al. (1988) Neuropsychobiology 20: 126–131.
13. Nielsen NP, Cesana B, Zizolfi S et al. (1990) Acta Psychiatr. Scand. 82: 366–371.

14. Bartholini G, Lloyd KG, Scatton B et al. (1985) Psychopharmacol. Bull. 21: 285–388.
15. Scatton B, Lloyd KG, Sanger DJ et al. (1990) In: Leonard B and Spenser P (eds.) Antidepressants: Thirty Years On. CNS Publishers, London, pp. 349–357.

Biological Psychiatry, Volume 1. G. Racagni et al., editors.

Do pharmacokinetic factors affect the rapidity of antidepressant actions?

A.C. Altamura and S.R. Bareggi

Institut of Clinical Psychiatry and Department of Pharmacology, School of Medicine, State University, Milan, Italy

The slow gradual onset of therapeutic effect of antidepressants (AD) is difficult to explain in view of their facilitating effects on neuronal activity (reuptake-blocking, MAO inhibiting, presynaptic α_2-adrenergic receptor blocking properties) because these effects occur acutely, shortly after a single dose. Research into the mechanism of action of AD has been focused on the chronic modifications of various transmitter receptors, mainly subsensitivity of postsynaptic β-adrenergic receptors and supersensitivity of α_1-adrenergic receptors.

These time-dependent adaptive phenomena may partially explain the therapeutic delay in AD treatment. There are, however, differences in the time of onset of therapeutic effects of different drugs and/or treatment settings (dosage regimen, route of administration, type of patients) which suggest that there may be additional factors that influence the time of onset.

How do pharmacokinetic factors influence this?

Route of administration and dose schedule

After oral administration, tricyclic (TC) AD undergo extensive pre-systemic metabolism which decreases their bioavailability and produces relatively large amounts of metabolites (active or inactive) that may interfere with the activity of parent drug. Intravenous infusion of TCADs into rats, in contrast to oral administration, produces a rapid and dose-dependent down-regulation of β-adrenergic receptors [1]. There are conflicting findings in patients: some studies report quicker onset after infusion of doxepin, clomipramine and maproptiline [2,3] whereas other studies report no differences between oral and i.v. infusion clomipramine (CHI) [4,5]. In these latter studies, doses were either very variable (25–300 mg, [4]) or rather low and increased slowly [5], with plasma levels not at the steady-state at the end of the study [5]. It has been shown, on the other hand, that either i.v. or oral loading doses (200 mg) of CHI, with which therapeutic levels can be rapidly attained, produce acute and lasting decreases of the "core" items of depression [6]. Response was also delayed observed in patients with lower levels of nortriptyline [7]. Therefore, it seems that both β-receptor down-regulation and the therapeutic response may be influenced considerably by the quantity of drug administered initially or, to put it differently, by rapidly reaching maximal levels.

Which brings us to the second point: half-life of elimination. In fact the shorter the half-life, the quicker maximal steady-state levels are reached.

Half-life

Most of the typical AD, including TCAD, have rather long half-lives ranging from 17 h (doxepin, desipramine) to over 70 h (protriptyline), whereas many atypical AD have short half-lives (Table 1). For these short half-life atypical AD (e.g., amoxapine, zimelidine), there have been reports of shorter lag-times for the onset of action than those of several typical AD (8–13), but there are also other reports that do not agree. Moreover, since some of the new atypical AD also have lesser adverse effects (e.g., the new RIMA, moclobemide and the new uptake inhibitor, venlafaxine), treatment can be started with full doses, avoiding the slow scaling-up of dosage used for most TCAD.

Age

An early response to TCAD treatment in elderly patients has been observed by several investigators [14]. Whether this early response is due to altered kinetics or to other factors is not clear. Higher steady-state levels of AD (e.g. imipramine, amitriptyline, clomipramine, mianserin, viloxazine, dothiepin [15–18]), possibly due to reduced clearance, have been found by many groups, but not by some others [15]. In the elderly there may be a problem of assessment even more important than in younger adults: in a controlled study [19] comparing trazodone, mianserin and amitriptyline, early effects on Hamilton Rating Scale for Depression (HRS-D) could be seen but not on Geriatric Depression Scale (GDS) due to the anxiolytic effects of these drugs which are overweighted by HRS-D but not by GDS, which is more sensitive for depressive symptoms. Therefore the early response observed in the elderly can be due not only to pharmacokinetic but also to other factors (pharmacodynamic, type of depression, assessment).

Table 1. Elimination half-lives of atypical antidepressants

Intermediate-long		Short	
Drug	Half-life (h)	Drug	Half-life (h)
Citalopram	23–75	Amoxapine	8
Fluoxetine	48–96	Moclobemide	2– 3
Fluvoxamine	15	Nomifensine	2– 4
Maprotiline	27–58	Trazodone	6–13
Mianserin	20–40	Venlafaxine	3– 5
		Viloxazine	2– 5
		Zimelidine	4– 6

Drug combinations

The delay of onset of action has been found to be shorter for some drug combinations: fluoxetine has been shown to reduce the delay of the therapeutic effects of desipramine, and there was significant improvement within 48 h after the addition of lithium to the treatment of patients who did not respond to 3 weeks of TCAD [20,21]. Whether or not these effects are due to different AD levels was not established.

Conclusions

High plasma levels in the first days of treatment seem to produce rapid, or even acute, therapeutic effects. To obtain such high levels, drugs should have short half-lives and (or) primarily be very safe in order to start with full or even loading doses of the drug (e.g, clomipramine among TCAD and venlafaxine or moclobemide among second generation AD).

The importance of high levels in the first days for obtaining a rapid response is substantiated by experimental findings of rapid adaptive changes of adrenergic receptors with high doses of various AD.

Some caution must be used because many studies use the total score to evaluate the therapeutic effect and, therefore, non-specific effects might mask the specific effects on depressive symptoms leading to misleading conclusions. This is of particular importance for the elderly, but can be also a problem in younger adults.

The biological and clinical heterogeneity of patients can be a major obstacle in studies attempting to identify the time factors for the therapeutic effects of antidepressants.

References

1. Sethy VH, Day JS and Cooper MM (1988) Prog. Neuro-Pschopharmacol. Biol. Psychiatry 12: 673–682.
2. Laux G, Konig W, Lesch KP and Stein A (1989) Wien Med. Wochenschr. 139: 525–529.
3. Kielholz P (1990) Zh. Nevropatol. Psikhiatr. 90: 53–56.
4. Escobar JI, Flemembaum A and Schiele B (1973) Psychopharmacologia 33: 111–116.
5. Faravelli C, Broadhurst AD, Ambonetti A, Ballerini A, De Biase L, La Malfa G and Das M (1983) Biol. Psychiatry 18: 695–706.
6. Pollock BG, Perel JM, Nathan RS and Kupfer DJ (1989) Arch. Gen. Psychiatry 46: 29–35.
7. Georgotas A, McCue RE, Cooper TB, Nagachandran N and Friedhoff A (1989) Psychiatr. Res. 28: 1–9.
8. McNair DM, Kahn RJ, Frankenthaler LM and Faldetta LL (1984) Psychopharmacology 83: 129–133.
9. Fabre LF (1985) J. Clin. Psychiatry 46: 521–524.
10. Montgomery SA, Montgomery DB, McAuley R, Rani SJ and Roy D (1982) In: Costa E and Racagni G (eds.) Typical and Atypical Antidepressants: Clinical Practice. Raven Press, New York, 35–42.
11. Casacchia R and Rossi A (1989) Pharmacopsychiatry 22: 152–155.

12. Lecrubier Y and Guelfi JD (1990) Acta Psychiatr. Scand. 360 (Suppl.): 18–23.
13. Venlafaxine (1991) Wyeth, Internal Report.
14. Plotkin DA, Gershon SC and Jarvik LF (1987) In: Meltzer HY (ed.) Psychopharmacology: The Third Generation of Progress. Raven Press, New York, pp. 1149–1158.
15. Rundorfer MV and Potter WZ (1987) In: Meltzer HY (ed.) Psychopharmacology: The Third Generation of Progress. Raven Press, New York, pp. 1353–1363.
16. Altamura AC, Melorio T, Invernizzi G and Gomeni R (1982) Psychopharmacology 78: 380–385.
17. Altamura AC, Melorio T, Invernizzi G, Colacurcio F and Gomeni R (1983) Psychopharmacology 81: 281–285.
18. Bareggi SR, Cavallaro R, Pirola R and Altamura AC (1990) Prog. Neuro-Psychopharmacol. Biol. Psychiatry 14: 163–170.
19. Altamura AC, Mauri MC, Rudas N et al. (1989) Clin. Neuropharmacol. (Suppl. 1) 12: S25–S33.
20. Eisen A (1989) Pharmacopsychiatry 22: 272–273.
21. DeMontigny C, Cowinoyer G, Marissette R et al. (1983) Arch. Gen. Psychiatry 40: 1327–1334.

Biological Psychiatry, Volume 1. G. Racagni et al., editors.

Some biological correlates of acute antidepressant activity in affective illness

P. Linkowski, M. Kerkhofs, P. Hubain and J. Mendlewicz
Department of Psychiatry, Hôpital Erasme, Université Libre de Bruxelles, Route de Lennik 808, 1070 Brussels, Belgium

A number of neuroendocrine abnormalities are associated with major depression. Twenty-four-hour hypersecretion of cortisol [1,2] diurnal hyposecretion of growth hormone [3] as well as 24-h normal levels of prolactin [4] have been reported in careful chronobiological studies of depressed patients, along with sleep recordings. In addition, a chronobiological abnormality in the rhythms of ACTH and cortisol secretion, consisting of a phase advance of the nocturnal quiescent period and a subsequent increase toward the morning maximum, has been consistently found in a subset of depressed patients suffering from endogenous depression in parallel with the observation that in the majority of the patients studied a large pulse of GH occurred before, rather than shortly after sleep onset, a finding also suggestive of a phase advance of the circadian timing [3].

In the present study we report 24-h profiles of ACTH, cortisol, GH and PRL in eleven male endogenously depressed patients studied before and after treatment with either amitriptyline or electroconvulsive therapy.

Subjects and Methods

Eleven men, aged 31–62 years, suffering from endogenous depression (6 unipolar and 5 bipolar) were studied after a drug wash-out of at least 15 days and after giving informed consent. Each patient was studied twice, first during the untreated acute episode of depression and subsequently after antidepressant treatment (6 patients had electroconvulsive treatment and 5 amitriptyline up to 250 mg). The patients were studied in the sleep laboratory of the University of Brussels and underwent a blood sampling (at 15-min intervals) protocol starting around 12:00 h and lasting 25 h. Sleep was polygraphically recorded. ACTH, GH, PRL and Cortisol levels were measured by radioimmunoassay. The circadian variations of all hormones were evaluated by building a best-fit curve obtained by repeated periodogram calculations as extensively described elsewhere [5]. The acrophase and nadir are, respectively, the times of occurrence of maxima and minima in the best-fit curve. Significant pulses of the hormones were identified and characterized using a computer program previously described [6].

Results

Sleep

The sleep abnormalities most common in the acute state were an increase in the amount of time spent awake, a decrease in the amount of slow-wave sleep and a shortening of the REM latency. Successful treatment resulted in a correction of these abnormalities, such that the distribution of sleep in the patients did not differ from normals. The difference in the times of the sleep onset before and after treatment was not significant. On the average REM latencies were significantly lengthened after treatment ($P < 0.05$).

ACTH and cortisol [1]

Before treatment, compared to normal subjects, endogenous depressed patients had increased 24-h mean plasma cortisol levels and decreased relative amplitude of the cortisol rhythm. An advance of the nadir of cortisol, paralleled by an advance of the nadir of ACTH was present ($P < 0.05$). The 24-h mean ACTH level was elevated when compared to normal subjects ($P < 0.01$). After treatment the cortisol concentration normalized ($P < 0.05$) and the nadir of cortisol was delayed by an average of 3 h ($P < 0.01$) resulting in a normal timing of the rhythm. A similar delay of the nadir of ACTH was present. Before treatment, the hypercortisolism in depressed patients was associated with an increase in the magnitude ($P < 0.05$) but not in the number of significant cortisol secretory pulses. During remission, the magnitude of the pulses was reduced compared to pretreatment values ($P < 0.05$) but remained significantly higher than that in normal subjects ($P < 0.05$). There was no significant effect on the magnitude of ACTH pulses [7].

GH [3]

During acute depression, the endogenous patients hypersecreted GH ($P < 0.05$) as compared to controls, this hypersecretion being confined to wakefulness hours ($P < 0.05$). The elevation in diurnal GH secretion was primarily due to an increase in the number of secretary pulses ($P < 0.05$) rather than an increase in their magnitude. The total amount of GH secreted over the 24-h span as well as during wakefulness decreased significantly after treatment ($P < 0.05$ and $P < 0.001$, respectively) and did not differ from normal values. The decline in diurnal GH secretion was associated with a decrease in the number of significant GH pulses ($P < 0.05$) which remained however, more frequent than that in normal subjects ($P < 0.05$) [7].

Prolactin [4]

Mean PRL secretion over the 24-h span was not diminished in men with endogenous depression as compared with healthy age and sex-matched subjects. However, an early timing in nocturnal PRL secretion and damping in night-time PRL elevation was found in depressed men.

No significant difference could be found between pretreatment and post-treatment secretory and circadian parameters [7].

Comment

During the acute phase of the illness, elevated 24-mean levels of cortisol, diurnal hypersecretion of GH and normal 24-h levels of PRL were observed in men with endogenous depression. An early timing of the hormonal rhythms was observed for all hormones. After successful treatment with either ECT or amitriptyline, these abnormalities (with exception of those found in the PRL study) were corrected. The normalization of the timing of hormonal secretions was accompanied by a correction of sleep abnormalities and, in particular, a lengthening of the REM latencies. Normalization of cortisol secretion was associated by a decrease in the magnitude of episodic cortisol pulses while normalization of GH secretion was due to a diminished number of secretory pulses. In conclusion, a disorder of circadian time keeping characterizes acute episodes of major depression. This abnormality, as well as the associated increases in adrenocorticotropic and somatotropic activities are state- rather than trait-dependent.

References

1. Linkowski P, Mendlewicz J, Leclercq R, Brasseur M, Hubain P, Golstein P and Van Cauter E (1985) J. Clin. Endocrinol. Metab. 61: 429–438.
2. Sachar EO, Hellman L, Roffwarg H, Halpern F, Fukushima D and Gallagher D (1973) Arch. Gen. Psychiatry 28: 19.
3. Mendlewicz J, Linkowski P, Kerkhofs M, Desmedt D, Golstein J, Copinschi G and Van Cauter E (1985). J. Clin. Endocrinol. Metab. 60: 505–512.
4. Linkowski P, Van Cauter E, L'Hermite-Baleriaux M, Kerkhofs M, Hubain Ph, L'Hermite M and Mendlewicz J (1989) Arch. Gen. Psychiatry 46: 813–819.
5. Van Cauter E (1979) Am. J. Physiol. 237: E255–E264.
6. Van Cauter E (1981) In: Van Cauter E and Copinschi G (eds.) Human Pituitary Hormones: Circadian and Episodic Variations. Nyhoff, The Hague, The Netherlands, pp. 1–25.
7. Linkowski P, Mendlewicz J, Kerkhofs M, Leclercq R, Golstein J, Brasseur M, Copinschi G and Van Cauter E (1987) J. Clin. Endocrinol. Metab. 65: 141–152.

Biological Psychiatry, Volume 1. G. Racagni et al., editors.

Pharmacological effects of antidepressants: Their chronology and potential clinical relevance

Alain J. Puech
Département de Pharmacologie, Groupe Hospitalier Pitié-Salpêtrière, 47, Bd de l'Hôpital, 75651 Paris Cedex 13, France

Introduction

Because in animals, some effects of the antidepressants occur only after chronic administration and thus mimic the chronology of clinical effects, most people focus on pharmacodynay to explain the onset of action of antidepressants in patients. This paper reviews the acute effects of antidepressants and the chronology of the adaptative changes after chronic administration.

Biochemical effects after acute administration

The primary biochemical effect of antidepressant occurs already after acute administration whatever the mechanism is: uptake inhibition (NE, 5-HT or DA) MAO inhibition, 5-HT_{1A} stimulation, α_2-adrenergic antagonism, β-adrenergic stimulation.

Biochemical effects after chronic administration

The adaptative changes observed after chronic administration are the following:
1. the NE stimulation cAMP is blunted;
2. β-adrenergic receptor down-regulation;
3. α_2-adrenergic receptor down-regulation;
4. 5-HT_{1A}-related pharmacological effects are increased;
5. presynaptic DA-related pharmacological effects are decreased;
6. postsynaptic DA-related pharmacological effects are increased;
7. α_1-adrenergic-related pharmacological effects are increased.

All these effects are not observed with all antidepressants. But all these effects are observed with a variety of antidepressants with different primary mechanisms of action.

Electrophysiological effects

After chronic administration, all antidepressants (whatever the primary effect) induce a facilitation of 5-HT transmission by 3 different mechanisms:

1. 5-HT_{1A} postsynaptic receptor facilitation;
2. 5-HT_1 presynaptic (terminals) receptor desensitization;
3. 5-HT_{1A} autoreceptor desensitization.

Chronology of the effects and net consequence on transmission

After acute administration, the noradrenergic transmission is increased with only some antidepressants (or putative antidepressants): NE uptake inhibitors, MAOI, α_2-adrenergic antagonists, β-adrenergic agonists.

After chronic administration, with the same drugs, the NE transmission is still facilitated, at least for α_1-adrenergic receptors and the same effect is observed with drugs without direct primary effect on NA transmission. It is difficult to speculate on the level of transmission at the β-adrenergic receptor site. Does the down-regulation of these receptors blunt the NE concentration increase?

The same phenomenon is observed on 5-HT and DA transmission. Facilitation of the transmission is observed after both acute and chronic administration, but only some antidepressants increase 5-HT or DA transmission after acute administration when most antidepressants seem to be able to facilitate this transmission after chronic administration. The conclusion is that most antidepressants induce a quite selective change after acute administration, while chronic administration induces a pattern of change, quite similar for most antidepressants.

Behavioural effects

Behavioural effects are observed with antidepressants after acute administration (forced swimming test, olfactory bulbectomy) subacute administration (4–5 days – learned helplessness) or chronic administration (>1 week chronic non-predictable stress). The predictivity of these tests is not very different and it is difficult to say today if chronic tests are really better from a purely pharmacological point of view.

Pharmacodynamic approaches to reduce onset of action of antidepressant activity

Different specific primary mechanisms have now been identified, leading to antidepressant activity and delayed action. In the pattern of changes described after chronic administration, nobody knows which are useful, which are harmful. Different strategies can be proposed to reduce the onset of action:

1. accelerate the adaptative changes (e.g. combination of a NE uptake inhibitor and an α_2-adrenergic receptor antagonist);
2. induce directly one effect observed after chronic but not after acute administration (e.g. α_1-adrenergic stimulation);
3. induce directly the pattern of change observed after chronic administration with a drug combination.

Factors delaying antidepressant effect

The onset of action of antidepressant could not only be related to the drug but also the patients. In rats, weight loss, hypothyroidism, diabetes delay the action of antidepressants. These factors are sometimes present in patients. Moreover, dysfunction of β-adrenergic and 5-HT_{1A} receptors have been described in depressed patients. These 2 targets seem very relevant for antidepressant activity. For each antidepressant, some of these factors could delay the activity, resulting in an overall delay of action for all antidepressants.

Biological Psychiatry, Volume 1. G. Racagni et al., editors.

Strategies for confirming the rapid onset of antidepressants

John P. Feighner and William F. Boyer
Feigner Research Institute, San Diego, California, U.S.A.

The delay in onset of antidepressant medications is a pressing clinical issue. Patients with major depression typically present with significant emotional distress and impairment. Waiting 2 or more weeks before the prescribed antidepressant starts to help requires much from a patient and family which are already extremely stressed. The delay may allow the depression to wreak further havoc with the patient, his or her livelihood, and family. The patient may even commit suicide. Therefore medications which relieve depression rapidly are crucially needed. In the recent past several antidepressants have been introduced with claims of rapid onset of action. Unfortunately these have not withstood the scrutiny of clinical experience. New antidepressant compounds continue to be developed and it is likely that one or more of them will have more rapid onset of action. However, to show this requires rigorous methodological considerations. It is our purpose to briefly review several of the most important considerations in this type of study. We will outline several of the features of an "ideal" or nearly ideal study designed to assess whether an investigational antidepressant truly does have more rapid onset of action.

Patient selection

Patient eligibility requirements should be designed to include patients who are likely to improve with medication and to exclude probable placebo responders. To this end, patients should have unipolar non-psychotic major depression, with melancholia, of at least one month's duration. Unipolar depression is suggested as it will reduce the need for concomitant psychotropic medications and avoid some potential complications in symptom scoring, including the possibility of rating drug-induced hypomania as treatment response. It is also helpful to set specific rating scale criteria. A 21-item HAMD total score of 26 or more is suggested. A minimum sample size of 25 to 50 patients per group should be sufficient to show clinically meaningful differences.

Patients with active alcohol or drug abuse or unstable medical conditions should not be included. Treatment-refractory patients should also be excluded. Refractoriness can be defined as a patient who has failed two or more adequate trials of antidepressants for the present episode. Patients with prominent Axis II diagnoses, especially of the "dramatic-erratic" type (e.g. borderline, histrionic, antisocial) should also be excluded, as they frequently are relatively treatment-refractory.

Study design

The study should utilize random assignment of patients to parallel groups. The treatment groups should include a placebo group and possibly an established antidepressant. A placebo group is essential to control for the natural course of the illness. If efficacy is already well established for the investigational antidepressant, then a standard antidepressant is not absolutely necessary. However, such a reference group will also allow comparison of the rate of improvement with an established treatment. In other words, a placebo group allows one to comment on whether there is early onset; a reference compound allows one to state whether there is earlier onset.

In a study dealing with early onset the greatest interest will, of course, be in the first few weeks of the trial. However the duration of the study should still approximate the 6-week standard. This is an important issue as a number of early improvers may in fact be placebo responders. Many of these will then relapse near the end of the study and this can be taken into account in the statistical analyses.

Concomitant medications should be closely controlled. Use of hypnotics, if allowed, should be recorded. Their use may be related to side-effect profile, such as activation-sedation as well as therapeutic effects. Concomitant medications that can influence depressive symptoms or the pharmacokinetics of the research compound should be avoided.

Patients should be withdrawn from previous psychotropics in a single-blind placebo washout period. This period will also allow for identification of some or most of the placebo responders. The absolute minimum period for tricyclic antidepressants (TCAs) should be one week, but a longer period will reduce the chance of TCA withdrawal effects masquerading as depressive symptoms. Patients should be off monoamine oxidase inhibitors for a minimum of two weeks and fluoxetine for one month for pharmacokinetic reasons.

Rating scales

Physician, patient and nursing scales should be utilized. Physician scales should include the Hamilton Depression Rating Scale (HAMD) [1], Montgomery-Asberg Depression Rating Scale (MADRS) [2] and Clinical Global Impressions (CGI). Patient scales may include the Beck Depression Inventory, one of the several forms of the Symptom Checklist (SCL) such as the SCL 90-R, or a global rating such as the Patient Global Evaluation. Nursing ratings may also include the CGI, NOSIE or equivalent.

Research setting

Given the need for frequent symptom ratings and safety monitoring, the need to control dosage times, as well as the severity of the patients' depression, the ideal initial setting will be inpatient. Outpatient setting or a day hospital may be used once initial response to medication has been assessed and if the patient's condition allows. The length of time required until hospital discharge may be one of the secondary efficacy variables.

Frequency of assessments

The baseline measurement should be taken at day one of the active treatment phase. Efficacy should be measured every 2–3 days for the first 2 weeks and then weekly for the remainder of the study. Patient ratings may be taken even more frequently. Clinical global assessments should be made daily for the first 2 weeks, then weekly. Observer-rated scales should be completed by the same raters and at the same time of day. The frequency of safety evaluations may vary pending any suspected problem e.g. cardiovascular side-effects, liver or bone marrow toxicity. A minimum would be laboratory and physical examinations at the beginning and end of the study with frequent inquiry concerning subjective adverse effects. Pharmacokinetic data should be obtained if possible to assess serum levels and clinical response. The "blind" must be maintained and these tests run in a separate laboratory.

Dosing schedule

Oral dosing should be utilized. Depending on pharmacokinetic and bioavailability data, a parenteral form may be utilized in a separate study to allow for the potential of even more rapid onset of action. The time of the dose will vary depending upon the profile of the investigational compound, i.e. a.m. versus p.m. for activating or sedating drugs. Dosage schedule may also vary according to the pharmacokinetics and tolerability of the research compound. For example, it may be given one to three times a day. Equal doses may be given at these times or more may be given in the morning or evening, again depending on the sedating-activating effects of the compound. There should be rapid dosage titration depending on how the patients tolerate the compound. A clinically effective and stable daily dose should be established as soon as possible. A fixed-flexible design, i.e. minimum and maximum allowed dosages, should be utilized. Unfortunately this may make interpretation of the serum concentration-response data more difficult, as non-responders are typically given higher doses which may create the false impression of a "therapeutic window."

Statistical considerations

There are 2 primary ways of managing the data from the main outcome measures. One is a "visit-wise" (VW) analysis. In a VW analysis the data from every patient remaining in each treatment group at each visit is compared with data from patients in the other treatment group(s) who are still in the study. This method has the advantage of accurately reflecting what the investigators see at each time point in the study. It is subject to dropout bias, however. For example, placebo-treated patients are more likely to drop out due to lack of efficacy. Therefore placebo patients who remain in the study are likely to be placebo responders. A VW analysis may therefore overestimate placebo response.

Another method is the "last observed carried forward" (LOCF) analysis. If a patient drops out of the study his or her last valid data is "carried forward" to each time point until the end of the study. This avoids the dropout bias, but is prone to another type of distortion. Patients on active medication are more likely to drop out due to adverse effects. These dropouts typically occur while the patient is significantly depressed, but their data still appears in the endpoint analyses. Therefore the LOCF analysis may underestimate drug response. The best compromise at present is to examine the data with both methods. Fortunately, a study designed specifically to look for early onset of action will be most concerned with the first few weeks. During this time the difference between VW and LOCF analyses will be smallest.

A third method is available but not yet as commonly used. "Pattern analysis" involves comparing the number of patients with persistent, or delayed-persistent, response with those who do not respond or who respond and then relapse. The persistent pattern is thought to represent "true" drug response, while the latter describes placebo response [3]. The advantage of this method is that it provides a consistent way of identifying placebo responders and eliminates some of the "noise" in the data. The main disadvantage is that defining "true" drug response as delayed is not consistent with a study designed to learn about early onset of action.

The data should be examined with statistical tests which are appropriate for the type of data. For example, CGI scores are categorical in nature. Tests such as χ^2, Fisher's Exact Test or Logit analyses are most appropriate. Scores on the HAMD and MADRS are ordinal in nature. With such data it is acceptable to use tests such as analysis of variance (ANOVA). Although the ANOVA assumes that the data is normally distributed, it is relatively "robust" and yields accurate results if the data only approximates this.

In addition to total scores on the rating scales, it is often valuable to examine factor scores, cluster scores and individual items. Factors are groups of items which are statistically derived so that items within each factor correlate highly with each other. Clusters are groups of items which are grouped together by "common sense." For example, insomnia, weight loss and suicidal ideation may logically cluster together while the items in a comparable factor may be somewhat different.

The advantage of examining these subscores is that it may provide information about special properties of a drug, such as effects on sleep, energy level, or libido.

The disadvantage is that scores based on individual items or small numbers of items are more subject to random variation than are total scores, in which the random variations are more likely to cancel each other. One also faces the situation that the larger the number of statistical tests performed, the greater the chance of finding a "significant" result by chance.

Some other variables may also provide useful information. It is often worthwhile to examine dropout data, such as the numbers of patients who discontinue due to lack of efficacy and/or side-effects. The need for and number of concomitant medications, such as prn hypnotics, may also be used as a dependent variable.

Summary

This discussion highlights some of the important methodological concerns in antidepressant studies designed to assess early onset of action. Perhaps the most important methodological consideration is replication and replicability. Single reports of quick onset of action are important, but cannot establish that a compound is truly quick-acting. Findings of rapid antidepressant onset in one study must be replicated before they can be accepted. Replicability can best be accomplished by adherence to a standardized methodology, such as that presented here.

References

1. Hamilton M (1960) J. Neurol. Neurosurg. Psychiatry 23: 56–62.
2. Montgomery SA and Asberg M (1979) Br. J. Psychiatry 134: 382–389.
3. Quitkin FM, Rabkin JG, Ross D et al. (1984) Arch. Gen. Psychiatry 41(8): 782–786.

Biological Psychiatry, Volume 1. G. Racagni et al., editors.

Clinical aspects of onset of action of antidepressant efficacy

S.A. Montgomery[1] and G. Magni[2]
[1]*St Mary's Hospital Medical School, London, U.K.; and* [2]*Wyeth-Ayerst, Paris, France*

The delay in the response to antidepressants is well known. Large multicentre studies have consistently found that a period of 4 to 6 weeks is required before a significant drug placebo difference can be demonstrated reliably. European regulatory authorities recognise this, requiring a minimum 4-week study to demonstrate efficacy against placebo.

The time lag in treatment response is of particular concern in depressive illness where the illness itself reduces the motivation to continue with treatment. The delay in response also carries with it an increased risk of suicide which is more likely during the acture treatment phase. Apart from adding to the risk inherent in the illness, the delay in response substantially increases the secondary effects of depression on social and occupational performance and the costs to the individual from loss of income and to society at large with the costs of care. Producing treatments which act faster is therefore an important aim. For recurrent brief depression, which is as common as major depression and as dangerous, only treatments which act fast have a chance of aborting the attack.

There is evidence that some patients do respond early to antidepressant treatment. There is, however, a methodological problem in identifying this phenomenon. An early symptomatic response, e.g. on sleep disturbance or the anxiety symptoms of depression, does not necessarily reflect a response of the depression unless this response is accompanied by a response on the core symptoms of depression. The response to antidepressants varies between individuals to such an extent that very large studies are required to detect what is a response to placebo and what is a pharmacological effect, particularly in the early phases of treatment. Some depression scales contain items that reflect full rehabilitation which occurs some time later than the remission of the depression. The use of sensitive scales which concentrate on the core symptoms of depression are more likely to reflect the course of illness and improves the chance both of detecting response to treatment and particularly of detecting early response. The Montgomery and Asberg Depression Rating Scale (MADRS), for example, which was constructed for sensitivity to change was able to detect a drug placebo difference at 1 week where the less sensitive Hamilton Rating Scale (HRS) was only able to detect the difference at 2 weeks in a 700-patient study (Dunbar et al., 1990). In this study on paroxetine the significant early difference was not clinically important.

The early response, detected by the MADRS, may be statistically significant in large studies but clinically not important. The statistically significant difference has still to be quantitatively large enough to be of clinical significance. One widely used measure is a difference of 4 points on the HRS or the MADRS.

Recent studies with venlafaxine have provided some important findings on early response to treatment. In the efficacy studies both high and low doses of venlafaxine were shown to have antidepressant efficacy at the end of the acute treatment period. The reports of a significant response at 1 week and 4 days with high doses but not with the low doses is of considerable theoretical and practical interest. In the high dose placebo controlled study carried out in the U.S.A. a significant difference was reported at the earliest assessment point, i.e. 1 week, suggesting an early onset of antidepressant response. In the European study, this finding was replicated with a significant difference observed on the MADRS after 4 days of treatment with a drug placebo difference of 22.3. At 1 week this was both statistically significant and clinically important with a drug placebo difference of 4.3.

The early response is likely to be clinically relevant and useful since it is registered even on less sensitive scales. The early response to venlafaxine suggests that its mechanism of action is likely to be more direct than that of other antidepressants which produce a delayed response. Quite why this is so is unclear; however, it may be relevant that venlafaxine is reported to functionally down-regulate the β-adrenoceptors after a single dose.

Early response appears to be seen best with high doses of venlafaxine, which suggests that the abrupt challenge of the high initial dose may be the important factor. If this is true a new approach to treatment becomes appropriate. Instead of starting with a low dose and raising the dose gradually, it may be more effective if a high dose is used initially to obtain a rapid response and the dose is subsequently lowered to sustain response.

Biological Psychiatry, Volume 1. G. Racagni et al., editors.

Venlafaxine: A new potent antidepressant agent with putative fast onset of action

Karl Rickels

Department of Psychiatry, University of Pennsylvania, 203 Piersol Building, 3400 Spruce Street, Philadelphia, PA 19104-4283, U.S.A.

Venlafaxine, a new antidepressant, inhibits or blocks neuronal uptake of serotonin, norepinephrine and dopamine, but has no MAO inhibitory activity, and no affinity for rat brain muscarinic, cholinergic, or histaminergic receptors. Preclinical evidence for a possible early onset of action is the rapid and prolonged desensitization of the noradrenergic system. Venlafaxine reduces cAMP responsiveness in the pineal gland model after both acute and chronic administration, while standard antidepressants such as desipramine do so only after chronic administration [1].

A large venlafaxine development program was conducted in the U.S. which included 5 positive double-blind controlled studies and 1 uninterpretable study in which the response to venlafaxine, imipramine and placebo was identical. Three studies were placebo-controlled and 3 studies were placebo- and active drug-controlled, 2 using imipramine and 1 trazodone as the standard agent. Based on 1,902 venlafaxine patients (Wyeth-Ayerst NDA submission, 1991), side-effects reported most frequently were nausea, drowsiness, insomnia, dry mouth, sexual dysfunction, sweating, dizziness, nervousness and constipation. Major side-effects reported by imipramine patients (n = 240) were dry mouth, constipation, drowsiness, sweating, dizziness and nervousness. Venlafaxine produced more nausea and sexual dysfunction than imipramine and imipramine produced more dry mouth and constipation. Headaches were equally frequently reported with all three treatments (28%).

In one multi-center dose response study, venlafaxine in daily doses of 375 mg/day, but not in daily doses of 225 mg/day or less caused a significant increase in pulse and diastolic and systolic blood pressure [2]. Most likely this increase in blood pressure is related to the noradrenergic effects of venlafaxine. All subsequent studies were conducted with a dose range not exceeding 225 mg/day and no significant increase in pulse and diastolic and systolic blood pressure were observed. For example, one 2-center double-blind study compared venlafaxine (179 mg/day) with imipramine (175 mg/day) and placebo over a 6 week period observed a response rate, assessed as at least a 50% reduction on the Hamilton Depression Scale, of 47% for placebo, 61% for imipramine and 77% for venlafaxine ($P < 0.05$). On the global improvement assessment, the respective percentages were 53%, 79% and 90% ($P < 0.05$). (Rickels K. et al., unpublished data).

Evidence for some possible fast onset of action was derived from the multi-center dosage range U.S. study [1] and from a study conducted with French inpatients (Guelfi J.D. and Bourgeois M., unpublished data). In the French study, at a mean daily dose of 169 mg/day, after only 4 days of treatment, venlafaxine was already found to produce significantly more improvement than placebo in the HAM-D item sleep disturbance and depressed mood, and in the total MADRS score. At a mean dosage of 230 mg/day, significant treatment differences were observed in all outcome measures after 1 week of therapy. Similar findings were observed in the U.S. multi-center dose response outpatient study where, however, outcome was assessed after only 1 week of treatment. At a mean dosage of 200 mg/day, venlafaxine was favored significantly over placebo in all HAM-D measures, including total score, MADRS total score, CGI severity and global improvement scales. In patients on a daily venlafaxine dose of 140 mg/day, this difference was observed only for the HAM-D depressed mood and cognitive disturbance items, and for the CGI global improvement, and no differences between venlafaxine and placebo were seen in the lowest dosage group (69 mg/day venlafaxine). Whether or not a similar fast onset of antidepressant action can also be achieved with such standard antidepressants as imipramine or amitriptyline for example without experiencing unacceptable side-effects, should be a subject of further research.

In conclusion, the U.S. NDA program and the French inpatient study demonstrated that venlafaxine is significantly more effective than placebo in relieving symptoms of depression. The lowest daily dose used (75 mg/day) was the least effective dose. The highest daily dose (250–375 mg/day) was the most effective dose, producing significantly more improvement than placebo already after only one week of therapy; this high dose group produced, however, the most adverse events and was associated with increases in blood pressure and pulse. Based on these data, one may make the following recommendations for the use of venlafaxine:

1. Optimum dose range is 75–225 mg/day and provides the most acceptable balance between efficacy and adverse event incidents.
2. Use of a high dose (250–375 mg/day) schedule during the first 1–2 weeks of therapy, if early onset is desired, even at the expense of higher incidents of adverse events, to be followed by a decrease in daily dosage for the remainder of therapy.
3. Use of a gradual dosing schedule (gradual increase in daily dosages up to 225 mg/day) if gradual onset of improvement and lower level of adverse events are desired, and early onset is not the major goal of therapy.

References

1. Muth EA, Haskins JT, Moyer JA, Husbands GE, Nielson ST and Sigg EG (1986) Biochem. Pharmacol. 35: 4493–4497.
2. Derivan A, Entsuah R, Rudolph R and Rickels K (1990) Early Response to Venlafaxine Hydrochloride, A Novel Antidepressant. Poster presented at the ACNP meeting in San Juan, Puerto Rico, December 1990.

Biological Psychiatry, Volume 1. G. Racagni et al., editors.

Lithium enhancement of brain 5-HT function in resistant depression: Relation to clinical outcome

Philip J. Cowen
Psychopharmacology Research Unit, Littlemore Hospital, Oxford OX4 4XN, U.K.

Introduction

Several recent clinical studies have shown that the addition of lithium to tricyclic antidepressant (TCA) treatment can produce a useful therapeutic effect in patients who have previously been unresponsive to the TCA alone [1]. The pharmacological mechanism of this effect has aroused much interest and it has been suggested by de Montigny et al., on the basis of animal studies, that a synergistic action of the 2 drugs on brain 5-hydroxytryptamine (5-HT) pathways might be responsible [2]. Lithium is known to produce marked effects on brain 5-HT function in animals: there is much evidence, for example, that it facilitates 5-HT release and, in addition, behavioural studies suggest that it may also increase the sensitivity of post-synaptic 5-HT_{1A} receptors [3].
The studies described here were undertaken to answer the following questions:
a) Does lithium increase brain 5-HT function in healthy volunteers?
b) Does the mechanism involve increased sensitivity of postsynaptic 5-HT_{1A} receptors?
c) Does lithium increase brain 5-HT function in depressed patients receiving tricyclic antidepressants?
d) Does the change in brain 5-HT function in these latter subjects correlate with clinical outcome?

Materials and Methods

Subjects

We studied healthy male volunteers and depressed patients. The 23 depressed patients met DSM III criteria for major depression and had been on a maximum tolerated dose of a tricyclic antidepressant for at least 3 weeks; this drug treatment was kept constant throughout the period of lithium augmentation. Clinical response to lithium augmentation was defined as a 50% decrease in pre-lithium Hamilton Depression Scores (HAMD).

5-HT neuroendocrine testing

We assessed brain 5-HT function by measuring the increase in plasma prolactin (PRL) that follows administration of drugs that increase brain 5-HT function by different mechanisms (Table 1). We also assessed the effect of lithium treatment on the PRL response to thyrotropin releasing hormone (TRH) and haloperidol. All subjects were tested before and following a defined period of lithium treatment (see Table 1).

Results

In healthy volunteers sub-acute lithium treatment (4–7 days) significantly increased the PRL response to LTP and clomipramine but did not alter the PRL increase that followed TRH and haloperidol (Table 1). The PRL response to gepirone was similarly unaltered. In the depressed patients the addition of lithium to TCA treatment significantly increased the PRL response to LTP after both 1 and 4 weeks of treatment. Ten of the 23 patients were clinical responders after 4 weeks of lithium treatment, but the increase in PRL produced by lithium did not differ between responders and non-responders. However, when the responders were considered alone there was a modest but significant correlation between change in HAMD score and increase in PRL response (rho = 0.673; $P = 0.03$).

Discussion

Our findings suggest that lithium treatment in humans increases brain 5-HT function, as measured by 5-HT-mediated PRL release. It is of interest that the increase in PRL response occurred with drugs that facilitate brain 5-HT function through actions on presynaptic 5-HT neurones [4,5] but not with gepirone which increases plasma PRL through a direct action on post-synaptic 5-HT_{1A} receptors [6]. This suggests that lithium does not increase 5-HT-mediated PRL release

Table 1. Effect of acute lithium on PRL responses to drug challenge

Drug	Mechanism	PRL response
LTP (100 mg/kg i.v.)	5-HT precursor	Increased
Clomipramine (0.1 mg/kg, i.v.)	5-HT uptake inhibitor	Increased
Gepirone (20 mg orally)	5-HT_{1A} receptor agonist	No change
Haloperidol (2.5–5 μg/kg, i.v.)	Dopamine receptor antagonist	No change
Metoclopramide (5 μg/kg, i.v.)	Dopamine receptor antagonist	No change
TRH (6.25 μg, i.v.)	Direct lactotroph stimulant	No change

See references [4] and [5].

through increasing the sensitivity of post-synaptic 5-HT_{1A} receptors and its ability to increase 5-HT-mediated PRL release is therefore presumably mediated via increased presynaptic release of 5-HT [3,5]. It is also important to note that lithium did not facilitate the PRL responses to metoclopramide, haloperidol or TRH, suggesting that its ability to increase 5-HT-mediated PRL release is not caused by an action on dopamine neurones or through a primary alteration in the pituitary release of PRL [4,5].

Lithium also increased the PRL response to LTP in depressed patients receiving TCAs [7]. Because TCAs themselves increase the PRL response to LTP, it is possible that the addition of lithium to TCA treatment does produce a further increase in brain 5-HT function as suggested by animal studies [2]. However, the increase in PRL response to LTP produced by lithium occurred equally in those depressed patients who appeared to respond to lithium treatment and those who did not. This suggests that there is not a straightforward relationship between lithium-induced changes in brain 5-HT function and clinical outcome [7].

We did, however, find a modest correlation between change in PRL response and change in HAMD in the responder group. From this it is possible to speculate that in patients who respond clinically to lithium augmentation, the antidepressant effect of lithium treatment may be mediated in part through increased brain 5-HT function.

Acknowledgement

These studies were supported by the Medical Research Council.

References

1. Price LH (1989) In: Extein IL (ed.) Treatment of Tricyclic-Resistant Depression. American Psychiatric Press, Washington, pp. 51–79.
2. de Montigny C, Grunberg F, Mayer A and Deschenes JP (1981) Br. J. Psychiatry 138: 252–256.
3. Wood AJ and Goodwin GM (1987) Psychol. Med. 17: 579–600.
4. McCance SL, Cohen PR and Cowen PJ (1989) Psychopharmacology 99: 276–281.
5. Cowen PJ, Cohen PR, McCance SL and Friston KJ (1990) J. Neurosci. Methods 34: 201–205.
6. Anderson IN, Cowen PJ and Grahame-Smith DG (1990) Psychopharmacology 100: 498–503.
7. Cowen PJ, McCance SL, Ware CJ, Cohen PR, Chalmers JS and Julier DL (1991) Br. J. Psychiatry (in press).

Biological Psychiatry, Volume 1. G. Racagni et al., editors.

Lithium supplementation therapy in refractory depression: Clinical aspects and neuroendocrine challenge effects

Baruch Shapira[1], Mohammed J. Yagmur[1], Michael E. Newman[2] and Bernard Lerer[2]

[1]*Depression Treatment Unit, Herzog Hospital-Ezrath Nashim; and* [2]*Department of Psychiatry, Hadassah University Hospital, Jerusalem, Israel*

Clinical aspects

Lithium (Li) supplementation has become an extensively used therapeutic intervention in depressed patients who fail to respond to treatment with tricyclic (TCA) and other antidepressants [1]. Further findings relevant to therapeutic efficacy and clinical correlates of response are presented in this chapter.

Forty-five depressed patients hospitalized in the depression treatment unit were administered Li (for at least 3 weeks, blood level 0.6 ± 0.17 mmol) after they failed to respond to 4 weeks of antidepressant treatment. The antidepressants supplemented by Li were: clomipramine (n = 24), imipramine (n = 10), maprotiline (n = 4), amitryptiline (n = 2), (median dose of TCA: 200 mg/day), maprotiline (n = 4, 150 mg/day), fluvoxamine (n = 2, 150 mg/day), fluoxetine (n = 1, 20 mg/day). Two patients who were delusionally depressed received the antidepressant in combination with an antipsychotic agent. Global clinical outcome was as follows: 27 patients (60%) achieved complete remission (enabling discharge from hospital without additional antidepressant intervention), 5 (11%) had a partial response and 13 (29%) minimal or no response. Twelve of the patients who remitted on Li supplementation had failed to respond to ECT during the current depressive episode.

In order to identify clinical characteristics associated with response to Li supplementation, patients who remitted (R) were compared to those with partial or no improvement (NR). Li blood levels were similar (0.68 ± 0.04, 0.62 ± 0.03 mmol) in the two groups. There was a trend towards better response in males than in females ($\chi^2 = 3.4$, $P = 0.06$), in the 8 bipolar patients ($\chi^2 = 3.5$, $P = 0.06$) and in patients receiving a higher TCA dose (R = 204 ± 7.81 mg/day; NR = 177.9 ± 10.47 mg/day; t = 1.97, $P = 0.05$). The sex difference in response is explained by polarity since 27% of the male patients were bipolar compared to 11% of the females. The effect of TCA dose raises the possibility that continuation beyond 4 weeks of TCA treatment alone (at higher dose levels) might have led to remission without Li supplementation in some of the subjects.

Table 1. δ-prolactin response to fenfluramine challenge (ng/ml)

	Pretreatment (1)	Clomipramine (2)	Clomipramine + Li (3)
Fenfluramine[a]	4.6 ± 1.08	11.6 ± 3.58	12.1 ± 4.02
Placebo	2.3 ± 0.85	3.3 ± 0.89	3.2 ± 2.05

[a]$F = 3.58$; df 16,2; $P = 0.05$ (ANOVA with repeated measures); (1) vs. (2), $P = 0.04$; (1) vs. (3), $P = 0.03$; (2) vs. (3), P = N.S. (by *t*-test).

Neuroendocrine challenge effects

The therapeutic mechanism of Li supplementation has been linked to enhanced serotonergic neurotransmission resulting from increased release of this neurotransmitter from presynaptic neurons [1]. As an index of central serotonergic function, prolactin (PRL) response to fenfluramine (FF) challenge was examined in 8 depressed patients who were medication-free for at least 2 weeks, following 4 weeks of treatment with clomipramine (CMI, 203 ± 11.01 mg/day) and after Li supplementation for a further 3 weeks (blood level 0.64 ± 0.04 mmol). The challenge test involved randomised, double-blind, oral administration of FF (60 mg) or placebo (separated by at least 48 h) as previously described [2]. Plasma PRL levels were measured prior to each challenge and then hourly for 6 h.

CMI treatment resulted in a significant enhancement of baseline PRL levels, as has been previously reported [3]. The data were therefore analysed by comparing peak minus baseline (delta) PRL levels in response to FF and placebo challenge. As we have observed for imipramine [2], CMI treatment significantly enhanced the PRL response to FF challenge but not to placebo. Li supplementation did not result in any further change in PRL release.

Previous reports using intravenous L-tryptophan as the challenge agent have noted an enhancement by short and long-term Li administration of serotonergically mediated PRL release in normal subjects [4] and also in depressed patients treated with TCA and receiving Li supplementation [5]. However, other authors have found that in depressed patients long-term (>3 weeks) Li administration does not enhance the PRL response to tryptophan [6]. The absence of a Li effect in the present study could result from a ceiling phenomenon due to maximal increase in PRL response following CMI treatment. Re-evaluation at lower FF dose is therefore indicated.

Acknowledgement

Supported in part by NIMH Grant No. 43873.

References

1. De Monigny D, Grunberg F, Mayer A and Deschenes JP (1981) Br. J. Psychiatry 138: 252–256.
2. Shapira B, Reiss A, Kaiser N, Kindler S and Lerer B (1989) J. Affective Disord. 16: 1–4.
3. Zohar J, Insel R, Zohar-Fadouch RC, Hill J and Murphy DL (1988) Arch. Gen. Psychiatry 45: 167–172.
4. Glue PW, Cowen PJ, Wutt DJ, Kolakowska T and Grahame-Smith DG (1986) Psychopharmacology 90: 398–402.
5. Cowen PJ, McClance SL, Cohen PR and Julier DL (1989) Psychopharmacology 99: 230–232.
6. Price LH, Charney DS, Delgado PL and Heninger GR (1989) Arch. Gen. Psychiatry 46: 13–19.

Biological Psychiatry, Volume 1. G. Racagni et al., editors.

Lithium potentiation of bupropion and fluoxetine: Theory and practice

Paul J. Goodnick
D79, Department of Psychiatry, University of Miami, Suite 304A, 1400 NW 10 Avenue, Miami, FL 33136, U.S.A.

Introduction

In 1983, de Montigny et al. [1] described a controlled study of depressed patients who only achieved remission of symptoms upon the addition of lithium carbonate to their antidepressant regimen. Although not all studies have supported the utility of lithium as a successful adjunctive treatment for depression [2], the results have been replicated on numerous occasions with various antidepressants. De Montigny explained his results on the basis of the serotonergic action of lithium. As recently reviewed [3], acute administration of lithium carbonate leads to alterations which could reflect enhancement of CNS serotonin function.

Two specific antidepressants released recently in the U.S.A. are fluoxetine (Prozac, Dista) and bupropion (Wellbutrin, Burroughs-Wellcome). Fluoxetine has specific action as a 5-HT reuptake blocker; it has relatively little effect in other CNS models, including post-synaptic D_1 and S_2 5HT receptors [4]. The mechanism of bupropion, by contrast, is relatively unknown; however, it appears to have significant effect on dopamine reuptake and may act as postsynaptic dopamine agonist [5].

This report summarizes available data on use of lithium as an adjunctive agent for patients who have not fully responded to either fluoxetine or bupropion.

Material and Methods

Background

At this time, there have been two series of case reports on adjunctive lithium treatment with fluoxetine [6] and with bupropion [7]. Data from the two case reviews is combined with that from the University of Miami (UM) for a total of 21 patients. All fluoxetine patients (8/8) had some degree of added response to lithium; this was true of 11/13 of the bupropion patients ($\chi^2 = 1.36$, P = N.S.). Of the two non-responders to the combination of bupropion and lithium [6], one only attained a clearly nontherapeutic concentration of lithium (0.04 meq/l), and the other had no response at all with a lithium level of 0.5 meq/l. The rest of this report will focus on the nature and course of responders to combined treatment.

Subjects

Overall, there were 10 women and 9 men, with a mean age of 42.9 ± 15.2 years. According to DSM III-R, all met criteria for major depressive disorder.

Methods

The points evaluated for each patient were before and after adjunctive lithium treatment. Note was made of dosage of the antidepressant, dosage of lithium, and lithium blood level at close of treatment period. For non-UM patients, percentage of improvement was based upon Hamilton Depression Rating Scale (HDRS) scores and, where a range of lithium levels were given, an average level was applied for statistical analysis. For UM patients, Beck Depression Inventory (BDI) scores were applied, with specifically available lithium concentrations at close of evaluation period. Duration of treatment until response was determined based upon presented case report information [6,7] or specifically available data for UM patients.

Results

Entire group

The degree of improvement of depression was 66.9 ± 21.8% from the time of the addition of lithium. This improvement required 3.9 ± 3.4 weeks to achieve at a mean lithium level of 0.74 ± 0.21 meq/l. Lithium level tended to correlate with rate of response ($r = 0.45$, $P = 0.07$) but not with degree of response ($r = 0.01$, P = N.S.).

Bupropion vs. fluoxetine

Rate of response did not differentiate significantly between the two groups, although patients on bupropion with lithium had fewer mean weeks until response (see Table 1). However, the bupropion group showed a greater percentage of improvement than the fluoxetine group on the addition of lithium (1-way ANOVA: $F = 5.12$, $P = 0.03$) (see Table 1).

Discussion

Overall response

Lithium adjunctive therapy was successful in improving response to both fluoxetine

Table 1. Response to lithium adjuctive therapy in depression: bupropion vs. fluoxetine

Treatment group	(n)	Lithium level (meq/l)	Time to response (weeks)	% Improved
Bupropion	11	0.64 ± 0.15	3.4 ± 2.0	75.6 ± 20.4
Fluoxetine	8	0.89 ± 0.20	4.6 ± 4.8	55.0 ± 18.4
Total	19	0.74 ± 0.21	3.9 ± 3.4	66.9 ± 21.8

and bupropion. Consistent with a previous review of lithium adjunctive treatment with antidepressants [2], this response took weeks; the time-course closely parallels that previously estimated for alterations of post-synaptic receptor sensitivity. As might be expected, higher lithium levels were associated with more rapid responses. Thus, the bupropion non-responders can be explained by their lithium levels of 0.04 meq/l and 0.5 meq/l.

Bupropion vs. fluoxetine

The response to adjunctive lithium therapy appears to have been significantly greater and perhaps slightly sooner in the bupropion patients than in the fluoxetine patients. As blood levels of lithium were higher in the fluoxetine group (1-way ANOVA: $F = 9.05$, $P = 0.009$) (see Table 1), the earlier onset of the bupropion group response becomes more significant when the lithium level effect is taken into account. The differential in response may be explained in the hypothesized lithium effect via the 5-HT system: bupropion has no 5-HT effects, whereas fluoxetine blocks 5-HT reuptake but does not influence 5-HT receptors [4,5]. Bupropion easily acts synergistically with lithium, but fluoxetine may overlap in biochemical effect with lithium since they both decrease 5-HT reuptake.

Conclusion

The addition of lithium to fluoxetine and bupropion may be clinically effective, as found in early reports. Perhaps if lithium's effect is via the 5-HT system, this may explain why the clinical response to a combination of lithium with a totally-non-5-HT medication (bupropion) acting synergistically, may be greater and perhaps sooner than with a 5-HT-uptake blocker (fluoxetine). Clearly, this hypothesis requires more testing under randomized, double-blind conditions with larger sample sizes. Also, although generally safe in combination, one should monitor the combination of lithium with either fluoxetine or bupropion, especially in the early weeks of treatment.

References

1. de Montigny C, Cournoyer G, Morissette R et al. (1983) Arch. Gen. Psychiatry 40: 1327–1334.
2. Schou M (1990) Lithium 1: 3–8.
3. Goodnick P (1990) Lithium 1: 65–73.
4. Lemberger L, Bergstrom RF, Wolen RL et al. (1985) J. Clin. Psychiatry 46: 14–19.
5. Ferris RM, Cooper BR and Maxwell RA (1983) J. Clin. Psychiatry 44 (Sect. 2): 74–78.
6. Pope HG Jr, McElroy SL and Nixon RA (1988) Am. J. Psychiatry 145: 1292–1294.
7. Apter JT and Woolfolk RL (1990) Ann. Clin. Psychiatry 2: 7–10.

Biological Psychiatry, Volume 1. G. Racagni et al., editors.

Effect of treatment with a lithium-imipramine combination on components of adenylate cyclase in the cerebral cortex of the rat

Arne Mørk and Arne Geisler

Department of Pharmacology, University of Copenhagen, Juliane Maries Vej 20, 2100 Copenhagen, Denmark

Lithium (Li^+) ex vivo reduces isoprenaline-induced stimulation of the activity of adenylate cyclase by GTP in the cerebral cortex of the rat, without affecting the enzyme stimulated by GTP alone. However, despite the lack of effect of Li^+ ex vivo, on the stimulation of the enzyme by GTP, the activity stimulated by Gpp(NH)p was reduced. These apparently contrasting observations were, at least, not due to different assay conditions. The inhibitory effect of lithium ex vivo on stimulation by Gpp(NH)p may be attributable to the fact that Gpp(NH)p is a more potent activator of adenylate cyclase. The stimulatory effect of Gpp(NH)p on N_S may thus mimic agonist stimulation of the receptor. The Ca^{2+}-dependent activation of adenylate cyclase by calmodulin is assumed to occur by a direct effect on the catalytic subunit. The reduced activity of Ca^{2+}-stimulated adenylate cyclase, observed in membranes from Li^+-treated animals, supports the assumption that lithium ex vivo can affect the catalytic subunit of adenylate cyclase. A marked decrease in the synergistic effect of Ca^{2+} and GTP after the treatment with Li^+ may largely be due to the effect of Li^+ on Ca^{2+} activation but may also indicate that the facilitated interaction of the N_S-catalytic subunit is highly sensitive to Li^+ ex vivo.

After chronic treatment with imipramine, isoprenaline-induced stimulation of the activity of adenylate cyclase by GTP was reduced, but no effect was found on the activity of the enzyme stimulated by GTP alone. This observation resembles that of lithium ex vivo. However, imipramine ex vivo did not affect the activity of adenylate cyclase activated through N_S or the catalytic subunit, by Gpp(NH)p and Ca^{2+}, respectively. Observations concerning effects of imipramine ex vivo on the activity of adenylate cyclase, stimulated distal to the receptor, are somewhat inconsistent. The present study, using the physiological activator Ca^{2+}, did not demonstrate any effect of imipramine ex vivo on the catalytic subunit of adenylate cyclase. Thus, treatment with imipramine did not impair the activity of either N_S or the catalytic subunit.

After the combined treatment with Li^+-imipramine, reduced activity of adenylate cyclase, activated by Ca^{2+}, Ca^{2+}/GTP and Gpp(NH)p was observed. However, this activity was not different from that in membranes of animals treated with Li^+ alone, suggesting that concurrent treatment with imipramine did not influence the post-receptor effects of Li^+.

The inhibitory effect of Li^+ and imipramine on receptor agonist-induced stimulation of adenylate cyclase by GTP, may be due to effects of the two drugs on the N proteins. The conformation of the N proteins induced by an endogenous regulator, such as GTP alone, is unaffected by Li^+ and imipramine ex vivo but the conformation induced by endogenous activators such as neurotransmitters is influenced. However, the reduced activation of the receptor agonist may also be explained by an impairment of the coupling between the receptor and the N_S proteins. This can be stated, since receptors are substrates for several protein kinases. Thus it might be speculated that uncoupling of receptors, after treatment with Li^+ and imipramine, could be due to alterations in activity of protein kinases.

Administration of Li^+ and imipramine together led to a greater decrement in isoprenaline-induced stimulation by GTP than that observed with separate treatment with Li^+ and imipramine, indicating that a greater down-regulating effect of the β-adrenergic adenylate cyclase could be achieved with the combined treatment. The precise mechanisms by which Li^+ and imipramine reduce isoprenaline-induced stimulation by GTP is unknown. In contrast to Li^+ ex vivo imipramine ex vivo did not impair the activity of N_S or the catalytic subunit. Furthermore, lithium ex vivo exerted its post-receptor effects on the adenylate cyclase, independent of a concurrent treatment with imipramine.

In conclusion, the addition of Li^+ to treatment with tricyclic antidepressant resulted in further inhibition of the synthesis of cAMP, due the additional receptor and post-receptor effects of Li^+ on adenylate cyclase. If a decrease in the number or sensitivity of β-adrenergic receptors is involved in the therapeutic effects of the antidepressants, the actions of Li^+ and imipramine on the activity of adenylate cyclase could partly explain the efficacy of this combined treatment in the treatment of refractory depression.

Biological Psychiatry, Volume 1. G. Racagni et al., editors.

Plasma/serum concentration of antidepressants and clinical response: State of the art

Lars F. Gram

Department of Clinical Pharmacology, IMB, Odense University, School of Medicine, J.B. Winsløws Vej 19, DK-5000 Odense C, Denmark

Introduction

More than 30 years after the introduction of imipramine, the tricyclic antidepressants (TCA) are still the first choice drug for treatment of depressions in most European countries. This is so in particular because the therapeutic efficacy of TCA is well established. *Dose/effect* studies with TCA occurred only sporadically through the 1960s [1] and only recently has this problem received some renewed attention [2]. The demonstration in the late 1960s of pronounced interindividual variations in the steady state levels on standard doses with TCA [3] created the basis for a series of studies aiming at linking this variability to the variability in clinical outcome. Several hundred papers on the *concentration/effect* relationship have been published [4]), but a series of questions remains open.

Methodological problems

Quite a large fraction of the studies on concentration/effect relationships for TCA have failed to define a clear relationship, whereas a smaller number of studies established a relationship between blood concentration of TCA and, in particular, the antidepressant response [5]. Obviously, a considerable type-2-error problem exists in this field and several variables not sufficiently controlled may explain the negative findings [5]. Diagnostic heterogeneity, high rate of spontaneous response, complex activity of metabolites, pronounced variations in protein-binding are some of the factors discussed [5]. An inherent problem is the time factor in antidepressant response to TCA which has to be accounted for as a third dimension. Furthermore, the therapeutic effect is gradual and often not reversible, and concentration/effect studies thus cannot be performed in patients, but only within groups of patients. Finally, it should be stressed that even the studies showing a concentration/effect relationship, with one exception, have been retrospective in design [1]. Therefore, they have been hypothesis-generating rather than hypothesis-testing and prospective controlled studies comparing different drug levels should ideally be required. However, the time it takes to establish stable steady-state levels may, in the light of the time factor in antidepressant response, make it impossible to find a valid and feasible design for this type of study.

Clinical applications

The general rationale for drug level monitoring: large pharmacokinetic variability relative to the therapeutic index and the lack of reliable clinical measures (response, side-effects, biological effects) for dose adjustment, is clearly fulfilled for TCA. Drug level monitoring of TCA should thus serve to improve efficacy and decrease risk of toxicity. What may be debated, however, is the certainty by which the recommended therapeutic concentrations have been established. For imipramine, nortriptyline and to a lesser extent amitriptyline and desipramine different research groups have reached some agreement [5] and this has created the basis for routine application of drug level monitoring in many clinical centers. Preskorn [6] has stressed the occurrence of CNS-toxicity (confusion and delirium), in particular in the elderly, as the first toxic reaction that can be avoided by TCA drug level monitoring. On the basis of the existing knowledge about several TCA compiled from various studies [5–7], a generalized scheme for various concentration/effect relations can be worked out with imipramine as an example (Table 1).

The common side-effects such as dry mouth, blurred vision, orthostatism etc. often occur at subtherapeutic levels and cannot be avoided by drug level monitoring. Such effects should not be used as guidance for dose adjustment because they are variable and poor indicators of the therapeutic concentration, and such a procedure may lead to therapeutic failure.

The recommended therapeutic range for imipramine (+ desipramine) of 600–1000 nM aims at optimizing the therapeutic effect and at the same time avoiding the more severe toxic reactions. However, side-effects such as orthstatism in elderly may be so severe at these effective concentrations that the treatment cannot be carried through.

A further development within the last decade has been the demonstration of the important *role of the sparteine/debrisoquine oxidation polymorhism* for the overall elimination of most TCA [6]. A simple phenotype test can identify the poor metabolisers of sparteine/debrisoquine (constituting 7% of European populations) who on standard doses of tricyclic antidepressants will develop nearly toxic blood levels. This procedure thus might become a useful supplement to drug level monitoring and allow more precise selection of an appropriate starting dose and thus reduce the time to reach the target concentration [9]. This technique may also make prospective concentration/effect studies feasible.

Several new antidepressants with a different structure and experimental profile have been introduced over the last 20 years. So far, there are few conclusive data on the concentration/effect relationships for these drugs, but in several cases this may be related to their uncertain therapeutic effect. *Dose/effect* studies are now generally required for new antidepressants, and such studies may offer a unique opportunity to establish the *concentration/effect* relationships. Indeed, this may also be a feasible strategy for further prospective studies of concentration/effect relationships of TCA.

References

1. Gram LF (1990) Clin. Neuropharmacol. 13 (Suppl. 1): 35–43.
2. Quitkin FM (1985) Br. J. Psychiatry 147: 593–597.
3. Hammer W and Sjöqvist F (1967) Life Sci. 6: 1895–1903.
4. de Oliveira IR, do Prado-Lima PAS and Samuel-Lajeunesse B (1989) Psychiatr. Psychobiol. 4: 43–60.
5. Gram LF (1977) Clin. Pharmacokinet. 2: 237–251.
6. Preskorn SH (1989) In: Dahl SG and Gram LF (eds.) Clinical Pharmacology in Psychiatry. Springer-Verlag, Heidelberg, pp. 237–243.
7. Gram LF, Pedersen OL, Kristensen CB, Bjerre M and Kragh-Sørensen P (1982) Ther. Drug Monit. 4: 17–25.
8. Brøsen K and Gram LF (1989) Eur. J. Clin. Pharmacol. 36: 537–547.
9. Gram LF and Brøsen K (1990) In: Alvan G et al. (eds.) European Consensus Conference on Pharmacogenetics. Commission of European Communities, Brussels-Luxembourg, pp. 87–96.

Biological Psychiatry, Volume 1. G. Racagni et al., editors.

Plasma monitoring of antidepressants: Clinical relevance of the pharmacogenetic of metabolism and of α_1-acid glycoprotein binding

P. Baumann and C.B. Eap
Unité de Biochimie et Psychopharmacologie Clinique, Département Universitaire de Psychiatrie Adulte, CH-1008, Prilly-Lausanne, France

Introduction

Both environmental and genetic factors contribute to the wide interindividual variability in the plasma levels of psychotropic drugs in patients examined in steady-state conditions. Plasma protein binding and extensive metabolism of the drugs by enzymatic systems in the liver constitute important mechanisms for regulating their fate in the organism. Recently, genetic polymorphisms have been described which concern the binding of basic drugs to plasma α_1-acid glycoprotein [1] and their metabolism by liver cytochrome P-450IID6 and cytochrome P-450IIC9 [2,3].

Genetic polymorphism of metabolism of antidepressants

About 5–10% of the Caucasian population have a genetic deficiency of cyt P-450IID6 and 3–5% have a genetic deficiency of cyt P-450IIC9 [2,3]. Today, patients can be genotyped for P-450IID6 using molecular biology techniques, but phenotyping is still the method of choice for characterising a patient's pharmacogenetic status, using sparteine, debrisoquine or dextromethorphane as test probes for the former and mephenytoin for the latter polymorphism.

Tricyclic antidepressants (TAD) of the tertiary amine type are metabolised mainly by N-demethylation, but also by hydroxylation, which represents the most important metabolic pathway for tricyclic antidepressants of the secondary amine type. Therefore, as this pathway is under the genetic control of P-450IID6, adverse effects have been observed in case studies with poor metabolisers of debrisoquine treated with TAD [4]. In a pilot study, the (dextromethorphane)-PM phenotype was artificially induced in healthy volunteers after premedication with the strong P-450IID6 inhibitor quinidine. In these conditions, not only was the elimination of trimipramine decreased but the EEG effects produced by the antidepressant were enhanced and prolonged as well (Eap et al., this meeting). On the other hand, several studies with groups of patients have shown that amitriptyline-treated patients lacking active P-450IID6 may have higher steady-state levels of amitriptyline plus nortriptyline than extensive metabolisers, but these levels do not reach those commonly associated with excessive side-effects [5,6].

The N-demethylation of these tertiary amines seems to be at least partially co-regulated by P-450IIC9, and consequently, their metabolism has found to be modified in poor metabolisers of mephenytoin [5,7]. This finding explains the recent gain of interest of this enzyme in psychiatry, in addition to those reports which point to an impaired metabolism of moclobemide (and also of diazepam) [8] in healthy subjects presenting a genetic deficiency of P-450CII9, but not of P-450IID6 [9].

In consequence, the available data reviewed together allow us to conclude that it may be clinically relevant to combine plasma level monitoring of these drugs with pharmacogenetic tests in patients suspected to be non-responders to the treatment.

The present knowledge about the specific mechanisms responsible for the metabolism of these psychotropic drugs helps us to understand some of their pharmacokinetic interactions with other drugs, e.g. thioridazine, which reportedly increases plasma levels of TAD, being itself a substrate [10] and potent inhibitor of cyt P-450IID6. Very recently, many reports have dealt with a metabolic interaction between TAD and the 5-HT uptake inhibitors fluoxetine or fluvoxamine, in that a combined treatment leads to an important increase in the plasma levels of TAD (cf. Vandel et al., Baumann, this volume). It is not known whether these newer antidepressants act specifically on the above-mentioned two enzymes or whether they inhibit rather generally but potently several cytochromes P-450.

Genetic polymorphism in the binding of drugs in plasma to α_1-acid glycoprotein (AAG)

AAG is a plasma protein which may arise several times following various illnesses such as cancer or inflammation. One of its polymorphisms is characterised by genetically determined variants which differ by amino acid substitutions in the peptide chain [11]. In fact, two genes code for two slightly different proteins (22 amino acid substitutions among a total of 181) in a human haploid genome [12].

AAG is the main basic drug binding protein in plasma and it therefore constitutes a factor which influences their pharmacokinetics [13]. Our studies show that various TAD and other drugs, especially methadone, show selectivity in the binding to AAG variants [14]. Using methadone as a model drug, its in vitro binding in plasmas of 45 healthy volunteers was studied while taking into account the role of other plasma constituents [15]. The results confirmed the importance of AAG in the binding of basic drugs, in particular the predominant role for the ORM2 A variant which is associated with the high affinity binding site of methadone and possibly of other drugs. Due to the fact that the ORM2 A variants represent only a fraction of the total AAG concentration, this may explain the decrease in binding observed in plasma when methadone concentrations are in the higher clinical range [15]. It is hypothesized that patients with "silent alleles" of the

ORM2 locus (no ORM2 bands detectable) may have a reduced drug binding capacity. Of possible clinical importance may also be the fact that the percentage of the ORM2 variant is genetically highly variable (17% to 48%) interindividually and even intraindividually in acute phase conditions [16,17].

In conclusion, among the genetic factors contributing to the high interindividual variability in the disposition of psychotropic drugs in the organism, genetic polymorphisms of drug binding and biotransformation have to be considered.

References

1. Baumann P and Eap CB (1989) In: Baumann P, Eap CB, Müller WE and Tillement JP (eds.) α_1-Acid Glycoprotein: Genetics, Biochemistry, Physiological Functions and Pharmacology. A.R. Liss, Inc., New York, pp. 379–397.
2. Eichelbaum M and Gross AS (1991) Pharmacol. Ther. 46: 377–394.
3. Meyer UA (1990) Fundam. Clin. Pharmacol. 4: 595–615.
4. Brosen K, Gram LF (1989) Eur. J. Clin. Pharmacol. 36: 537–547.
5. Baumann P, Jonzier-Perey M, Koeb L, Küpfer A, Tinguely D and Schöpf J (1986) Int. Clin. Psychopharmacol. 1: 102–112.
6. Schnyder C, Baumann P, Jonzier-Perey M, Koeb L and Wertheimer J (1985) Schweiz. Med. Wochenschr.. 115: 1128–1134.
7. Skjelbo E, Brosen K, Hallas J and Gram LF (1991) Clin. Pharmacol. Ther. 49: 1823.
8. Bertilsson L, Henthorn TK,. Sanz E, Tybring G, Säwe J and Villén T (1989) Clin. Pharmacol. Ther. 45: 348–355.
9. Schoerlin MP, Blouin RA, Pfefen JP and Guentert TW (1990) Acta Psychiatr. Scand. (Suppl.) 360: 98–100.
10. Meyer JW, Woggon B, Baumann P and Meyer UA (1990) Eur. J. Clin. Pharmacol. 39: 613–614.
11. Eap CB and Baumann P (1989) In: Baumann P, Eap CB, Müller WE and Tillement JP (eds.) α_1-Acid Glycoprotein: Genetics, Biochemistry, Physiological Functions and Pharmacology. A.R. Liss Inc., New York, pp. 111–125.
12. Dente L, Ciliberto G and Cortese R (1985) Nucleic Acids Res. 13: 3941–3952.
13. Kremer JMH, Wilting J and Janssen LHM (1988) Pharmacol. Rev. 40: 1–47.
14. Eap CB, Cuendet C and Baumann P (1988) Naunyn Schmiedeberg's Arch. Pharmacol. 337: 220–224.
15. Eap CB, Cuendet C and Baumann P (1990) Clin. Pharmacol. Ther. 47: 338–346.
16. van Dijk W, Pos O, van der Sfelt ME et al. (1991) Biochem. J. (in press).
17. Eap CB, Fischer JF and Baumann P (1991) (submitted).

Biological Psychiatry, Volume 1. G. Racagni et al., editors.

Plasma levels of amitriptyline during treatment of depression: Influence of combined treatment with dibenzepine

A. Saria, R. Neumann, C. Humpel, F. Lieder, G. Dosser and H. Oberbauer
Department of Psychiatry, University of Innsbruck Medical School, Anichstr. 35, A-6020 Innsbruck, Austria

Introduction

The tricyclic antidepressants are powerful agents used in monotherapy of major depression. In addition, a combination of antidepressants is occasionally used in practical medicine. At our hospital, monotherapy with tricyclic antidepressants is commonly used although in some cases a combination of dibenzepine (DIB) and amitriptyline (AMI) may be applied. In our laboratory, drug monitoring of antidepressants and antipsychotic agents is routinely performed. As a result, we observed apparent low levels of amitriptyline and nortriptyline (NOR), the major metabolite, when administered together with DIB. Therefore, we investigated plasma levels of DIB, AMI and NOR in a prospective study and compared the therapeutic efficacy of DIB treatment with combined DIB/AMI therapy.

Material and Methods

Patients suffering from major depression according to DSM III criteria were selected from a randomized list to be treated with either 7 mg/kg DIB [1] or 7 mg/kg DIB plus 1.5 mg/kg AMI after a washout period of 3 days. Dibenzepine was administered intravenously daily in the morning for 2 weeks. Thereafter, the same dose was given daily p.o. AMI was administered p.o. daily in the evening. A control group consisting of patients with insomnia or depressive neurosis received 1.5 mg/kg AMI daily p.o. The Hamilton Depression Scale (HAMD) was evaluated on days 0, 7, 14, 21 and 28 after commencement of the study in the two patient groups. Plasma levels of DIB, AMI and NOR were determined in the morning and in the evening before administration of the next dose of the respective drug in heparinized plasma by reversed phase high performance liquid chromatography with ultraviolet detection at 254 nm.

Results

The results are summarized in Table 1. HAMD scores were not significantly different in both patient groups before the therapy on day 0. The HAMD score gradually decreased during the 4-week observation period to a value which was not significantly different in both groups. However, the HAMD scores determined on days 7, 14 and 21 were significantly lower in the DIB group compared to the patient group receiving DIB and AMI. The plasma level determinations were

Table 1. Plasma concentrations of antidepressants and HAMD score. Plasma levels of AMI, NOR and DIB (ng/ml plasma) in the morning (m) and in the evening (e) at certain days during treatment and the corresponding HAMD scores

Day	Amitriptyline	Nortriptyline	Dibenzepine	HAMD
Patient group receiving DIB alone:				
0/m	–	–	–	29.0 ± 1.5
7/m	–	–	140 ± 46	19.0 ± 2.5[a]
14/m	–	–	153 ± 51	14.0 ± 2.6[a]
21/m	–	–	199 ± 58	10.0 ± 2.3[a]
28/m	–	–	264 ± 73	11.0 ± 2.6
0/e	–	–	–	–
7/e	–	–	458 ± 105	–
14/e	–	–	608 ± 178	–
21/e	–	–	467 ± 95	–
28/e	–	–	480 ± 89	–
Patient group receiving DIB and AMI:				
0/m	–	–	–	33.0 ± 2.0
7/m	37 ± 11	21 ± 7	193 ± 56	28.5 ± 2.4
14/m	26 ± 8	12 ± 2	58 ± 20	24.2 ± 2.9
21/m	16 ± 5	7 ± 5	93 ± 39	19.4 ± 2.7
28/m	11 ± 3	14 ± 6	152 ± 62	15.3 ± 1.4
0/e	–	–	–	–
7/e	15 ± 4	28 ± 15	318 ± 60	–
14/e	18 ± 8	19 ± 8	270 ± 65	–
21/e	15 ± 5	34 ± 17	352 ± 82	–
28/e	20 ± 9	9 ± 4	247 ± 97	–
AMI control group:				
0/m	–	–	–	–
7/m	59 ± 10	47 ± 18	–	–
14/m	58 ± 15	49 ± 20	–	–
21/m	54 ± 18[a]	77 ± 43[a]	–	–
28/m	–	–	–	–
0/e	–	–	–	–
7/e	30 ± 10	49 ± 19	–	–
14/e	30 ± 7	40 ± 20	–	–
21/e	50 ± 25[a]	83 ± 48[a]	–	–
28/e	–	–	–	–

[a]$P < 0.05$ vs. corresponding data in group 2 (DIB plus AMI treatment). Values are means ± S.E.M., n = 4–12, since not all parameters could be determined in several patients.

scheduled to represent steady state levels. Since in this case, the determinations took place before the next administration of a particular substance and the time difference between the administration of DIB and AMI was 12 h, we monitored plasma levels every 12 h. The plasma concentrations of DIB were not significantly different in the two patient groups, either in the morning or in the evening, though there was a tendency for DIB levels in the patient group receiving the combination therapy to be lower in the evening compared to the group receiving DIB alone. Interestingly, the levels of AMI and NOR were only about half of those in the control group, reaching statistical significance at day 21. This difference was evident 12 h as well as 24 h after administration of a particular dose of AMI.

Summary

The plasma levels of AMI and NOR are lower in combination with DIB compared with the same dose of AMI alone, indicating a drug interaction which seems to increase drug metabolism. The therapeutic efficacy of AMI in this combination can therefore be questioned. Evaluation of HAMD scores indicate that the combination of DIB plus AMI for treatment of major depression does not have an advantage over monotherapy with DIB, where a therapeutic effect could be observed even earlier.

Reference

1. Christensen H and Felby S (1975) Acta Pharmacol. 37: 393–401.

Biological Psychiatry, Volume 1. G. Racagni et al., editors.

Pharmacokinetics of antidepressants: Fluoxetine and fluvoxamine in daily clinical practice

S. Vandel[1], S. Bouquet[2], B. Bonin[1], G. Bertschy[1] and P. Baumann[3]

[1]Laboratoire de Pharmacologie Clinique et Service de Psychiatrie, Chu Besançon, 25030 Cedex; [2]Laboratoire de Pharmacocinétique, Chu Poitiers, 86021 Cedex, France; and [3]Unité de Psychopharmacologie Clinique, Clinique de Psychiatrie Universitaire, 1008 Prilly, Lausanne, Switzerland

Introduction

During the past 15 years, selective inhibitors of serotonin uptake have been developed for therapeutic purposes, especially fluoxetine and fluvoxamine. Due to a wide prescription, reports of side-effects and interactions appear in the literature.

After a review of their main pharmacokinetic properties, we will present our own results concerning some pharmacokinetic problems.

Pharmacokinetic review

Fluoxetine and fluvoxamine pharmacokinetic data were mainly obtained in healthy volunteers.

Absorption. Following oral administration, fluoxetine and fluvoxamine are well absorbed, peak plasma concentrations: 6 to 8 and 2 to 8 h respectively after ingestion. No important difference between fasted and fed states. Steady state after 2 to 4 weeks for fluoxetine and after about 10 days for fluvoxamine.

Distribution. Apparent volume of distribution : fluoxetine (20 to 42 l/kg), fluvoxamine (5 l/kg). Protein binding: 94% of fluoxetine and 77% of fluvoxamine in plasma are protein bound.

Metabolism. Fluoxetine is demethylated in norfluoxetine, which is a specific serotonin re-uptake inhibitor and may contribute to the clinical activity. Eleven metabolites of fluvoxamine are known, produced mainly by oxidative demethylation. None of them is likely to possess psychotropic activity.

Excretion. About 60% of fluoxetine and 94% of fluvoxamine were recovered in urine. Mean elimination half-life ($t_{1/2}$) of the terminal phase of fluvoxamine excretion: 14.6 h. Fluoxetine elimination half-life: 2 to 7 days after multiple doses, desmethylfluoxetine half-life: 7 days. In rat the apparent elimination $t_{1/2}$ of fluoxetine markedly increased with higher dose, possibly because of transient saturation of fluoxetine metabolism. The possibility of dose-dependent kinetics in man must be considered. The available data today suggest that there is no effect of age on the pharmacokinetics of these 2 drugs. No abnormality in fluoxetine elimination or binding has been noted in the presence of renal dysfunction, but in alcoholic cirrhosis, its elimination is significantly reduced. Schenker suggests a 50% reduction of the dose in these patients.

Tricyclic/fluoxetine or fluvoxamine interaction

We would like to present data concerning tricyclic antidepressant (TCA) interaction with fluoxetine or fluvoxamine. Recently we published a report on 3 cases of fluvoxamine/TCA interaction of the same type that prompted us to seek additional cases and to compare the importance of the TCA interaction obtained with fluoxetine or fluvoxamine.

Figure 1 shows the fluvoxamine/TCA interaction. The TCA plasma levels were obtained before and after the fluvoxamine association (100 to 300 mg/day). In all the cases the TCA dose and other drug associations remained unchanged. There was an increase in the metabolic ratios (MR) after fluvoxamine addition, due to the important increase in the tertiary amine and the decrease in the secondary amine plasma levels.

Figure 2 shows the fluoxetine/TCA interaction. The TCA plasma levels were obtained before and after the fluoxetine addition (20 to 40 mg/day). The amitriptyline (AMT)/fluoxetine interaction seems to be absent or insignificant in comparison with that of clomipramine (CL) and imipramine (IMI). The variation in

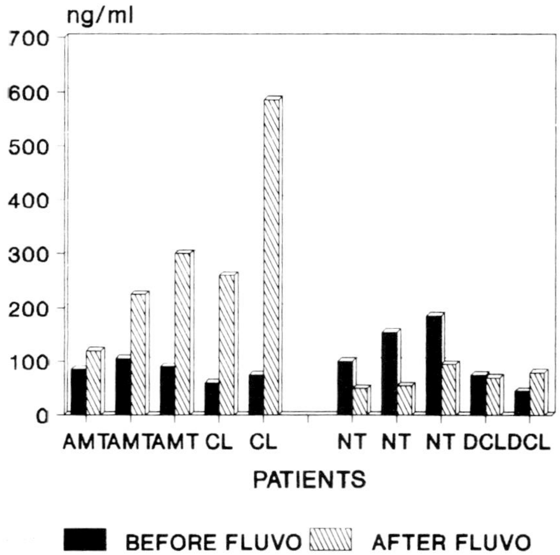

Fig. 1. Fluvoxamine/TCA interaction; TCA plasma levels.

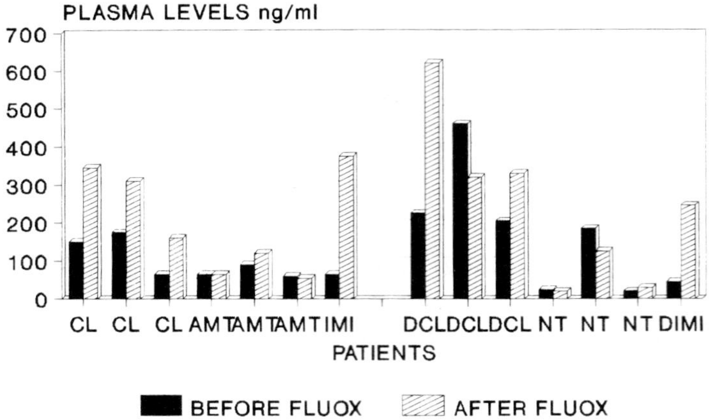

Fig. 2. Fluoxetine/TCA interaction.

the metabolic ratios after the association is not always in the same direction and of lesser importance in comparison with fluvoxamine.

In three patients it was possible to compare the fluoxetine and fluvoxamine/TCA interaction. The results are shown in Fig. 3. The treatment for the first patient was: firstly, CL alone (150 mg/day), secondly, CL (75 mg/day) with fluvoxamine (150 mg/day), and finally, CL (75 mg/day) with fluoxetine (20 mg/day). The second patient received firstly, AMT alone (125 mg/day), with secondly, fluvoxamine

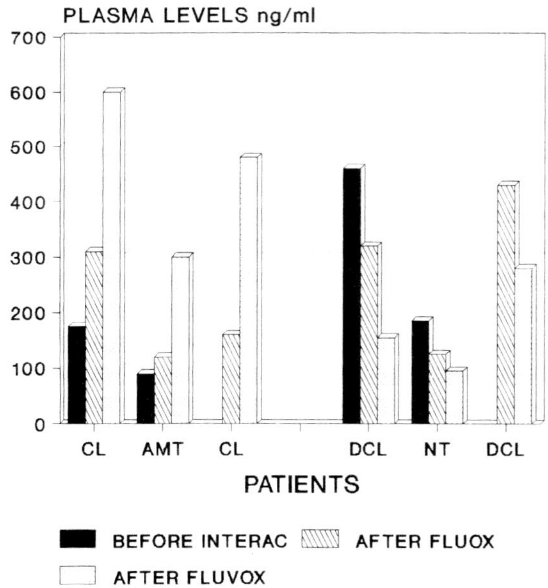

Fig. 3. Comparison between TCA/fluoxetine or fluovoxamine interaction.

(300 mg/day), and finally, fluoxetine (20 mg/day). The third patient received 150 mg/day of CL on two occasions: the first time with fluvoxamine (50 mg/day) and the second time with 10 mg/day of fluoxetine. In the three cases the interaction is quantitatively more important with fluvoxamine than with fluoxetine.

Discussion

Our experience confirms that the fluvoxamine/TCA interaction is quantitatively more important than that of fluoxetine, and that it is, in addition, more constant. The metabolic interaction seems to be particularly at the demethylation level with fluvoxamine, and inhibition of hepatic hydroxylation and demethylation may be involved with fluoxetine. Confirmation of this hypothesis could be given using dextromethorphan and mephenytoin phenotyping in treated patients, before and after the drug association.

Another problem is the length of the fluoxetine interaction, after discontinuation of this drug due to the prolonged half-life of fluoxetine and its metabolite.

The clinical implications of these pharmacokinetic drug-drug interactions may be important in increasing TCA toxicity risk. Plasma level monitoring could be of interest in this regard.

Biological Psychiatry, Volume 1. G. Racagni et al., editors.

Pharmacokinetics of reversible MAO-A inhibitors (RIMA)

G. Laux[1], M.P. Schoerlin[2], W. Classen[1], T. Becker[1], K.P. Lesch[1] and G. Carl[1]
[1]*Department of Psychiatry, University of Wuerzburg, Fuechsleinstr. 15, 8700 Wuerzburg, Germany; and* [2]*Department of Clinical Pharmacology, F. Hoffmann-La Roche Ltd, 4002 Basel, Switzerland*

Introduction

Knowledge of the pharmacokinetic properties of the new reversible inhibitors of MAO-A (RIMA) gives the dose recommendations a rationally justifiable foundation. The present review thus aims to give a pharmacokinetic evaluation of reversible MAO-A inhibitors already being registered or in pre-registration phase at present.

Pharmacokinetic properties of various reversible MAO-A inhibitors

In contrast to the irreversible MAOIs, RIMAs show different pharmacokinetic properties especially regarding elimination half-lives and plasma protein binding (Table 1) [1-5].

Plasma concentration/time profiles of five RIMAs presented in Fig. 1 reveal considerable differences regarding absorption (t_{max}) and elimination ($t_{1/2}$) the latter varying from a few hours (moclobemide, toloxatone) to more than 10 h (brofaromine, cimoxatone) [5].

Table 1. Pharmacokinetic parameters of reversible inhibitors of MAO-A (RIMA)

Drug	Absorption				Elimination	
	F	t_{max} (h)	f_b (%)	$t_{1/2}$ (h)	Cl (l/h/kg)	fe
Moclobemide	0.5–0.8	0.5–2.0	50	1.0– 3.0	0.2 –1.0	<0.01
Toloxatone	0.5–0.6	0.5–1.0	50	0.9– 2.5	0.46 –0.86	<0.01
Brofaromine		1.8–4.0	98	12.0–15.0	0.26 –0.29	<0.01
Climoxatone		1.0–5.0	95	8.9–16.0	0.023–0.045	n.d.
Amiflamine		2.0	23	4.9–12.0	0.42 –0.83	0.002

t_{max}: Time of maximum concentration; F: Bioavailability; f_b: Fractions of the substance bound in plasma; fe: Renally-excreted dose fraction (unchanged substance); Cl: Clearance; n.d.: Not detectable; $t_{1/2}$: Elimination half-life.

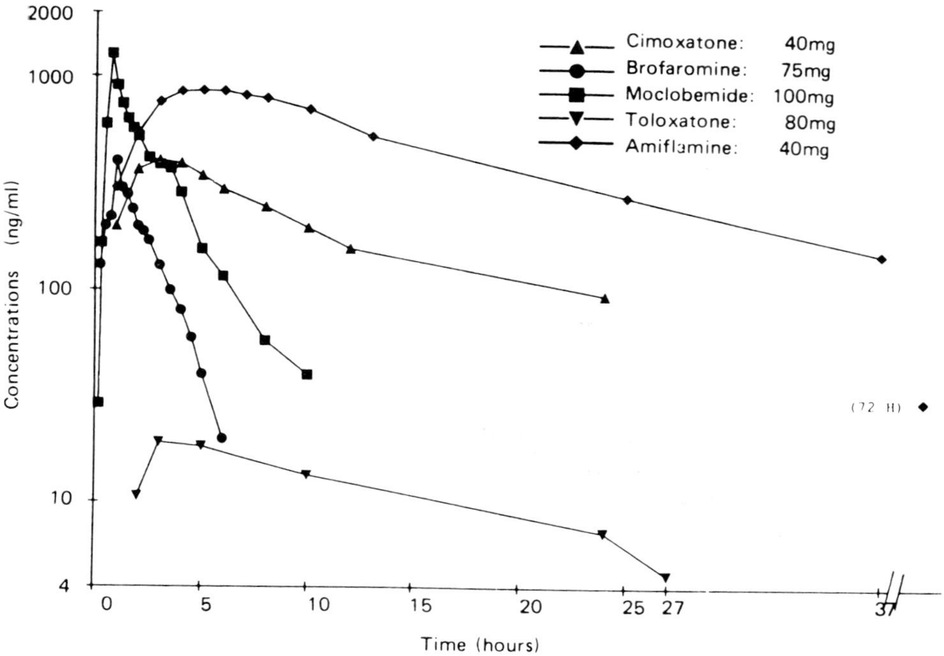

Fig. 1.

Own results

Twenty severely depressed inpatients suffering from predominantly endogenous depressions have been treated with 100 mg moclobemide 3 times daily after an initial wash-out period within the scope of a double-blind study [6]. Considerable variations in plasma concentrations of moclobemide, its active and main metabolite could be measured (Table 2).

Under long-term outpatient conditions moclobemide plasma levels tended to be

Table 2. Plasma levels of moclobemide, its active and main metabolite under moclobemide treatment; (average dosage 287 mg on day 14, 327 mg on day 28)

	Moclobemide (ng/ml)	Active metabolite (ng/ml)	Main metabolite (ng/ml)
x̄ Day 14[a] (n = 13)	226.2 (198.2)	80.4 (55.7)	164.5 (117.6)
x̄ Day 28[a] (n = 12)	272.4 (392.1)	74.5 (27.2)	159.5 (90.6)

[a]Plasma sampling 3 h after morning dose; ( ) = S.D.

Table 3. Plasma levels of moclobemide, its active and main metabolite under long-term treatment; (2–17 months average dosage 309.2 mg/d)

	Moclobemide (ng/ml)	Active metabolite N-oxide (ng/ml)	Main metabolite lactam (ng/ml)
1.5–2.5 h after last dose (n = 7)	1097.0 (808.0)	308.0 (282.1)	565.4 (283.4)
3–5 h after last dose (n = 8)	591.0 (402.9)	236.7 (125.5)	474.9 (172.7)
12–16 h after last dose (n = 5)	183.3 (178.8)	99.4 (71.4)	254.1 (197.4)

( ) = S.D.

higher; 12–16 h after last dose, distinct decline of moclobemide plasma concentrations could be detected (Table 3) [7].

Possible clinical implications of pharmacokinetic properties including risk populations (old age, reduced kidney and/or liver function, [8]) indicated.

References

1. Amrein R, Allen SR and Guentert TW et al. (1989) Br. J. Psychiatry 155 (Suppl. 6): 66–71.
2. Hengen N, Jedrychowski M and Hoffmann E (1984) In: Tipton KF, Dostert P and Benedetti MS (eds.) Monoamine Oxidase and Disease. Academic Press, London, pp. 185–191.
3. Strolin-Benedetti M, Rovei V, Dencker SJ et al. (1982) Arzneim. Forsch. Drug Res. 32: 276–280.
4. Antonin KH, Jedrychowski M and Bieck PR (1990) Muench. Med. Wochenschr. 132 (Suppl. 1): S13–S17. 5. Schoerlin MP, Guentert TW (1990) Psychiatr. Prax. 17: 8–16.
6. Laux G, Beckmann H, Classen W and Becker T (1989) J. Neural Transm. (Suppl.) 28: 45–52.
7. Carl G, Laux G (1990) Psychiatr. Prax. 17: 26–29.
8. Stoeckel K, Pfefen JP, Mayersohn M et al. (1990) Acta Psychiatr. Scand. 82 (Suppl. 360): 94–97.

Biological Psychiatry, Volume 1. G. Racagni et al., editors.

Clinical utility of antidepressants' plasma level assessment: Methodical aspects

Bruno Müller-Oerlinghausen

Laboratory of Clinical Psychopharmacology, Department of Psychiatry, Free University of Berlin, Eschenallee 3, D-1000 Berlin 19, Germany

Everyday therapeutic practice in psychiatry does not generally seem to be guided by sound clinical-pharmacological principles. Cases of fatalities related to inadvertent overdosing of psychiatric patients and which have sometimes resulted in malpractice suits illustrate this situation.

This often struck me when I had to certify in court that many doctors use psychotropic drugs as some kind of "unidirectional" tool without having the slightest idea of their pharmacokinetic properties. Negative attitudes towards the clinical significance of individual pharmacokinetic data prevail among clinicians. In my view, clinical indications for therapeutic monitoring (TDM) of antidepressants do exist, and can be summarized as follows:

- adverse drug reactions;
- fatalities;
- non-response;
- compliance problems;
- patients at special risk;
- co-medication (e.g. neuroleptics);
- long-term medication.

In the following, I will discuss the necessary criteria to be fulfilled in order to draw useful information from TDM. Certainly, this starts with a meaningful clinical question. In this context, I should mention the findings of a recent study by one of the speakers in the symposium, Dr. P. Baumann. He and his co-workers scrutinized the quality of requests for antidepressant monitoring in their hospital. The average rate of inappropriate requests varied between 41 and 26% [1].

The appropriateness of a request does not only depend on a clear notion, why monitoring is to be done now in this individual patient, but also requires the transfer of necessary information about the patient to the laboratory, or to the person in charge of interpreting the data delivered by the analytical machinery. Information is required on the following items:

- total duration of AD treatment;
- time of last dose change;
- time of ingestion of last tablet;
- co-medication;
- patient's age, body weight;
- exact blood sampling time.

As I just learnt during a national consensus conference on TDM of antidepressants, the often malfunctioning communication between the clinic and the laboratory appears to be one of the most frequent causes of learned helplessness symptoms or even paranoid behaviour among persons in charge of the analytical procedures.

There are also, of course, requirements concerning the quality of the laboratory: quantitative, substance-related methods rather than immunological or radio receptor methods should be used, allowing the separation of parent drug and metabolites. External quality control (legally required in many countries) should be supplemented by regular internal controls, possibly comparing findings obtained by different methods in the same laboratory. One person in the hospital, preferably a clinical pharmacologist rather than a clinical chemist, should be assigned to comment on the daily data on the basis of sufficient information provided by the physicians in charge of the patient.

Problems in interpreting TDM data have been indicated in several good reviews in the past [2]. Apart from the many apparent controversies about the relationship of blood level and clinical outcome, which can partly be explained by insufficient methodology, and the potential relationship of blood levels to toxicity, where only a few studies are available, the clinical significance of metabolites, the existence of non-linear kinetics in some patients, and the potential significance of drug binding to albumin and α_1-acid glyco-like protein dominate the discussion. Regarding protein binding, the recent consensus conference in Germany on TDM of antidepressants has decided that routine assessment of the protein binding is not meaningful, since appropriate reference data are not available.

Also some understanding of the many technical problems and pitfalls of antidepressant blood level assessments will be helpful for more valid data interpretation. Some frequently discussed problem areas are for example:

- should plasma or serum be used? (how to handle extremely lipaemic sera);
- what are the most appropriate extraction procedures? (very important);
- what is the optimal matrix for spiked calibrators? (e.g., human or bovine material?);
- how to handle samples from patients with a lot of co-medication?;
- how to speed up the turnaround time for results? (very important);
- how to perform the assessment in an economical way? [3].

Let me add some items of information which doctors in hospitals or private practice should be free to ask of laboratories selling their service to psychiatrists:

- preferable matrix, optimal transportation?
- method? (specificity – sensitivity – inter-/intra-assay variance)
- simultaneous determination of metabolites?
- range of linearity?
- quality control?

To conclude, I would like to contribute my personal view on the question, whether in fact more frequent TDM of antidepressants will improve the general quality of our drug treatment. My answer would be "Yes", but only if at the same time we improve the knowledge of our medical students and colleagues in general clinical pharmacology – and this may take a while.

References

1. Vuille F, Amey M and Baumann P (1991) Pharmacopsychiatry (in press).
2. APA Task Force on the Use of Laboratory Tests in Psychiatry (1985) Am. J. Psychiatry 142: 155–162.
3. Müller J, Hertrampf R and Müller-Oerlinghausen B (1985) Pharmacopsychiatry 18: 48–49.

Biological Psychiatry, Volume 1. G. Racagni et al., editors.

Direct and indirect actions of monoamine oxidase

Keith F. Tipton, John M. McCrodden and Eimear M. O'Brien
Department of Biochemistry, Trinity College, Dublin 2, Ireland

Introduction

The role of the monoamine oxidases in terminating the actions of the amine neurotransmitters and dietary amines has been extensively reviewed in the past [1]. Less attention has been paid to the potential toxicity of the products formed; hydrogen peroxide, an aldehyde and ammonia. The more recent discoveries that the B-form of the enzyme may also play a role in the toxification of compounds such as I-methyl-4-phenyl-1, 2, 3, 6-tetrahydropyridine (MPTP) [2,3] and, perhaps in the activation of the anticonvulsant pro-drug 2-n-pentylaminoacetamide (milacemide) [4] suggests that the functions of MAO may be broader than was thought.

Specificities

Although earlier studies indicated the specificity of MAO to be restricted to primary amines and secondary amines bearing a small substituent on the nitrogen, the enzyme has, more recently, been found to be active towards a wider range of amine derivatives, including appropriately-substituted secondary and tertiary amines. It also appears that the enzyme is sensitive to mechanism-based inhibition by a number of its substrates. Time-dependent inhibition of MAO-B has been observed with milacemide [4], MPTP [5], high concentrations of 2-phenylethylamine [6] and some long-chain aliphatic amines. MAO-A appears to be less susceptible to substrate inhibition of this type. Some newer data on inhibition by such substrates will be presented. The possible significance of this phenomenon in vivo has yet to be assessed.

It has been proposed that the action of MAO-B initiates the anticonvulsant actions of milacemide by oxidative cleavage to form glycinamide, which is subsequently hydrolysed in the brain to form glycine [4]. However, we have recently found an analogue of this compound, α-methylmilacemide:

$$CH_3(CH_2)_3CH_2NHCH_2CONH_2$$

Milacemide

$$CH_3(CH_2)_3\underset{}{\overset{\displaystyle CH_3}{\overset{|}{C}}}HNHCH_2CONH_2$$

α-methylmilacemide

to be an anticonvulsant although, in common with other α-methyl-substituted amines [7], it is not a substrate for MAO-B [8]. Furthermore, unlike milacemide itself, its administration does not result in any significant glycinamide formation in the mouse [8]. Although the similarity between the anticonvulsant valproate and α-methylmilacemide might be interpreted as indicating that the latter compound might act in a different way from milacemide, the most parsimonious explanation of the results is that the action of MAO-B is to terminate, rather than to initiate the neurotoxic actions of milacemide.

Although it has been suggested that this broader specificity may be a peculiar property of MAO-B, the A-form of the enzyme also shows activity towards several such substrates, including MPTP. There may, however, be considerable species differences in the interactions of such compounds with MAO.

Products

The products formed in the MAO-catalysed reaction are all potentially toxic. The hydrogen peroxide may act as a source of reactive oxygen radicals and it can also act as a substrate for potentially damaging reactions involving peroxidase, which themselves involve radical intermediates [9]. Aldehydes may react to form condensation products with proteins [10] and other cellular components and subsequent reactions of such adducts may generate compounds with distinct pharmacological activities [11]. The toxicity of ammonia is well known, but rather little is known about its specific effects in the brain. Similarly, the extent to which the inhibition of the production of such toxic metabolites may be involved in the protective actions claimed for the selective MAO-B inhibitor (–)-deprenyl(selegiline) remains to be evaluated.

References

1. Tipton KF (1975) American Physiological Society Handbook of Physiology (6), pp. 667–691.
2. Kinemuchi H, Fowler CJ and Tipton KF (1987) Neurochem. Int. 11: 359–373.
3. Singer TP, Castagnoli N, Ramsay RR and Trevor AJ (1987) J. Neurochem. 49: 1–8.
4. Janssens de Varebeke P, Pauwels G, Buyse C, David-Remacle M, De Mey J, Roba J and Youdim MBH (1989) J. Neurochem. 53: 1109–1116.
5. Tipton KF, McCrodden JM and Youdim MBH (1986) Biochem. J. 240: 279–285.
6. Kinemuchi H, Arai Y, Oreland L, Tipton KF and Fowler CJ. Biochem. Pharmacol. 31: 959–964.
7. Mantle TJ, Tipton KF and Garrett NJ (1976) Biochem. Pharmacol. 25: 2073–2077.
8. O'Brien EM, Tipton KF, Strolin Benedetti M, Bonsignori A, Marrari P and Dostert P (1991) Biochem. Pharmacol. 41: 1731–1737.
9. Valoti M, Della Corte L, Tipton KF and Sgaragli G (1988) Biochem. J. 250: 501–507.
10. Maunch TJ, Donohue TM, Zetterman RK, Sorrell MF and Tuma DJ (1986) Hepatology 8: 263–269.
11. Tipton KF (1988) Neurochem. Int. 13: 301–305.

Biological Psychiatry, Volume 1. G. Racagni et al., editors.

Comparison between the pharmacology of reversible and irreversible inhibitors of MAO-A

John P.M. Finberg

Rappaport Institute and Faculty of Medicine, Technion – Israel Institute of Technology, POB 9697, Haifa, Israel

Introduction

The major clinical indications for the use of MAO inhibitors are for the treatment of affective disorders and Parkinson's disease. In the case of affective disorders, selective inhibition of MAO-A rather than MAO-B has been associated with therapeutic effectiveness [1]. In Parkinson's disease, only (–)-deprenyl has so far been used therapeutically [2] and non-selective or MAO-A selective inhibitors would cause dangerous potentiation of the cardiovascular side-effects of L-DOPA.

The introduction of reversible inhibitors of MAO has been the major advance in the pharmacology of this class of drugs in recent years, in an attempt to produce MAO inhibitors devoid of "cheese effect". The rationale for use of these drugs can be stated as follows:

1. Since tyramine concentrations will be highest in the lumen of the GI tract, some tyramine will still be metabolised during absorption across the intestine, because of competitive displacement of the inhibitor.
2. Following build-up of tyramine within the sympathetic nerve, some tyramine will be metabolised by intraneuronal MAO-A.
3. If a tyramine reaction does occur, it will be limited in time, since the enzyme itself is not permanently inactivated, as in the case of irreversible inhibitors.

Although reversibility of action may be advantageous from the point of view of limiting a tyramine reaction, it may be disadvantageous if inhibition of neurotransmitter metabolism does not develop to a sufficiently high degree. It is therefore of particular interest to study the effect of reversible inhibitors of MAO-A on both tyramine-induced responses and on neurotransmitter release.

Potentiation of tyramine pressor responses in the rat

The effect of treatment with reversible or irreversible MAO-A inhibitors on tyramine-induced pressor responses in the rat was studied by prior implantation of arterial catheters, and subsequent blood pressure recording in the conscious unrestrained animal. Tyramine was administered either intravenously (i.v.) [3] or orally [4]. Pressor responses to tyramine given i.v. were potentiated by the reversible MAO-A inhibitors moclobemide, amiflamine, cimoxotone and CGP-11305A (all given intra-peritoneally), albeit to a lesser degree than clorgyline. When the oral route of tyramine administration was used, virtually no potentiation of the pressor effect could be detected following moclobemide, at a dose of 30 mg/kg p.o. By contrast, the same dose of moclobemide caused marked potentiation of the pressor effect of i.v. tyramine, to a similar extent to that produced by tranylcypromine [5].

No clear explanation is presently available as to why moclobemide potentiates i.v. but not oral tyramine responses. Following either route of administration, the plasma tyramine concentration would be expected to bear some relationship to the pressor response. Tyramine is extensively metabolised in intestine and liver following oral administration, but that proportion of an oral dose which enters the blood circulation should act on the sympathetic nerve ending in a similar way to that fraction injected directly into the venous system. One possibility may be that the metabolites of tyramine formed following extensive hepatic metabolism may exert their own moderation of the pressor effect. Another explanation relates to the more rapid tyramine uptake following i.v. as opposed to oral administration [5].

The mechanism of tyramine's pressor response is mediated by its ability to release noradrenaline from the sympathetic nerve ending, which is then available for interaction with post-synaptic α- and β-adrenoceptors. Possible sites of action for interference with tyramine's pressor effect therefore include antagonism of a) neuronal membrane uptake; b) vesicular release; and c) post-synaptic adrenoceptors. Pharmacological investigation of moclobemide using in vitro techniques is limited by its metabolism to active compounds. Ability of the compound to antagonise α-adrenoceptors was investigated in conscious rats, by examining antagonism of pressor responses to the selective α_1-agonist phenylephrine injected i.v. Pressor response to a submaximal dose of phenylephrine (2 μg/kg) was unchanged (102 ± 12% control) after moclobemide (10 mg/kg p.o.). Lack of tyramine pressor potentiation, therefore, cannot be explained by an α_1-antagonist effect.

Effects on neuronal monoamine release

Tyramine induces release of noradrenaline by a non-exocytotic process. Neuronal transmission is mediated, however, by exocytotic release. Noradrenaline release was determined in cardiovascular system of pithed rats and in isolated rat vas deferens 2 h after a single dose of clorgyline (2 mg/kg) or 24 h after the last of 21 daily doses of clorgyline (1 mg/kg), which caused the same degree of MAO inhibition. In neither case was there any increase in release following the acute treatment, whereas release increased after the chronic treatment [6,7]. These studies indicate that the vesicular store of noradrenaline may increase in a time dependent fashion with MAO inhibition.

The ability of antidepressant drugs to increase noradrenaline release in the CNS following chronic treatment is reflected by down-regulation of β-adrenoceptors. Such down-regulation also develops after chronic treatment with reversible MAO inhibitors, albeit to a lesser extent than that produced by irreversible inhibitors [8]. This result is therefore in agreement with other studies showing that reversible inhibitors are capable of enhancing synaptic levels of amine neurotransmitters in the CNS.

References

1. Murphy DL, Lipper S, Pickar D, Jimerson D, Cohen PM, Garrick NA, Alterman IS and Campbell IC (1981) In: Youdim MBH and Paykel ES (eds.) Monoamine Oxidase Inhibitors – The State of the Art. Wiley, Chichester, pp. 189–205.
2. Birkmayer W, Riederer P, Youdim MBH and Linauer W (1975) J. Neural Transm. 36: 303.
3. Finberg JPM and Youdim MBH (1988) J. Neural Transm. (Suppl.) 26: 11.
4. Da Prada M, Kettler R, Burkard WP and Haefely WE (1984) In: Tipton KF, Dostert P and Strolin Benedetti M (eds.) Prospects for Therapy with Reversible Inhibitors. Academic Press, London, pp. 137–154.
5. Da Prada M, Zurcher G, Wuthrich I and Haefely WE (1988) J. Neural Transm. (Suppl.) 26: 31.
6. Finberg JPM and Kopin IJ (1985) Naunyn Schmiedeberg's Arch. Pharmacol. 332: 236.
7. Finberg JPM, Ari G, Lavian G and Hovevey-Sion D (1990) J. Neural Transm. 32: 405.
8. Dupont H, Rumigny JF and Strolin Benedetti M (1984) In: Tipton KF, Dostert P and Strolin Benedetti M (eds.) Prospects for Therapy with Reversible Inhibitors. Academic Press, London, pp. 629–630.

Biological Psychiatry, Volume 1. G. Racagni et al., editors.

Neurotransmitter turnover in neurodegenerative disorders of the CNS

Peter Riederer[1], Wieland Gsell[1], Christine Konradi[1], Ludwig Käsbauer[1], Emin Sofic[1], Gunther Moll[1], Gert Hebenstreit[2] and Kurt Jellinger[3]

[1]Clinical Neurochemistry, Department of Psychiatry, University of Würzburg, Füchsleinstraße 15, D-8700 Würzburg, Germany; [2]Niederösterreichisches Landeskrankenhaus, Mauer; and [3]LBI-Clinical Neurobiology, Lainz-Hospital, Vienna, Austria

Neuropathology

Parkinson's disease (PD) and Alzheimer's disease (AD)/senile dementia of the Alzheimer type (SDAT) are neuropathologically characterized each by a clear rank order of neuronal degeneration. While in PD substantia nigra (SN) is severely damaged (about 80% neuronal cell loss as compared to age-matched controls [1–3]), nucleus basalis of Meynert (NBM) is the most prominent area affected by degeneration in AD (about 70% neuronal cell loss as compared to age-matched controls [4–6]) and SDAT (about 60% neuronal cell loss as compared to age-matched controls [4–8]). Locus coeruleus (LC) and dorsal raphe nucleus (DRN) are both moderately degenerated in both diseases (58 to 83% neuronal loss as compared to age-matched controls [1,9–14]). Weak neuronal degeneration is observed in NBM of patients with PD (about 38% neuronal loss as compared to age-matched controls [15–17]) and in SN of patients with AD/SDAT [12,18–20], although unpublished investigations of our group reveal that it can reach up to 50% of the neurons within the latter area or up to 55% of dopaminergic neurons from ventral tegmental area (VTA) in AD [21].

Neurochemistry

Dopaminergic system

About the same picture is seen when looking at neurotransmitter systems arising from these areas. As a consequence of prominent neuronal loss in SN of patients with PD dopamine (DA) levels in basal ganglia in PD decline [22]. But as long as about 30% of DAergic neurons survive, DA loss is functionally compensated by an increase in DA turnover, as it is approximately expressed by an increase in homovanillic acid (HVA)/DA-ratio [23]. In cortical regions slightly reduced concentrations of DA have been found [24], while the limbic system seems to be unaffected [25,26]. In contrast, no significant changes in DA concentrations have been found in basal ganglia, cortical regions and limbic systems of brains from patients with AD/SDAT [24], which coincides with the moderate cell loss in VTA and SN. HVA levels in AD/SDAT do not alter in basal ganglia, while they decrease significantly in limbic and cortical areas [24].

Noradrenergic system

Results in noradrenaline (NA) levels in AD/SDAT brains equal those found for DA. The slight decrease of NA levels in basal ganglia, limbic system and cortical areas, which in most areas is not significant, resembles those of the moderate degeneration of LC [24]. In contrast, a significant loss in NA concentrations is observed within the 3 areas in brains from patients with PD [24] and parallels the degeneration of the LC in PD. The NA metabolite 3-methoxy-4-hydroxyphenylglycol (MHPG) is decreased significantly inasmuch as NA in PD [27], indicating no enhanced NA metabolism as compared to DA in PD.

Serotoninergic system

The moderate loss of neurons in DRN is reflected by little changes in serotonin (5-HT) content in limbic system and basal ganglia in SDAT, while in cortical regions it reaches 70% for 5-HT and 50% for its metabolite 5-hydroxyindoleacetic acid (5-HIAA) [24]. In PD a significant loss of 5-HT is found in many regions [23] and 5-HIAA levels are reduced in cortical areas [24].

Neurobiochemistry

Biogenic amines are deactivated and metabolized by monoamine oxidases (MAO-A and B type), catecholamine-O-methyltransferase (COMT), aldehyde dehydrogenase (ALD-DH), DA additionally by dopamine-β-hydroxylase (DβH) and NA additionally by phenylethanolamine-N-methyltransferase (PNMT) [28]. Interaction between enzymes and regulation by intermediate levels regulates the overall metabolization. In PD, MAO and COMT are mostly unchanged (a possible exception being SN with an increase in MAO-B activity of up to 125% of controls) in advanced stages when compared to normal aging [29]. A significant increase (127% of age-matched controls) in ALD-DH activity was found in the putamen of patients with PD, when stimulated with indole acetaldehyde. It is uncertain whether this may account in part for the increased DA turnover, because short-chain aldehydes fail to stimulate ALD-DH of patients with PD. Increased ALD-DH activity is also observed in putamen of patients with SDAT (130% of age-matched controls) and reaches about the level of increase in putamen of younger alcoholics (146%). Additionally to the increase of ALD-DH, MAO activity increases in a number of brain regions in AD/SDAT [30,31], although an increased neurotransmitter turnover as judged by HVA/DA-ratios in degenerating dopaminergic neurons in PD has not been observed either in the dopaminergic or in the serotoninergic system in AD/SDAT.

References

1. Mann DMA and Yates PO (1983) Neuropathol. Appl. Neurobiol. 9: 3–19.
2. Gibb WRG and Lees AJ (1987) Acta Neuropathol. 73: 195–201.
3. Hirsch E, Graybiel AM and Agid YA (1988) Nature 334: 345–348.
4. Etienne P, Robitaille Y, Wood P, Gauthier S, Nair NPV and Quirion R (1986) Neuroscience 19: 1279–1291.
5. Ichimiya A, Arai H, Kosaka K and Iizuka R (1986) Acta Neuropathol. 70: 112–116.
6. Jellinger K (1986b) Adv. Neurol. 45: 1–18.
7. Mann DMA, Yates PO and Marcyniuk B (1985) Neurosci. Lett. 56: 51–55.
8. Jellinger K (1987c) Neurobiol. Aging 8: 556–561.
9. Tomlinson BE, Irving D and Blessed G (1981) J. Neurol. Sci. 49: 419–428.
10. Bondareff N, Mountjoy CQ and Roth M (1982) Neurology 32: 165–168.
11. Tomonaga M (1983) J. Neurol. 230: 231–240.
12. Mann DMA, Yates PO and Hawkes J (1983) Clin. Neuropathol. 2: 1–7.
13. Jellinger K (1987) In: Marsden CD and Fahn S (eds.) Movement Disorders. Butterworth, London, pp. 124–165.
14. Ingram VM, Koenig JH, Miller CH, Moore HE, Blanchard B and Perry DE (1987) In: Wurtman RJ, Corkin SH and Growden JH (eds.) Alzheimer's Disease: Advances in Basic Research and Therapy. Cambridge, pp. 435–440.
15. Gaspar P and Grey F (1984) Acta Neuropathol. 64: 43–52.
16. Whitehouse PJ, Hendreen JC, White CL and Price DL (1983) Ann. Neurol. 13: 243–248.
17. Jellinger K (1986) In: Fahn S, Marsden CD, Jenner P and Teychenne R (eds.) Recent Developments in Parkinsonism. Raven Press, New York, pp. 33–66.
18. Jellinger K (1987) J. Neural Transm. 24 (Suppl.): 109–129.
19. Mann DMA, Tucken CM and Yates PO (1987) Neuropathol. Appl. Neurobiol. 13: 123–139.
20. Gibb WRG (1988) In: Jankovic J and Tolowa E (eds.) Parkinson's Disease and Movement Disorders. Urban and Schwarzenberg, Baltimore, pp. 205–223.
21. Uhl GR, Hedreen JC and Price DL (1985) Neurology 35: 1215–1218.
22. Ehringer H and Hornykiewicz O (1960) Klin. Wochenschr. 38: 1236–1239.
23. Bernheimer H, Birkmayer W, Hornykiewicz O, Jellinger K and Seitelberger F (1973) J. Neurosci. 20: 415–455.
24. Riederer P, Sofic E, Moll G, Freyberger A, Wichart I, Gsell W, Jellinger K, Hebenstreit G and Youdim MBH (1990) In: Dostert P, Riederer P, Strolin Benedetti M and Roncucci R (eds.) Early Markers in Parkinson's and Alzheimer's Diseases. Springer-Verlag, New York, pp. 221–232.
25. Birkmayer W and Riederer P (1975) J. Neural Transm. 37: 175–182.
26. Scatton B, Javoy-Agid F, Rouqier L, Dubois B and Agid Y (1984) In: Usdin E, Carlsson A, Dahlström A and Engel J (eds.) Catecholamines: Neuropharmacology and Central Nervous System – Therapeutic Aspects. A.R. Liss, New York, pp. 43–52.
27. Riederer P, Birkmayer W, Seemann D and Wuketich S (1977) J. Neural Transm. 41: 241–251.
28. Birkmayer W and Riederer P (1989) Understanding the Neurotransmitters: Key to the Workings of the Brain. Springer-Verlag, Vienna.
29. Birkmayer W and Riederer P (1985) Die Parkinson-Krankheit. Springer-Verlag, Vienna.
30. Danielczyk W, Streifler M, Konradi C, Riederer P and Moll G (1988) Acta Psychiatr. Scand. 78: 730–736.
31. Adolfsson R, Gottfries CG, Oreland L, Wiberg A and Winblad B (1980) Life Sci. 27: 1029–1034.

Biological Psychiatry, Volume 1. G. Racagni et al., editors.

Effects of MAO inhibition on age-induced changes in tissue amino acid levels in mice and rats

Margherita Strolin Benedetti[1] Pietro Marrari[1], Massimo Cini[1], Mose' Da Prada[2] and Philippe Dostert[1]

[1]Farmitalia Carlo Erba, R&D-Erbamont Group, Via Imbonati 24, 20159 Milan, Italy; and [2]F. Hoffmann-La Roche Ltd., Pharmaceutical Research Department, 4002 Basel, Switzerland

Introduction

Age-related changes in rat brain amino acid concentrations have previously been discussed mainly as a possible consequence of the increase in brain MAO activity with ageing [1]. The effects of lifelong treatment with the selective and short acting MAO-A and -B inhibitors moclobemide and Ro 19-6327, respectively, on amino acid levels in the rat brain have also been studied [2].

The purpose of the present study was to further investigate the effects of lifelong administration of both MAO inhibitors on amino acid levels in mouse brain and rat and mouse heart. In the rat heart, a marked increase (500–600%) in MAO-A concentration [3] and no change in glutamine synthetase activity [4] have been shown to occur with ageing.

Material and Methods

Four groups of female Wistar rats (KFM-HAN) and 4 groups of female C57 B1/6J mice were used. In both rats and mice, group 1 was composed of young animals (2 months), group 2 of 28-month-old animals and groups 3 and 4 of 28-month-old animals having received moclobemide and Ro 19-6327 in the diet for their whole life-span respectively. In rats doses were approximately 13 and 2 mg/kg/day and in mice 48 and 6 mg/kg/day for moclobemide and Ro 19-6327 respectively.

The animals were sacrificed after injection of 3-mercaptopropionic acid, tissues were removed, the different brain areas were dissected and the analysis of amino acids was carried out according to [1]). Inhibition of MAO activity was measured in cerebellum and liver at the end of treatment as previously described [5].

Old control animals and animals treated with moclobemide or with Ro 19-6327 were compared to young control animals using Dunnett's test.

Results and Discussion

Comparison between the young and the old control groups

By contrast with rats, in which the levels of amino acids have been shown to significantly change with ageing in all of the 9 brain structures examined except hypothalamus [1,2], no changes in amino acid concentrations were found in 4 (accumbens, hippocampus, hypothalamus and cerebellum) out of the 7 brain regions of old mice compared to young animals. Whenever significant changes in amino acid concentrations were observed in old mice, they were always a decrease, with the exception of a significant increase of glutamine (Gln) in the cortex and of taurine (Tau) in the pons-medulla (Table 1). In mice brain, no decrease in Tau levels was observed with ageing, in contrast to rats where, however, brain Tau concentrations are lower than in mice [1,2].

No age-related changes in GABA concentrations were found, whereas serine (Ser) and glycine (Gly) concentrations were lower in the cortex of old mice as compared with young animals. A significant decrease in glutamic acid (Glu) and

Table 1. Amino acid levels (μmol/g wet tissue) in brain and heart from young and old mice and rats

Tissue	Group	Asp	Glu	Ser	Gln	Gly	Tau
Mouse striatum	1	3.37	12.25	1.10	6.61	1.30	14.98
	2	2.63[a]	9.62[a]	0.92	8.71	1.03	12.40
	3	2.78	10.45	0.91	7.79	1.03	14.11
	4	2.76	10.04	1.04	7.61	1.09	12.98
Mouse pons-medulla	1a	5.12	8.80	0.41	4.78	4.62	3.94
	2	4.22[b]	7.59[a]	0.37	5.94	4.13	4.82[b]
	3	4.33[a]	7.73	0.36	4.95	4.25	5.02[b]
	4	4.00[b]	7.07[b]	0.38	4.65	3.58	4.63[a]
Mouse cortex	1	4.57	14.26	1.07	6.53	1.27	11.45
	2	4.29	13.00[a]	0.90[b]	8.61[a]	1.09[a]	10.43
	3	4.34	13.40	0.90[b]	7.20	1.06[b]	11.24
	4	4.34	13.31	0.96	7.30	1.07[a]	10.77
Mouse heart	1	1.45	5.71	0.66	5.56	0.57	38.37
	2	1.75	5.52	0.49[b]	6.69[b]	0.47[b]	36.51
	3	1.60	5.39	0.45[b]	6.55[a]	0.42[b]	37.93
	4	1.64	5.00	0.51[a]	6.06	0.47[b]	34.52
Rat heart	1	2.54	5.44	0.60	7.18	0.26	28.11
	2	1.74	4.84	0.32[b]	5.90[a]	0.23[a]	28.01
	3	1.56[a]	4.84	0.29[b]	6.31	0.26	28.32
	4	1.74	4.78	0.33[b]	6.27	0.24	28.25

Data are expressed as means from 8 or 7 (a) animals; [a]$P < 0.05$; [b]$P < 0.01$: Dunnett's test; Groups 1 to 4: see Material and Methods.

aspartic acid (Asp) levels was found in striatum and pons-medulla in old mice, while Glu concentrations were also lower in cortex.

In the heart of both rats and mice, statistically significant decreases in Ser and Gly levels were found with ageing, whereas Tau concentrations remained unchanged. Compared to the brain, Tau concentrations are high in the heart. This might explain why heart Tau levels do not reflect the enhanced formation of H_2O_2, which accompanies the large increase in MAO activity with ageing. The content of Tau in the heart has been shown to remain relatively constant in many pathologic and metabolic states and may be regulated by hormonal factors [6]. Furthermore, since in the rat heart, contrarily to the brain, Tau concentrations are much lower in mitochondria than in cytosol [7], the increased activity of the mitochondrial enzyme MAO might affect heart Tau levels considerably less than brain Tau levels.

Despite the large increase in heart MAO activity with ageing, slightly but significantly lower Gln concentrations were found in the heart of old rats compared to young animals. Detoxication of NH_3 in the heart proceeds mainly through the α-ketoglutarate-glutamate-glutamine pathway, but urea formation is an additional pathway of NH_3 removal, which might be favoured in pathological situations [8]. Gln levels were higher in the heart of old mice compared to young animals, but the influence of age on the activity of MAO and glutamine synthetase has to be determined before suggesting any hypothesis.

Effects of MAO inhibitors

In the cerebellum of mice a higher (187%) MAO-B activity was found in ageing, in keeping with previous results [9]. Inhibition of mice liver and cerebellum MAO-A activity was at least 75% and that of MAO-B activity at least 90% after lifelong administration of moclobemide and Ro 19-6327 respectively, compared to age-matched controls.

Moclobemide restored Asp and Glu concentrations in the striatum, Glu concentrations in pons-medulla and cortex and Gln levels in cortex to values not statistically different from those of young controls (Table 1). The effects of Ro 19-6327 were rather similar.

Moclobemide and Ro 19-6327 brought Gln and Gly, but not Ser, concentrations in rat heart back to the same values as in young rats. In mice heart, the only significant effect on age-induced amino acid modifications was that caused by Ro 19-6327 on Gln levels.

References

1. Strolin Benedetti M, Cini M, Fusi R, Marrari P and Dostert P (1990) J. Neural Transm. 29: 259–268.

2. Strolin Benedetti M, Kettler R, Marrari P, Cini M, Da Prada M and Dostert P (1990) J. Neural Transm. 2: 239–248.
3. Cao Danh H, Strolin Benedetti M and Dostert P (1984) In: Tipton KF, Dostert P and Strolin Benedetti M (eds.) Monoamine Oxidase and Disease. Prospects for Therapy with Reversible Inhibitors. Academic Press, London, pp. 301–317.
4. Cao Danh H, Strolin Benedetti M and Dostert P (1985) Gerontology 31: 95–100.
5. Da Prada M, Kettler R, Keller HH, Burkhard WP, Muggli-Maniglio D and Haefely WE (1989) J. Pharmacol. Exp. Ther. 248: 400–414.
6. Reibel DK, Shaffer JE, Kocsis JJ and Neely JR (1979) J. Mol. Cell. Cardiol. 11: 827–830.
7. Macaione S, Tucci G and Di Giorgio RM (1975) Ital. J. Biochem. 24: 162–174.
8. Smirnov VN, Asafov GB, Cherpachenko NM, Chernousova GB, Mozzhechkov VT and Krivov VI (1974) Circ. Res. 34–35: III-58–III-69.
9. Wiener HL, Hashim A, Lajtha A and Sershen H (1988) Res. Commun. Psychol. Psychiatr. Behav. 13: 305–308.

Biological Psychiatry, Volume 1. G. Racagni et al., editors.

Safety of the RIMA antidepressant moclobemide: Minimal interactions with dietary tyramine and 5-HT uptake blockers

Erico Pietro Bonetti, Richard Scherschlicht and Mosé Da Prada
F. Hoffmann-La Roche Ltd., Pharma Division, Preclinical Research, CH-4002 Basel, Switzerland

Introduction

Moclobemide (Aurorix®) is the prototype of a new generation of non-hydrazine reversible inhibitors of MAO (monoamine oxidase) type A (RIMA). Compared to the classical irreversible MAO inhibitors (MAOI), moclobemide has the advantage of lacking hepatotoxic liability and of producing a much weaker increase of the tyramine pressor effect [1]. Detailed information on the amount of tyramine in European foodstuffs as a rational basis for providing advice to patients treated with moclobemide have been published recently [2,3]. Relevant pressor effects are highly unlikely if less than 100–150 mg of tyramine is ingested during therapy with moclobemide [2,3] (a large European and Far Eastern meal averages 36 and 21 mg tyramine, respectively).

In clinical treatment of depressive disorders, the combination of irreversible MAOIs with 5-hydroxytryptamine (5-HT) uptake inhibitors has been reported to present some hazards [4]. Adverse events have included increased muscle tone, myoclonic movement, hyperthermia, convulsions, coma and possibly even death. So far, studies to reproduce these interactions in animals have been carried out only with irreversible MAOIs. Here we present acute experiments using gross behavioural observation of mice or rats and body temperature measurements in rabbits to study the interaction of moclobemide or the irreversible MAOI phenelzine with two 5-HT uptake inhibitors.

Materials and Methods

One or 2 h after administration of a MAOI or vehicle to mice, a 5-HT uptake inhibitor or vehicle was given and the animals thereafter observed for at least 1 h. In rats, a single i.p. injection of the 5-HT reuptake inhibitor fluoxetine on 2 successive days was followed 16 h later by either phenelzine i.p. or moclobemide i.p. Immediately after the injection of these MAOIs the rats were observed for changes in gross behaviour, particularly for the appearance of serotoninergic signs. For studying body temperature male rabbits were used. Rectal temperature was measured in °C. Phenelzine or moclobemide (a single dose on 2 successive days)

Table 1. Observation of gross behaviour in mice. 5-HT uptake inhibitors fluoxetine and clomipramine given p.o. once 1 or 2 h after phenelzine or after moclobemide. Doses are mg/kg p.o.

Phenelzine	Hours	Clomipramine	Putative 5-HT signs
30	1	10,100	L
30	2	10,100	+[a]
		Fluoxetine	
30	1	30,100	+[a]
30	2	30,100	+[a]
Moclobemide		Clomipramine	
100,180,300	1	10,100	L
100,180,300	2	10,100	L
		Fluoxetine	
100,180	1	10,30,100	L
100,180	2	10,30,100	L
300	1	10,30,100	L
300	2	10,30,100	+[b]

[a]Twitches, [b]tremor; L = lack of 5-HT signs.

were injected. Two hours after each dose of the MAOI the rabbits received a single i.v. injection of clomipramine or fluoxetine.

Results (Tables 1, 2 and 3)

In mice and rats, in contrast to the irreversible MAOI phenelzine, moclobemide did not induce a serotoninergic syndrome, even when given in huge doses before or after the 5-HT inhibitor.

In rats, phenelzine but not moclobemide showed an interaction even 16 h after the very long-lasting 5-HT uptake inhibitor fluoxetine [5].

Moclobemide, in contrast to phenelzine, did not induce hyperpyrexia or even lethality when given before 5-HT inhibitors in rabbits.

Table 2. Observation of gross behaviour in rats. Phenelzine or moclobemide were given once daily, on 2 successive days, after the 5-HT uptake inhibitor fluoxetine. Doses are mg/kg i.p.

Fluoxetine	Hours	Phenelzine	Putative 5-HT signs
10	16	10	+++[a]
10	16	30	+++++[b]
		Moclobemide	
10	16	30	L
10	16	100	L

[a]Wet dog shakes, reciprocal forepaw treading, hypersalivation.
[b]As above and, in addition, twitches and Straub tail; L = lack of 5-HT signs.

Table 3. Rectal temperature of rabbits. Phenelzine or moclobemide were given once daily, on 2 successive days, followed by clomipramine or fluoxetine

MAOI (mg/kg i.p.)	5-HT inhibitor (mg/kg i.v.)	Difference to the initial value, in °C, at time indicated after the 5-HT inhibitor (min)				
		–5	15	30	60	120
Phenelzine	Clomipramine					
10	4	0	0.25	0.1	0	0.25
20	4	0	0.75	1.75	5.2	#
40	4	0	3.75	4.75	#	
80	4	0	#			
Phenelzine	Fluoxetine					
10	15	0	#			
20	15	0	#			
40	15	0	#			
Moclobemide	Clomipramine					
100	4	0	0.25	0.25	0.25	0
200	4	0	–0.45	0	0.1	–0.1
400	4	0	0.25	0	–0.35	–
800	4	0	0.25	0	0.2	0.15
Moclobemide	Fluoxetine					
200	15	0	0.27	0.05	0	–0.1
400	15	0	0.3	0.25	–0.55	–0.75

n = 1 per dose; #: death of the animal.

Conclusion

Patients treated with moclobemide can safely consume average types and amounts of European as well as Far Eastern foods. Given before (in mice and rabbits) or after (in rats) 5-HT uptake inhibitors, moclobemide showed an interaction liability which was clearly lower than that exhibited by the irreversible MAOI phenelzine.

References

1. Da Prada M, Kettler R, Burkard WP, Lorez HP and Haefely W (1990) Acta Psychiatr. Scand. (Suppl.) 360: 7–12.
2. Da Prada M, Zürcher G, Wüthrich I and Haefely WE (1988) J. Neural. Transm. (Suppl.) 26: 31–56.
3. Da Prada M and Zürcher G (1991) Psychopharmacology (Suppl.) (in press).
4. Lader M (1989) J. Clin. Psychiatry 44: 20–24.
5. Wong DT, Bymaster FP, Horng JS and Molloy BB (1975) J. Pharmacol. Exp. Ther. 193: 804–811.

Biological Psychiatry, Volume 1. G. Racagni et al., editors.

Brofaromine and 5-HT uptake inhibition: Structure-activity relationship of congeners

Peter Waldmeier, Raymond Bernasconi and Walter Schilling
Research Department, Pharma Division, Ciba-Geigy Ltd., CH-4002 Basle, Switzerland

Introduction

The reversible monoamine oxidase A (MAO-A) inhibitor brofaromine is a member of the benzofuranylpiperidine series, in which MAO-A inhibition is combined with serotonin (5-HT) uptake inhibition in varying proportions. Brofaromine was originally selected because of its effects on MAO-A; its 5-HT uptake inhibitory properties were considered too weak to be of importance. However, with growing knowledge about the compound this judgement seemed questionable. Here we compare the MAO-A and 5-HT uptake inhibitory properties in different models in the rat in vivo or ex vivo. Moreover, we describe the effects of variations in the substitution of the benzofuranylpiperidine structure on these two parameters.

Methods

MAO-A activity was determined in vitro in whole brain homogenates [1] from rats orally pretreated for 2 h with the drugs to be tested, using [^{14}C]5-HT as the substrate. Uptake of [^{3}H]5-HT into midbrain synaptosomes prepared from rats pretreated for 1 h were determined as described previously [2]. In the in vivo binding experiments, brofaromine was administered 30 min after [^{3}H]brofaromine or 30 min before [^{3}H]cyanoimipramine. The animals were decapitated 4 or 2 h after the i.v. injection of radioactivity, respectively. For details of the methods for the determination of specific binding of the two ligands, see Waldmeier and Stöcklin [3,4].

Results and Discussion

Figure 1 compares the effects of brofaromine on MAO-A activity in the rat whole brain and on 5-HT uptake into rat midbrain synaptosomes determined ex vivo with those on the in vivo binding of [^{3}H]brofaromine to MAO-A and of [^{3}H]cyano-imipramine to the 5-HT transporter in the rat hypothalamus. The data of the respective in vivo and ex vivo paradigms agree closely and suggest that, in this species, brofaromine inhibits 5-HT uptake with a 10–30-fold lesser potency than

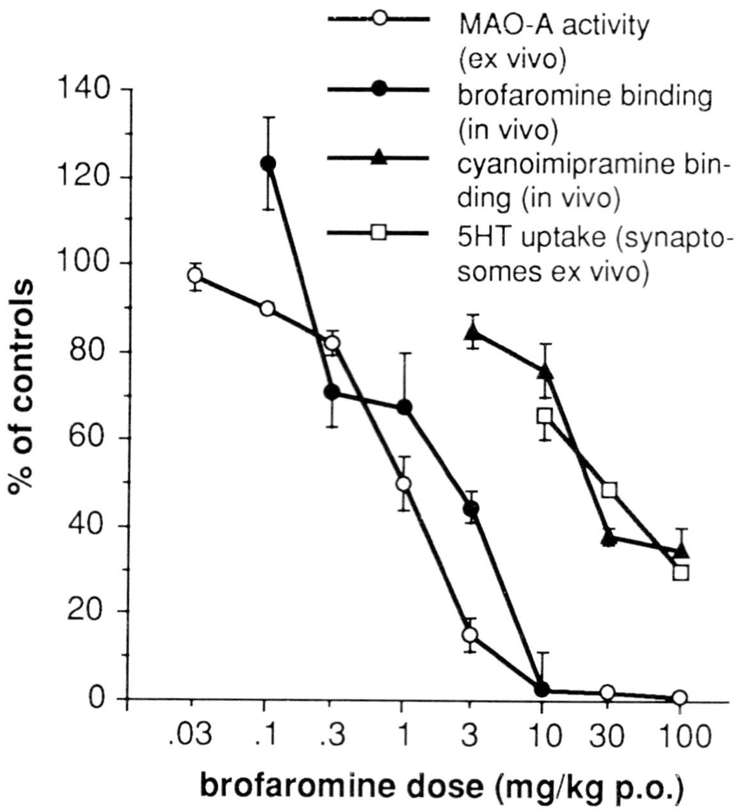

Fig. 1.

MAO-A. In Fig. 2, the ED_{50} values of a number of structural analogs of brofaromine with respect to inhibition of MAO-A in rat brain and of 5-HT uptake into rat brain synaptosomes ex vivo are plotted against each other. This demonstrates the wide range of proportions in which MAO-A and 5-HT uptake inhibition occur in the benzofuranylpiperidine series. A few pieces of information not contained in this graph may be of interest: replacement of piperidine by pyridine yielded inactive compounds; N-alkylated compounds were always less active than the secondary amines; piperidones were inactive; with a few exceptions the compounds preferentially inhibited MAO-A as compared to MAO-B; the parent unsubstituted compound also inhibited noradrenaline uptake, but this property was weaker or lost in all derivatives.

In the absence of suitable methodologies to measure cerebral 5-HT uptake inhibition in humans, only extrapolations based on animal experiments and comparative reasoning can be made with respect to the question of whether such an effect occurs with brofaromine under clinical conditions. Whereas brofaromine in rat brain synaptosomes in vitro only has one-third of the 5-HT uptake inhibitory

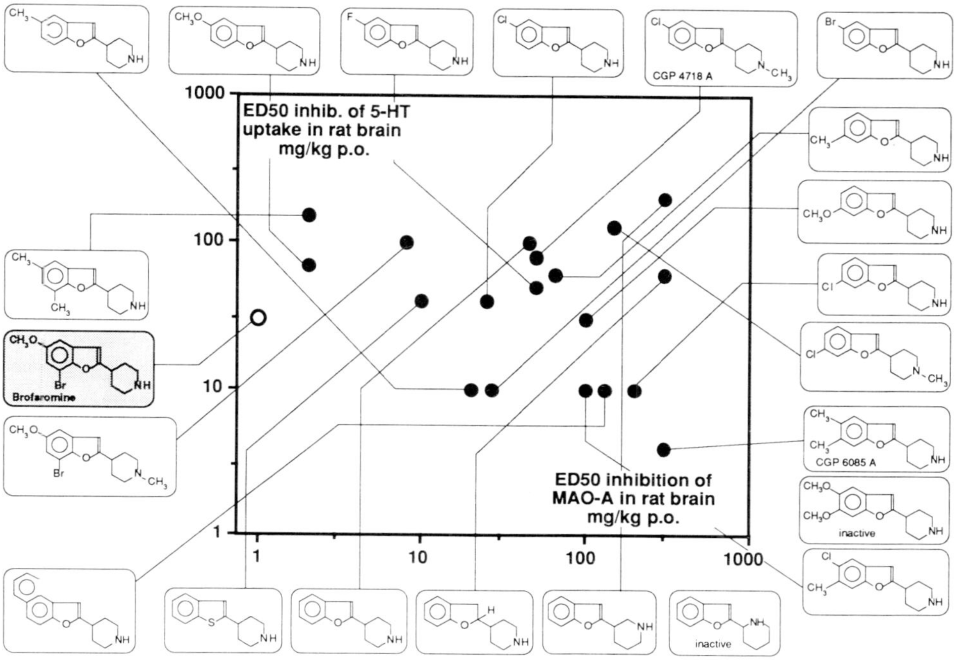

Fig. 2.

potency of imipramine, it is about twice as potent in vivo or ex vivo models [2,4]. Clinical daily doses as well as the order of magnitude of the plasma levels of the two drugs are similar. 5-HT uptake into thrombocytes of patients treated with daily doses of 50–300 mg imipramine was clearly inhibited [5,6]. On the other hand, in the rat in vivo imipramine is more potent in inhibiting cerebral than thrombocyte 5-HT uptake, which probably reflects the fact that its brain levels are higher than those in blood. Since this also holds for brofaromine, cerebral 5-HT uptake inhibition may occur to a certain extent at clinical doses. Even a small inhibition by 20–30% may be expected to enhance the effect of MAO-A inhibition on 5-HT transmission. This in turn might explain why therapeutic efficacy of brofaromine seems to increase between 50 and 150 mg daily [7], whereas the extent of MAO-A inhibition does not. An experimental verification must probably await the availability of a suitable PET ligand for the 5-HT transporter. Studies on thrombocytes are problematic in view of the high plasma protein binding (>98%) of brofaromine.

References

1. Waldmeier PC, Felner AE and Tipton KF (1983) Eur. J. Pharmacol. 94: 73–83.
2. Waldmeier PC and Baumann PA (1983) Naunyn-Schmiedeberg's Arch. Pharmacol. 324: 20–26.

3. Waldmeier PC and Stöcklin K (1989) Eur. J. Pharmacol. 180: 297–304.
4. Waldmeier PC and Stöcklin K (1989) Eur. J. Pharmacol. 169: 197–204.
5. Arora RC and Meltzer HY (1983) Psychiatr. Res. 9: 29–36.
6. Tuomisto J, Tukiainen E and Ahlfors UG (1979) Psychopharmacology 65: 141–147.
7. Schiwy W, Heath WR and Delini-Stula A (1989) J. Neural Transm. (Suppl. 28): 33–44.
8. Waldmeier PC, Antonin KH, Feldtrauer JJ, Grunenwald C, Paul E, Lauber J and Beck P (1983) Eur. J. Clin. Pharmacol. 25: 361–368.

Biological Psychiatry, Volume 1. G. Racagni et al., editors.

Modulatory actions of steroid hormones on MAO-A but not MAO-B activities

Moussa B.H. Youdim
Technion-Bruce Rappaport Faculty of Medicine, Department of Pharmacology, Haifa, Israel

Introduction

There is ample pharmacological and clinical evidence suggesting neuropsychotropic actions of steroids. In some cases the action of steroids has been attributed to their effects on aminergic receptors, catecholamine metabolism and the enzymic reaction involved in metabolism of catecholamines. Among the steroids, estrogen has received much prominence because of the latter's antidepressant activity on women in the postmenopause period [1]. This assumption has been attributed to the ability of estrogen to inhibit monoamine oxidase (MAO) since studies have clearly demonstrated changes in brain MAO activity during rat oestrous cycle and in human endometrium during the menstrual cycle [2]. Furthermore, in in vivo experiments, when rats were injected chronically with low doses of estrogen or progesterone, MAO activity in uterus, ovary and adrenal gland was either decreased or increased respectively [2,3]. The suggestion was made that the steroids have their action on the synthesis of the enzyme since in vitro no such effects were observed.

If we are to understand the action of sex steroids on MAO activity and attribute their effects to this enzyme, it is important not only to establish a direct link with the changes in the enzyme activity, but also to establish which of the two MAO forms is altered. This is rather important since intraneuronal MAO is type A [4], and this enzyme regulates the metabolism of dopamine, noradrenaline and serotonin within the cytoplasm of their respective neurons [4]. The only exception is the presence of MAO-B within the serotonin neurons of raphe nucleus. The function of the latter enzyme in the raphe nucleus is not known. Animal studies, at least, have shown that inhibition of MAO-B does not alter raphe nucleus serotonin. Therefore, a change in MAO-A activity may be pertinent to psychotropic action of steroids.

Results and Discussion

The availability of specific cell types having as their origin the neural crest and being endowed with only MAO-A or MAO-B activity has allowed us to study the action of steroids on the enzyme activities in culture under controlled conditions.

We have established that while isolated bovine adrenal chromaffin cells contain only MAO-B [5], phaechromacytoma (PC12) cells are endowed with only MAO-A [6], a phenomenon also observed in adrenal medullary capillary endothelial cells [7]. These cells were cultured as described previously [7] in the presence of 1 and 10 M of estrogen, progesterone, dexamethasone, testosterone and hydrocortisone for up to 17 days. At intervals MAO activity and incorporation of [^{14}C]-leucine and [^{14}C]-thymidine were also determined. Our studies showed that the MAO-B activity in the adrenal chromaffin cell was unresponsive to steroids. Indeed, long culture time (>3 days) resulted in loss of enzyme activity. However, the MAO-A activity in both PC12 [8] and capillary endothelial cells [7] was influenced by the steroids, whereas much as progesterone, dexamethasone and hydrocortisone greatly induced the enzyme activity, estradiol treatment reduced the activity of MAO-A. The induction and diminution of MAO-A activity in these cell types is parallel to the synthesis of protein as demonstrated by the incorporation of [^{14}C]-leucine and [^{14}C]-thymidine. The direct regulation of MAO-A synthesis by the above steroids was established by binding studies with the irreversible MAO inhibitor pargyline. This inhibitor binds covalently mol/mol to the enzyme active site at N-5 of the cofactor FAD [7].

The present findings demonstrate for the first time that steroids have the ability to induce and diminish the activity of MAO-A and not of MAO-B in cell types possessing a single enzyme form. PC12 cells have been used as models of adrenergic neurons since they possess the ability to synthesize, store and release catecholamines in response to K^+ and tyramine. Furthermore, similarly to their potentiate tyramine-induced release of catecholamines from these cells [6,9]. While PC12 cells may not be absolutely representative of adrenergic nerve endings, they do have antigenic and other properties similar to those of adrenergic neurons. These properties acquire a special significance from the fact that the MAO-A activity in cells can be modulated by steroids, as suggested originally for the MAO in the adrenergic nerve ending. The relevance of alteration in MAO-A activity in response to neuroendocrine input is obvious, considering that MAO-A is located in the adrenergic neuron and selective inhibitors of this enzyme have been shown to have significant antidepressant property. Obviously the central role of MAO-A modulation by steroids cannot be ignored in psychotherapy of depressive illness with steroids. The response to drugs may very well be dependent on the state of the MAO-A activity in the nerve ending. If estrogens do indeed have antidepressant action, the mechanism of which is not well understood, its ability to reduce MAO-A activity in the serotonergic and adrenergic nerve ending cannot be ignored.

References

1. Holzboer F, Benkert O and Demisch L (1983) Mod. Probl. Pharmacopsychiatry 19: 321–327.
2. Youdim MBH and Holzbauer M (1976) J. Neural Transm. 38: 193–229.

3. Collins GGS, Pryse-Davies J, Sandler M and Southgate J (1970) Nature 226: 642–643.
4. Youdim MBH, Finberg JPM and Tipton KF (1989) In: Trendelenburg U and Weiner N (eds.) Catecholamine II. Springer-Verlag, Berlin, pp. 119–192.
5. Youdim MBH, Banerjee DK and Pollard HB (1984) Science 224: 619–621.
6. Youdim MBH, Heldman E, Polard HB, Fleming P and McHugh E (1986) Neuroscience 19: 1311–1318.
7. Youdim MBH, Banerjee DK, Kelner K, Offut K and Pollard HB (1989) FASEB J. 3: 1753–1759.
8. Youdim MBH (1991) Eur. J. Pharmacol. 192: 201–202.
9. Youdim MBH (1990) J. Neurochem. 54: 411–414.

Biological Psychiatry, Volume 1. G. Racagni et al., editors.

The role of MAO inhibitors in the treatment of affective disorders

E.S. Paykel
Department of Psychiatry, University of Cambridge, Addenbrooke's Hospital, Cambridge CB2 2QQ, U.K.

Atypical depression

MAO inhibitors (MAOIs) were introduced into therapy before tricyclics, but still have a much more limited place. A view of their selective clinical place was first crystallised by West and Dally [1]. Patients responding to iproniazid were found to show an absence of self-reproach, morning worsening and early wakening, presence of evening worsening, hysterical symptoms, tremor and a history of having been worsened by ECT. They described a syndrome with additional features of anxiety and fatigue.

In the many subsequent papers, three different meanings have been assigned to the term atypical depression [2]. One is the idea of marked anxiety and phobic symptoms, either accompanied by depression, or alone. The second meaning is what is now usually referred to as reversed vegetative symptoms, i.e. depression with a diurnal pattern of evening worsening, initial insomnia, increased sleep, increased appetite and weight, all in the direction opposite to the physiological changes said to characterise endogenous depression. A third meaning, at one time common and probably closest to the original, but now rarely used, was that of non-endogenous depression in general.

These three meanings identify different groups of patients. We found little overlap among patients assigned by the three different criteria [2]. The concept of atypical depression is imprecise and it is better to specify which aspect is to be emphasized.

Evidence from controlled trials

The best evidence on the efficacy of MAOIs is for phenelzine. Among seventeen controlled trials against placebo in depression [3] ten were positive, three doubtfully positive and four negative. In these studies there was not a very strong relationship between response and defined subtype, but most of the positive studies were in outpatient samples, with studies on inpatients being mostly negative. Outpatients tend to be less severely ill and more neurotic in symptom pattern. Some re-evaluation may be needed since most of the inpatient trials were early studies, using doses and treatment periods that were relatively low by modern standards. There have also been four positive studies against placebo in anxiety disorders with one doubtful study and one negative study. However, there is also good evidence that tricyclics are superior to placebo in anxiety disorders [4].

In a controlled trial of phenelzine, amitriptyline and placebo in outpatient depressives and mixed anxiety depressives, we found clear drug effects for both drugs with surprisingly little difference between them [5,6]. On anxiety measures and in initially anxious subjects, phenelzine was minimally superior to amitriptyline and on depression measures and predominantly depressed subjects amitriptyline was minimally superior to phenelzine. Neither of the other two views of atypical depression gave significant interactions with drug response. Overall the findings of this study suggested some selectivity of MAOIs in patients showing anxiety, but the difference was weak.

These weak differences are consistent with other studies. Ravaris et al. [7] found phenelzine to be weakly superior to amitriptyline on anxiety measures. Davidson et al. [8] found weak trends for better effects of MAOIs rather than tricyclic, where a precipitant was present and, contrary to expectation, in the absence of agoraphobia. There were also some differences between the two sexes. Georgotas et al. [9] found only weak differences in elderly depressives, as did Sheehan et al. [10] in younger subjects with phobic anxiety. The Columbia group have found stronger differences [11–15]. Selecting patients with reversed vegetative symptoms, they found phenelzine most effective; imipramine was less so, although better than placebo. What is most striking in their studies is the limited response of patients with reversed vegetative symptoms to imipramine. No studies have yet been published on responsive groups to the new MAO-A selective drugs.

It remains possible that a biochemical variable, rather than clinical subtype, predicts response. Most clinicians have some patients under their care who respond only to MAOIs. Pare and Mack [16] compared patients who in successive episodes had received antidepressants of the same type or of different type, and found significantly consistent response to the same type of drug and divergent responses across different kinds of drug.

European study of MAOIs

A general conclusion for MAOIs would therefore be that they are weakly selective for anxiety and reversed vegetative symptoms, but the differences from tricyclics are not sufficiently strong to guide treatment choice. Since tricyclics are safer and easier to use, the logical place for MAOIs is as a second choice where tricyclics have failed and ECT is not indicated.

This is the way they are in fact used. We carried out a survey study of psychiatrists' views in Europe [17]. Psychiatrists regarded the literature as demonstrating efficacy for MAOIs. However, when asked how they would treat various kinds of disorder in practice, only a minority endorsed MAOIs, even for second choice in atypical depression. There were considerable cross-national differences in use. Two views were found as to the significance of retardation. Psychiatrists in one group of countries regarded it as a facet of endogenous depression and a contraindication for MAOI use; those from the other, an aspect of fatigue and therefore an indication.

The major problem in use has been not efficacy but side-effects, particularly interactions with tyramine and other amines. The new generation of MAO-A selective rapidly reversible drugs could very much change the current picture and bring the MAOIs into widespread use.

References

1. West ED and Dally PJ (1959) Br. Med. J. 1: 1491–1499.
2. Paykel ES, Parker RR, Rowan RR, Rao BM and Taylor CN (1983) Psychol. Med. 13: 131–139.
3. Paykel ES (1990) In: Hawton K and Cowen P (eds.) Dilemmas and Controversies in the Management of Psychiatric Patients. Oxford University Press, Oxford.
4. Marks I and O'Sullivan G (1988) Br. J. Psychiatry 153: 650–658.
5. Paykel ES, Rowan PR, Parker RR and Bhat AV (1982) Arch. Gen. Psychiatry 39: 1041–1049.
6. Rowan PR, Paykel ES and Parker RR (1982) Br. J. Psychiatry 140: 475–483.
7. Ravaris CL, Robinson DS, Ives JO, Nies A and Bartlett D (1980) Arch. Gen. Psychiatry 37: 1075–1080.
8. Davidson J, Pelton S, Krishnan RR and Allf B (1986) J. Affective Disord. 11: 51–61.
9. Georgotas A, McCue RE, Friedman E and Cooper TB (1987) Br. J. Psychiatry 151: 102–106.
10. Sheehan DV, Ballinger J and Jacobsen G (1980) Arch. Gen. Psychiatry 37: 51–59.
11. Liebowitz MR, Quitkin FM, Stewart JW, McGrath PJ, Harrison WM, Markowitz JS, Rabkin JG, Tricamo E, Goetz DM and Klein DF (1988) Arch. Gen. Psychiatry 45: 129–137.
12. Quitkin FM, Stewart JW, McGrath PJ, Liebowitz MR, Harrison WM, Tricamo E, Klein DF, Rabkin JG, Markowitz JS and Wager SG (1988) Am. J. Psychiatry 145: 306–311.
13. Stewart JW, McGrath PJ, Quitkin FM, Harrison W, Markowitz J, Wager S and Leibowitz MR (1989) Arch. Gen. Psychiatry 46: 1080–1087.
14. Quitkin FM, McGrath PJ, Stewart JW, Harrison W, Wager SG, Nunes E, Rabkin JG, Tricamo E, Markowitz J and Klein DF (1989) Arch. Gen. Psychiatry 46: 787–793.
15. Quitkin FM, McGrath PJ, Stewart JW, Harrison W, Tricamo E, Wager SG, Deepek-Welikson K, Nunes E, Rabkin JG and Klein DF (1990) Arch. Gen. Psychiatry 47: 935–941.
16. Pare CMB and Mack JW (1971) J. Med. Gen. 8: 306–309.
17. Paykel ES and White JL (1989) Br. J. Psychiatry 155(6): 9–17.

Biological Psychiatry, Volume 1. G. Racagni et al., editors.

Significance of reversibility as a safety factor of MAO-A inhibitors: Preclinical data

Keith F. Tipton and Mary C. Anderson
Department of Biochemistry, Trinity College, Dublin 2, Ireland

Introduction

The first generation of monoamine oxidase inhibitors were irreversible inhibitors of both forms of the enzyme. Aside from problems that arose from hepatotoxicity, because of their chemical nature (for review see [1]), they gave rise to strong hypertensive responses following the ingestion of some foods and beverages. This was shown to be a result of the relatively high concentrations of amines, often tyramine, in the ingested material (see [1–4]). Since some cheeses are particularly rich in tyramine, this effect has become known as the "cheese reaction". However, many other foods and beverages contain amines which can interact in this way, and because of the nature of some of the foods involved and the lack of any legislation controlling the tyramine contents, the quantities present can be extremely variable (see [2–4]).

The discovery of selective irreversible MAO inhibitors led to hopes that it might be possible to have effective antidepressants that were free from the cheese reaction. The observations that tyramine was a substrate for both forms of MAO, as were dopamine and noradrenaline, whereas 5-hydroxytryptamine (5-HT) was a substrate only for MAO-A (for reviews see [1,5]) led to the belief that a selective inhibitor of either form of the enzyme might only impair the ability to oxidase ingested tyramine by about 50%. It has been shown that inhibitors of MAO-A, such as clorgyline are effective antidepressants, whereas those of MAO-B, such as l-deprenyl (selegyline), are apparently not (see [1]). However, MAO-A inhibitors precipitate a cheese reaction which appears to be no less pronounced than that caused by the earlier non-selective inhibitors. In contrast, the selective MAO-B inhibitors do not give a cheese reaction.

This has been shown to be a result of MAO-A being the predominant form of the enzyme present in the human intestine [6,7]. A similar situation exists in the rat intestine [6,8]. Studies on tyramine transport in everted rat intestine have shown that little free tyramine is transported, since almost all is metabolized during passage through the intestinal cells. MAO-B inhibitors have little effect on this process, whereas MAO-A inhibitors result in a greatly enhanced transport of unchanged tyramine at the expense of its metabolites [6]. Although the intestine is often regarded as the first line of defence against ingested amines, some metabolism may also occur in the cells of the stomach. However, it has been shown that the relative activities of the 2 forms of MAO in human stomach are similar to those in the intestine [9].

Reversible selective inhibitors

The behavior of reversible selective inhibitors of MAO will differ in several respects from those of the irreversible inhibitors. In the former case the duration of their effects in vivo will be dictated solely by the pharmacokinetics of drug elimination, since as the concentration of free drug in the tissues falls, it will dissociate from the enzyme. In contrast, the recovery from the effects of an irreversible inhibitor will require the synthesis of new enzyme to replace that which will remain inhibited even after the complete elimination of free drug. Measurements of the rates of recovery of MAO activity after administration of a single dose of a selective inhibitor have given similar values for the half-times of MAO-A and -B, of about 2.5–3.5 and 10–13 days for rat liver and brain, respectively [10,11] but a very much longer half-life (30 days) has been reported for primate brain [12]. The turnover rates of MAO-A and -B have been reported to be different in the rat intestine, with values of 2.2 and 7.7 days, respectively, being determined for the half-lives [13]. Such rates of recovery imply a risk of loss of inhibitor selectivity as a result of repeated dosage.

A competitive reversible inhibitor should not completely prevent the enzyme from metabolizing ingested tyramine, unless present at very high concentrations. The relationships between the inhibitor concentration causing 50% inhibition (IC_{50}) and the percentage inhibition with the substrate and inhibitor concentrations will be:

$$IC_{50} = (1 + [S]/K_m)K_i \text{ and } \% \text{ inhibition} = [I]/\{K_i(1 + [S]/K_m) + [I]\}$$

where [S] and [I] are the substrate and inhibitor concentrations and K_m and K_i are the Michaelis and inhibitor constants, respectively. These relationships show that the effective inhibition at any given inhibitor concentration will decrease as the substrate concentration increases. In the case of tyramine (K_m = about 100 μM) it can be seen that the extent of inhibition by a concentration of inhibitor equal to the K_i value will be 50% at very low tyramine concentrations and that this will decrease as the substrate concentration is increased. This ability to displace inhibitor does not apply to all reversible inhibitors, since the degree of inhibition will actually increase with the substrate concentration in the case of an uncompetitive inhibitor or be unaffected by the concentration if inhibition is of the true noncompetitive type. A mixed-noncompetitive inhibitor will show both competitive and uncompetitive effects [see 14]. Should an inhibitor be tight-binding, showing time-dependence in association with the enzyme and in dissociation from it, the above analysis will remain valid if the inhibitor binds to the same site on the enzyme as the substrate (i.e. it is competitive). Thus it should be applicable to brofaromine, which has been shown to behave in this way [15].

In tissue preparations there is considerable non-specific binding of brofaromine to components other than the active site of MAO [15]. This might dilute its action in vivo, necessitating the use of higher concentrations than would be expected from its K_i value. Alternatively, however, non-specifically-bound material might act as a reservoir of inhibitor, prolonging its actions in the cell as it dissociates and becomes available to interact with MAO-A. The situation with the reversible MAO-A inhibitor moclobemide might be expected to be more complicated; this compound appears to act as a pro-drug, being converted to the active inhibitor enzymically [see 16].

The behavior of the reversible MAO-A inhibitors brofaromine and moclobemide on tyramine transport in vitro has been examined using everted intestinal preparations by procedures previously used to investigate the effects of irreversible inhibitors [6]. Results will be presented to show that their behavior is in accord with these predictions, suggesting that this type of inhibitor will indeed offer a margin of safety not obtainable with irreversible inhibitors. However, the possibility of interindividual variations in intestinal MAO activity, together with the wide variations in the tyramine contents of foods and beverages suggests that the unrestricted use of such inhibitors should be considered with caution.

References

1. Tipton KF (1989) In: Tipton KF and Youdim MBH (eds.) Biochemical and Pharmacological Aspects of Depression. Taylor and Francis, London, pp. 1–24.
2. Da Prada M, Zürcher G, Wüthrich I and Haefely WE (1988) J. Neural Transm. (Suppl.) 26: 31–56.
3. Wheatley AM and Tipton KF (1987) J. Food Biochem. 11: 133–142.
4. Dostert P (1984) In: Tipton KF, Dostert P and Strolin Benedetti M (eds.) Monoamine Oxidase and Disease. Academic Press, London, pp. 9–24.
5. Youdim MBH, Finberg JPM and Tipton KF (1988) In: Trendelenburg U and Weiner N (eds.) Handbook of Experimental Pharmacology, Vol. 90. Springer Verlag, Berlin, pp. 119–192.
6. Hasan F, McCrodden JM, Kennedy NP and Tipton KF (1988) J. Neural Transm. (Suppl.) 26: 1–9.
7. Squires RF (1972) Adv. Biochem. Psychopharmacol. 5: 355–370.
8. Strolin Benedetti M, Boucher T, Carlsson A and Fowler CJ (1983) Biochem. Pharmacol. 32: 47–52.
9. Biek PR, Kemmler H, Antonin K-H and Tipton KF (1988) Pharmacol. Res. Commun. (Suppl. 4) 20: 129–130.
10. Della Corte L and Tipton KF (1980) Biochem. Pharmacol. 29: 811–815.
11. Neff NH and Goridis C (1972) Adv. Biochem. Psychopharmacol. 5: 307–323.
12. Arnett CD, Fowler JS, MacGreggor RR, Schyler DJ, Wolf PP, Långström B and Halldin CJ (1987) J. Neurochem. 49: 522–527.
13. Callingham BA, Mazel P and Porter JC (1985) Br. J. Pharmacol. 86: 553P.
14. Tipton KF and Fowler CJ (1984) In: Tipton KF, Dostert P and Strolin Benedetti M (eds.) Monoamine Oxidase and Disease. Academic Press, London, pp. 27–40.
15. Anderson MC, Waldmeier PC and Tipton KF (1991) Biochem. Pharmacol. (in press).
16. Da Prada M, Kettler R, Keller HH, Cesura AM, Richards JG, Saura Marti J, Mugli-Maniglio D, Wyss P-C, Kyburz E and Imhof R (1990) J. Neural Transm. (Suppl.) 29: 279–292.

Biological Psychiatry, Volume 1. G. Racagni et al., editors.

Clinical pharmacology of selective and reversible MAO-A inhibitors: Comparison with the first generation of MAO inhibitors

Peter R. Bieck, Karl-Heinz Antonin and Rainer Schulz
Human Pharmacology Institute Ciba-Geigy, Waldhörnlestr. 22, D-7400 Tübingen, Germany

The older clinically used monoamine oxidase inhibitors (MAOI) phenelzine and tranylcypromine non-selectively inhibit MAO-A+B. MAO-A is selectively inhibited by clorgyline. These drugs are irreversible MAOI with long-lasting effects and with an enhanced liability to tyramine-related hypertension (cheese effect). A second generation of MAOI was developed with the goal of obtaining selective and reversible inhibition. To this group belong the 2 MAO-A inhibitors brofaromine and moclobemide. There is a large body of evidence that drugs which affect MAO-A are more effective antidepressants than inhibitors of MAO-B [1,2].

Immediately following MAOI treatment, there is an increase of the concentrations of noradrenaline and serotonin (preferential substrates of MAO-A), dopamine (preferential substrate of MAO-B) and tyramine (substrate of both MAO-A+B). All indices of sympathetic outflow are diminished by MAOI treatment. In contrast, the pressor and catecholamine release responses to tyramine show there is increased stored noradrenaline available for release. The dampening effect on the sympathetic activity is more pronounced with MAO-A inhibition [1]. We examined the dose-response relationship of parenteral amines and of oral tyramine and cheese during administration with several MAOI (for review see [3]).

Interaction studies

From separate dose-response curves the amine doses to raise systolic blood pressure by 30 mmHg were estimated as pressor dose 30 (=PD_{30}). The intensity of the tyramine effect was assessed by quantal dose-response curves. The median effective doses (ED_{50}) give indirect information about the functional state of the adrenergic nerve terminal. The time for normalization of pressor sensitivity after stopping treatment is an index for the reversibility of MAO inhibition.

MAO-A inhibition in peripheral neurons can be assessed by *parenteral tyramine* administration. For tranylcypromine and brofaromine a 10- and 5-fold potentiation – compared to untreated subjects – was found (Table 1). The sum of MAO inhibition in the gastrointestinal tract and the effect on peripheral neurons can be assessed after *oral tyramine* intake. Potency of MAOI in this test is highest for the non-selective tranylcypromine (ED_{50} ratio of 55) and phenelzine (ED_{50} ratio of

Table 1. Extent and duration of tyramine pressor sensitivity enhancement

Treatment	MAO-type	ED_{50} i.v. tyramine (mg)	ED_{50} ratio	ED_{50} p.o. tyramine (mg)	ED_{50} ratio	Normalization time
None	–	4.0	1	437	1	
First generation MAOI						
Tranyl-cypromine	A+B	0.4	10	8	55	4 weeks
Phenelzine	A+B	1.8	2	33	13	>11 weeks
Selective irreversible MAOI						
Clorgyline	A			43	10	>15 weeks
Selegiline	B	1.9	2	96	5	3 days
Second generation MAOI						
Brofaromine	A	0.8	5	44	10	8 days
Moclobemide	A			63	7	3 days

13). Selective inhibition by clorgyline, selegiline, brofaromine and moclobemide causes a 5- to 10-fold increase of oral tyramine pressor sensitivity. Normalization after stopping the drugs took place within 1 week after the 2 reversible MAO-A inhibitors and after the MAO-B inhibitor selegiline. After stopping the irreversible inhibitors of the first generation and after clorgyline this took up to 15 weeks or longer (Table 1).

Tyramine absorption and metabolism

Hypertensive episodes following ingestion of foodstuffs with high tyramine content have been well documented in patients treated with MAOI [4]. Inactivation of tyramine has been attributed to first-pass intestinal and hepatic metabolism. To evaluate the contribution of decreased gastrointestinal deamination to the pressor effects of oral tyramine, metabolism before and during MAO inhibition by different drugs was compared. For this, the amounts of unconjugated and conjugated tyramine and of the metabolite p-hydroxyphenylacetic acid (HPAA) in plasma were measured [5]. Expressed as a percentage of the total AUC/dose, the contributions of unconjugated tyramine, conjugated tyramine and HPAA in untreated subjects are 0.4%, 12.7% and 86.9%. During subchronic treatment with MAOI, deamination to HPAA becomes impaired and sulfate conjugation is enhanced. The relative bioavailability (BAV_{rel}) of conjugated tyramine after treatment with different MAOI is significantly correlated with their potency in the oral tyramine pressor test (Fig. 1).

Cheese containing the PD_{30} of tyramine was given to 10 subjects treated with brofaromine. Bioavailability was enhanced only 4-fold instead of 6.8-fold and

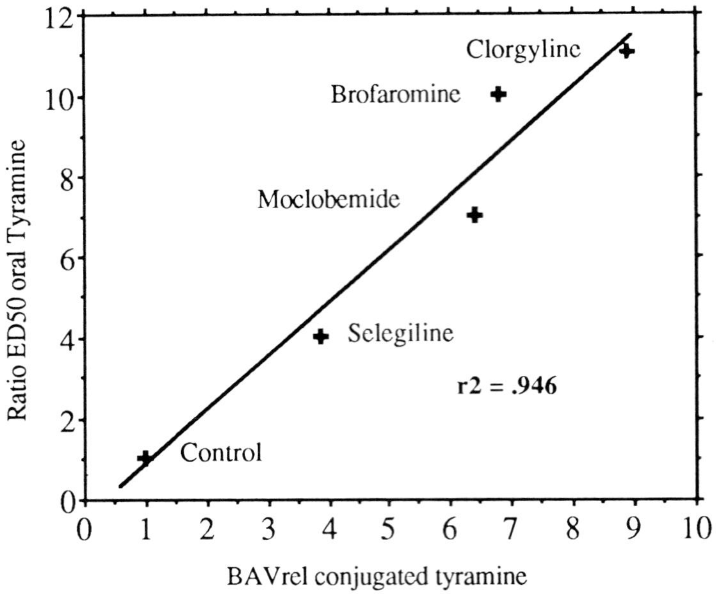

Fig. 1. Correlation between relative bioavailability (BAV_{rel}) of conjugated tyramine and oral tyramine pressor sensitivity (ratio ED_{50}) during treatment with different MAOI drugs.

blood pressure increase was on the average only 10 mmHg in 10 subjects. In plasma, conjugated tyramine was measurable for at least 7 h, but no tyramine peaks occurred. This can be explained by slow absorption of tyramine during digestion [6].

Amine metabolite excretion

With MAOI treatment, reductions in CSF, plasma and urinary concentrations of MPG (3-methoxy-4-hydroxyphenylglycol) occur. MHPG is a major metabolite of noradrenaline and is produced in the neurons of the peripheral nervous system by the action of MAO-A. During treatment of healthy volunteers with different MAOI drugs, 24 h urine was collected and analyzed for MHPG. The MAO-A inhibitors clorgyline, brofaromine and moclobemide, which interfere more markedly with neuronal MAO-A activity than nonspecific MAOI, diminish MHPG excretion significantly. There is a significant correlation (n = 7; r = 0.77; $P < 0.05$) between decreased MHPG excretion and potentiation of parenteral tyramine pressor sensitivity (PD_{30}). The results from healthy volunteers agree well with those from clinical studies [7,8].

Like the pressor sensitivity to tyramine, MHPG excretion normalized quickly within one week after stopping the reversible MAO-A inhibitors brofaromine and moclobemide. Normalization was slow and took several weeks after the irreversible inhibitors clorgyline, phenelzine and tranylcypromine.

Tolerability

Non-specific biochemical or pharmacological effects have not been found either with brofaromine or moclobemide. Generally, their clinical tolerability seems to be better than those of the older compounds and the liability of hypertensive reactions is lessened. In particular, edema, weight gain and sexual dysfunction as seen with the older MAOI are not observed.

References

1. Murphy DL, Aulakh CS, Garrick NA and Sunderland T (1987) In: Meltzer HY (ed.) Psychopharmacology, The Third Generation of Progress. Raven Press, New York, pp. 545–552.
2. Mann JJ, Aarons SF, Wilner PI et al. (1989) Arch. Gen. Psychiatry 46: 45–50.
3. Bieck PR, Antonin KM and Schulz R (1991) In: Yasuhara H, Parvez SH, Sandler M, Oguchi K and Nagatsu T (eds.) Monoamine Oxidase; Basic and Clinical Aspects. VSP Press, Zeist, The Netherlands (in press).
4. Marley E and Blackwell B (1970). Adv. Pharmacol. Chemother. 8: 185–239.
5. Bieck PR, Aichele G, Schick C, Hoffmann E and Nilsson E (1988) In: Boulton AA, Juorio AV and Downer RGH (eds.) Trace Amines, Comparative and Clinical Neurobiology. Humana Press, Clifton, New Jersey, pp. 309–320.
6. Bieck PR and Antonin K-H (1988) J. Clin. Psychopharmacol. 8: 237–245.
7. Hauger RL, Schenin M, Siever LJ, Linnoila M and Potter WZ (1988) Clin. Pharmacol. Ther. 43: 32–38.
8. Murphy DL, Aulakh CS and Garrick HA (1986) In: Antidepressants and Receptor Function. Ciba Foundation Symposium 123, Wiley, Chichester, pp. 106–125.

Biological Psychiatry, Volume 1. G. Racagni et al., editors.

General efficacy and safety of brofaromine in depression

Hans-Jürgen Möller
Department of Psychiatry, University of Bonn, D-5300 Bonn, Germany

The development of brofaromine [1] appears to mark an important milestone on the way towards better tolerated MAO inhibitors. The greater safety is guaranteed by the following mechanisms: selective blockade of MAO-A, reversible inhibition with a short pharmacodynamic half-life and competitive inhibitory mechanism [2]. Brofaromine has a new chemical structure which is unrelated to that of any other known substance. The aim of the following presentation is to summarize the most relevant clinical findings with respect to safety and tolerability.

Results from inpatient studies

Among others, two large multicenter studies on hospitalized patients with "major depressive disorders" (according to DSM III) were performed. In one of these studies brofaromine was compared to tranylcypromine, in the other to imipramine. The design of both studies was quite similar. The therapeutic response and unwanted accompanying effects were evaluated at weekly intervals with the aid of standardized rating instruments, including the Hamilton Depression Scale and a self-rating scale – the Adjective Mood Scale. To shed further light on the tolerability of the medication, the patients' blood pressure, heart rate, body weight and a series of laboratory parameters were measured at regular intervals. In this short review we cannot go into detail.

In the first study 100 to 150 mg brofaromine per day was compared to 20 to 30 mg tranylcypromine per day. The data on about 70 patients showed that, in terms of the observer rating and the self-rating, a comparably good effect had been achieved. There were also hardly any differences with respect to the global assessment of efficacy and of tolerability. Eighty-three of the patients in the brofaromine group, 79% of the tranylcypromine group were judged to have shown a good or very good improvement. In nearly all cases the tolerability of the medication was assessed as good or very good. It should be mentioned that because of the administration of tranylcypromine, a tyramine-restricted diet had to be adhered to. The profile of adverse reactions to brofaromine was very similar to that of tranylcypromine [3].

In a similar study, 100 to 150 mg brofaromine was compared to 100 to 150 mg imipramine per day. The data on about 120 patients demonstrated a marked improvement during the trial period in both treatment groups, as well on the basis of observer ratings as on self-rating basis. The treatment effect was very similar in both treatment groups. The global assessment of efficacy showed no differences: 57% of the patients in the brofaromine group and 60% of those in the imipramine group were judged to have shown a good or very good improvement. The global assessment of tolerability revealed no statistically significant distinction between the treatment groups, although as regards the number of patients with unwanted side-effects (27 in the brofaromine group and 36 in the imipramine group) there was a trend in favor of brofaromine. The spectrum of side-effects differed with respect to the higher incidence of anticholinergic side-effects (particularly dryness of mouth) in the imipramine group. In this study a low tyramine diet was not imposed [4].

Results from outpatient studies

To recruit a higher number of patients and to test brofaromine under outpatient conditions, double-blind multicenter studies on outpatients treated by privately practicing psychiatrists were performed. These studies followed a similar design as the inpatients studies, apart from the longer duration of the treatment period (8 weeks) and the 2:1 randomization. The dosage was flexible: 25 mg to 150 mg brofaromine or imipramine per day.

In the first study on 143 analyzable brofaromine and 72 imipramine patients, the two primary target parameters, Hamilton Depression Scale and Adjective Mood Scale, demonstrated a slight superiority of brofaromine's therapeutic efficacy over imipramine which reached statistical significance. Brofaromine and imipramine were administered at comparable dosages which rules out that different dosage behaviours account for the difference in efficacy. The mean dosage amounted to about 90 mg brofaromine or imipramine, respectively. The therapeutic superiority of brofaromine was also demonstrated by the global assessment data on efficacy. With respect to tolerability, brofaromine was rated as "very good" more often than imipramine (54% vs. 41%); correspondingly the categories "moderate" and "poor" were given more often in the imipramine group (18% vs. 28%). The difference is statistically significant. The profile of side-effects showed similar differences to those in the inpatient study. Although a low tyramine diet was not prescribed, no case of hypertensive crisis occurred.

In a similar study on 127 analyzable brofaromine and 62 imipramine patients (older than 60 years) no difference in the therapeutic efficacy could be found. In this study there was no discrepancy between the two treatments with respect to the therapeutic results. As to the global evaluation of tolerability, again a certain advantage for brofaromine was demonstrated: a very good or good tolerability was noted for 88% of the brofaromine group, but only for 72% of the imipramine group, which is statistically significant.

Both these studies, beside the acute treatment period, included a long-term investigation. Outpatients for whom a long-term antidepressive treatment seems to be indicated according to the judgement of the doctor in charge of the patient should be included in this long-term trial. The special intention was to evaluate the tolerability of brofaromine under long-term treatment conditions. The analysis of the data from these studies is still ongoing.

Conclusion

All in all, the results of these clinical studies together with other studies on brofaromine not reported here, indicate that brofaromine seems to show no differences in antidepressive efficacy as compared to tranylcypromine and especially imipramine. At an oral dosage which is therapeutically effective, it is well tolerated. Apparently, brofaromine offers the opportunity for dietary restrictions to be radically relaxed, especially as it has been found that the tyramine content of food has hitherto been grossly overestimated [5]. This prospect should increase the use of brofaromine in clinical practice.

References

1. Waldmeier PC, Baumann PA, Delini-Stula A, Bernasconi AR, Sigg K, Büch O and Felner AE (1983) Mod. Probl. Pharmacopsychiatry 19: 31–52.
2. Möller HJ, Wendt G and Waldmeier P (1991) Pharmacopsychiatry 24: 50–54.
3. Zapletálek M, Faltus F, Svestka J, Molán J, Binz U and Wendt G (1990) Münch. Med. Wochenschr. 132 (Suppl. I): 18–20.
4. Fischer EK, Heim M, Möller HJ, Uebelhack R, Wolfersdorf M, Binz U and Wendt G (1990) Münch. Med. Wochenschr. 132 (Suppl. I): 21–24.
5. Da Prada M, Zürcher G, Wüthrich I and Haefely WE (1988) J. Neural Transm. 26 (Suppl.): 31.

Biological Psychiatry, Volume 1. G. Racagni et al., editors.

Evaluation of brofaromine in geriatric depressed patients

P.A.F. Jansen and P.M.J. Haffmans

Geriatric Department, Psychiatric Centre Bloemendaal, P.O. Box 53002, 2505 AA, The Hague, The Netherlands

Introduction

Depression is the most common psychiatric disorder in elderly patients aged 60–80 years [1]. Prevalence rates range from 2 to 18% [2]. Diagnosis is sometimes difficult; symptoms of depression may be less prominent and atypical features can predominate. Depressive symptoms may be attributed to co-existent physical disease. Otherwise somatic diseases present sometimes with symptoms of depression.

In the depressed geriatric patient a thorough physical, neurological and psychiatric examination as well as blood analysis is therefore warranted.

Antidepressant treatment is more difficult in the elderly because adverse events are less tolerated and more severe. Drugs of first choice are antidepressants like nortriptyline and trazodone with little chance for orthostatic hypotension and anticholinergic side-effects. Lithium addition in elderly depressed patients may be of value [3]. Serious side-effects, however, should be taken into account.

In the Netherlands electroconvulsive therapy is not general accepted and only a few patients are treated with it each year. The need for an alternative remains. Monoamine-oxidase (MAO)-inhibitors have proven to be powerful antidepressants, in the elderly also. However, these drugs result in severe side-effects and interactions with drugs and food. The use of the classical MAO-inhibitors is therefore limited. With the development of a new class of selective and reversible MAO-A inhibitors an alternative may be found [4,5]. We performed an open study with brofaromine in geriatric inpatients with major depression, resistant to cyclic antidepressants.

Patients and Methods

After an informed consent procedure 13 patients with major depression according to DSM III-R entered the study. For inclusion a score of ≥18 points on the Hamilton Rating Scale for Depression (HRSD; 17 items) was required. All patients were still depressed after treatment with a cyclic antidepressant in a dosage of at least 75 mg/day during at least 4 weeks. After a wash-out period of 1 week brofaromine was started in a dose of 25 mg twice daily. In case of no or insufficient response, the brofaromine dose was increased on day 8 and 15 to 50 mg and 75 mg twice daily respectively. The treatment period was 4 weeks. Pulse rate and blood pressure were checked 3 times a week; weight, ECG and laboratory assessments at weekly intervals. A 48-h ECG-registration (Holter) was performed at the end of the wash-out period and in the third week of the treatment period. The efficacy and tolerability were assessed with HRSD and the side-effects and symptoms list. Response was defined as a decrease of 50% or more of the HRSD score.

Results

At the end of the wash-out period one patient recovered completely. The remaining group consisted of 9 women and 3 men with mean age 76.5 (range 67–88) years. Three patients dropped out before the end of the treatment period: 1 because of a pneumonia, 1 because of severe orthostatic hypotension and 1 because of addition of unallowed medication. All other patients were treated with a brofaromine dose of 75 mg twice daily at day 28. Two patients recovered completely, 2 had a moderate response and 5 a poor response.

As side-effects, severe orthostatic hypotension was seen in 1 patient. In the wash-out period, blood pressure was 130/70 mmHg in the recumbent and standing position in this patient. With a dosage of 75 mg brofaromine twice daily, blood pressure was 105/55 mmHg recumbent and 70/45 mmHg at standing measured after 1 min. Pulse frequency increased from 76 to 92 beats per min. The patient complained of severe dizziness. Three days after cessation of brofaromine, blood pressure was 110/60 mmHg recumbent and 100/60 mmHg at standing; dizziness disappeared. In 2 other patients, mild and transient orthostatic hypotension was found. Sleep disturbances hardly occurred. Brofaromine had no significant effects on weight and no significant changes occurred in various laboratory and ECG-parameters.

In 11 patients Holter-monitoring could be analysed. All patients showed a sinus-rhythm. In 3 patients a consistent decrease of heart rate was seen during the treatment period. In all patients supraventricular extrasystoles were seen, ventricular extrasystoles were present in 7 patients and doublets in 6. No significant differences could be detected between the baseline and treatment values. Supraventricular tachycardia occurred in 9 patients. In 1 patient a significant 10-fold decrease and in another a significant 20-fold increase was seen during brofaromine treatment. No relation with concomitant conditions were present. Ventricular tachycardia was seen in 3 patients at the baseline phase and did not change during treatment with brofaromine.

Discussion

We performed an open study in a few geriatric severely depressed inpatients, all resistant to cyclic antidepressants. No definite conclusions can be drawn about efficacy. In general brofaromine was well tolerated, although orthostatic hypo-

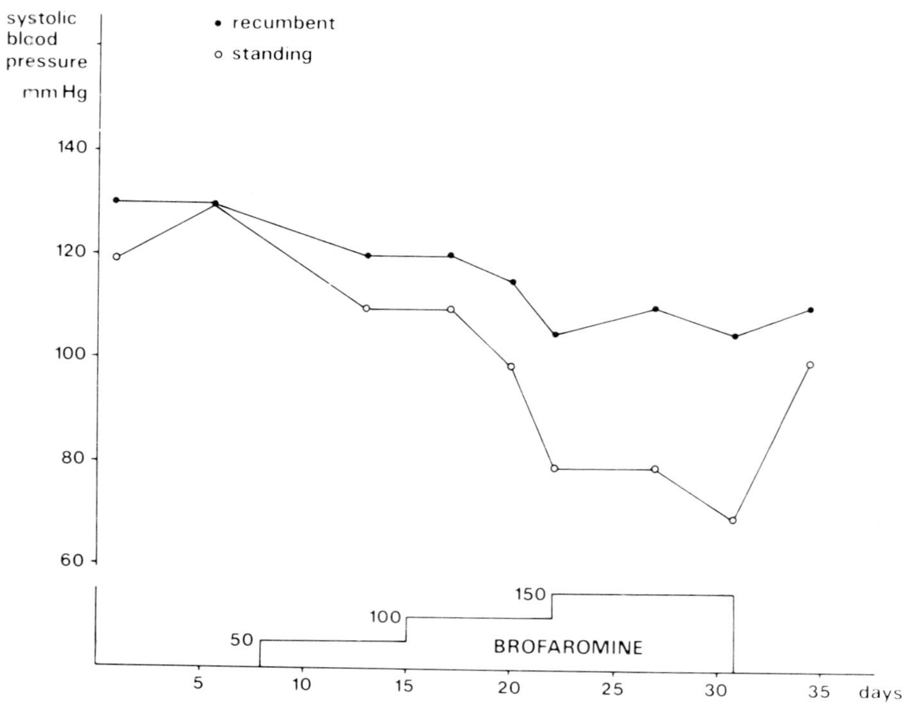

Fig. 1.

tension was found to be a serious side-effect in 1 case. During 48 h ECG-registration, 1 out of 11 patients showed a significant increase of supraventricular tachycardia periods, which maybe defined as an arrhythmogenic effect. The patient did not report any complaints during this period. In all other patients no arrhythmogenic effects of brofaromine could be detected.

References

1. Georgotas A (1983) Age Ageing 12: 1–10.
2. Blazer D (1989) N. Engl. J. Med. 320: 164–166.
3. Marwijk van HWJ, Bekker FM, Nolen WA, Jansen PAF, Nieuwkerk van JF and Hop WCJ (1990) J. Affective Disord. 20: 217–223.
4. Snaith JA and Knaevelsrod OP (1991) Efficacy and safety of brofaromine, a reversible inhibitor of monoamine-oxidase-A versus imipramine in elderly depressed out-patients. Abstr. 5th World Congress of Biological Psychiatry, Florence.
5. Versiani M, Nardi AE, Figueira ILV and Stabl M (1990) Acta Psychiatr. Scand. (Suppl.) 360: 24–28.

Biological Psychiatry, Volume 1. G. Racagni et al., editors.

New findings in child psychiatry

Gerhardt Nissen

Klinik und Poliklinik für Kinder- und Jugendpsychiatrie, Julius-Maximilians-Universität Würzburg, Füchsleinstr. 15, D-8700 Würzburg, Germany

Children and adolescents should only be given psychopharmaca, as indeed is the case for all medicaments, after stipulated particularly strict measures. However, the prejudice that we sometimes encounter of never giving children psychopharmaca, if they are suffering from a psychic illness, would be unintentionally inhuman. Beside that, however, there is also the danger of not recognising schizophrenic or affective psychoses among children or, as occasionally happens, of intentionally avoiding this diagnosis. By diagnostic labelling a prognosis is of course not improved but continues to deteriorate, because no suitable therapy has been introduced. Nobody, neither opponents nor advocates, holds the opinion that chemical substances can solve family conflicts or social crises. The question of whether psychopharmaca are causally effective or not is also controversial. However, it is of no doubt that among children and adolescents there are also indications with unbeatably high rates of improvement by psychotropic substances. From this point of view, psychopharmaca are not works of the devil but rather those which condemn psychopharmaca.

The chemical substances that are at our disposal today have a wide effective range. At the experimental stage, it is often not known whether the desired main effect is only an undesirable side-effect or vice-versa. Desirable or undesirable effects are often opposed and contribute to the fact that medicaments are not lightly prescribed. Yet, whoever ignores the clearly favourable effect of certain psychopharmaca, such as in the case of severe hyperkinetic syndromes, depressive or paranoid illness, would act just like a doctor, who rejects the therapy for bacterial encephalitis by pointing out that because of possible side-effects, the treatment of a child could on principle not be considered.

In the last decade there has also been a gradual paradigmatic change in child and juvenile psychiatry after the dominating causal genetic and therapeutic concepts had not fulfilled the expectations that had been placed in them. It became clear that a considerable biological defect was not only present with regard to the normal psychic development of the child (such as development-dependent changes in neurochemical metabolic processes), but also for psychic disorders in childhood and an age and development-specific psychopharmacology. Almost all clinical findings of the effect-bases of psychopharmaca and their pharmacokinetics, pharmacogenetics, pharmacodynamics, receptor behaviour of and towards psychopharmaca etc. are based on research on adults. For the clinic and pediatric practice that does not have age-specific metabolic research on physical illnesses at its disposal, this would mean that they would be forced to adopt the findings in adult medicine without testing them. Unfortunately, this signifies the actual situation in which child and adolescent psychiatry lies at present, with regard to the neurochemical and psychopharmacological research.

The existing accounts should convey an impression of the use of specifically effective known and new psychopharmaca among children with psychic disorders. The lecturers are scientists who for many years have tried to find precise indications and to reveal the effect-mechanisms of psychotropic medicaments in children, in particular in illnesses that have proved refractory towards other therapeutic methods. These experts and their colleagues not only dispose of special experience in medicamentous and non-medicamentous treatment: they know that with regard to the further psychic and physical development of the child, everything must be omitted that could possibly impede this process. We must not only consider acute and direct side-effects but also the indirectly caused disorders in further development. For these and other manifest reasons it is an urgent task for the future to create the necessary conditions for an independent biological child and adolescent psychiatry, that besides a condition-free basic research should clarify urgent child and adolescent specific problems in psychopharmacology. A start to this has been made in recent years.

Biological Psychiatry, Volume 1. G. Racagni et al., editors.

Psychopharmacological treatment of stuttering in children

A. Rothenberger[1], H. Johannsen[2], H. Schulze[2] and H. Amorosa[3]

[1]Central Institute of Mental Health, Child and Adolescent Psychiatry, 0-6800 Mannheim 1; [2]University of Ulm, Phoniatric, 0-7900 Ulm; and [3]Max-Planck-Institute of Psychiatry, 0-8000 Munich 40, Germany

Objectives

The moment of stuttering can be viewed, at least partially as a CNS disorder of movement regulation [1,2]. It is assumed that the automatic feedback loops of motor timing during speech exceed their limits of variability. This may disturb the system of articulation and thus interfere with fluent speech, leading either to oscillations or standstill – especially, if there is not enough capacity for voluntary and controlled speech sequencing available to compensate this deficit [3]. Thus, we initiated a study with the D_2-blocker tiapride, since our clinical experience suggested that this drug may allow a child to better tune his movement sequences during speech.

Method

Thirteen children of normal intelligence with chronic stuttering participated in a 20-week open controlled treatment program with tiapride (Fig. 1), including evaluation of psychopathology by parent questionnaires (e.g. CBCL) and speech performance (parent ratings, Stuttering Severity Index on the basis of video rating, phonetic-sonagraphic analyses of speech probes). Eleven children completed the trial (8 boys, 3 girls, mean age 13.6 years, range 10–17 years).

Preliminary results

There were only few side-effects of the drug (slight fatigue in 1 child, transient amenorrhea in another, slight and transient elevation of liver phosphatase in 3 children). Group data are presented in Tables 1 and 2. Case examples can be seen in Figs. 2 and 3. Figure 2 reflects a tendency of the whole group. Concerning sonagraphic data of voice onset time (VOT) and length of the syllables /tá ta/ there were no significant differences, either between the different points of time of investigation or the 2 syllables. So far, spectrograms for the vowel /a/ of only 1 boy could be evaluated (Fig. 3) and showed a positive drug effect.

```
                                         Tiapride
        Baseline            Phase 1                 Phase 2                 Monitoring
/------------/----------------/-----------------/---------------/
 (no treatment)  (low dose; 3mg/kg)  (high dose; 10mg/kg)    (no treatment)

    1 W     1 W            6 W                    6 W                  6 W
/-----/------/----------------/-----------------/---------------/
To/0   To/1    To/2                    T1                       T2                    T3

CBCL                              CBCL                 CBCL                 CBCL
Conners       Conners             Conners              Conners              Conners
F-scales                          F-scales             F-scales             F-scales
PRS           PRS                 PRS                  PRS                  PRS
SSI           SSI                 SSI                  SSI                  SSI
SPS           SPS                 SPS                  SPS                  SPS
```

CBCL: Child Behavior Checklist
Conners: Conners scale for hyperkinetic behavior
F-scales: Frontal lobe functioning scales
PRS: Parent Rating Stuttering
SSI: Stuttering Severity Index
SPS: Speech Probes Sonagrams
W: Duration in weeks
T: points of time of investigation

Fig. 1. Stuttering and tiapride (nil = 10–17 years) Design of the study.

Table 1. Psychopathology of children with chronic stuttering at different points of time of investigation (n= 11; mean values). In addition the values of a normal control group (matched for age and sex) are given (Norm.). IC: Impulse control

Parameter	Point in time					Norm.
	T_0	T_1	T_2	T_3	*P*-value[a]	
CBCL (T-value)						
Total score	59.9	55.4	58.0	53.5	*	50.9
Externalizing	60.0	57.9	60.5	56.0	T	51.5
Internalizing	59.0	53.4	57.4	51.5	T	50.7
Conners (score; max. 33)	11.8	10.0	11.1	7.2	N.S.	3.9
F-scales (% deficit)						
Sequential planning	31.0	18.4	18.0	26.2	N.S.	17.1
Cognitive IC	30.5	18.8	18.3	23.5	N.S.	15.7
Emotional IC	38.5	32.8	30.8	36.0	N.S.	23.2
Cognitive flexibility	37.2	30.7	31.5	36.2	N.S.	22.7
Speech control	39.5	33.8	32.8	35.2	N.S.	14.0

[a]Friedman rank variance analyses for patient data; *: $P < 0.05$; T: $P < 0.10$. In general, values of the control group differ significantly from stutterers (Mann-Whitney U-tests).

Table 2. Results of global stuttering in the Stuttering Severity Index (% of non-fluent syllables). So far: n = 6; mean values (standard deviations)

Situation	Points in time			
	$T_{0/2}$	T_1	T_2	T_3
Reading	16.8 (13.2)	11.0 (8.4)	7.6[a] (5.6)	14.0[b] (10.6)
Describing picture	24.5 (11.5)	23.3 (14.0)	17.0[c] (8.0)	22.5[c] (14.0)
Speaking spontaneously	20.4 (10.8)	17.0 (9.2)	13.6[c] (5.2)	21.2[c] (10.4)

Wilcoxon-test: T_0 vs. T_2 (positive drug effect); T_2 vs. T_3 (rebound effect); [a] $P \leq 0.05$; [b] $P \leq 0.10$. ;[c] $P \leq 0.22$.

Discussion

There is a long history of efforts to improve the speech of chronic and severe stutterers with pharmacological agents. However, adequately controlled clinical trials have almost always shown such treatments to be largely ineffective or to produce intolerable side-effects. On the other hand, there may be some help for stutterers by certain drugs, but the compliance of the patients over longer periods seems to be rather poor [4]. Nonetheless, as seen in Brady's and our study, some of the stutterers decided to continue with the medication. Thus, a psychopharmacological treatment of severe chronic stuttering seems only to be useful as 1 component (probably limited over time) within a broad program of speech training and psychosocial support. Our preliminary results of an open controlled study with tiapride suggest that this agent could be helpful within such a context. Tiapride was found to be superior to no medication (before and after drug phase) and tended to be more effective in higher vs. lower dosage mainly with the reading measure. This is in concordance with the double-blind data of Brady et al. [4] for verapamil. To explain our findings, we assume that tiapride may provide the stuttering patient with a better motor control, which implicates the supplementary motor area [1,3],

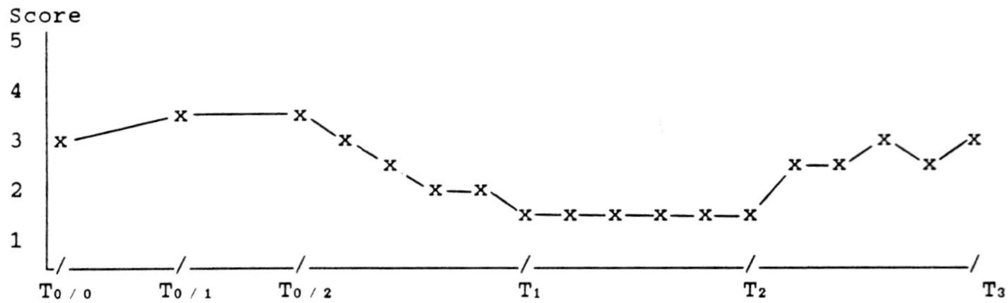

Fig. 2. Boy (12.8 years) with severe chronic stuttering. Parent rating of stuttering severity in daily situations (PRS). Each value represents global impression of 1 week of observation on a scale from 1 (no disfluency) to 6 (very high rate of disfluency). Low scores while taking tiapride (T_0 vs. T_1/T_2) and rebound effect (T_2 vs. T_3) can be seen.

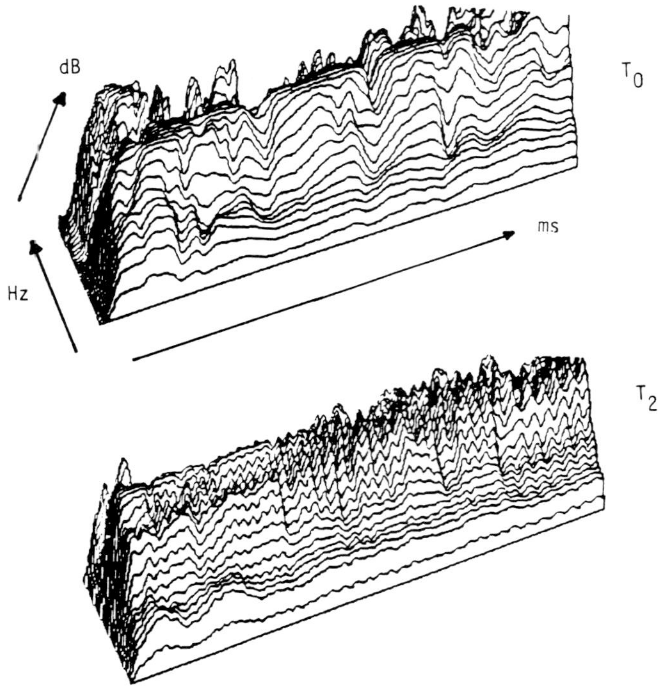

Fig. 3. Boy, 17 years old, severe chronic stuttering. Three-dimensional representation of 2 wide band spectrograms (duration 2 s, Formant 1 and 2, set of 400 256-point FFTs extending over 8 ms each) of the vowel /a/, which had to be produced continuously over a period of 5 s. The reduced variability of the amplitudes during medication (T_0 vs. T_2) indicates that the respiration-guided movements of the vocal cords were more stable with tiapride. T_0: no medication T_2: 10 mg/kg of tiapride.

by reducing the variability of cortical-subcortical tuning of motor timing/sequencing during speech and therefore allowing the patient to increase speech fluency. Unfortunately, our data cannot exclude the possibility that during spontaneous speech emotional and cognitive interferences, which are obviously higher in stutterers than in normals, may reduce the benefit of drug treatment.

Acknowledgements

Supported by a grant from Schürholz Arzneimittel, Munich, Germany. Spectrographic evaluations with the assistance of Prof. Dr. Eric Keller, Signalyze-TM, Neuchâtel, Switzerland.

References

1. Webster WG (1988) Brain Lang. 33: 226–244.
2. Johannsen HS and Schulze H (1990) In: Rothenberger A (ed.) Brain and Behaviour in Child Psychiatry. Springer, Berlin, pp. 190–204.
3. Rothenberger A (1990) In: Rothenberger A (ed.) Brain and Behaviour in Child Psychiatry. Springer, Berlin, pp. 34–58.
4. Brady JP, Price TRP, McAllister TW and Dietrich K (1989) Biol. Psychiatry 25: 626–630.

Biological Psychiatry, Volume 1. G. Racagni et al., editors.

Pharmacotherapy of conduct disorders in children and adolescents

Jovan G. Simeon

Conduct disorders (CD) (disruptive behaviors) are a major public health concern due to their high prevalence, chronicity, poor long-term outcome and cost to society. No single treatment modality specific to CD has been shown to be effective, probably because these conditions are not a true diagnostic entity, but rather heterogenous conditions associated with a variety of complex biological, family and social factors. Certain psychotropic drugs (such as lithium, stimulants, antidepressants, antipsychotics, propranolol, clonidine) are useful for some patients, but not for others. World-wide there are large differences in the percentage (from zero to 80%) of CD children receiving a variety of drugs [1].

The role of psychostimulants in the therapy of CD has been a controversial issue, and the data inconclusive. To investigate the efficacy of methylphenidate in boys with conduct disorders (CD) in contrast to those with attention deficit hyperactivity disorders (ADHD), differences between responders and nonresponders and predictors of response, a placebo controlled cross-over study was undertaken in boys 7.4 to 12.7 years old (mean 10.1 years) [2]. Of 83 patients, 75 completed the study: (ADHD 39; CD 36). All CD patients also had histories and DSM III-R symptoms of ADHD. The 10-week study design consisted of 2 weeks pre-drug placebo, and methylphenidate and placebo therapy four weeks each. The results (Table 1) indicate that three-quarters of both ADHD and CD patients showed marked or moderate clinical global improvement with methylphenidate.

Marked improvements, however, were 2.7 times greater for the ADHD than for the CD groups. In contrast, with placebo only 13% of ADHD and 30% of CD patients showed marked or moderate improvements. As compared to admission, about one-half of ADHD and one-third of CD patients showed no change after

Table 1. Percent of patients showing clinical global change compared to admission

		Very much improved	Much improved	Minimally improved	No change	Worse	Total
MPH	ADHD	46	28	18	5	3	100
4 weeks	CD	17	56	22	6	–	101
Placebo	ADHD	5	8	26	51	10	100
4 weeks	CD	8	22	25	31	14	100

placebo therapy. These findings clearly indicate that: 1) methylphenidate has a significant therapeutic effect not only in ADHD patients, but also in those with CD, though the effect is greater in the former group; and 2) psychosocial factors (social learning) play a greater role in the treatment of CD patients than in those with ADHD. Following the discontinuation of methylphenidate, significant clinical deterioration (rebound) to levels worse than those at baseline was evident in about 12% of all the patients after 4 weeks of placebo therapy. This rebound was more marked during the first and second weeks after methylphenidate discontinuation. These findings indicate the importance of a comprehensive approach – pharmacotherapy and psychosocial interventions – the former more evident with ADHD, the latter with CD. Pharmaco-EEG investigations demonstrated statistically significant effects after single dosages as well as chronic administration of methylphenidate; δ reduction and α augmentation was related to behavioral improvement in both ADHD and CD patients [2].

In ongoing clinical trials, the therapeutic efficacy of buspirone has been investigated in chronic adolescent psychiatric patients with various diagnoses. These adolescents had shown partial or no clinical response to prior therapies, including pharmacotherapy. Thirteen adolescents 12 to 20 years old (mean, 16 years), with diagnoses of attention deficit and/or conduct disorders (n = 4), anxiety and/or depressive disorders (n = 5), obsessive-compulsive disorders (n = 2), and psychosis (n = 2), received buspirone alone or in combination with other drugs in daily dosages from 10 to 40 mg (mean 25 mg) from one to four months (mean 2.5 months). With the addition of buspirone, clinical global improvement was marked in seven cases, moderate in three, mild in two and not at all in one. Regardless of diagnosis the greatest improvement occurred in mood (n = 9), anxiety (n = 6), social interaction (n = 6) sleep (n = 4), aggression (n = 3), concentration (n = 3) and irritability (n = 1). These preliminary single case trials suggest the usefulness of buspirone in the treatment of various adolescent psychiatric disorders including conduct disorders, and controlled trials with buspirone are recommended.

These findings, as well as those of a large number of drug trials in conduct disorders suggest that a more useful and rational approach to the pharmacotherapy of CD should focus on more clearly defined dysfunctions and symptoms related to temperament, impulsivity, aggression, mood, affect, anxiety, cognition, learning etc., independent of diagnosis.

References

1. Simeon JG and Wiggins DM (1990) Childhood disruptive behaviours – world wide investigation. In: Stefanis CN, Soldatos CR and Rabavilas AD (eds.) Psychiatry: A World Perspective, Vol. I. Elsevier Science Publishers B.V., (Biomedical Division), Amsterdam.
2. Simeon JG, Ferguson HB, Knott VJ, Davidson SI, Dubois C and Wiggins D (1991) Investigation of methylphenidate effect and predictors in attention deficit and conduct disorders (in preparation).

Biological Psychiatry, Volume 1. G. Racagni et al., editors.

Moclobemide, a new MAO-inhibitor in hyperkinetic children

G.E. Trott, H.J. Friese, M. Menzel and G. Nissen

Hospital for Child and Adolescent Psychiatry of the University of Würzburg, Füchsleinstraße 15, D-8700 Würzburg, Germany

Recently research results have shown evidence of a "mono-amino-oxidase hypothesis" for ADHD [1,2]. Cloriglyne, a MAO-A inhibitor, was given by Zametkin [3] at NIMH to 6 children, tranylcypromine, a MAO-A and B blocker to 8 children and deprenyl, a MAO-B blocker to 14 children. Already after a few days the children who had been treated with cloriglyne and tranylcypromine showed dramatic improvement, whereas the children treated with deprenyl hardly showed any change.

The new selective MAO-A blocker Ro 11-1163 moclobemide has proved to be very effective in the former studies among adult patients and with a low rate of side-effects compared to the classic drugs. Due to the latter aspect our aim was to test the effectiveness of the substance among children and adolescents.

After gaining the consent of the control-register of the Ethics Commission of the University of Würzburg, in a 4-week study we examined children aged between 6–14 years among whom the criteria ADHD according to DSM III-R were present. Of course the principles of the Declarations of Helsinki kept in line with the addenda of Tokyo and Venice and the patients and their parents were extensively informed.

Initially we gave moclobemide after a 3-day placebo phase with 100 mg corresponding to 2.3 mg/kg up to 5 mg/kg weight, distributed in 2 doses (07.00 and 13.00 h). The dose was increased after 8 and 14 days by 50 mg to 200 mg. Besides regular internal and neurological control examinations with blood chemical analyses, ECG and EEG, we carried out a quantitative EEG analysis (brain-mapping, CATEEM system, 10/20 system, real time-on-line, test with eyes closed for 15 min each, 16 channel-digitalisation, interpolation and finally "fast Fourier transformation" on 99 points from 1–35 Hz) at the beginning and end of the treatment.

For the evaluation of the therapeutic efficacy at the beginning of the treatment, after the placebo-phase and then weekly intervals, we followed the points on the Conners Scale (parents and teachers), Clinical Global Impression (CGI) as well as Dose Record and Treatment Emergence Symptom Scale (DOTES). The neuropsychological running examinations comprised the d 2 test or rather DLKG among children under 9 years as well as the neuropsychological test-battery with the computer-based instrument Cognitrone.

Up to now we have treated 17 patients (16 male, 1 female) with a mean age of 9.1 years. All patients had been previously treated with methylphenidate (ritalin) (4–80 weeks) and had been drug-free for at least 10 days.

The use of methylphenidate was stopped among these patients because of undesirable side-effects such as sleeping problems (n = 9), depressive moods (n = 5), tics (n = 1) or ineffectiveness (n = 2).

The 4-week term of treatment was observed in 17 patients; 1 patient dropped out after 3 weeks due to low therapeutic effectiveness on the request of the parents. All the patients found the medication agreable to take. Only in the case of 2 patients in the first week, slight unspecific gastrointestinal complaints occurred. The ECG-results showed no pathological findings before or after the treatment.

As considerable parameters for the assessment of therapeutic effectiveness the Conners Scale of parents and teachers were included.

Among the 11 outpatients and 6 inpatients on day 0 in the abbreviated Conners Scale [4] there was an average score of 19.2 points (S.D. ± 4.0) that decreased after 28 days to 11.8 (S.D. ± 4.6). The improvement was statistically significant ($P < 0.001$).

An analysis of the single items of the Conners Scale parents among outpatients reveals that these were described as less whiny (Item 8), more tolerant of frustration (Item 7) and less restless (Item 5). The impulsive behaviour (Item 2) and unrest (Item 1) receded at almost the same rate.

The CGI brought a recession of 7.05 = seriously ill to 5.1 (S.D. ± 0.65) = moderately ill. The change in condition was assessed as "much better" (3.4) (S.D. ± 0.9), the therapeutic efficacy as a clear improvement with particular remission of the symptoms.

In the concentration test on d 2 an increase was shown from the percentage-rating 28.9 (S.D. ± 26.2) to percentage-rating 85 (S.D. ± 35) after 28 days. The increase was significant ($P < 0.001$).

In a computer-based process to objectively assess attentiveness and memory function among the 14 patients examined here, there was also a significant decrease ($P < 0.004$) in the discrimination time from 245 ms (S.D. ± 46.8) to 194 ms (S.D. ± 48.1) and in the recognition time from 103.8 (S.D. ± 31.3) to 92.4 (S.D. ± 15.8). The number of errors was reduced ($P < 0.05$) from 9.3 (S.D. ± 3.4) to 6.3 (S.D. ± 3.7).

By means of brain-mapping 8 patients before treatment and 6 patients on day 0 and on the 28th day of treatment could be examined. With the tests of 15 min each, a maximum of δ-activity above the frontal sectors could be found among 8 patients. Above the frontal electrodes (F3 – F8) with reference to the total δ-activity an average frontal result of 149% could be found. After 28 days under medication the relative δ-activity among 3 of 6 patients decreased on average by 35%.

The preliminary results show that the therapy with moclobemide may offer an acceptable alternative to the classical stimulant-treatment. At the same time the efficiency of moclobemide enables confirmation of the "mono-amino-oxidase-hypothesis" of the hyperkinetic syndrome, as there is no amphetamine-like activity in moclobemide [5].

References

1. Brown GL, Murphy DL, Langer DH, Ebert MH, Post RM and Bunney WE (1984) Monamine Enzymes in Hyperactivity: Response to d-Amphetamine. Paper presented at the Annual Meeting of the American Academy of Child Psychiatry, Toronto.
2. Shekim WO, Bylund DB and Alexon J (1986) Psychiatr. Res. 18: 179–188.
3. Zametkin A, Rapoport JL, Murphy DL, Linnoila M and Ismond D (1985) Arch. Gen. Psychiatry 42(10): 962–966.
4. Conners CK (1969) Am. J. Psychiatry 126: 884–888.
5. Porsolt RD, Pawelec C, Roux S and Jalfre M (1984) Neuropharmacology 23: 566–573.

Schizophrenia and related disorders: Clinical and biological studies

Biological Psychiatry, Volume 1. G. Racagni et al., editors.

Schizophrenia: Gender and age
Why is the onset of schizophrenia later in women?

Heinz Häfner, Stephan Behrens, Jean de Vry and Wagner F. Gattaz
Central Institute of Mental Health, P.O. Box 122120, 6800 Mannheim 1, Germany

Introduction

The numerous studies of the influence of gender and age on the onset of schizophrenia were based on first admissions or operationalized estimates of onset, which may explain the considerable variation in their results. The influence of gender and age on symptomatology and course of schizophrenia prior to first admission has not yet been systematically investigated.

Material and Methods

Our representative sample included all 392 first hospital admissions for schizophrenia – broad definition – in a 2-year period, drawn from a population of 1.5 million. We assessed the true onset and the early patterns of course of the psychoses. We operationally defined "onset" as age: 1) at the manifestation of the first-ever symptom of a mental disorder; 2) at the first manifestation of a characteristic schizophrenic symptom; and 3) at the first hospital admission. For assessing "onset" we developed and used a semistructured patient interview schedule, "IRAOS", and additionally supplemented the patients' statements by an interview with the closest relative and by the collection of objective data.

Results

Starting out from the occurrence of the earliest sign of a mental disorder, males show an early steep increase and reach their maximum value between 15 and 24 years of age. Under the age of 25 two-thirds of all male schizophrenics have become manifest. Beyond this age, first onset rates for males rapidly and monotonously decrease towards zero. Females show a slower increase and reach a flat peak in the age-group 20–29 years. After a rapid decrease, a second smaller peak is observed in the age-group 45–49 years, covering about 15% of female first-onset schizophrenia.

Independent of the operational definition of onset, the mean age at onset reveals a significant gender difference of 3.2 to 3.9 years. However, the cumulative

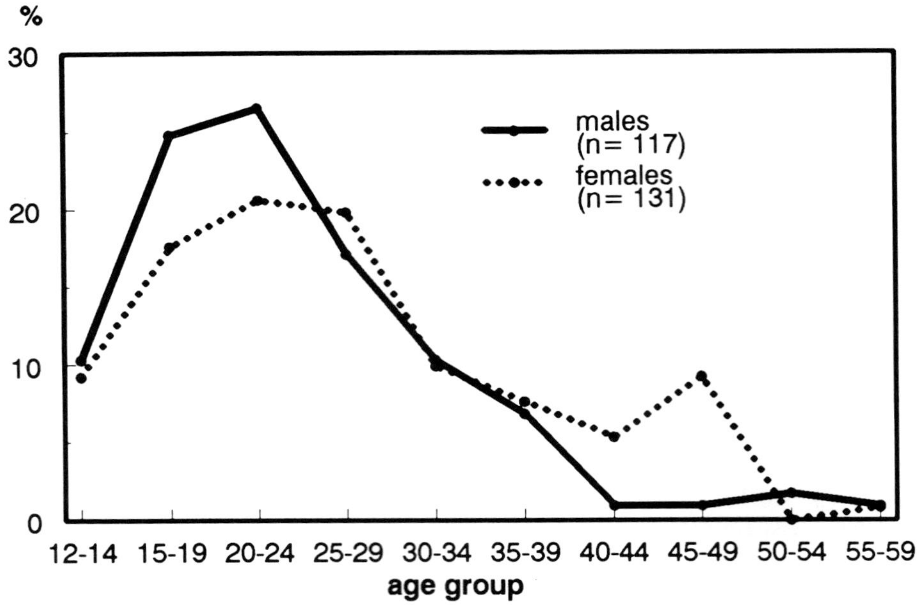

Fig. 1. Sex-specific age distribution at time of earliest signs of the psychosis (based on the first sign of a mental disorder).

lifetime risk up to the age of 60 years is virtually the same for both sexes, both for a restrictive and a broad definition of schizophrenia.

After having excluded competitive explanations, we tested the hypothesis: estradiol enhances the vulnerability threshold for schizophrenia by acting as an early structural effect on the development of the brain. From puberty to menopause this effect is enhanced by a functional effect of estrogen. We examined the effect of estradiol (17-β-E_2) on dopamine-induced behaviour in an animal model consisting of three groups of neonatal and adult Wistar rats, two groups of which were ovariectomized and received estrogen or placebo injections and implants, the third group being sham-ovariectomized and placebo-treated.

Estradiol significantly reduced both dopamine-agonist- and dopamine-antagonist-induced behaviour. Effects were stronger in neonatal rats. Since estradiol caused the DA receptor affinity for sulperid to be 2.8 times lower, we assumed that the behavioural changes due to estradiol were accounted for by a down-regulation of the DA_2 receptor sensitivity. The delay in the onset of female schizophrenia may therefore be due to the effects of estrogens. Those females with a predisposition to schizophrenia who did not fall ill until menopause, account for the second peak of first onsets to be attributed to the dropping of the estrogen level and, as a result, the lowering of the vulnerability threshold.

The comparison of symptomatology between the sexes at the time of first admission, based on 38 CATEGO syndromes, revealed only few significant differences. All of them are more likely to be ascribed to variations in illness behaviour – e.g. frequent obsessive symptoms, alcohol abuse and self-neglect in males, social overadjustment in females – than to the core symptom of schizophrenia itself. A comparison over three age-groups (12–24, 25–34, 35–39 years) did not show any differences in negative symptoms, whereas in positive symptoms all of the significant differences found were accounted for by the influence of the personality development on the differentiation and the complexity of symptoms. An analysis at the single-item level confirmed this result.

Non-characteristic symptoms like anxiety and depressiveness had their maximum value in the same age-groups as reported in the studies of the total population.

The early patterns of the course of the psychosis are also surprisingly equal in both sexes and in the age-groups. The predominance of negative symptoms and their prolonged course in females compared to males at the age of 35 and over at onset contradicts traditional assumptions.

Our findings support the vulnerability hypothesis under the assumption that within certain limits neurohormones have an effect on the vulnerability threshold over lifetime. They also support the assumption of a relative uniform, almost age- and sex-invariant reaction pattern of schizophrenia, the etiology of which is heterogeneous, but not heterosomal. Dichotomous disease concepts of schizophrenia scarcely tally with our findings.

Biological Psychiatry, Volume 1. G. Racagni et al., editors.

Molecular genetics and the epidemiology of schizophrenia: Emerging research issues

Peter McGuffin

Department of Psychological Medicine, University of Wales College of Medicine, Heath Park, Cardiff CF4 4XN, U.K.

Schizophrenia as a complex phenotype

There is widespread acceptance of the idea that schizophrenia has a genetic basis. This view, once unfashionable because of its supposed pessimistic determinism, has now prevailed because of the overwhelming amount of supporting evidence from "old" genetics, family, twin and adoption studies [1]. In addition, the success of the "new genetics" of recombinant DNA technology in elucidating the molecular basis of various physical diseases and providing important insights into methods of prevention and treatment has meant that the science of genetics is now viewed in a much more optimistic light by most clinicians including psychiatrists. However, most of the phenotypes which have been successfully tackled so far using molecular genetic approaches have simple mendelian patterns of inheritance and include diseases such as Huntington's chorea, an autosomal dominant, Duchenne's muscular dystrophy, an X-linked recessive and cystic fibrosis, an autosomal recessive. Although none of these is rare in Western European populations, all have lifetime incidences which are very low in comparison with schizophrenia. Here the lifetime risk is about 1% and both the pattern of distribution within families and the definition of the phenotype itself are complex.

Schizophrenia, therefore, cannot be classified along with simple mendelian traits and has more in common with other comparatively high frequency diseases such as diabetes, coronary heart disease and certain common forms of familial cancer. There is evidence of genetic influences in all of these conditions but the environment probably also plays a part. Furthermore, the genes involved may reside at more than one locus and the environmental influences are likely to be multiple, playing a greater part in some cases than in others. In short, schizophrenia is one of those conditions which is almost certainly multifactorial in aetiology and it could be very misleading to approach a search for its causes as if it were a simple single factor condition.

However, this still leaves open the possibility that at least some forms of schizophrenia are transmitted via a major locus with other genes of smaller effect and/or family environmental factors also contributing to the correlation in liability between relatives.

The search for major genes

Recent studies which have applied the techniques of complex segregation analysis to family data on schizophrenia have been somewhat disappointing because they have been unable to produce convincing evidence either for or against a major gene effect [2–4]. An alternative and potentially more powerful means of detecting major gene effects is to study not just the segregation of the disease within families but the cosegregation of the disease and genetic markers, in other words to perform linkage studies. Applying linkage analysis in studies of schizophrenia usually means that the following 3 assumptions have to be made:

1. There is major gene inheritance at least in a proportion of cases.
2. Even if heterogeneity is possible in schizophrenia as a whole, within families with multiple members affected it is probable that homogeneity will be found.
3. The mode of transmission of the disease can be specified "approximately".

This last condition means that an educated guess is made after careful inspection of the pedigrees in which linkage analysis is to be performed and indeed most researchers in studying complex diseases tend to apply a range of plausible models rather than just one. This is defensible on the grounds that misspecification of the mode of transmission may bias the estimate of the recombination fraction and may even cause the researcher to overlook linkage when it exists. It will not, however, usually result in the spurious detection of linkage when linkage is not in fact present [5].

Loci of current interest

The early promise of positive findings in the HLA complex located on the short arm of chromosome 6 unfortunately was unfulfilled. The combined results of several family genetic linkage studies effectively exclude a major gene for schizophrenia from this region [6]. More recent attention has focused on 3 different parts of the genome, the so-called pseudo-autosomal region of the sex chromosomes, the D_2 dopamine receptor locus and adjacent parts of chromosome 11q and the short arm of chromosome 5, the 5q11-q13 region.

The report of linkage between a schizophrenia susceptibility gene and markers on chromosome 5q provoked particular interest [7] but unfortunately could not be replicated and combining the data across studies effectively excludes linkage in this region [8]. Despite this, researchers remain optimistic about the prospects of future positive findings and collaborative programmes have been established both in Europe and in the United States with the aim of mounting a systematic search throughout the genome. It is likely that if major genes (and not just polygenes) exist, they will be detected and localized within the next 4–5 years. It will then be a matter of applying the techniques of "reverse genetics" to elucidate the pathogenesis of the disorder.

References

1. Gottesman II and Shields J (1982) In: Schizophrenia: The Epigenetic Puzzle. Cambridge University Press.
2. Carter CL and Chung CS (1980) Psychol. Med. 8: 387–398.
3. Risch N and Baron M (1984) Am. J. Hum. Genet. 36: 1039–1059.
4. Vogler GP, Gottesman II, McGue MK and Rao DC (1990) Behav. Genet. 20: 461–472.
5. Clerget-Darpoux F, Bonaiti-Pellie C and Hochez J (1986) Biometrics 42: 393–399.
6. McGuffin P and Sturt E (1986) Hum. Hered. 36: 65–88.
7. Sherrington P, Brynjolfsson J, Petursson H, Tuddleston K, Barraclough B, Wasmuth J, Dobbs M and Gurling H (1988) Nature 336: 164–167.
8. McGuffin P, Sargeant M, Hett G, Tidmarsh S, Whatly S and Marchbanks M (1990) Am. J. Hum. Genet. 47: 524–535.

Biological Psychiatry, Volume 1. G. Racagni et al., editors.

Certain aspects of epidemiology in biological schizophrenia research

Fini Schulsinger

Institute of Population Research (formerly Psykologisk Institut), Kommunehospitalet, DK-1399 Copenhagen K, Denmark

This presentation consists of a compilation of brief descriptions from a variety of studies. The purpose is to illustrate that epidemiological thinking and methodology are indispensable in large areas of contemporary psychiatric research.

Research on etiology

In a study on the possible heredity of suicide [1], the present author was surprised to learn that results from studies of psychiatric precursors of suicide could not be replicated in a population-based sample. The most prominent studies of psychiatric suicide precursors showed that psychiatric illness was a precursor in 75–94% of retrospectively well-studied cases. When sampling cases of completed suicides from a geographically well-defined area, the author found that only 50% of the suicides ascertained had shown signs of a psychiatric condition – hospitalized as well as non-hospitalized. Only 10 years later, during an update of the original study, the present author found another study [2], which confirmed that epidemiological sampling methods resulted in a larger number of "non-psych" cases of suicide than expected. This again validated the genetic results from the first study: that "non-psych" suicide runs in families – also among the family members who were reared in non-biologically related adoptive homes since early childhood.

In another study at our institute, 207 children of schizophrenic mothers and their 104 matched controls were studied from 1962–1964 [3] and followed-up until 1989. Certain psychophysiological deviations were found in the high-risk sample at the first assessment. In a subsequently organized prospective study of children at high-risk for schizophrenia [4], these psychophysiological deviations were not replicated. This difference might have been due to Berkson's fallacy [5], insofar as the inclusion criteria in the second study also stipulated that the children should be living in non-broken homes. Mednick [6] was able to demonstrate that if the children of schizophrenic mothers in his own study [3], who grew up in a broken home were excluded from his sample, the psycho-physiological results resembled those from the second study. In other words, it is advisable to conceptualize the meaning of inclusion/exclusion criteria. The reported problems show that the price of the ideal study of non-broken family rearing results in the loss of a considerable number of *representative* cases.

A third illustration of the utilization of an epidemiological approach comes from the International Pilot Study of Schizophrenia [7]. The report on the 5-year follow-up of the original sample showed that the prognosis for schizophrenia was best within the areas studied in developing countries, e.g. India, Colombia. First and foremost, a hypothesis on the supportive and protective family networks in the mainly rural areas has to be tested. The outcome of such testing will probably be positive. However, one should be careful not to leave it at that. Other factors may contribute towards a seemingly favourable prognosis. It is generally accepted that schizophrenia with a sudden and dramatic onset has a more favourable prognosis than is the case for the more insidious and less dramatic onset types. In the developing countries, the hospitalization threshold must be very high due to the limited number of hospital beds. This may very well result in a relatively high number of admissions of the acute and dramatic onset patients who have a relatively good prognosis in most cases anyhow.

Should that be the case, it will have implications for the clinical assessment instruments. The PSE, 9th edition, which was used in the reported study, is not especially designed to discriminate between the poor prognosis and bad prognosis schizophrenias.

This section will be concluded by another example from the above-mentioned study on children at high risk from schizophrenia at our institute [3]. Over the years, the children developed in accordance with general genetic expectations into several diagnostic outcome groups [8]. As a result of a mid-way assessment in 1972–1974, half of the expected number of schizophrenias were diagnosed [9]. Machón et al. [10] found that even in this limited sample the generally assumed seasonal variation in births of future schizophrenics was confirmed. It turned out, however, that the first trimester of the year surplus came exclusively from births in Copenhagen, the metropolitan city of Denmark.

Speculations about this were eventually affected by the ever-increasing speculations about virus as an etiological agent in the development of schizophrenia. Obviously, people in a metropolitan city would have more infections those in rural areas. In a thoroughly designed and controlled study of offspring which were fetuses during the neurotoxic Asiatic influenza epidemic of 1957–1958, Mednick found [11] that there was a surplus of schizophrenics born in Helsinki after the epidemic there. The surplus came from the pregnancies which were in the second trimester during the peak period of the epidemic in Helsinki.

The results were replicated by Chris Barr et al. [12] through a study in Denmark using monthly reports on contagious diseases from county health commissioners over a 40-year period, and information from the Danish National Register of Psychiatric Hospital Admissions. A merging of these two data sets showed that each influenza epidemic peak period was accompanied by an excess number of births of future schizophrenics.

It is obvious that without an epidemiological approach in several directions (sampling, seasonal variation, epidemiology of infectious diseases, etc.), it would hardly be possible to situate the results from studies carried out with fascinating new biotechnological means at our disposal within a meaningful context.

Research on treatment

It may be worthwhile to consider the possible influence of deinstitutionalization on the assessment of psychopharmacological drugs such as neuroleptics and antidepressants. After the 1950s and 1960s, relatively few neuroleptics have been marketed. Looking back on the clinical assessments referred to by the pharmaceutical industry for approval and for marketing purposes, one may feel vaguely perplexed. Is one drug really more effective than another? Of course, a few drugs stand out as having rather few, or as having rather many unwanted side-effects. A considerable number of neuroleptics have been compared through clinical assessments with chlorpromazine. Most of them were found to be equal to chlorpromazine, but rarely better with regard to therapeutic effect.

But, how is it that neuroleptics belonging to very different chemical groups are so uniform with regard to efficacy? Is this similarity real or apparent? An elegant paper by Cohen and Cohen [13] convincingly suggests that such a similarity might be due to sampling errors, i.e. insufficient consideration of basic epidemiological principles.

Cohen and Cohen describe how the probability of including, e.g. a schizophrenic patient in a research sample is proportional to the duration of the patient's illness. A patient whose illness has lasted for 10 years is 10 times as likely to be present in the hospital as a patient whose illness has lasted for one year only. This correlation, though very logical, may not be as dramatic when the increasing deinstitutionalization is taken into consideration. Along with deinstitutionalization, there is a development of community mental health services – at least in Europe – which reduces the likelihood of hospitalization, and especially rehospitalization. This phenomenon does not invalidate the type of arguments presented by Cohen and Cohen. As long as duration of illness differs, it has to be accounted for by those methods suggested by the authors. They list an intriguing variety of other pitfalls of an epidemiological nature, all resulting in misinterpretations of findings.

In order to make a long story short, the ideal sampling for assessment of drugs – or other treatments, would be to sample on an incidence basis rather than on a prevalence basis, i.e. it is justified to aim at drug assessments on samples of new cases; but a demanding task to have a sample of new cases from a variety of sources and areas. On the other hand, it would certainly clarify the effects of the drug under assessment.

Conclusions

Epidemiology has to do with populations. In order to maximize utility of population studies, it is necessary to select the right populations. Compromises, however, are unavoidable. If they are accounted for in detail, useful results are unavoidable as well.

References

1. Schulsinger F, Kety SS and Wender PH (1979) In: Schou M and Strömgren E (eds.) Origin, Prevention and Treatment of Affective Disorders. Academic Press, London, U.K., pp. 277–287.
2. Mitterauer B and Pritz WF (1984) Wiener Med. Wochenschr. 134: 37–43.
3. Mednick AS and Schulsinger F (1965) In: Methods and Goals in Human Behavior Genetics. Academic Press, New York, U.S.A., pp. 255–295.
4. Erlenmeyer-Kimling L (1972) In: Ehrman L, Omenn GS and Caspari E (eds.) Genetics, Environment and Behaviour. Academic Press, New York, U.S.A., pp. 181–208.
5. Berkson J (1955) In: Proc. Staff Meetings Mayo Clinic 1955, pp. 319–348.
6. Mednick SA (1978) In: Wynne LC, Cromwell RL and Matthysse S (eds.) The Nature of Schizophrenia. Wiley, New York, U.S.A.
7. World Health Organization (1979) "Schizophrenia - An International Follow-Up Study." John Wiley and Sons, Chichester, U.K.
8. Schulsinger F, Mednick SA and Parnas J (1990) In: Stefanis CN, Sodatos CR and Rabavilas AD (eds.) Psychiatry: A World Perspective. Excerpta Medica, Amsterdam, The Netherlands, Vol. 2, pp. 53–65.
9. Schulsinger H (1970) Acta Psychiatr. Scand. 53: 371–386.
10. Machón RA, Mednick SA and Schulsinger F (1987) Br. J. Psychiatry 151: 122–124.
11. Mednick SA, Machón RA, Huttunen MO and Bonett D (1988) Arch. Gen. Psychiatry 45: 189–192.
12. Barr C, Mednick SA and Machón RA (1991) Exposure to influenza epidemics during gestation and adult schizophrenia: A 40-year study (submitted for publication).
13. Cohen P and Cohen J (1984) Arch. Gen. Psychiatry 41: 1178–1182.

Biological Psychiatry, Volume 1. G. Racagni et al., editors.

Long-term neuroleptic treatment of schizophrenia: A review of follow-up studies

Cesario Bellantuono

Servizio di Psicologia Medica, Istituto di Psichiatria, Università di Verona, Ospedale Policlinico, 37134 Verona, Italy

In a recent review of the literature on long-term neuroleptic (NL) treatment of schizophrenia, Tantam and McGrath [1] summarize the results of 10 discontinuation studies with follow-up of a year or more. The 1-year relapse rate in these studies varied from 41% to 87% in the untreated group and from 0% to 38% in the NL-treated group (Table 1).

The difference in the results of these trials can be, at least in part, explained taking into account that different methodological procedures have been adopted: in particular the *definition of relapse* (hospitalization, exacerbation of schizophrenic symptoms, increase in dosage etc.) and *the criteria of case selection* (diagnostic criteria, duration of previous medication exposure, when the trial is begun in the course of treatment etc.). Despite the possible differences in the methodology, on average these data provide an estimated percentage of relapse rate of 20% for drug-treated patients and 65% for patients withdrawn from NL. More information on the efficacy of long-term NL treatment derives from 3 studies with a longer follow-up period [2–4] (Table 2).

These studies indicate that about half the patients on NL will eventually relapse, although the rate of relapse declines with time. They also show the decrease in

Table 1. Relapse rates in the first year of prolonged neuroleptics compared to no active treatment

	Percentage relapse:	
	Drug	No drug
Cheung, 1981	13	62
Engelhardt et al., 1963	26	52
Hirsch et al., 1973	12	73
Hogarty et al., 1973	31	67
Johnson, 1976	21	60
Kane et al., 1982	0	41
Leff and Wing, 1971	33	83
Rifkin et al., 1977	10	87
Johnson et al., 1983	16	65
Crow et al., 1986	38	63

From: Tantam and McGrath (1989).

Table 2. Longer-term relapse and survival rates

	Percentage of subjects relapsing up to and during time period		Percentage of subjects at risk relapsing during time period	
	Drug	No drug	Drug	No drug
First year				
Hogarthy et al., 1973	31	67	31	68
Johnson, 1979	21	51	21	60
Crow et al., 1986	38	63	38	63
Second year				
Hogarty et al., 1977	48	80	25	43
Johnson, 1979	36	59	23	23
Crow et al., 1986	46	63	20	7
Third and fourth years				
Johnson, 1979	43	66	14	22

From: Tantam and McGrath (1989).

risk of relapse which occurs with time especially in patients not on NL. The convergence of relapse rates of treated and untreated patients over the course of several years has been explained by the hypothesis that neuroleptics delay, but do not prevent relapse.

Summarizing, the results of the most significant follow-up studies so far published indicate that on average: a) about half (43% to 48%) the schizophrenic patients relapse whether they are on NL or not ("non-responders"); b) about a quarter (from 20% to 40%) do not require NL treatment to prevent relapse ("good prognosis"); and c) about a quarter (from 17% to 32%) would have relapsed without medication.

A number of relevant questions concerning a maintenance programme arise from these findings. For example: how to identify patients who do not require treatment with NL (patients with a "good prognosis"); when can medication be stopped? Which dosage (standard vs. low) and NL preparation (oral vs. depot) should be preferred? How to improve the outcome of patients who, despite prolonged NL treatment, relapse ("non-responders")? Unfortunately, these and some other questions concerning the long-term NL management of schizophrenic patients are still unresolved (or at least partially resolved), so that further clinical and epidemiological investigations are needed to fully clarify this topic.

In the present paper, I wish only to present some data concerning the patients who might be considered for drug withdrawal and the possible clinical guidelines derived from these studies. Several studies have attempted to find characteristics associated with a reduced rate of relapse in withdrawal studies. The following have been identified: first illness, acute florid onset, good premorbid personality, good social adjustment, late onset in life, "low expressed emotion" in family. However, these are the characteristics of a good prognosis, irrespective of treatment. In particular the high significance of family environment in influencing the relapse rate has been shown by a series of well known publications from the MRC Social Psychiatry Unit (see [5]). Tantam and McGrath, however, underline that good prognostic characteristics should not be considered reliable predictors of patients who do not require neuroleptics.

Apparently those patients who do not relapse over a long period are candidate to stop drug-treatment, but this is not often the case, as suggested by the results of the following two studies. Denker et al. [6] selected 32 patients from 200 successfully maintained for years and especially selected to come off maintenance medication because they wished to stop: 92% relapsed in two years (81% in the first year). Wistedt [7] also found that 94% of a cohort of schizophrenic patients (well established on NL) relapsed in two years. It is clear from these studies that patients who have remained well (or stable) on NL for long time should not be considered for drug withdrawal simply because they have remained well.

Since there are no available criteria for the identification of patients who should be considered for drug withdrawal, the alternative is thus to proceed by trial and error. A rational approach in these patients, as indicated by Carpenter and Heinrich [8], could be the so-called "*targeted strategy*" which is based on careful empirical withdrawal aiming at dose reduction and intermittent use of NL as required. However, it must be stressed that this procedure is only effective when deployed within the context of a highly responsive case-management system that involves patients, their family, care-givers and general practitioners, as well as mental health professionals [9]. The targeted strategy should be avoided in a minority of patients: a) those with continuous severe psychosis worsening on drug withdrawal; and b) those whose relapses are acute and catastrophic. It seems inevitable that this method might increase the risk of relapse, but this risk has to be set against the side-effects of a prolonged NL medication which makes it an unacceptable form of treatment for many patients with schizophrenia.

According to Hirsch [10] we believe that "the social cost of relapse for a large population of schizophrenic patients does not seem high so that the venture, to follow such strategy, may be worthwhile".

References

1. Tantam D and McGrath G (1989) Int. Clin. Psychopharmacol. 4: 167–194.
2. Hogarty GE and Ulrich RF (1977) Arch. Gen. Psychiatry 34: 297–301.
3. Crow TJ, MacMillan JF, Johnson AL and Johnstone EC (1986) Br. J. Psychiatry 148: 120–127.
4. Johnson DAW (1979) Br. J. Psychiatry 135: 524–530.
5. Leff JP, Kupers L, Berkowitz R, Eberlein-Vries R and Sturgean D (1983) Psychol. Med. 13: 799–806.
6. Denker SJ, Lepp M and Malm U (1980) Acta Psychiatr. Scand. (Suppl.) 279: 64–74.
7. Wistedt B (1981) Acta Psychiatr. Scand. 64: 65–84.
8. Carpenter WT and Heinrichs DW (1983) Schizophr. Bull. 9: 34–43.
9. Falloon IRH and Shanahan NJ (1990) Br. J. Hosp. Med. 43: 62–66.
10. Hirsch SR (1986) In: Bradley PB and Hirsch SR (eds.) The Psychopharmacology and Treatment of Schizophrenia. Oxford University Press, Oxford, pp. 286–339.

Biological Psychiatry, Volume 1. G. Racagni et al., editors.

Schizophrenia and neuroleptic prescribing patterns: A survey on a representative sample of mental health services in Piedmont

C. Munizza, E. Pirfo, F. Punzo and G. Tibaldi

Centro Studi e Ricerche in Psichiatria, Ospedale Giovanni Bosco, Piazza del Donatore di Sangue 3, 10154 Turin, Italy

Introduction

Recent international research on neuroleptic (NL) prescribing patterns has revealed some phenomena which move away from previously formulated guidelines [1–3]. In particular the following have been observed: prescriptions with more than one NL (polypharmacy); high dose prescriptions, with an increased risk of short- and long-term side-effects; the use of NL in patients with neurotic and depressive disorders. Recent research carried out in Italy, besides revealing prescribing patterns that are different from those of other countries like the U.S.A., has demonstrated that the type of treatment offered to psychiatric patients is influenced by the setting, by various socio-demographic factors relating to the patients (e.g., age, education, marital status), as well as by the potency of the NL used [4–7]. The aim of this survey is to analyze the relationships between NL dosage and the socio-demographic characteristics of a group of patients with diagnoses of schizophrenia or delusional disorder (DSM III-R), who form part of a larger sample of psychiatric patients, most of them in treatment at Community Mental Health Centers (CMHC) in the region of Piedmont.

Materials and Methods

In 1990 a cross-sectional survey of patients in treatment with the psychiatric services was carried out in Piedmont. All patients, treated at inpatient or outpatient care level, during 4 index days, with a month interval (unduplicated) were included. The data presented here refer to 60 CMHC which participated in the survey; because the sample involved over 75% of the CMHC in Piedmont, it is probably highly representative. Socio-demographic and diagnostic data were collected, as well as information on the patients' psychiatric history. The type and dose of the psychotropic drugs being prescribed at the time of survey were also recorded. This survey examined patients with diagnoses of schizophrenia or delusional disorder on NL treatment (1109, 37.5% of the total at CMHC). The prescribed NL doses were converted to an estimated equivalent amount of chlorpromazine using standard potency ratio tables. The active components were then

Table 1. Characteristics of the CMHC users with DSM III-R diagnosis of schizophrenia or delusional disorder

	No.	%		No.	%
Sex			*Education (years)*		
Males	589	53.1	0–5	519	48.8
Females	520	46.9	6–8	377	35.4
			>8	168	15.8
Age (years)					
16–30	192	17.3	*Length of psychiatric history (years)*		
31–60	754	68.0	0–3	158	15.4
>60	163	14.7	4–7	190	18.5
			8–12	233	22.7
Marital status			>12	447	43.5
Not married	864	78			
Married	243	22			

subdivided into two groups: those with low to intermediate potency, and those with high potency. Chi-square statistic and multiple regression were used to evaluate the relationship between NL dose and patient characteristics.

Results

The principal results of the data analyzed are presented in Tables 1–4.

Discussion

Like other surveys which have been carried out in Italy, this one reveals that the average dose of NL prescribed by CMHC in Piedmont is not high, even though the sample only considered patients with diagnoses of schizophrenia or delusional

Table 2. Prescribing patterns

	No.	%		No.	%
No. of NL drugs			*Chlorpromazine equivalent daily dose*		
1	743	67.0	10–100 mg	383	34.5
2	305	27.5	101–200 mg	286	25.8
3 or more	61	5.5	201–300 mg	173	15.6
			301–500 mg	132	11.9
Potency			>500 mg	135	12.2
Low-intermediate	101	9.1			
High	791	71.3			
Mixed (L or I + H)	217	19.6			

Table 3. Distribution of chlorpromazine equivalent daily dose according to patient characteristics

	10–300 mg		301–600 mg		>600 mg		χ^2	DF	*P*-value
	No.	%	No.	%	No.	%			
Sex									
Males	412	69.9	109	18.5	68	11.6	24.6	2	< 0.0001
Females	430	82.7	57	11	33	6.3			
Age (years)									
16–30	133	69.3	36	18.7	23	12	16.52	4	< 0.005
31–60	567	75.2	115	15.2	72	9.6			
>60	142	87.1	15	9.2	6	3.7			
Education (years)									
0–5	413	79.6	70	13.5	36	6.9	9.16	4	= 0.057
6–8	271	71.9	62	16.4	44	11.7			
>8	124	73.8	29	17.3	15	8.9			
Marital status									
Not married	637	73.7	140	16.2	87	10.1	10.92	2	< 0.005
Married	204	83.9	25	10.3	14	5.8			
Length of psychiatric history (years)									
0–3	134	84.8	17	10.8	7	4.4	11.84	6	= 0.066
4–7	145	76.3	27	14.2	18	9.5			
8–12	178	76.4	35	15	20	8.6			
>12	321	71.8	75	16.8	51	11.4			
No. of NL drugs									
1	667	89.8	58	7.8	18	2.4	298.47	4	< 0.0001
2	164	53.8	86	28.2	55	18			
3 or more	11	18	22	36.1	28	45.1			

disorder (with elective indications for NL treatment). About 75% of the patients treated with NL receive up to 300 mg per day (the average dose for the whole sample was 267 mg of chlorpromazine equivalent). Age and, only partially, length of psychiatric history were the only patient characteristics linked to the NL dose, while the other variables (sex, education, marital status) did not seem to influence the dose prescribed, once adjusted for other factors in the linear regression analysis. Drug-related factors, NL polypharmacy, and the type of drug used, also seemed to play a major independent role in determining the amount of drug prescribed. Two or more NLs were associated in about one-third of our cases. Regarding the type of NL used, our research shows that prescriptions with low potency NL are not very frequent (9.1%), and that there is a marked prevalence in the use of high potency NL, whether on their own (73.3%) or in association with other low potency NL (19.6%). Our results also confirm that NL doses prescribed in Italy are significantly lower than those prescribed in the U.S.A., where a large number of studies have been carried out on prescribing patterns, particularly for schizophrenic patients. In order to improve prescribing habits by better preparation

Table 4. Multiple linear regression results of patient characteristics on neuroleptic daily dose

	b	S.E. of b	*t*-test	*P*-value
Sex				
Females	–20.28	20.088	–1.01	0.31
Age (years)				
16–30	140.05	39.762	3.52	<0.0005
31–60	92.61	29.217	3.17	<0.005
Education (years)				
0–5	–21.27	28.604	–0.74	0.46
6–8	11.65	29.096	0.40	0.69
Marital status				
Not married	–0.63	24.753	0.03	0.98
Length of psychiatric history (years)				
0–3	–77.28	30.958	–2.50	<0.05
4–7	–24.89	28.311	–0.88	0.37
8–12	–54.15	25.163	–2.15	<0.05
No. of NL drugs				
1	–426.20	51.191	–8.33	<0.0001
2	–295.63	44.838	–6.59	<0.0001
Potency				
Low-Int	96.35	33.304	2.89	<0.005
Mixed	188.82	34.949	5.40	<0.0001

regarding the problems linked to NL potency and to polypharmacy the following strategies might be useful in:

a) the monitoring of prescriptive habits [8,9];
b) academic detailing, or information given to the individual doctor on the scientific knowledge relating to a given drug or group of drugs, by experts independent of the pharmaceutical market;
c) the elaboration, starting with research similar to that presented here, of guidelines agreed on at consensus conferences that involve experts as well as staff working in the CMHC of a given area.

References

1. Carpenter WT and Heinrichs DW (1983) Schizophr. Bull. 9: 533–541.
2. Kane JM (1983) Schizophr. Bull. 9: 528–531.
3. Baldessarini RJ and Davis JM (1980) Psychiatr. Res. 3: 115–122.
4. Muscettola G, Casiello M, Bollini P, Sebastiani G, Pampallona S and Tognoni G (1987) Acta Psychiatr. Scand. 75: 55–61.
5. Muscettola G, Bollini P and Pampallona S (1990) Factors associated with neuroleptic prescribing patterns in Italian mental health services. Drug Intell. Clin. Pharm. (in press).

6. Hemminki E (1975) Soc. Sci. Med. 9: 111–121.
7. Baldessarini RJ, Katz B and Cottom P (1984) Am. J. Psychiatry 141: 748–752.
8. Barton JL (1978) J. Clin. Psychiatry 39: 690–692.
9. De Girolamo G, Williams P and Cappiello V (1987) Psychol. Med. 17: 989–997.

Biological Psychiatry, Volume 1. G. Racagni et al., editors.

Clinical and neurobiological heterogeneity of schizophrenic psychoses*

Tetsuo Fukuda
Osaka Institute of Clinical Psychiatry, Osaka Takatsuki, and Doshisha University, Kyoto 602, Japan

In his clinico-genetic study about half a century ago, Mitsuda [1] presented the data strongly arguing in favor of the clinical and nosological heterogeneity of schizophrenia. The concept of atypical psychoses came into being as a result. It is the group of psychoses that had been variously labelled since about the same time when kraepelinian dichotomy was established; schizoaffective psychosis (Kasanin), oneirophrenia (von Meduna), schizophreniform psychosis (Langfeldt), degenerationspsychose (Bonhoeffer, Kleist), mixed psychosis (Gaupp et al.), cycloid psychosis (Leonhard), oneiroide emotionspsychose (Störring), Bouffée délirante polymorphe (Magnan), psychose délirante aiguë (Ey), endogene pseudoschizophrenie (Rümke), schizophrenie-ähnliche emotionspsychose (Labhardt), reactive or psychogenic psychosis (Wimmer, Strömgren), to name only some of them.

Of the comprehensive studies subsequently conducted to substantiate the core issue by Mitsuda and associates, the one that may be appropriate to briefly remark upon at this symposium is what Fukuda and Matsuda [2] found in both chronic schizophrenia and fresh cases of typical and atypical schizophrenia. It was a longitudinal study employing EEG mecholyl-test prior to and during ECT and subsequently followed-up. What was impressive in their findings through this study were the significant and unequivocal differences in terms of the response to the successively given mecholyl test and the EEG change, both being measured in parallel with a total of 10 ECT at 3 per week, as well as for 1 month following the ECT treatment. Full remissions were seen exclusively in atypical schizophrenia while the contrary was the case for typical schizophrenia. Changes in reactivity to mecholyl were explained by Gellhorn and Kiely [3] in terms of hypothalamic trophotropic-ergotropic balance; Fukuda and Matsuda interpreted them in more general terms, i.e. reactivity of the central autonomic system and reversibility thereof, which are easily variable for better in atypical schizophrenia and rather resistant or inflexible. EEG slowing was pronouncedly recognizable in atypical schizophrenia, lasting for some weeks at the minimum following ECT treatment, while practically the opposite was the case for the typical schizophrenia. In conclusion then, the 2 groups of schizophrenia are identifiable not only at the phenotypic but also the phenogenetic level as having differential cerebral pathology at the autonomic function level as measurable with mecholyl by successive-

*This symposium is held in memory of H. Mitsuda (1910–1979).

longitudinal testings. Such was the work done during the 1960s. During the past decade, new techniques and a variety of new strategies became available and cerebral pathology of schizophrenic psychoses are intensively investigated, some of them allowing direct clinical applications. Hence, the core issue of this symposium has indeed been reexamined, however diverse the disease concept of schizophrenia may be for different investigators. Nevertheless, the work of Hayashi et al. [4] is consistent with the aforementioned core issue, providing more accurate and subtle differences at various brain structure sites including the laterality aspect. Some of the more recent works by Andreasen and Crow [5,6], for example, also seem to be concerned with the core issue here at clinical-neurobiological levels although their clinical descriptive psychopathology makes use of somewhat uncomfortable terminology; we have repeatedly emphasized that clinical description, course and outcome or prognosis are inseparable from diagnosis [7–9]. And the "positive-negative symptom", seemingly popular to many investigators, should suffer the blame of oversimplification at times, requiring definitive reservations, not to mention the otherwise superb description of clinical picture and/or type (but not disease entity) by Leonhard [10,11].

One more work of Fukuda and Hirota [12,13] also deserves a mention. It dealt with a paraphrenic group of schizophrenia, or chronic paranoid-hallucinatory psychoses, differentiating non-affective from affective or affect-laden paraphrenia in the sense of Leonhard. In brief, differential diagnosis by means of psychopathological analysis, psychological batteries and EEG was found quite possible. The cases have been followed-up about 2 decades so far, in the same manner as in the aforementioned work of Fukuda and Matsuda. The work of Retterstöl and Opjordsmoen [14] seems partly, at least, in agreement with that of Fukuda and Hirota in that some chronic paranoid-hallucinatory psychoses, usually considered as schizophrenia, may better be identified under categories different from the typical schizophrenia, some as atypical psychoses and the others as paraphrenias more or less in the sense of Leonhard; affective or affect-laden paraphrenia seems to be closer to our atypical psychoses.

The title of this symposium has deliberately been chosen for certain reasons. Obviously, it aims at nosological heterogeneity. Current trends in neuroscience and molecular biology, which are so rapidly progressing, combined with descriptive psychopathology accumulated by our predecessors, should shed more light on the problem under debate in the not too distant future.

References

1. Mitsuda H (1942) Psychiatr. Neurol. Jpn. (in Japanese with German summary) 46: 298–362 (English version by Fukuda, 1967).
2. Fukuda T and Matsuda Y (1969) Int. Pharmacopsychiatry 3: 13–41.
3. Gellhorn E and Kiely WF (1973) In: Mendels J (ed) Biological Psychiatry. John Wiley and Sons, New York, U.S.A., pp. 235–261.
4. Hayashi T et al. (1991) This volume.

5. Andreasen NC (1991) This volume.
6. Crow TJ (1987) In: Häfner H, Gattaz WF and Janzarik W (eds.) Search for the Causes of Schizophrenia. Springer, Berlin, Germany, pp. 260–266.
7. Mitsuda H (1967) In: Mitsuda H (ed.) Clinical Genetics in Psychiatry. Igaku-Shoin, Tokyo, Japan, pp. 49–90.
8. Mitsuda H (1975) In: Mitsuda H and Fukuda T (eds.) Biological Mechanisms of Schizophrenia and Schizophrenia-like Psychoses. Thieme, Stuttgart, pp. 1–9.
9. Mitsuda H (1979) In: Fukuda T and Mitsuda H (eds.) World Issues in the Problems of Schizophrenic Psychoses. Igaku-Shoin, New York, U.S.A., pp. 121–124.
10. Leonhard K (1986) Aufteilung der endogenen Psychosen und ihre differenzierte Ätiologie. Akademie, Berlin, Germany.
11. Fukuda T (1989) Seishin-Igaku (Clin. Psychiatry) 31: 553–555.
12. Fukuda T, Hirota Y, Iida N and Miyazaki S (1976) In: Huber (ed.) Therapie, Rehabilitation und Prävention schizophrener Erkrankungen. Schattauer, Stuttgart, pp. 207–215.
13. Fukuda T (1979) In: Obiols J et al. (eds.) Biological Psychiatry Today. Elsevier, Amsterdam, The Netherlands, pp. 325–334.
14. Retterstöl N and Opjordsmoen S (1991) This volume.

Biological Psychiatry, Volume 1. G. Racagni et al., editors.

Multivariate analyses of brain imaging data from typical and atypical schizophrenic psychoses

T. Hatashi, H. Kitou, T. Kachi, H. Suga and M. Ohara

Department of Neuropsychiatry, Aichi Medical University, 21, Yazako-Karimata, Nagakute-cho, Aichi-ken, 480-11 Japan

Introduction

Mitsuda [1] studied the heterogeneity of the schizophrenic psychoses from the standpoint of phenotype and genotype and suggested the existence of separate atypical psychoses. To verify his important works various studies have been pursued including the aspects of pathogenesis. For example, Hatotani [2] carried out endocrinological research on periodic psychoses (atypical psychosis) and concluded that functional vulnerability of the diencephalo-hypothalamo-pituitary system can be postulated as a predisposing factor in this group of psychoses. Furthermore, Fukuda and Matsuda [3] conducted pathophysiological studies using EEGs and Mecholyl test and indicated a characteristic instability of autonomic function in atypical psychosis.

The present communication deals with some attempts of our own in which the heterogeneity concept of schizophrenia was further examined by means of brain imaging technique, such as CT scan and ^{123}I-IMP-SPECT.

Results and Discussion

First, Hayashi [4] examined the brain CTs of 68 endogenous psychosis patients, who were under 40 years of age and had been admitted to the psychiatric ward of Aichi Medical University Hospital from 1982 to 1986: these were compared with 20 controls. Applying Mitsuda's classification system, the cases were divided into 41 schizophrenics and 27 atypical psychotics. In order to investigate variation in CT findings between the 2 patient groups and the controls. Twelve different CT scan indices were determined.

The schizophrenics had larger values for 9 of the CT scan indices: inter-hemispheric fissure (IHF) index, VBR, 2 lateral ventricle (L-V) and 3rd ventricle (3-V) indices and 4 sylvian fissure (SF) indices, while the atypical psychotics had larger values for 3 SF indices, especially the right side compared to controls. Moreover, the schizophrenics had greater 3-V and L-V indices than the atypical psychotics.

When the correlation matrix of CT indices for all the psychotics was examined in detail, it was found that the VBR correlated with the left SF indices and also the 3-V index correlated well with the other CT indices, whereas the VBR, IHF and right SF indices did not correlate with one another. Such findings led us to the speculation that there might be 3 subgroups, each with a main focus of an alteration in the above-mentioned regions.

Subsequently, all the cases were divided by cluster analysis into 4 clusters and a residue group. The first (I) group, which contained mainly normal controls, had no abnormal CT findings. The second (II) group had almost normal CT findings, and the third (III) group had right SF enlargement. Groups II and III, which comprised mainly atypical psychosis patients, had no ventricular enlargement. The fourth (IV) group had significant IHF enlargement and the residue group (V) had left SF enlargement. Group IV and V, which consisted mostly of schizophrenics, had significantly greater ventricular enlargement than the other groups.

The schizophrenics in groups II and III more frequently exhibited positive family histories and comprised paranoid subtypes including paraphrenia as compared to those in groups IV and V, suggesting that paraphrenia is closely related to atypical psychosis. In addition, the atypical psychotics in group III had a significantly higher family history rate than in group II, indicating that further subclassification of atypical psychotics is warranted.

The attenuation values of brain density were then investigated in 14 schizophrenics, 9 atypical psychotics and 9 controls. Density values, given in Hounsfield units (HU), were measured in 14 selected regions of interest (ROI) in the gray and white matters of the frontal and parietal regions, the temporal regions, the thalami and heads of the caudate nucleus in each hemisphere. In each ROI, no statistically significant difference in density was found among the three groups, but the schizophrenics in groups IV and V showed significantly higher density in the frontal regions and the caudate nucleus in contrast to atypical psychotics.

Furthermore, ^{123}I-IMP-SPECT was studied on 13 schizophrenics, 8 atypical psychotics and 16 controls. These subjects were all under 40 years of age. The regional cerebral (RU) and cerebellar uptakes (CU) of ^{123}I-IMP in ROIs were measured in transverse sections at 5 cm and 2 cm above the OM-line and the regional cerebral uptake rates (RU/CU) were calculated.

On early imaging, the schizophrenics showed significantly decreased uptake rates in the bilateral frontal regions. The atypical psychosis patients, on the other hand, showed no findings in frontal regions, but a significantly decreased rate in right basal ganglia compared to controls. On late imaging, the schizophrenics displayed a significantly decreased rate not only in the frontal region, but also in left occipital and basal ganglia regions. The atypical psychosis patients, however, had no significantly decreased uptake rate in any of these regions.

If one was to assume that ^{123}I-IMP uptake in early imaging indicates regional cerebral blood flow and in late imaging retention in the brain, the decreased uptake on early imaging might reflect functional brain disorders and on late imaging some organic brain changes. Therefore, atypical psychotics might have functional disorders in the right basal ganglia as Fukuda once suggested. Since frequent recurrence of the disease might finally result in irreversible organic alteration, such SPECT findings in atypical psychosis may be related in some way to that of right SF enlargement in CT studies.

Are there 3 distinct types of schizophrenia – frontal, basal ganglia, left temporal lobe illness – with possibly different etiology? Or are there various degrees of a deficit in a single frontal-striatal temporal neural system? Recently, Buchsbaum [5] has discussed this subject on the basis of the evidence from brain imaging, post-mortem and psychopharmacological studies. According to our CT studies, VBR, IHF and right SF indices did not correlate with one another. Therefore, we identified 3 types of schizophrenia and divided all the cases into several subgroups by cluster analysis. Indeed, the patients in the groups and had no significant abnormal CT findings, but the 3 characteristic patient groups were differentiated. Group III, as stated above, corresponds to the "right SF-basal ganglia type", consisting mainly of atypical psychotics and paranoid-type schizophrenics including paraphrenia. Group IV was the "IHF-frontal lobe type" and group V corresponds to the "VBR-left SF type", in other words, "left temporal lobe type". The "VBR type" and the "IHF type" comprised almost entirely typical schizophrenics. So far, these 2 types of schizophrenia could not be differentiated from one another on the basis of clinical features or hereditary traits.

Conclusion

The results of our brain imaging studies employing Mitsuda's classification system can be summarized as follows: schizophrenic psychosis is a more or less heterogeneous disease. Since there are significant brain morphological and/or functional differences between typical and atypical schizophrenia, it seems justifiable to divide them into 2 groups at least: typical schizophrenia on the one hand, and atypical psychosis on the other. Moreover, each of the 2 psychosis groups might be further dividable into distinct subgroups.

References

1. Mitsuda H (1968) In: Mitsuda H (ed.) Clinical Genetics in Psychiatry. Igaku-Shoin, Tokyo, pp. 3–21.
2. Hatotani N (1983) In: Hatotani N and Nomura J (eds.) Neurobiology of Periodic Psychoses. Igaku-Shoin, Tokyo, pp. 1–14.
3. Fukuda T and Matsuda Y (1969) Int. Pharmacopsychiatry 3: 13–41.
4. Hayashi T (1989) J. Aichi. Med. Univ. Assoc. 17: 609–625.
5. Buchsbaum MS (1990) Schizophr. Bull. 16: 379–389.

Biological Psychiatry, Volume 1. G. Racagni et al., editors.

Clinical heterogeneity of schizophrenia: Perspectives from neuroimaging

Nancy C. Andreasen[1], Michael Flaum[1], Delwyn Miller[1], James Ehrhardt[2], Karim Rezai[2], Gregg Cohen[1] and Daniel S. O'Leary[1]

[1]The University of Iowa, Department of Psychiatry, 500 Newton Road, Iowa City, IA 52242; and [2]The University of Iowa Hospitals and Clinics, Department of Radiology, Iowa City, IA 52242, U.S.A.

Research in schizophrenia is often difficult to replicate, and samples of schizophrenic patients typically have a larger standard deviation for most variables that are measured than do normal controls. In addition to these persistent clues concerning the heterogeneity of schizophrenia from the research literature, the clinical picture of schizophrenia also suggests the likelihood of heterogeneity. Symptoms, course, and outcome are quite variable across patients. In all likelihood, the illness that we refer to as "schizophrenia" should more properly be called "the group of schizophrenias" (as Bleuler has done) [1,2].

Investigators frequently pay lip service to the possibility that schizophrenia is heterogeneous, but most studies still combine all patients given a diagnosis of schizophrenia, without attempting to tease apart possible confounders that affect our ability to detect potential etiologic heterogeneity in schizophrenia. These confounders include age, gender, stage of illness and effects of medication. One strategy for coping with these confounders is to do parallel studies in which they are examined separately, e.g. first-episode vs. chronic patients, males vs. females, or medicated vs. unmedicated. In addition, patients may also be subdivided in terms of presenting phenomenology, e.g. patients with prominent positive vs. negative vs. mixed symptoms.

In CT and MR studies, we have explored the effects of both gender and stage of illness on ventricular enlargement. We have measured VBR in two CT studies and two MR studies. CT-1 included a sample of 50 schizophrenic patients and 46 normal controls; CT-2 had sample sizes of 80 and 63 respectively; MR-1 had a sample of 38 schizophrenics and 49 normal volunteers; and MR-2 included 43 and 50 respectively. Data from these studies are summarized in Table 1.

As Table 1 indicates, we have noted prominent gender effects in 3 out of 4 of these studies. Males have consistently tended to have more prominent ventricular enlargement than females. Since males are more vulnerable to birth defects and early childhood mental illnesses (e.g. increased rate of spontaneous abortion, increased rate of learning disabilities), these results may suggest that ventricular enlargement in schizophrenia represents an interaction between a group of genetic and environmental factors that produce neural injury in males and make them

Table 1. Simple main effects of gender and diagnosis on ventricle-brain ratio in four studies

Study	t-Value				df
	Diagnosis[a]		Gender[b]		
	Male subjects	Female subjects	Control subjects	Schizophrenic subjects	
CT-1 [3]	1.29	−2.05[c]	1.31	0.52	92
CT-2 [4]	−2.89[d]	−0.25	−1.38	1.18	139
MRI-1 [5]	−2.55[d]	−0.52	−1.13	0.45	81
MRI-2 [6]	−3.08[d]	−0.47	−0.88	1.21	92

[a]Differences between genders within diagnosis; [b]differences between diagnosis within genders; [c]$P < 0.051$; [d]$P < 0.01$.

subsequently more vulnerable to the development of schizophrenia and to a more malignant course of illness.

In the CT and MR studies, we have explored the possibility of reducing heterogeneity by examining phenomenologic subtypes of schizophrenia using the positive vs. negative distinction [8–12]. This strategy was pursued in CT-1, CT-2 and MR-2 [4,6,9]. A significant relationship was observed between ventricular enlargement and prominent negative symptoms in 2 out of 3 of these studies (CT-1 and MR-2). In these studies, patients were classified into 1 of 3 groups using predefined diagnostic criteria: positive, negative, and mixed. In addition to having more prominent ventricular enlargement, the negative patients also tended to have other indicators of “malignant” schizophrenia, such as poor premorbid adjustment, cognitive impairment and lower educational and occupational achievement. Negative patients also tended to be predominantly male.

In recent studies using SPECT, we have focused primarily on the effects of medication and stage of illness [13]. In these studies, we have used a tomomatic 64 and the xenon inhalation method. Although a variety of cognitive challenges have been explored, we chose to use the Tower of London in several large samples because it appeared to be a particularly promising prefrontal activator. We have used the Tower of London in 13 drug-naive patients, 23 chronic patients, and 15 healthy normal volunteers. The baseline task consists of watching undulating colors on a video monitor, while the cognitive challenge consists of performing the Tower of London by manipulating a joy stick to move colored balls from one spot to another using a locally developed program that is run on the same video monitor. When performing this cognitive challenge task, healthy normal volunteers display a marked increase in perfusion to the left medial prefrontal cortex and to the right parietal cortex. Both never medicated and chronic patients (evaluated after being withdrawn from medications for 3 weeks) fail to show this activation affect and are instead “hypofrontal”. In addition, hypofrontality appears to be associated with prominent negative symptoms. Thus, it appears that hypofrontality is neither an effect of stage of illness nor of medication. Instead, it is characteristic of young first-episode patients as well as chronic patients. These results suggest that hypofrontality and schizophrenia may be in some sense fundamental to the illness, rather an epiphenomenon produced by chronicity or medication effects.

These studies represent examples of an approach to teasing apart the potential heterogeneity of schizophrenia. While they make a contribution, they do not solve the problem. Ongoing efforts are needed to develop new approaches and strategies at both the clinical and technical levels. At the clinical level, we are exploring new approaches to subtyping. One that appears to be particularly promising involves subdividing positive patients into 2 groups (floridly psychotic and disorganized), with the negative subtype representing a third group. In addition, we are continuing to look at correlates of symptoms in addition to subtypes. At the technical level, we are exploring new approaches to providing cognitive challenges and integrating information from multiple modalities (e.g. MRI, SPECT and electrophysiology). Analyses of gender effects are also continuing.

References

1. Andreasen NC, Shore D, Burke JD Jr, Grove WM, Lieberman JA, Oltmanns TF, Pettegrew J, Pulver AE, Siever LJ, Tsuang MT and Wyatt RJ (1988) Schizophr. Bull. 14: 345–363.
2. Andreasen NC (1987) Schizophr. Bull. 12: 9–22.
3. Andreasen NC, Smith MR, Jacoby CG, Dennert JW and Olsen SA (1982) Am. J. Psychiatry 139: 292–296.
4. Andreasen NC, Swayze VW, Flaum M, Yates WR, Arndt S and McChesney C (1990) Arch. Gen. Psychiatry 47: 1008–1015.
5. Andreasen NC, Nasrallah HA, Dunn V, Olson SC, Grove WM, Ehrhardt JC, Coffman JA and Crossett JHW (1986) Arch. Gen. Psychiatry 43: 136–144.
6. Andreasen NC, Ehrhardt JC, Swayze VW, Alliger R, Yuh WTC, Cohen G and Ziebell S (1990) Arch. Gen. Psychiatry 47: 35–44.
7. Flaum M, Arndt S and Andreasen NC (1990) Am. J. Psychiatry 147: 1327–1332.
8. Andreasen NC, Olsen SA, Dennert JW and Smith MR (1982) Am. J. Psychiatry 139: 297–302.
9. Andreasen NC (1982) Arch. Gen. Psychiatry 39: 789–794.
10. Andreasen NC (1989) Br. J. Psychiatry (Suppl. 7) 155: 93–98.
11. Andreasen NC (1982) Arch. Gen. Psychiatry 39: 784–788.
12. Andreasen NC (1987) Psychiatr. & Psychobiol. 11: 240–251.
13. Andreasen NC, Rezai K, Alliger R, Swayze VW, Flaum M, Kirchner P, Cohen G and O'Leary DS (1991) Arch. Gen. Psychiatry (submitted).

Biological Psychiatry, Volume 1. G. Racagni et al., editors.

Long-term course in schizophrenia: Neurobiology and psychopathology

Gisela Gross and Gerd Huber

University of Bonn, Department of Course Psychiatry (Research Unit), D-5300 Bonn 1, Venusberg, Germany

There are not very many facts consistently found in schizophrenia research. In the following we comment mainly upon some results of our group as to course and outcome (Huber et al., 1979; Gross and Huber, 1986; Huber, 1990).

Most frequently the disorder begins in the 3rd decade of life, followed by the 2nd and the 4th decade. The age of onset is lower in men than in women: 70% of men but only 47% of women fell ill before the age of 30. The outcome in males is poorer but without significance. There is no over-representation of the lower social levels. Psychological precipitants are favorable as to the long-term outcome. The intra- and interindividual variability of schizophrenia is very marked, especially also with respect to course and outcome. Patients with onset of the illness before the psychopharmacological era have a poorer prognosis than those who became ill later. Patients who were somatically treated within 1 year after onset including the prodromes have a much better long-term prognosis than those treated only later or never at all (Huber et al., 1979; Gross et al., 1983).

Angst, Fukuda and we have shown the impact of the variability of concepts of schizophrenia on the results of long-term and other studies. Because the European long-term studies of Bleuler (1972), Ciompi and Müller (1976) and our group (Huber et al., 1979) made the diagnosis independently of outcome according to the definitions of Schneider and Bleuler, they allow comparisons between studies. As prognostically favorable factors, the following were found: normal primary personality, psychoreactivity and peracute and acute onset of the 1st psychotic phase, prevalence of catatonic, cenesthetic and endogenous-depressive initial syndromes; as unfavorable factors abnormal psychopathic primary personality, elementary school failure, chronic onset, hebephrenic initial syndromes and auditory hallucinations. Several prognostically favorable factors are identical to criteria used to classify atypical, schizoaffective or cycloid psychoses, e.g. acute onset, depressive syndromes, precipitating life events and not abnormal primary personality. Long-lasting prodromes (more than 2 years) before the 1st psychotic phase are unfavorable because these usually not recognized precursor states of schizophrenia delay the beginning of treatment. At the beginning of the illness no secure prediction is possible. According to the findings obtained with univariate (Huber et al., 1979) and multivariate statistical methods (Stassen et al., 1990), reliable predictions exist only for extreme outcome subgroups, i.e., for full remissions vs. typical schizophrenic defect psychosis or fully employed on premorbid level vs. unemployed (see in Huber, 1990).

Twenty-two percent of the Bonn and the Zurich study showed complete psychopathological remissions; 43% more or less non-characteristic types of remission, mainly slight pure deficiency syndromes ("pure defect"), determined by dynamic and cognitive basic symptoms (BS); 35% characteristic schizophrenic defect psychoses. Ninety percent were permanently living at home at the last follow-up; 56% were fully employed yet with only 38% at previous occupational level and 18% below the premorbid level.

There are 4 groups of course types each embracing about a quarter of the whole sample: a favorable (with nearly 100% social remissions), a relatively favorable, a relatively unfavorable and an unfavorable group (with a social recovery rate of only 2% in course type XII). These results show very clearly the great heterogeneity of course and outcome of schizophrenia defined according to Bleuler and Schneider and lead to a revision of the doctrines of incurability, incessant progression and numinous singularity of schizophrenia. The long-term outcome is largely independent of the duration of the illness. Most of the schizophrenics are for most time of the course psychopathologically not schizophrenic in the conventional sense. According to Zubin the results of the European studies, confirmed in the U.S.A. by the Vermont study, mean a revolution in our knowledge about schizophrenia, a proclamation of emancipation for schizophrenia from the joke of inevitable chronicity.

In view of the far-reaching overlapping of the symptomatology of the pre- and postpsychotic basic stages, the Bonn Schedule for the Assessment of BS (BSABS) could be constructed for the standardized documentation of all types of basic stages (Gross et al., 1987). Certain basic symptoms form the basis of certain schizophrenic 1st rank symptoms (Klosterkötter, 1988). In a prospective study of 338 patients we could show that it is possible to single out of seemingly neurotic and personality disorders with the help of BSABS a group with increased risk of transition into 1st rank psychosis. These patients, 30% of the whole group, had shown a significantly higher rate of thought-, perception- and motor-BS at the time of index examination that took place on average 7 years before catamnesis. These cognitive BS can be considered as psychopathological predictors or vulnerability markers that indicate a high risk of transition into schizophrenic psychosis, whereas other potential predictors do not reveal correlations with the criterion "transition into 1st rank psychosis" (Gross et al., 1990; Klosterkötter et al., 1990). Thus we have the chance to improve the long-term prognosis of schizophrenia by early recognition and therefore by early treatment already at the frequently pseudoneurotic precursor states of the illness.

Many data support the assumption that BS are closer to the hypothesized somatic substrate as the complicated and fixed psychotic "end-phenomena" and that BS or certain BS are the consequence of disorders of information processing and biochemical abnormalities in the limbic system (see in Huber, 1990)): pure deficiency syndromes show a decrease of performance in psychological tests that correlates with the subjectively experienced BS; abnormal rhythmicity (theta- or alpha-parenrhythmia) in EEG related to the limbic system in process-active basic stages; EEG signs of schizophrenia described by Kornhuber and Koukkou; a slight ventricular enlargement in a subgroup with irreversible pure deficiency syndromes ("pure defect"; Huber, 1957); quantitative-morphometric findings of Bogerts et al. pointing to an atrophy in areas of the limbic system; the observations that transition-relevant cognitive basic deficiencies and cenesthesias occur in organic brain diseases preferentially of the limbic system; symptomatic schizophrenias in temporal lobe epilepsy. The list of aura symptoms reported by Wieser (see in Huber, 1990) in stereoelectroencephalographic studies seems largely identical with BS described in the Bonn Schedule (BSABS; Gross et al., 1979).

In this context belongs the hypothesis that the primary cause of schizophrenia is not a hyperfunction of dopaminergic but a hypofunction of glutamatergic systems. The paroxysmal occurrence of certain BS may also reflect an instability of neurochemical parameters. We found in 178 drug-free schizophrenics that process-active patients showed higher levels of dopamine and especially norepinephrine and 5-HT (compared to healthy controls); against this, patients with inactive stages showed a hypoactivity of catecholaminergic and possibly also serotoninergic systems. Glutamate was on the contrary to the most other amino acids, significantly decreased in serum (Huber et al., 1990) and in CSF (Kornhuber, 1985).

Our opinion (1981) that the separation into positive and negative, type-I and type-II schizophrenia (Crow, 1980; Andreasen, 1982) cannot be maintained, has to be defined exactly: negative symptoms are not the same as BS; the transition from negative into positive symptoms really means the development of productive-psychotic 1st rank symptoms out of BS that are already positive symptoms "in nascent state". We must differentiate BS, positive and negative symptoms as stages of the same disorder that develop in schizophrenia frequently in this chronic sequence too. As a rule BS precede the positive and the negative symptoms. As to the problem of heterogeneity of schizophrenia, we have elsewhere named the arguments speaking for the continuum-hypothesis of idiopathic psychosyndromes. Studies that compare the most important course models of schizophrenia established that the models of Kraepelin, Crow and Andreasen cannot be confirmed, whereas the results are compatible with the basic symptom concept (Häfner and Maurer, 1990).

References (to be found in following volumes)

Gross G, Huber G, Klosterkötter J and Linz M (1987) BSABS. Bonn Scale for the Assessment of Basic Symptoms. Springer, Berlin.

Huber G (ed.) (1990) Idiopathische Psychosen: Psychopathologie, Neurobiologie, Therapie. Schattauer, Stuttgart.

Biological Psychiatry, Volume 1. G. Racagni et al., editors.

Different responsiveness of negative symptoms to pharmacotherapy

Kazutoyo Inanaga and Masahiro Kuniyoshi
Chikusuikai Institute for Neuroinformation, Chikusuikai Hospital, 1191 Yoshida, Yame, Fukuoka-Ken, 834 Japan

Introduction

In 1971 we observed remarkable improvement in 3 schizophrenic patients by the administration of levodopa in addition to the conventionally used neuroleptics [1]. These cases led us to make an extensive trial of levodopa treatment of schizophrenia [2,3]. Two double-blind studies confirmed the effectiveness and safety of levodopa in the treatment of negative symptoms of schizophrenia [4,5].

These clinical experiences indicated that the dose of levodopa to be used concomitantly with neuroleptics in the treatment of schizophrenia is reasonably small.

The therapeutic effect of DA agonists in schizophrenia was explained to be mediated by the stimulation of presynaptic DA autoreceptors, thus lowering the activity of enzyme tyrosine hydroxylase and, consequently, the DA synthesis and release [6].

B-HT920 (Talipexole) is a selective autoreceptor agonist. It has been reported that by stimulating the presynaptic dopamine receptors, Talipexole inhibits neuronal firing [7], dopamine synthesis [8], dopamine release [9] and lowers dopaminergic neuron activity.

With such action Talipexole is expected to prove to be a new type of therapeutic drug for schizophrenia, different from conventional neuroleptics.

We examined the clinical effects of Talipexole on schizophrenia in two steps and report the results thereof.

Step 1

Subjects and Methods

Twenty-two patients with schizophrenia were selected as the subjects. The test drug was administered at the starting dose of 0.05 mg 3 times a day, which was increased gradually and the dose giving therapeutic efficacy was employed as the maintenance dose. The test drug was administered for a period of 8 weeks. If some patients had been treated with neuroleptics before the start of study, they underwent a week wash-out period.

Also, after the start of the present study, concomitant use of neuroleptics and anti-depressants was prohibited. However, concomitant use with benzodiazepines was only permitted as a hypnotic. BPRS and SANS were used for evaluation of psychiatric symptoms.

Results

High improvement ratings were noted for psychiatric symptoms such as guilt feeling, depressive mood and suspiciousness, but aggravation was also seen at fairly high rates for the symptoms of tension, hostility, uncooperativeness and excitement. SANS symptom improvement ratings by global rating, slow improvement of such symptoms as affective flattening and avolition and apathy, whereas almost no aggravation was seen.

The above finding suggests that Talipexole is effective against negative symptoms, but as to positive symptoms it could bring about aggravation in some cases. The tendency of aggravation of positive symptoms was observed, especially in the cases which had been washed out the pretreatment with neuroleptics.

Step 2

Subjects and Methods

Since aggravation of positive symptoms was observed in step 1, we modified the study protocol. That is, the subject patients who had been treated with neuroleptics before the start of study, did not take the wash-out period, but they were administered the test drug as a direct switch from, or as concomitant use (add on) with the pretreatment of neuroleptics. Also the subjects were limited, as a rule, to those who show main psychotic states such as lowered spontaneity, neurotic state, or depressive state.

Results

High ratings of improvement were seen for symptoms such as the somatic concern, depressive mood, and motor retardation. Aggravation was not seen for any symptoms. As to the SANS symptom improvement rating by global rating, the results obtained were almost similar to those obtained in step 1.

Talipexole exclusive administration showed improvement of negative symptoms, whereas clear improvement of negative symptoms was not seen in the group of cases which had concomitant use with neuroleptics.

Discussion

Several dopamine agonists have been administered to schizophrenic patients with conflicting results. However, there is provocative evidence that low doses of dopamine agonists can produce transient improvement in some schizophrenic patients.

Exacerbation of psychotic symptoms may result from high doses of dopamine agonists [10]. The dose of dopamine agonists should be maintained low enough to preferentially and effectively stimulate dopamine autoreceptors. As Cutler et al. [11] have already mentioned, we can speculate that those schizophrenic symptoms that do not respond to postsynaptic dopamine receptor blockade by neuroleptics might improve with autoreceptor stimulation by low-dose dopamine agonists. Negative symptoms of schizophrenia may be due to the dysfunction of presynaptic dopamine receptors.

References

1. Inanaga K, Oshima M, Tachibana H, Nakamura K and Koketsu K (1971) Kurume Med. J. 18: 161–168.
2. Inanaga K, Inoue K, Tachibana H, Oshima M and Kotorii T (1975) Folia Psychiatr. Neurol. Jpn. 26: 145–157.
3. Inanaga K and Tanaka M (1973) In: Ban TA et al. (eds.) Psychopharmacology, Sexual Disorders and Drug Abuse. North Holland Publishing Co., Amsterdam, pp. 229–233.
4. Inanaga K, Nakazawa Y, Inoue K, Tachibana H, Oshima M and Kotorii T (1975) Folia Psychiatr. Neurol. Jpn. 29: 123–143.
5. Inanaga K, Nakazawa Y, Tachibana H et al. (1978) Clin. Psychiatry 20: 877–889.
6. Aghajanian GK and Bunney BS (1977) Naunyn-Schmiedeberg's Arch. Pharmacol. 297: 1–7.
7. Eriksson E, Svensson K and Clark D (1985) Life Sci. 36: 1819–1827.
8. Andén N-E, Golembiowska-Nikitzn K and Thornström U (1982) Naunyn-Schmiedeberg's Arch. Pharmacol. 321: 100–104.
9. Pichler L, Pifl C, Hornykiewicz O and Kobinger W (1987) Eur. J. Pharmacol. 135: 239–242.
10. Meltzer HY (1982) Pharmacol. Biochem. Behav. (Suppl. 1) 17: 1–10.
11. Cutler NR, Jeste DV, Kaufmann CA, Karoum F, Schran HF and Wyatt RJ (1984) Prog. Neuro-Psychopharmacol. Biol. Psychiatry 8: 277–283.

Biological Psychiatry, Volume 1. G. Racagni et al., editors.

Long-term course and outcome in delusional psychoses

Nils Retterstøl and Stein Opjordsmoen
University of Oslo, Gaustad Hospital, P.O. Box 24, Gaustad, N-0320 Oslo 3, Norway

Introduction

Delusional psychoses were defined as all psychoses accompanied by delusions, except bipolars and confusional states where the delusions faded as soon as the confusion cleared up. The long-term course and outcome (22–39 years personal follow-up, average 30 years) will be presented.

Material and Method

Included in the study, which started in 1958, were all first-time admitted patients consecutively admitted to the psychiatric department, University of Oslo, during 2 periods: 1946–1948 (the long-term group) and 1958–1961 (the short-term group). The patients were personally followed-up, usually in their homes. The short-term group was followed up twice by N.R.: after 2–5 years and after 5–8 years, the long-term group once by N.R. (after 15–18 years) [1, 2]. Both groups were again followed up by S.O. after 22–39 years [3]. In the last follow-up the patients were rediagnosed according to DSM III and ICD 9, course and outcome measured according to Global Assessment Scale, Strauss-Carpenter's and McGlashan's Scale.

Hospital diagnoses according to the Scandinavian tradition at the time of admission for the 301 patients were: reactive psychoses 163, schizophreniform psychoses 76, schizophrenia 52, other psychoses 10. The discharge diagnoses according to DSM III are shown in Fig. 1.

Clinical and social outcome in relation to the Scandinavian diagnostic tradition after 15–18 years revealed that no psychotic symptoms could be traced in 81% of the patients with reactive psychoses, in 61% of those with schizophreniform psychoses and only in 23% of those with schizophrenia. The percentage of self-supporting persons was 79, 67 and 30% respectively. There was a gradual development from the very favourable outcome in reactive psychoses to the unfavourable in schizophrenia, with the schizophreniform psychoses (Langfeldt) in between.

The outcome after 20 more years of observation in relation to DSM III demonstrated no diagnosis of psychotic disorder in 84 and 82% respectively of those with schizoaffective and affective disorders, 52% in those with paranoid and

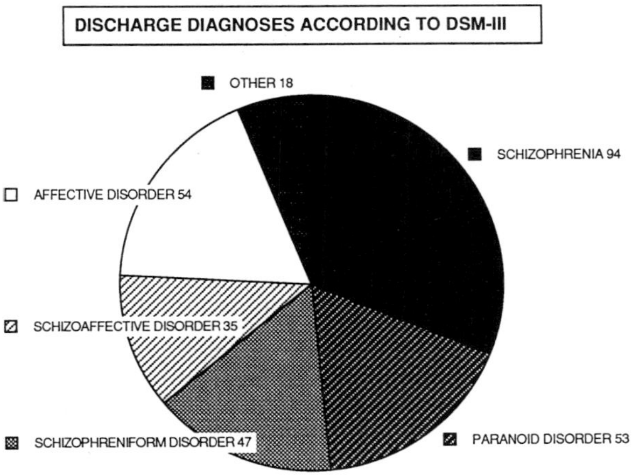

Fig. 1. Discharge diagnoses according to DSM III.

38% in those with schizophreniform disorder, and only 9% in those with schizophrenia.

The course of the cases diagnosed according to Scandinavian traditions, measured according to McGlashan's Scale (global), and evaluated at last follow-up demonstrated a score of 2.6 in reactive psychoses, 2.1 in schizophreniform psychoses and 1.0 in schizophrenia, similar differences in the more detailed scores: hospitalization 3.4, 2.9 and 2.2, in work 2.8, 2.3 and 1.0, psychopathology 2.6, 2.0 and 1.1.

The same differences were marked when the material was scored as to outcome with Strauss-Carpenter's Scale and GAS. In all dimensions the same differences were clear: patients with a diagnosis of reactive psychosis scored much better than the schizophrenics, the group with schizophreniform psychoses in between.

The differences between the GAS-scores on the basis of the first and the last follow-up were small: 65.5 and 62.8 in reactive psychoses, 57.7 and 54.2 in schizophreniform psychoses and 49.0 and 45.1 in schizophrenia.

Patients with paranoid (delusional) disorders, as defined in this study, were without psychotic symptoms in 65% after an average of 10 years, in 60% after an average of 30 years. There was in other words a small development to the worse as time passed. The most important predictor in our material was the *discharge diagnosis*.

There is hardly anything in our results which indicates that the new diagnostic tools given us in DSM III provide a more valuable prognostication than the diagnoses in use in Scandinavia in the 1960s. Of all prognostic factors the discharge diagnoses in both systems are the most important prognostic factor.

Using a multivariate technique at the follow-ups taking place on average 10 and 30 years later, the following significant predictors of outcome emerged: discharge diagnosis, according to Scandinavian traditions and DSM III, accounted for most of the total variance, marital status and Axis V at 10 years' outcome, and diagnosis, marital status and gender at 30 years' outcome. Women did slightly better than men at 10 years' follow-up, but at 30 years' follow-up men did slightly better, a new finding that should be confirmed in other studies before an explanation can be proffered.

Outcome of the predominant delusion

It was clearly demonstrated that the difference in outcome according to the type of delusion diminished as years passed. The favourable results for the patients with depressive delusions per se at index admission (found by Retterstøl at first follow-up) could not be confirmed at later follow-up.

Our results clearly demonstrated that *course and outcome are primarily dependent on the diagnostic category, not on the type of delusion.*

Paranoia

Let us then turn to the special group with original diagnosis of *paranoia*, the patients with systematized and encapsulated delusional ideas, as defined by Kraepelin. Following his strict criteria there were 26 paranoia patients in the material. Of these patients, 42% were without a diagnosis of psychosis at last follow-up, while the diagnosis paranoia was kept in 50% and changed in the remaining 8% (schizophrenia). In other words: the old maxim "once paranoia – always paranoia" is not correct.

Conclusion

The results clearly demonstrate that course and outcome are predominantly dependent on the diagnostic category, not on the type of delusion. There are clear differences in course and outcome for the different groups, both according to the Scandinavian diagnostic concepts and DSM III.

References

1. Retterstøl N (1966) Paranoid and Paranoiac Psychoses. Charles C. Thomas, Springfield, Illinois.
2. Retterstøl N (1970) Prognosis in Paranoid Psychoses. Charles C. Thomas, Springfield, Illinois.
3. Opjordsmoen S (1989) Delusional disorders. A personal 22–39 year follow-up study. Doctoral thesis, University of Oslo.

Biological Psychiatry, Volume 1. G. Racagni et al., editors.

Schizophrenia viewed as a neurotransmitter imbalance syndrome, involving dysregulation of sensory input and arousal

Arvid Carlsson, Maria Carlsson and Anders Svensson
Department of Pharmacology, University of Göteborg, P.O. Box 33031, 5-400 33 Göteborg, Sweden

Numerous clinical observations support the view that a disturbance of sensorimotor gating constitutes an important feature of the schizophrenic disorder. An oversensitivity to external stimuli, which may at least in part be due to defective habituation, appears to result in an overload of information, leading to cognitive fragmentation. An insufficiently controlled retrieval of stored information may add to this overload. Dopamine appears to play a crucial role in this regulation. Thus hyperdopaminergia is accompanied by a deficient habituation and an attenuated so-called prepulse inhibition of, for example, startle responses [1]. A similar disturbance can be demonstrated in schizophrenic patients and may at least partly account for the fact that dopaminergic agonists can provoke or aggravate, and dopaminergic antagonists alleviate schizophrenic symptomatology.

The precise mechanism underlying the abnormal sensorimotor gating in schizophrenia has not been established. The cognitive fragmentation indicates a cortical location, but an involvement of subcortical dopamine-rich structures, and especially the ventral "limbic" striatum, seems likely. To account for the apparently strong impact of dopamine on cortical cognitive mechanisms, the following hypothesis has been advanced [2].

The mesostriatal dopamine system serves to modulate a negative feedback loop, starting out in the cerebral cortex by the corticostriatal glutamatergic system and including both the dorsal and the ventral (limbic) striatum. The loop then proceeds via the dorsal and ventral pallidum, respectively, to thalamic nuclei and finally returns to the cerebral cortex. Also the mesencephalic reticular formation is proposed to be included in this feedback control, by means of which the cerebral cortex is proposed to be able to regulate the amount of sensory information relayed by the thalamus as well as the arousal. The dopaminergic system is proposed to be inhibitory on this negative feedback loop and will thus raise the amount of sensory information filtered through the thalamus as well as the arousal. It thus serves as an antagonist to the corticostriatal glutamatergic system, which enhances the inhibitory function of the striatum on the thalamus.

In line with this view, PCP (phencyclidine, "angel dust"), a glutamatergic antagonist acting on the ion channel of the NMDA receptor, is capable of mimicking schizophrenic symptomatology and of disrupting the prepulse inhibition of the startle reflex [1].

Our hypothesis predicts that the strong psychomotor inhibition induced by removal of dopaminergic function through depletion of dopamine or inhibition of dopamine receptors can be relieved by reducing the glutamatergic corticostriatal tone. To test this, we induced a severe depletion of dopamine in the brains of mice by treating the animals with reserpine plus α-methyltyrosine. The severe immobility thus produced could be reversed by treatment with a number of NMDA receptor antagonists [3–9]. Moreover, a partial NMDA-receptor inhibition, which in itself was insufficient to induce any psychomotor activity, resulted in a dramatic enhancement of the responsiveness of dopamine as well as α_2-adrenergic receptors to their respective agonists [7,10]. Pretreatment with antimuscarinic agents had a similar effect to NMDA antagonists in this regard.

Our studies support the view that the responsiveness of monoaminergic receptors to agonists can be dramatically influenced by manipulating NMDA receptors or cholinergic receptors. This opens up new perspectives on the problem of dopamine receptor sensitivity in schizophrenia.

References

1. Geyer MA, Swerdlow NR, Mansbach RS and Braff DL (1990) Brain Res. Bull. 25: 485–498.
2. Carlsson A (1988) Neuropsychopharmacology 1: 179–186.
3. Carlsson M and Carlsson A (1989a) J. Neural Transm. 75: 221–226.
4. Carlsson M and Carlsson A (1989b) J. Neural Transm. 77: 65–71.
5. Carlsson M and Carlsson A (1989c) J. Neural Transm. (Sect. P-D) 1: 317–322.
6. Carlsson M and Carlsson A (1990) Trends Neurosci. 13: 272–276.
7. Carlsson M and Svensson A (1990a) Pharmacol. Biochem. Behav. 36: 45–50.
8. Carlsson M and Svensson A (1990b) Life Sci. 47: 1729–1736.
9. Svensson A, Pileblad E and Carlsson M (1991) J. Neural Transm. (in press).
10. Carlsson M, Svensson A and Carlsson A (1991) Naunyn-Schmiedeberg's Arch. Pharmacol. (in press).

Biological Psychiatry, Volume 1. G. Racagni et al., editors.

Cognitive science- and neuropsychological aspects of schizophrenia research

Hinderk M. Emrich
Max Planck Institute for Psychiatry, Kraepelinstr. 10, W-8000 Munich 40, Germany

Binocular depth inversion-illusion and its disturbance in schizophrenia

The phenomenon of depth inversion is impressively documented in the "Haunted Mansion" at Disneyland in California, where visitors see a pair of human faces that appear to rotate precisely as they walk by. In reality, these faces are 3-dimensional outside-in (hollow) masks, which are perceived incorrectly as normal faces. This illusion of "depth inversion" had been investigated by von Helmholtz and Mach in the 19th century. Questions as to its basic mechanisms have been reconsidered by Gregory [1]. It has been demonstrated, especially in experiments by Yellott [2], that stereoscopic visual experience is the result of "a process in which the brain tests hypotheses about the 3-dimensional shape of objects against the evidence provided by their retinal images".

The three-component-hypothesis of perception [3] gives rise to the idea that an equilibrium between a constructivist and a correcting processor function is disturbed in psychosis. Thus, if the correction of preconceptions is impaired in psychosis and if the processor, which is relevant for visual perception, were disturbed in the way predicted above, an impaired binocular depth inversion should be observed in psychotic patients. Such experiments have in fact been performed [3], using a stereoscopic projection-device and linearly polarised light and demonstrated a highly pronounced impairment of the ability of the schizophrenic CNS to correct implausible hypotheses.

This finding appears to support the idea that schizophrenic psychoses are not primarily due to a deficiency of a "filter" [4] which protects the brain from an overload of information arising from the outer world [5], but results from a deficiency of an active correcting processor which interacts with both internal conceptualisation and external sensory input.

Though developed independently, this concept has some analogy to Huxley's [6] interpretation of the mode of action of psychedelic drugs, developed under the influence of Bergson and Broad, which states that these psychotogenic compounds tend to weaken an internal censuring function which is relevant for perception.

Also Malenka et al. [7] observed central error in the correcting behaviour of motor control in schizophrenic patients. The view of the basic deficiency in psychosis elaborated here appears to be in line with the concepts both of Huxley and Malenka et al., insofar as it is assumed that internal correcting systems are deficient or in imbalance in relation to conceptualisation during a psychotic state (cf. also Frith's important contributions in this regard [8–10]).

Neurobiology of censorship (comparator-systems)

During the recent past the concept of "modularity of mind" has become dominant in the field of concepts about the organizational structure of mind [11,12]. The main idea is that – in contrast to the classical concepts of neuropsychology – the processing in the brain is a "parallel" one. Different mental representations are performed by different "modules" which can interact with each other.

An important module in this concept is Gazzaniga's "interpretator", a module which coordinates and integrates the computations (the "votes") of other modules, and the result of such an "interpretator"-related computation has apparently the subjective quality of being "granted", being "true", being "real". This system may exert what the above-mentioned "censorship" has to be attributed to. The function of this system is to stabilize "reality-fictions" and one may – as a result of the present considerations as well as from the impaired inversion-illusion in psychosis – anticipate that this system in particular is defective or to an increased extent "vulnerable" in psychosis.

How might such a system be realised neurobiologically? Censorship certainly has great demands regarding long-term memory, since the question, as to what is "plausible", "senseful", "biologically meaningful at the present", can only be decided on the basis of a history of experience of failure and success which have been stored over longer periods of time. Thus, hippocampal structures may play a prominent role herein. Hippocampal structures thus may work as "comparators" [13,14] and calculate meaningful expectations in relation to sensory input. Recently, neurochemical data on GABA in hippocampus have been acquired which are in line with this concept [15]. Interestingly, dopamine also plays a functional role herein [15], a finding which may explain the therapeutic effects of antidopaminergic (neuroleptic) compounds.

Thus the censorship-systems described above may be characterized as "comparators", a concept which fits in with the idea that to have "consciousness" means to "compare" world-models with actual (sensory or imagined) intentional data. Comparison of actual data with sets of acquired world-models is a definition which may thus turn out to be an adequate description of the function of "zensorship" which is to stabilize "reality fictions".

References

1. Gregory RL (1973) In: Gregory RL and Gombrich EH (eds.) Illusion in Nature and Art. Freeman. Oxford, pp. 49–96.
2. Yellott JI Jr (1981) Sci. Am. 245: 118–125.

3. Emrich HM (1988) Nervenarzt 59: 456–464.
4. Broadbent DE (1958) Perception and Communication. Pergamon, New York.
5. Chapman LJ and Chapman JP (1973) Disordered Thought in Schizophrenia. Meredith, New York.
6. Huxley A (1954) The Doors of Perception. Chatte & Windus, London.
7. Malenka RC, Angel RW, Hampton B and Berger PA (1982) Arch. Gen. Psychiatry 39: 101–107.
8. Frith CD (1987) Psychol. Med. 17: 631–648.
9. Frith CD and Done DJ (1988) Br. J. Psychiatry 153: 437–443.
10. Frith CD and Done DJ (1989) Psychol. Med. 19: 356–363.
11. Fodor JA (1983) The Modularity of Mind. MIT Press, Cambridge.
12. Gazzaniga MS (1985) The Social Brain. Basic Books, New York.
13. Gray JA and Rawlins JNP (1986) In: Isaacson RL and Pribram KH (eds.) The Hippocampus, Vol. 4. Plenum Press, New York, pp. 159–201.
14. Olton DS (1989) In: Chan-Palay V and Köhler C (eds.) The Hippocampus: New Vistas. A.R. Liss, New York, pp. 411–424.
15. Bischoff S (1986) In: Isaacson RL and Pribram KH (eds.) The Hippocampus, Vol. 3. Plenum Press, New York, pp. 1–32.

Biological Psychiatry, Volume 1. G. Racagni et al., editors.

Brain systems and abnormal word generation in schizophrenia

Chris Frith

CRC Psychiatry, Northwick Park Hospital, Watford Road, Harrow HA1 3UJ; and MRC Cyclotron Unit, Hammersmith Hospital, Ducane Road, London W12 0HS, U.K.

Introduction

In order to link the signs and symptoms of schizophrenia with underlying brain abnormalities it is necessary to develop a firm theoretical and experimental basis for studying the cognitive processes that underlie signs and symptoms. It is these processes, rather than their behavioural manifestations that will map onto brain systems. I shall illustrate this approach to the study of schizophrenia with the example of the processes underlying word generation.

Speech disorders in schizophrenia

Speech disorders are commonly observed in schizophrenia. These can take the form of poverty of speech in which speech is reduced in quantity and complexity, or incoherence of speech in which the listener finds it difficult to perceive the connections between the words produced. In collaboration with my colleagues at the CRC (Eve Johnstone, John Leary and David Owens), I have studied word generation in a population-based sample of 283 schizophrenic patients and related their performance to clinical ratings of signs and symptoms [1]. Subjects were timed while generating 5 words in a specified semantic category (e.g. animals). In comparison to controls matched for pre-morbid IQ, schizophrenic patients took almost twice as long to generate 5 words ($P < 0.001$). Not unexpectedly, this slow rate of word production was significantly correlated with ratings of poverty of speech ($P < 0.01$). We also rated the quality of the words generated. Bafing and Montague [2] have provided norms indicating the words most likely to be produced in this sort of task. Thus, when asked for animals, most subjects will start by saying cat and dog. We counted the number of unlikely words generated (i.e. infrequent words in the category norms). We found a significant relationship between ratings of incoherence and the tendency to produce unlikely words ($P < 0.001$). Incoherent patients might start with words like aardvark or bison. Using these simple word generation tasks, it is possible to study experimentally some of the abnormalities of speech observed by clinicians in schizophrenic patients.

The cognitive basis of single word processing

Single word processing has been studied extensively in normal people and a number of accounts are available concerning the cognitive processes underlying access to and production of words. Most accounts are variants of the "logogen model" proposed by John Morton [3]. In this account every word is represented (this representation may well be distributed) as part of a network, such that when one word is activated this activation will spread to words that are similar in meaning (or sound or appearance). This process of "spreading activation" underlies the phenomenon of priming by which a word is more easily perceived when it is proceeded by a related word (bread – *butter*) or an appropriate context (coming in, he took off his *coat*). This model provides a suitable framework for considering the disorders of word generation observed in schizophrenia. Perhaps the simplest possibility is that schizophrenic patients have fewer words in their lexicon. This would result in the generation of fewer words and the more rapid appearance of unusual words for the category. Heidi Allen, Petter Liddle and I have investigated this possibility by asking 20 chronic schizophrenic patients to generate words from one category repeatedly. The overlap between these attempts permits an estimate of the size of the total word pool from which the words are being selected. We found that patients with poverty of speech and reduced verbal fluency nevertheless had a normal-sized pool of words from which they were selecting the words required. The abnormality must therefore lie with the way word representations in the network are activated. There are essentially two ways in which a word representation might be activated. First, the subject hears or sees a word and has to find the corresponding representation in his inner lexicon. Second, as in the verbal fluency task, the subject is given a category, such as animals and has to find the word in his inner lexicon most appropriate to that category. Karl Friston has developed a connectionist model for a network which can operate in these 2 different modes. A simple modulation of the network as a whole can optimise performance in each mode. Identifying words presented externally is best achieved when the network is easily activated. In contrast, identifying words prototypical of some category is best achieved when the network is damped down, so that its intrinsic structure can be revealed with minimal interference from external activation [4]. The abnormalities of word generation in schizophrenic patients would be consistent with a failure in the process which normally damps down the responsiveness of the lexicon to external stimuli. Having derived a detailed hypothesis about the cognitive basis of word generation, the next step is to map cognitive processes onto brain systems.

The brain systems underlying word generation

Along with Karl Friston, Peter Liddle, Richard Frackowiak and many other colleagues at the MRC Cyclotron Unit, I have used positron emission tomography

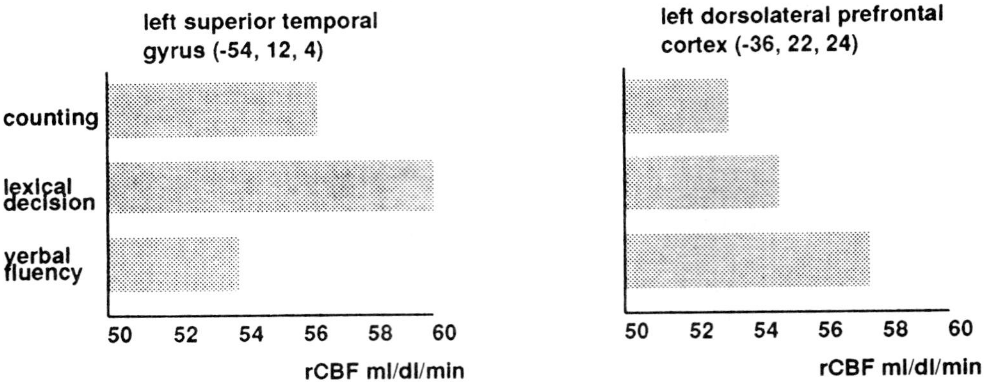

Fig. 1. Effects of verbal fluency and lexical decision on regional cerebral blood flow.

to study word generation in four normal volunteers. We measured changes in regional blood flow (rCBF) using $C^{15}O_2$ as a tracer. We compared word generation (saying words beginning with A) with a lexical decision task and simply counting aloud. Each of these tasks was carried out during the 2 min of the PET scan. We found that word generation was associated with increased rCBF in the dorsolateral prefrontal cortex on the left and decreased rCBF in superior temporal cortex bilaterally. In contrast, lexical decision was associated with no change in frontal cortex and increased rCBF in superior temporal cortex (see Fig. 1). This result is consistent with the theory that the lexicon is located in the superior temporal cortex. During word generation this area receives inhibitory modulation from dorsolateral prefrontal cortex. The abnormal word production seen in schizophrenic patients could be a consequence of an abnormality in this modulatory process.

References

1. Frith CD, Leary J, Cahill C and Johnstone EC (1991) Psychological test performance and demographic and clinical correlates. Br. J. Psychiatry (Spec. Suppl.) (in press).
2. Battig WF and Montague WE (1969) J. Exp. Psychol. Monogr. 80: 1–46.
3. Morton J (1970) A functional model for memory. In: Norman DA (ed.) Models of Human Memory. VH Winston, Washington, D.C.
4. Friston KJ, Frith CD, Liddle PF and Frackowiak RSJ (1991) Investigating a network model of word generation with positron tomography. Proc. R. Soc. Ser. B (in press).

Biological Psychiatry, Volume 1. G. Racagni et al., editors.

Event-related potentials in facial recognition task in schizophrenics

Noriko Tsuru, Eigoro Minami and Satoru Genda
Miyazaki Medical College, Miyazaki, Japan

Introduction

The endogeneous evoked potentials provide a means to evaluate the physiology of the human brain during cognitive processing. P300s elicited in a number of paradigms have been significantly smaller for schizophrenics than for controls. The prolonged N_2 latency of normal amplitude in unmedicated schizophrenics has been reported [1]. The decreased N_2 amplitude of normal latency at Cz to both deviant targets and deviant non-targets in schizophrenics has also been reported [2]. To elucidate the discrepancy of these results as to the N_2 change in schizophrenics, we investigated the event-related potentials (ERPs) in a facial recognition task in controls and schizophrenics.

Methods and Subjects

Eighteen normal, right-handed students, aged 20–33 years (25.3 ± 3.1 years) and 13 schizophrenics aged 18–31 years (27.9 ± 5.5 years) underwent the experiment. The mean BPRS score in schizophrenics was 26.7 years. Their neuroleptic doses were 75–1,225 mg (533.8 ± 341.5 mg) of a chlorpromazine equivalent. Mean duration of their psychiatric illness was 2–13 years (6.5 ± 3.8 years).

"Oddball" paradigm testing visual recognition for faces consists of 20% of target stimuli which is a picture of Mrs. Thatcher and 80% of non-target stimuli which is a picture of an actress. Stimuli were presented on a T.V. screen for a duration of 66 ms at a distance of 1.5 m from the eyes through an image memory board of the computer triggered by a stimulator. Visual evoked responses were collected from 12 electrode sites (Fp_1, Fp_2, F_7, F_8, C_3, C_4, T_5, T_6, O_1, O_2, Fz < Pz) with AG/AgCl electrodes referred to linked-ears and with a filter set between 0.53–60 Hz. Subjects were asked to count infrequent stimuli. Epochs were collected at 800-ms intervals, with a 16-ms pre-stimulus epoch (the average of which established baseline). Trials with artifacts including blink artifacts were rejected automatically. Forty-five trials were averaged for each subject to produce the infrequent-stimuli waveform. Baseline-to-peak-amplitudes and latencies were determined for the maximum and minimum within latency bins accounting for N_2 (200–400 ms post stimulus onset) and P_3 (300–600 ms) for T_5, T_6, O_1, O_2, Pz. Statistical analysis, comprised of ANOVA with repeated measure factors for the group (schizophrenics and controls) and electrode sites (T_5, T_6, O_1, O_2, Pz), and reduced electrode sites (T_5, T_6 or O_1, O_2) were used to examine the laterality.

Results

Grand-averaged waveforms associated with the target stimulus are displayed in Fig. 1. The ERPs to target stimuli at O_1 had a negative component of 319 ms (N_2) and positive component of 438 ms (P_3) in the controls and negative component of 308 ms (N_2) and positive component of 448 ms (P_3) in schizophrenics.

Comparison of overall ERPs in controls and schizophrenics

The overall amplitude of N_2 of the ERPs for the infrequent target in schizophrenics seemed to be larger than those in the controls. However, it was not significant ($F(1,29) = 3.847$, $P > 0.05$). The overall amplitude of P_3 in schizophrenics were almost the same as that of the controls ($F(1,29) = 0.573$).

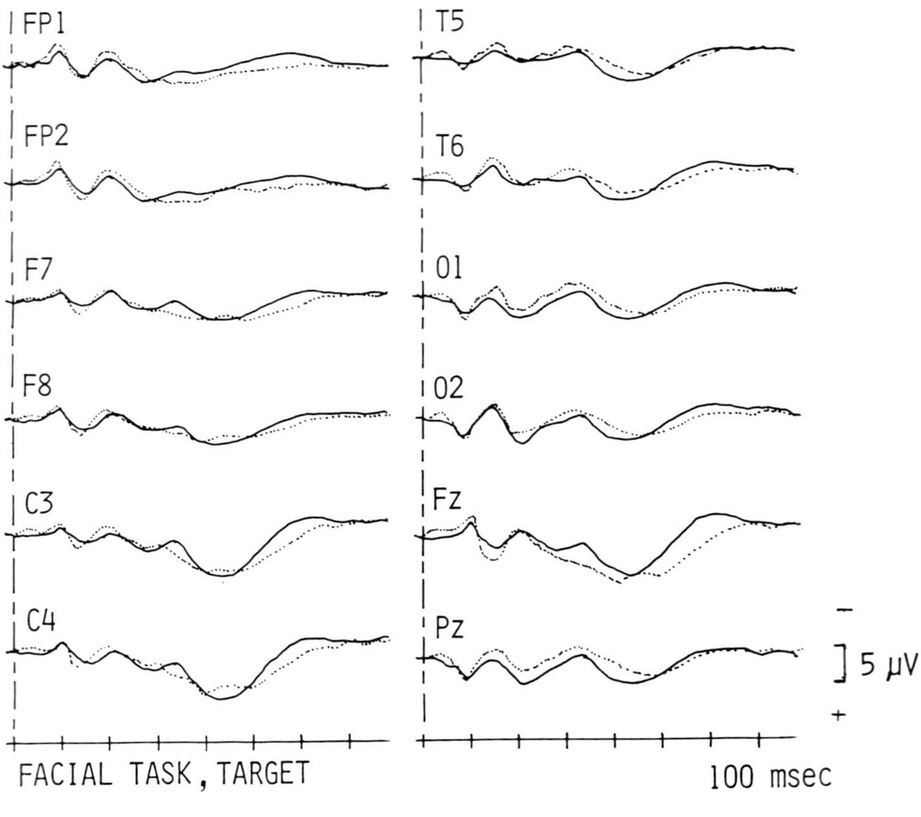

Fig. 1. Event-related potentials for target stimuli in controls (solid lines) and schizophrenics (dotted lines).

Laterality

The schizophrenics had almost the same P300 amplitudes at O_1, O_2 as the controls ($F(1,29) = 1.361$). However, there was a strong group-by-laterality interaction, indicating statistically significant topographic differences ($F(1,29) = 7.836$ $P < 0.01$), with the schizophrenics showing a strong left < right laterality and the controls showing a left > right laterality. As to the amplitude of P_3 at T_5, T_6 schizophrenics had the same P300 amplitude as the controls ($F(1,29) = 0.048$). There was no interaction ($F(1,29) = 1.596$).

As to the amplitude of N_2 at T_5, T_6 there was no significant interaction ($F(1,29) = 1.576$), indicating no significant left < right laterality with the schizophrenics. As to the amplitude of N_2 at O_1, O_2 there was no interaction ($F(1,29) = 0.038$).

The latencies of N_2 and P_3 in schizophrenics were the same as those in the controls ($F(1,29) = 1.191$, and $F(1,29) = 0.039$, respectively).

Discussion

These data imply that occipital left < right asymmetries of P300 amplitude are present in medicated schizophrenics. There were neither significant amplitude differences of N_2 nor significant latency differences of N_2 and P300.

Faux et al. [3,4] reported the auditory P300 asymmetries in medicated schizophrenics and unmedicated schizophrenics. Our results suggested that there are also visual P300 asymmetries in schizophrenics. In our previous studies we reported the existence of more errors in the right hemifield of the Benton Visual Retention Test in schizophrenics [5,6]. The existence of schizophrenic P300 asymmetries may imply the existence of a pathological neurophysiological asymmetries of cerebral function in schizophrenics. These data might be related the laterality of eye movement and more errors in the right hemifield of Benton Visual Retention Test in schizophrenics.

References

1. Brecher M, Porjesz and Begleiter H (1987) Electroencephalogr. Clin. Neurophysiol. 66: 369–375.
2. Pfefferbaum A, Winegrat BG, Ford JM, Roth WT and Kopell BS (1984) Electroencephalogr. Clin. Neurophysiol. 59: 104–124.
3. Faux SF, Torello MW, McCarley RW, Shenton MW and Duffy FH (1988) Biol. Psychiatry 23: 776–790.
4. Faux SF, Nestor PG, McCarly RW, Shenton ME, Horvath T and Davis K (1990) In: Brunia CVM, Gaillard AWK and Kok A (eds.) Psychophysiological Brain Research, Vol. 2, Tilburg University Press, Netherlands, pp. 209–212.
5. Fujiwara M and Tsuru N (1986) Jpn. J. Psychiatr. Neurol. 40: 583–594.
6. Tsuru N and Fujiwara M (1987) In: Takahashi R, Flor-Henry P, Gruzelier J and Niwa S (eds.) Cerebral Dynamics, Laterality and Psychopathology. Elsevier, The Netherlands, pp. 187–197.

Biological Psychiatry, Volume 1. G. Racagni et al., editors.

Brain glucose metabolism and clinical correlates in schizophrenia

Frits-Axel Wiesel[1] and Gustav Wik[2]
[1]Department of Psychiatry, Uppsala University, Ulleråker, S-750 17 Uppsala; and [2]Department of Psychiatry and Psychology, Karolinska Institute, Sweden

Introduction

Schizophrenia is a severe and in the majority of cases a disabling disease including psychosocial capabilities. There are many indirect findings supporting the view of schizophrenia as a brain dysfunction disease. Positron emission tomography (PET) makes it possible to directly study the brain. In comparison with other functional techniques PET enables the study of both cortical and subcortical brain regions with a high resolution and sensitivity. The interest in studying regional glucose metabolism comes from its close coupling to regional neuronal activity, thereby making it possible to investigate if psychopathology in schizophrenia can be related to changes in neuronal function.

Methods

Brain glucose metabolism could be determined with radiolabelled 2-deoxyglucose or glucose. Deoxyglucose can be labelled with the positron emitting isotopes ^{11}C or ^{18}F and glucose with ^{11}C. The radioactivity data are collected by the positron camera after the i.v. injection of the tracer. To obtain functional images the data must be analyzed according to a model developed for the biochemical process under investigation. It has been shown that a three-compartment model (tracer in plasma and tissue, metabolized tracer in tissue) describes the accumulation of radioactivity in brain tissue and from the kinetic parameters regional brain glucose metabolism can be calculated [1–3]. There are great differences among investigators in reported metabolic levels due to several factors like the use of different tracers and parameters when calculating the metabolic values and differences in camera resolution. However, it is still meaningful to evaluate and combine different studies since the results are interpreted in relation to the findings in respective control group.

Comments

Regional metabolic rates

Patients with schizophrenia have 10 to 20% lower metabolism in several parts of the brain during a resting condition (see [4]). Decreases in metabolism seem to be more pronounced in cortical than in subcortical regions. Altogether the results seem to indicate widespread changes in regional glucose metabolism and do not support the view of dysfunction in a specific region. It is therefore proposed that patients with schizophrenia suffer from a general dysfunction in the neuronal network influencing most brain regions. When studying relationships among regional metabolic rates in patients and healthy controls, distinctly different correlation patterns emerged [4]. In the patients all regions were highly intercorrelated, as if the activity of the regions were synchronized. The controls' association areas were intercorrelated but subcortical regions except the caudate were not correlated to other parts of the brain.

Lower metabolic rates were found in chronic patients but not in 1st episode patients [5,6]. The duration of neuroleptic treatment was not related to a lower metabolism. It seems as if first-episode patients do not have profound changes in the regional brain metabolism but that such changes become evident during the course of the disease. Several investigators have found relationships between metabolism and clinical symptomatology. Thus a low metabolism has been found to be correlated to autistic or negative symptoms in two studies (see [4,5]). In another study patients with negative symptoms had lower metabolic rates than those with more positive symptoms (see [4]). A relationship between higher metabolic rates and pronounced positive symptoms has also been reported in another study (see [4]). A positive correlation between the level of anxiety and metabolism both in normals and patients with schizophrenia has been reported [7]. However, results from PET studies and anxiety are inconsistent. It seems as if the type of anxiety influences its coupling to metabolism and blood flow. How the PET investigation is performed is also crucial [7].

Pattern of metabolism

Hypofrontality is one of the most discussed concepts in schizophrenia research (see [4]). This concept was originally based on the findings of a lower blood flow in the frontal part of the brain than in the posterior part, while the controls exhibited the opposite patterns, i.e. hyperfrontality. The hypofrontal pattern, however, was evident only in a group of older schizophrenic patients and not in younger patients. Investigations of first-episode young patients with schizophrenia have not demonstrated a hypofrontal pattern but rather a hyperfrontal pattern [5,6]. There is support for the opinion that hypofrontality is a state-dependent phenomenon which develops with time and is more evident in residual schizophrenic patients [8].

Regional relative rates have indicated that the function of subcortical areas are changed to a lesser degree than neocortical areas (see [4]). Regional relative rates have resulted in less consistent correlations to clinical symptoms than absolute rates. However, interesting findings have been obtained for left/right differences in hemisphere activity and clinical symptoms. Thus in two studies, a higher left hemisphere activity was associated with greater severity of psychopathology [9,10]. In our own study no correlations between clinical symptoms and regional relative rates were found except for anxiety [5,7]. The intensity of anxiety was found to be negatively correlated to the relative rates in the left thalamus and the right medial frontal cortex in the patients [7]. Patients without anxiety (8 of 20 patients) had higher relative rates in the left caudate than the anxious patients and the controls who all were anxious during the investigation. These findings may indicate that the right medial frontal cortex and the left thalamus are relatively inhibited in a state of anxiety or that processes of anxiety are modulated from these regions. In the healthy volunteers no regional relative rates were correlated to anxiety. However, positive correlations between anxiety and frontal/parietal ratios of the left hemisphere were found which was not the case in the patients. This may indicate that the processing of neuronal information in anxiety is different between patients and normals, suggesting that anxiety in patients with schizophrenia does not arouse the frontal cortex as in normals.

Conclusions

Schizophrenia seems to involve a widespread brain dysfunction. Patients with pronounced autistic behavior or negative symptoms seem to have lower metabolic rates. Positive symptoms may be coupled with higher left hemisphere activity.

Acknowledgements

Ms. A. Liberg is gratefully acknowledged for preparing the manuscript. The research project was supported by the Swedish Research Medical Council (B91-21X-08318-04A).

References

1. Phelps ME, Huang SC, Hoffman EJ, Selin C, Sokoloff L and Kuhl DE (1979) Ann. Neurol. 6: 371–388.
2. Reivich M, Alavi A, Wolf A, Fowler J, Russell J, Arnett C, MacGregor RR, Shiue CY, Atkins H, Anand A, Dann R and Greenberg JH (1985) J. Cereb. Blood Flow Metab. 5: 179–192.
3. Blomqvist G, Stone-Elander S, Halldin C, Roland PE, Widén L, Lindqvist M, Swahn C-G, Långström B and Wiesel F-A (1990) J. Cereb. Blood Flow Metab. 10: 467–483.
4. Wiesel F-A (1989) Psychiatr. Dev. 1: 19–47.

5. Wiesel F-A, Wik G, Sjögren G, Blomqvist G, Greitz T and Stone-Elander S (1987) Acta Psychiatr. Scand. 76: 628–641.
6. Cleghom JM, Garnett ES, Nahmias C, Firnau G, Brown GM, Kaplan R, Szechtman H and Szechtman B (1989) Psychiatr. Res. 28: 119–133.
7. Wik G and Wiesel F-A (1991) Biol. Psychiatry (accepted for publication).
8. Geraud G, Arné Bes MC, Guell A and Bes A (1987) J. Cereb. Blood Flow Metab. 7: 9–12.
9. DeLisi LE, Buchsbaum MS, Holcomb HH, Langston KC, King AC, Kessler R, Pickar D, Carpenter Jr WT, Morihisa JM, Margolin R and Weinberger DR (1989) Biol. Psychiatry 25: 835–851.
10. Gur RE, Resnick SM and Gur RC (1989) Psychiatr. Res. 27: 325–334.

Biological Psychiatry, Volume 1. G. Racagni et al., editors.

Locomotion and behaviour: The interaction of loops and transmitter

Peter Riederer and Wolfgang Berger
Department of Psychiatry, Division of Clinical Neurochemistry, University of Würzburg, Füchsleinstraße 15, D-8700 Würzburg, Germany

Introduction

For well-coordinated performance of motor and psychic actions, an intact balance of the neurotransmisson systems is essential. The basal ganglia play a crucial role in this concert and are regarded as an interface of different systems. They are part of a corticothalamo-cortical feedback-loop. To put together single motor programs so that they achieve a smooth and harmonic performance is the main task of the basal ganglia [1,2]. Many influences from the limbic system modulate the motor programs at this level. Therefore it is easy to imagine that disturbances of this complex balance lead to a variety of different disorders.

Motor loop

This is one of the most important and best characterized corticothalamo-cortical feed-back loops leading through the basal ganglia. Glutamatergic neurons from various regions in the cortex project to the putamen. Neurons using the inhibiting transmitter GABA and substance P (SP) as a modulator connect the putamen with the internal globus pallidus (GPI) and the substantia nigra pars reticulata (SNr). These neurons are modulated by dopaminergic cells situated in the substantia nigra pars compacta (SNc). From the SNr and GPI GABAergic axons terminate in the thalamus. Excitatory glutamatergic neurons leading to the cortex close this feed-back loop. A parallel way from the striatum leads via GABAergic neurons to the external globus pallidus (GPE) and to the subthalamic nucleus (STN), which sends excitatory glutamatergic axons to the SNr and GPI (Fig. 1) [1,3–6].

Papez loop

In 1937 Papez described a system connecting the parahippocampal gyrus, hippocampus, mammillar body, thalamus and back to the parahippocampal gyrus [7]. Influences from the cortex and septal region take part in this circuit. Recent research has revealed an even more complex picture [8,9]. The striatum and the thalamus are both used by the motor and the Papez loop. Therefore they are a place where many interactions between these systems are possible.

Parkinson's disease

A loss of dopaminergic cells in the SNc of at least 70% is necessary to cause symptoms in Parkinson's disease [10]. The main symptoms are akinesia, rigidity and tremor. The loss of dopaminergic input in the striatum has two effects within the motor loop. First it leads to a decrease in inhibition of the GPI and SNr. The second consequence is an increase of GABAergic inhibition of the GPE. Therefore the less inhibited STN stimulates the GPI and SNr in an increased manner by glutamate. The elevated activity of GPI and SNr leads to an increased GABAergic inhibition of the thalamus. A decrease of glutamatergic stimulation of the cortex is the result. Dopaminergic drugs are therefore the main therapeutic approach. Another possibility for the therapy of Parkinson's disease is perhaps NMDA-antagonist reducing the glutamatergic drive of the NST into the SNr and GPI and of the cortico-striatal glutamatergic activity [14] (Fig. 1).

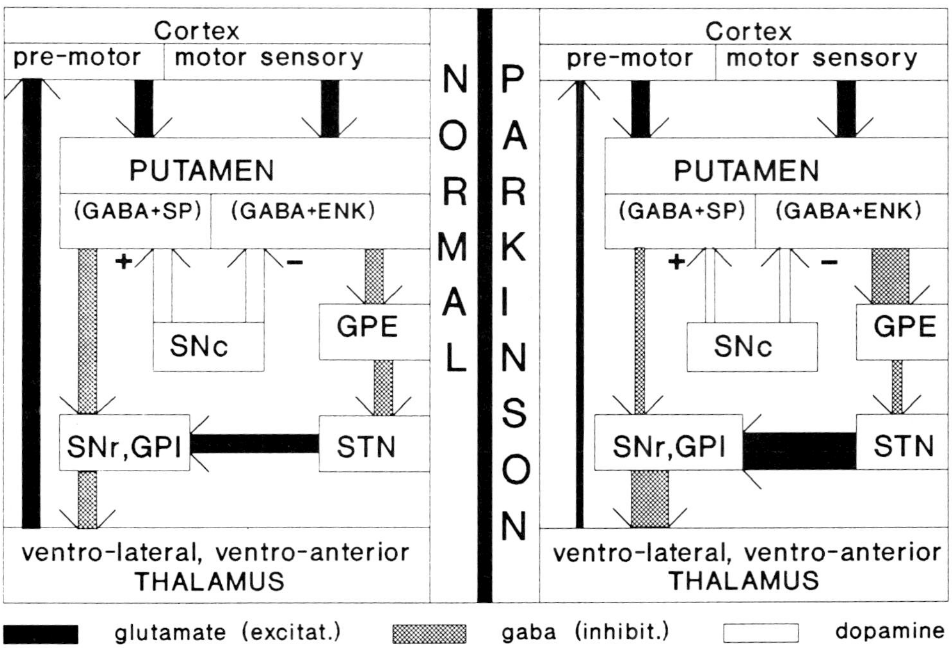

Fig. 1. Motor loop (modified according to [1,3,4,14]). STN: subthalamic nucleus; SNc/SNr: substantia nigra pars compacta/reticulata; GPI/GPE: globus pallidus internus/externus; SP: substance P; ENK: enkephalin.

Schizophrenia

As described above, the basal ganglia and especially the ventral portion seem to be an interface between the motor loop and the limbic system [6,9,11]. Some evidence indicates that in schizophrenia a glutamatergic deficit causes a dopaminergic overactivity. Drugs like phencyclidine acting as a non-competitive antagonist at the NMDA-glutamate receptor produce schizophrenia-like symptoms [6,8,12,13]. On the other hand, all dopamimetic substances can cause psychotic side-effects in Parkinson's disease. One possibility for this "psychotic" effect of dopamimetic substances could be a relative loss of glutamatergic stimulation of the striatum in Parkinson's disease due to dopaminergic overactivity. This causes reduced GABA-ergic inhibition of the dopaminergic pathways [14]. In addition, the loss of balance between dopaminergic and glutamatergic systems in limbic areas (e.g. perforant tract, etc.) might contribute to paranoid hallucinatory psychosis [12].

Future investigation should keep in mind that the variety of psychotic symptoms is probably the result of complex imbalances between different transmitter systems and brain regions of which cortical and striatal regions are highly addressed.

References

1. Carlsson M and Carlsson A (1990) Trends Neurosci. 13: 272–276.
2. Marsden CD (1982) Neurology 32: 514–539.
3. Albin RL, Young AB and Penney JB (1989b) Trends Neurosci. 12: 366–375.
4. Alexander GE, DeLong MR and Strick PL (1986) Ann. Rev. Neurosci. 9: 357–381.
5. DeLong MR (1990) Trends Neurosci. 13: 281–285.
6. Evarts EV, Nimura M, Wurtz RH and Hikosaka O (1984) Trends Neurosci. 7: 447–453.
7. Papez JW (1937) Arch. Neurol. Psychiatry 38: 725–743.
8. Kim JS, Kornhuber HH, Schmid-Burgk W and Holzmüller B (1980) Neurosci. Lett. 20: 379–382.
9. Nieuwenhuys R, Voogd J and Huijzen C (1989) The Human Central Nervous System. 3rd Edition. Springer-Verlag, Berlin, p. 348.
10. Bernheimer H, Birkmayer W, Hornykiewicz O, Jellinger K and Seitelberger F (1973) J. Neurosci. 20: 415–455.
11. Somogyi P, Bolam JP, Totterdell S and Smith AD (1981) Brain Res. 217: 245–263.
12. Kornhuber J, Mack-Burkhardt F, Riederer P, Hebenstreit GF, Reynolds GP, Andrews HB and Beckmann H (1989) J. Neural Transm. 77: 231–236.
13. Snyder SH (1980) Nature 285: 355–356.
14. Deutsch SI, Mastropaolo J, Schwartz BL, Rosse RB and Morihisa JM (1989) Clin. Neuropharmacol. 12: 1–13.
15. Heimer L (1983) The Human Brain and Spinal Cord. Springer-Verlag, New York, p. 327.
16. Nauta WJH, Smith GP, Faull RLM and Domesick VB (1978) Neuroscience 3: 385–401.

Biological Psychiatry, Volume 1. G. Racagni et al., editors.

Pathomorphological aspects of schizophrenia

K.A. Jellinger[1], H. Beckmann[2] and H. Heinsen[2]
[1]L. Boltzmann Institute of Clinical Neurobiology, Lainz-Hospital, A-1130 Vienna, Austria; and [2]Department of Psychiatry, University School of Medicine, D-8700 Würzburg, Germany

The search for an organic basis of schizophrenia has a long and controversial history and most changes observed in previous studies were regarded either as non-specific or substrates of mental impairment rather than of the primary psychosis [1]. The process of identifying consistent differences between schizophrenics and controls is made more difficult by a rather high incidence of unexpected identifiable brain pathology (e.g. vascular, degenerative and metabolic diseases, Alzheimer and Parkinson type lesions, tumor, etc.) in schizophrenics ranging from 14 to over 50% which is significantly greater than in age-matched controls [1-3]. Among 133 consecutive autopsy cases fulfilling Feighner's research criteria, we found identifiable brain pathology in 48.2% (28.6% organic lesions, 19.6% localized pathology, and 9% superimposed lesions). More recent neuroimaging and postmortem studies using standardized techniques have provided increasing evidence that brains of schizophrenic patients show consistent but subtle anatomical abnormalities and that some structural brain deficits may be associated with certain clinical subtypes.

Macroscopic changes

Macroscopic changes include a significant decrease in brain weight by 5.5 to 8% and 4 to 6% reduction in brain length for both hemispheres in both sexes [3,4]. Previous data indicating significant volume reduction of cerebral hemispheres, cortex, white matter or basal ganglia were not confirmed by recent volumetric studies [5,6]. Planimetric autopsy studies confirmed neuroimaging data of ventricular enlargement (13 to 33%) with preferential dilatation of the temporal horn (70%) [4,5], asymmetry being also observed in controls [7]. Brain atrophy and ventricular enlargement (ventricular:brain ratio) are significantly related to the severity of symptoms, while most studies have failed to show correlations between brain atrophy or ventricular enlargement and the duration of schizophrenia [2–4]. The structural changes preferentially affect the medial temporal lobe and morphometric MRI and autopsy studies show volume reduction of hippocampus, parahippocampal gyrus and amygdala by 3 to 30% that correlates significantly with increased area of the ventricular temporal horn [3–5,7–10], but is much less than in Alzheimer's disease (28 to 50%) [11].

Affected regions

Of the various brain areas believed to be related to schizophrenia, the limbic system, in particular the hippocampus, has recently become the subject of intense morphologic studies, since schizophrenia-like psychoses are seen in patients with temporal lobe epilepsy and various neurologic diseases with limbic system lesions [1,3]. Abnormalities reported in the hippocampus of schizophrenics include decreased volume, gliosis, structure asymmetry, decreased immunoreactivity and binding sites of neuropeptides, reduced cell numbers in some hippocampal areas, decreased density, disarrayed orientation of pyramidal cells and other cytoarchitectonic alterations in the entorhinal and parahippocampal cortex [3,4,10,12].

Anatomically, the cornu ammonis includes the hippocampus with the segments CA1-4, fascia dentata, prosubiculum, subiculum, pre- and parasubiculum, and parahippocampal gyrus (entorhinal area) showing a trilaminar cortical architecture. Hippocampal inputs from association areas (frontal, temporal, cingulate cortices) converge on the entorhinal cortex and reach the hippocampus via the perforant pathway. The hippocampal output is organized in a similar fashion from projection neurons within the subiculum. By virtue of this arrangement the parahippocampal gyrus and glutamatergic perforant pathway serve to "gate" all information entering and leaving the hippocampus [5,13]. Mesolimbic cortex and hippocampus are thought to be central in the integration of emotional responses, behavior and intellect, and lesions in these regions may alter the function and neurochemistry of other CNS systems [13].

In the hippocampus altered orientation of pyramidal cells, particularly at the CA 1/2 and CA 1-prosubiculum interface zones has been reported, suggesting defective patterns of neuronal migration [14]. The volume and cell density were reduced in all areas of the left cornu ammonis of schizophrenics, most pronounced in the CA4 region, but not accompanied by gliosis [10], while no changes were found in the size, shape and variability of orientation in the CA 1 region [12]. Among 64 autopsy cases of schizophrenia, Jakob and Beckmann [15] in two-thirds reported abnormal sulcogyral pattern of the temporal lobe cortex, with cell loss and cytoarchitectonic changes in parahippocampal gyrus and/or ventral insula (claustrocortex). Poorly developed structures in the second pre-α layer of the entorhinal region with heterotopic nerve cell clusters in the third layer pre-β and relative absence of neurons above these clusters are mainly present in the medial and central parts of the parahippocampal gyrus, while the lateral (transitional) region and other parts of the temporal cortex are not involved. These findings, confirmed by personal (unpublished) and other studies [16], suggest abnormal ontogenic development of a small part of the entorhinal region due to disturbances of neuronal migration in late phases of cortical development (around the 5th month of gestation) [15].

Other regions of the brain can be affected in schizophrenia but to a much lesser degree. Cytoarchitectonic changes in deep layers of the prefrontal, motor and cingulate cortex with increase in vertical axons were seen in the anterior cingulate cortex [17]. The results of morphologic studies of the corpus callosum have been contradictory, but recent MRI studies showed some disease-related distortion suggesting ventriculotomy rather than intrinsic abnormality of the corpus callosum [18]. Atrophy of superior cerebellar vermis is seen in some schizophrenic patients [19]. There are no changes in basal ganglia, mesocorticolimbic or nigrostriatal dopamine systems [6].

Increased incidence of cortical, white matter and periventricular gliosis often reported in schizophrenic brains [2,3,20] is often associated with various types of acquired or superimposed brain pathology, while "purified" groups (after removing cases with identifiable brain pathology) show no significant cerebral gliosis that might signal a degenerative disease process or other acquired exogenous lesions [2].

Conclusions

Recent neuropathologic research indicates that the brains of patients with schizophrenia show consistent but subtle structural abnormalities and may differ from normal controls. The changes involve mild reduction in brain weight (mean 6%), length and volume with mild, usually non-progressive enlargement of the lateral and third ventricles, smaller anterior hippocampi, prefrontal cortex and upper cerebellar vermis. Structural changes preferentially affect medial temporal lobe regions and cingulate cortex with neuronal loss and cytoarchitectonic changes unaccompanied by gliosis that suggest developmental abnormalities rather than a degenerative or other exogenous process. Changes in brain structure may differ in degree and may affect both hemispheres or prefer the left one. Most of the cerebral changes are probably genetic in origin, while environmental factors account only for a small minority of cases. In addition, the brains of schizophrenics show higher degrees of acquired neuropathologic damage which appears to be superimposed on the developmental structural changes the etiology of which remains unknown.

References

1. Jellinger K (1985) In: Beckmann H and Riederer P (eds.) Pathochemical Markers in Major Psychoses. Springer-Verlag, Berlin, pp. 1–23.
2. Bruton CJ, Crow TJ, Frith CD et al. (1990) Psychol. Med. 20: 285–304.
3. Roberts GW and Bruton CJ (1990) Neuropathol. Appl. Neurobiol. 16: 3–16.
4. Brown R, Colter N, Corsellis JAN et al. (1986) Arch. Gen. Psychiatry 43: 36–42.
5. Heckers S, Heinsen H, Heinsen Y and Beckmann H (1990) Arch. Gen. Psychiatry 47: 1016–1022.
6. Heckers S, Heinsen H, Heinsen Y and Beckmann H (1991) Biol. Psychiatry 29: 556–566.
7. Young AH, Blackwood DHR, Roxborough H et al. (1991) Br. J. Psychiatry 158: 158–164.
8. Bogerts B, Ashtari M, Degreef G et al. (1990) Psychiatr. Res. 35: 1–13.
9. Suddath RL, Christison GW, Torrey EF et al. (1990) N. Engl. J. Med. 322: 789–794.
10. Jeste DV and Lohr JB (1989) Arch. Gen. Psychiatry 46: 1019–1024.
11. Kesslak JP, Nalcioglu O and Cotman CW (1991) Neurology 41: 51–54.

12. Christion G, Casanova M, Weinberger D et al. (1989) Arch. Gen. Psychiatry 46: 1027–1032.
13. Hyman BD, Van Hoesen GW and Damasio AR (1987) Ann. Neurol. 22: 37–40.
14. Kovelman JA and Scheibel AB (1984) Biol. Psychiatry 19: 1601–1621.
15. Jakob H and Beckmann H (1986) J. Neural Transm. 65: 303–326.
16. Falkai P, Bogerts B and Rozumek M (1988) Biol. Psychiatry 24: 515–521.
17. Benes FM and Bird ED (1987) Arch. Gen. Psychiatry 44: 608–616.
18. Casanova FM, Sanders R, Goldberg T et al. (1990) J. Neurol. Neurosurg. Psychiatry 53: 416.
19. Sandyk R, Kay SR and Merriam AE (1991) Int. J. Neurosci. 56: 205–212.
20. Stevens CD, Altshuler LL, Bogerts B and Falkai P (1988) Biol. Psychiatry 24: 697–700.

Biological Psychiatry, Volume 1. G. Racagni et al., editors.

Markedly increased number of striatal D_2 dopamine receptors in human narcolepsy but without psychosis: Implications for the dopamine hypothesis of schizophrenia

Stephen J. Kish, Mortimer Mamelak, Anthony Lewis, Caroline Slimovitch, Lori M. Dixon, Linda Distefano and Oleh Hornykiewicz
Clarke Institute of Psychiatry, 250 College Street, Toronto, Ontario, Canada, M5T 1R8

Introduction

The dopamine hypothesis of schizophrenia is supported by the demonstration, in most postmortem human brain studies, of a markedly increased number of D_2 dopamine receptors in the striatum (caudate and putamen) of patients with schizophrenia [1]. Comparatively little information is available regarding the behaviour of the striatal dopamine receptor in autopsied brain of patients with other psychiatric and neurological disorders, leaving the specificity of the changes in schizophrenic brain uncertain. We have examined the levels of the D_1 and D_2 dopamine receptors in the autopsied striatum of three patients with narcolepsy, a sleeping disorder characterized by excessive daytime drowsiness, sleep attacks, and fragmented nocturnal sleep. We report that although all three patients were psychiatrically normal, the density of the striatal D_2 dopamine receptor was elevated (+125%) to a greater extent than that typically observed in schizophrenic brain.

Patients and Methods

Autopsied brain was obtained from 3 patients with narcolepsy (55 ± 9 years) and 7 controls matched with respect to age and postmortem time. The postmortem time interval was less than 24 h for all cases. Two of the 3 patients had been treated chronically with d-amphetamine (1 case up to 6 months before death; 1 case up to 1 month before death) whereas the third patient had not received any stimulant medications during the last 40 years of life. All 3 patients had been extensively followed clinically and were found to be psychiatrically normal. Dopamine D_2 receptor binding was measured with minor modification of a filtration binding assay [2] using ^{3}H-spiperone (20 to 1000 pM) and, for non-specific binding, 10 μM sulpiride. Dopamine D_1 receptor binding was determined by filtration binding using ^{3}H-SCH 23390 (0.2–5 nM) and, for non-specific binding, 10 μM + butaclamol.

Table 1. Dopamine D_1 and D_2 receptor density (B_{max}) in autopsied human brain: controls vs. narcolepsy

	Caudate nucleus		Putamen	
	Controls	Narcolepsy	Controls	Narcolepsy
^{3}H-SCH 23390 binding (D_1)	360 ± 34	356 ± 170	214 ± 20	205 ± 52
^{3}H-Spiperone binding (D_2)	93 ± 10	209 ± 24[a]	91 ± 9	206 ± 20[a]

Values (fmol/mg protein) represent mean ± S.E. of 5–7 controls and 3 patients with narcolepsy; [a] $P < 0.001$, student's two-tailed *t*-test.

Results

As shown in Table 1, mean ^{3}H-spiperone binding to the D_2 dopamine receptor was markedly and significantly elevated (+125% as compared with the controls, $P < 0.001$) in both caudate and putamen of the patients with narcolepsy. No overlap was observed between the range of the individual control and narcoleptic D_2 values. No significant differences were observed in these brain areas in the density of ^{3}H-SCH 23390 binding to the D_1 dopamine receptor, or in the affinity constants (K_d) for the D_1 and D_2 receptors (data not shown).

Discussion and Conclusion

The major finding of our study is a marked increase in the number of the D_2 dopamine receptors in the striatum of three patients with narcolepsy. We suggest that these data may have important implications for the dopamine hypothesis of schizophrenia. In this regard, we have observed that the magnitude of the increase (+125%) in number of the striatal D_2 dopamine receptors in narcolepsy was actually greater than that typically observed in the striatum of schizophrenic patients [1]. Our patients with narcolepsy, however, had never suffered from schizophrenia or any other psychiatric illness (all were extensively followed clinically). Our findings, therefore, demonstrate that an increase in the number of striatal D_2 dopamine receptors cannot be sufficient by itself to produce the symptoms of schizophrenia and argue against the specificity of this biochemical change in schizophrenia.

References

1. Seeman P (1987) Synapse 1: 133–152.
2. Seeman P, Ulpian C, Bergeron C et al. (1984) Science 225: 728–731.

Biological Psychiatry, Volume 1. G. Racagni et al., editors.

Amino acid transmitters and dopamine function in the brain in schizophrenia

Gavin P. Reynolds
Department of Biomedical Science, University of Sheffield, Sheffield S10 2TN, U.K.

Introduction

There is increasing evidence for neuropathological abnormalities in schizophrenia. The advent and development of tomographic imaging techniques and the application of morphometric and cytometric techniques in neuropathology has led to the identification of subtle, yet substantial, abnormalities indicative of neuronal deficits in the disease. This evidence is inevitably reflected by a neurochemical pathology in which changes in transmitters and transmitter-related biochemical measures, including receptors and synthetic enzymes, is apparent. These neuronal deficits and their corresponding biochemical markers have been observed particularly in the medial temporal lobe, and perhaps to a lesser extent in the frontal cortex.

Dopamine and antipsychotic effects

A full understanding of brain dysfunction in schizophrenia will depend not only on the description of brain pathology but also on the interaction of antipsychotic drugs with this pathology. Thus the amelioration of symptomatology brought about by these drugs must in some way rely on the reversal of the (eventual) effects of the neurotransmitter dysfunction in schizophrenia. The transmitter most strongly implicated in the effects of antipsychotic drug treatment is dopamine, the greatest support for which comes from the substantial evidence for dopaminergic antagonism being an action common to the neuroleptic drugs. Thus the dopamine D_2 receptor blockade induced by these compounds is the one pharmacological effect which clearly correlates with their clinical antipsychotic dosage. This, of course, points particularly well to the site of antipsychotic action but provides no direct evidence for a hyperactivity of dopaminergic transmission in the disease. Of the reports of changes in dopamine systems in the brain in schizophrenia it is only the finding of a lateralised increase in the transmitter in the amygdala [1] which cannot be readily explained by the effects of antipsychotic medication.

Temporal lobe neurochemistry

If the observed abnormality in amygdala dopamine is related to an atrophy or disorganization of other neuronal systems within the temporal lobe, then other identifiable neurochemical changes should reflect this more primary disturbance. Some other recent findings may provide clues. The reported diminished concentrations of CCK and somatostatin in the hippocampus and other temporal structures in some schizophrenic patients is consistent with a deficit of neurons containing these peptides [2]. Such neurons are likely to be GABAergic, since both these peptides coexist primarily with GABA. We have recently obtained more direct evidence for a deficit of GABAergic neurons in schizophrenia.

We have identified a deficit of [^{3}H]-nipecotic acid binding to GABA uptake sites in the hippocampus in schizophrenia [3]. Since we find the binding of this ligand to be diminished in Huntington's disease striatum, in which there is a loss of GABAergic neurons, it would appear that [^{3}H]-nipecotic acid binding is a marker for the integrity of these neurons in human postmortem brain tissue. Our results show a greater deficit in the left hemisphere in schizophrenia; there is also other evidence for a lateralised loss of hippocampal neurons. Kerwin et al. [4] found reduced kainate receptor binding in the left hippocampus in schizophrenia; they also showed decreased expression of the gene for this receptor [5]. This evidence is certainly suggestive of loss of neurons on which the receptors are found, or an abnormal regulatory process. How these abnormalities might interact with dopamine systems has been under investigation; the deficit of hippocampal GABAergic neurons could conceivably lead to a disinhibition of limbic dopamine systems, indicating a mechanism whereby neuroleptic drug treatment might ameliorate the effects of a neuronal deficit in schizophrenia.

Certainly the GABAergic deficit, with a more profound effect in the left hemisphere, is potentially related to the increased concentrations in dopamine in the amygdala. Only in the left hemisphere of schizophrenic patients is there a correlation between amygdala dopamine concentrations and the numbers of hippocampal GABA uptake sites. The result certainly suggests that the (lateralised) changes in dopamine may be induced by a deficit of hippocampal neurons and brings together the increasing evidence for neuronal deficits with the dopamine hypothesis of the disease and its drug treatment. In particular it relates the neurochemical pathology of the temporal lobe to the "positive" symptoms of schizophrenia that respond to treatment with dopamine antagonist drugs.

Frontal cortex neurochemistry

We have also been studying neurochemical abnormalities in the cortex. Although there are some indications of neuronal deficits in the frontal cortex [6], this has not been as extensively studied as the evidence for temporal lobe pathology. There are some indications of transmitter changes in the frontal cortex in schizophrenia. The

Table 1. Glutamate concentrations in cortical tissue

	Left	Right
Frontal cortex (area 11)		
Schizophrenics (14)	1434 ± 239	1362 ± 222[a]
Controls (15)	1153 ± 179	1203 ± 137
Temporal cortex (area 22)		
Schizophrenics (16)	1383 ± 319	1359 ± 210
Controls (14)	1295 ± 125	1280 ± 152

[a]$P < 0.01$ vs. controls; Values are mean ± S.D. in μg/g tissue.

increase in cortical concentrations of the dopamine metabolite HVA is well established and presumed to be an effect of chronic neuroleptic drug treatment. In an attempt to identify neurochemical correlates of the evidence, morphological and psychological, for neuronal dysfunction in frontal and/or temporal cortex in schizophrenia, we have also measured concentrations of transmitter amino acids directly. We have recently found an increase in the concentration of glutamate in the frontal, but not the temporal, cortex, a result consistent with some other reports of changes in glutamatergic systems in this area (Table 1). Thus Nishikawa et al. [7] first described an increase in kainate receptors in frontal cortex and more recent studies [8] have indicated changes in the density of ligand binding to frontal cortical glutamate uptake sites, suggesting that there might be an excess of glutamatergic innervation in this region. Our finding of a specific increase in glutamate concentration of approximately 25% in the schizophrenic patients certainly supports this interpretation, although as yet it is not possible to exclude the possibility that the result reflects a change in glutamate metabolism, reflecting glutamatergic activity.

In contrast to the hippocampal GABAergic deficit, these results have not been found to correlate with any marker of dopaminergic function, whether in the frontal cortex or in the temporal lobe. It is thus possible that the changes in glutamatergic systems observed in frontal cortex relate to the symptoms of schizophrenia that are less likely to respond to the antipsychotic dopaminergic antagonist drugs. There is other evidence that has related negative symptoms to the frontal cortex; imaging studies identifying a "hypofrontality" in schizophrenia indicate that this is associated with more negative symptoms [1]. The cortical glutamatergic abnormalities may well provide a neurochemical reflection of this "hypofrontality".

References

1. Reynolds GP (1983) Nature 305: 527–529.
2. Ferrier IN, Roberts GW, Crow TJ et al. (1983) Life Sci. 33: 475–482.

3. Reynolds GP, Czudek C and Andrews HB (1990) Biol. Psychiatry 27: 1038–1044.
4. Kerwin RW, Patel S, Meldrum BS, Czudek C and Reynolds GP (1988) Lancet i: 583–584.
5. Harrison PJ, McLaughlin D and Kerwin RW (1991) Lancet i: 450–452.
6. Benes FM, Davidson J and Bird ED (1986) Arch. Gen. Psychiatry 44: 1017–1021.
7. Nishikawa T, Takashima M and Toru M (1983) Neurosci. Lett. 40: 245–250.
8. Deakin JFW, Slater P, Simpson MDC et al. (1989) J. Neurochem. 52: 1781–1786.
9. Ingvar DH (1987) In: Helmchen H and Henn FA (eds.) Biological Perspectives of Schizophrenia. Wiley, Chichester, pp. 201–211.

Biological Psychiatry, Volume 1. G. Racagni et al., editors.

Glutamate and schizophrenia

Johannes Kornhuber and Peter Riederer
Department of Psychiatry, University of Würzburg, Füchsleinstrasse 15, 8700 Würzburg, Germany

Introduction

The "glutamate hypothesis" of schizophrenia proposes that a deficiency in glutamatergic neurotransmission and a resulting disturbed balance between glutamatergic and dopaminergic systems within the striatum and nucleus accumbens may play a key role in the pathophysiology of schizophrenia [1–4]. Glutamatergic drugs might thus be of therapeutic value in the treatment of schizophrenia. The balance between glutamatergic and dopaminergic systems might explain the therapeutic action of neuroleptic drugs. The "glutamate hypothesis" is compatible with the growing evidence for a dysfunction of glutamatergic neurotransmission in schizophrenia:

Indirect evidence:
- Centrally-acting NMDA antagonists like PCP or MK-801 seem to have psychotomimetic properties in man.
- Markers for glutamatergic neurotransmission are high in regions thought to be involved in the pathogenesis of schizophrenia (frontal and temporal cortex, area entorhinalis, hippocampus, amygdala).
- Since the major glutamatergic pathways in the brain originate in the cerebral cortex, the "glutamate hypothesis" is consistent with the cortical atrophy observed in schizophrenic patients and with the possible hypometabolism found in frontal cortex of schizophrenic patients.

Direct evidence:
- Veratridine-induced glutamate release is reduced in frontal and temporal cortex of schizophrenic patients [5].
- Increases in [^{3}H]kainic acid binding sites have been reported in the medial frontal cortex and eye movement area [6] as well as in the orbital frontal cortex [7] of schizophrenic patients.
- Cerebrospinal fluid glutamate levels were found to be reduced in schizophrenics [1].

The "thalamic filter dysfunction hypothesis" by Carlsson [8] is a more sophisticated version of the "glutamate hypothesis" incorporating the cortico-striatal projection into a feedback-loop running from the cortex via the striatum and thalamus back to the cortex.

Because of the possible relevance of the glutamate receptor, especially the NMDA receptor subtype, we have measured these sites in postmortem brain tissue from schizophrenic patients using [^{3}H]MK-801 as a ligand [2,9,10].

Methods

Brain tissue was taken at autopsy. Preparation of homogenates and binding assays was done essentially as previously described [9].

Results and Discussion

Firstly, we investigated the effect of several antemortem and postmortem factors on [^{3}H]MK-801 binding in the frontal cortex of 38 human control brains [10]. These factors included age, gender, laterality, postmortem delay, storage time of brain tissue and brain weight. Increased storage time of brain tissue at low temperature had a reducing effect on [^{3}H]MK-801 binding sites. However, they were still well detectable even after 8 years of storage and there was no change within the first year of storage. The second factor of influence was the age of the control persons. There was a transient increase in [^{3}H]MK-801 binding in the postnatal period reaching a maximum between age 1 and 2 years. After age 10 years, [^{3}H]MK-801 binding sites disappeared at about 6% per decade. There was no effect of gender, brain weight or postmortem time-interval (up to 72 h) and the binding sites were bilaterally symmetrically distributed in the frontal cortex.

Thereafter, we have measured these binding sites in postmortem brains from schizophrenic patients using a single concentration of [^{3}H]MK-801 [2]. The above-mentioned factors of influence did not significantly differ between schizophrenics and controls. Tissue samples from either side of the frontal cortex, putamen, amygdala, entorhinal region and hippocampus were analyzed. In schizophrenia [^{3}H]MK-801 binding values were increased in all brain regions investigated, reaching significance in the putamen (+44.4%, $P < 0.01$). This increase was significant in both sides of the brain and may be due to an upregulation of the density of binding sites mediated by a presynaptic dysfunction of the glutamatergic system [11].

Since a large portion of these patients will have received long-term antipsychotic drug treatment, it is conceivable that this may have had an effect on the NMDA receptor. However, haloperidol did not displace [^{3}H]MK-801 from postmortem human frontal cortex nor did it alter [^{3}H]MK-801 binding characteristics after an acute or long-term administration in the rat.

References

1. Kim JS, Kornhuber HH, Schmid-Burgk W and Holzmüller B (1980) Neurosci. Lett. 20: 379–382.
2. Kornhuber J, Mack-Burkhardt F, Riederer P, Hebenstreit GF, Reynolds GP, Andrews HB and Beckmann H (1989) J. Neural Transm. 77: 231–236.
3. Kornhuber J, Riederer P and Beckmann H (1990) In: Bunney WE, Hippius H, Laakmann G, Schmauß M (eds.) Neuropsychopharmacology. Springer, Berlin, Heidelberg, pp. 714–720.
4. Kornhuber J (1990) Trends. Pharmacol. Sci. 11: 357.
5. Sherman AD, Davidson AT, Baruah S, Hegwood TS and Waziri R (1991) Neurosci. Lett. 121: 77–80.
6. Nishikawa T, Takashima M and Toru N (1983) Neurosci. Lett. 40: 245–250.
7. Deakin JFW, Slater P, Simpson MDC, Gilchrist AC, Skan WJ, Royston MC, Reynolds GP and Cross AJ (1989) J. Neurochem. 52: 1781–1786.
8. Carlsson A (1988) Neuropsychopharmacology 1: 179–186.
9. Kornhuber J, Mack-Burkhardt F, Kornhuber ME and Riederer P (1989) Eur. J. Pharmacol. 162: 483–490.
10. Kornhuber J, Mack-Burkhardt F, Konradi C, Fritze J and Riederer P (1989) Life Sci. 45: 745–749.
11. Samuel D, Errami M and Nieoullon A (1990) J. Neurochem. 54: 1926–1933.

Biological Psychiatry, Volume 1. G. Racagni et al., editors.

Postmortem investigations of *sigma* and PCP receptors in psychosis

Arthur D. Weissman[1] and Errol B. de Souza[2]
[1]*National Institute on Drug Abuse, Baltimore, MD 21224; and* [2]*The Du Pont Merck Pharmaceutical Co., Wilmington, DE 19880, U.S.A.*

Introduction

The psychotomimetic effects of certain drugs that interact with phencyclidine (PCP) and/or *sigma* binding sites have suggested that these sites may be important in the etiology of schizophrenia. In individuals abusing PCP, prolonged psychotic episodes that resemble schizophrenia can extend beyond the detection of significant quantities of PCP in the blood [1], and PCP exacerbates some symptoms in schizophrenic patients [2]. A compelling role for the *sigma* site in schizophrenia may be indicated by the high affinity of many antipsychotic drugs, including haloperidol, for the *sigma* site [3]. PCP [4] and *sigma* [5] receptors have been identified and characterized in human postmortem brain areas implicated in the generation of schizophrenic symptoms. Our studies were directed at a postmortem assessment of the regional brain PCP and *sigma* binding sites in a population of schizophrenics [6] and PCP drug abusers [7]. Our rationale was that psychosis generated either endogenously or by exogenous drug use may be related to alteration in either regional PCP and/or *sigma* receptor properties.

Materials and Methods

Autopsy samples were from St. Elizabeth's Hospital, Washington D.C. or from cases referred from the Washington D.C. Medical Examiner. An independent confirmation of the psychiatric diagnosis was made from retrospective chart reviews according to DSM III-R criteria. Two groups of schizophrenics, paranoid and undifferentiated, were included in the study as well as a group of schizo-affectives. The addict population was comprised of individuals who had a history of repeated exposure to PCP and who had detectable blood levels of the drug after death. Control brains were obtained from individuals who had died of natural or accidental causes and had no history of neurological or psychiatric disease. Gross pathology of the control brain at death appeared normal. An additional group of suicide victims who had no history of neurological disease or schizophrenic symptoms was included to control for "non-specific" effects of neuropsychiatric illness, drug treatment and manner of death. No significant differences in age or postmortem delay were evident between groups. The brain regions were dissected from frozen tissue and included the frontal, temporal, parietal and anterior cingulate cerebral cortex as well as the dentate nucleus, caudate, putamen, hippocampus, cerebellum and thalamus.

Sigma receptors in brain homogenates were labelled with [^{3}H]haloperidol in the presence of 50 nM spiperone (to preclude [^{3}H]haloperidol binding to D_2 dopamine receptors) and PCP receptors were labelled with [^{3}H]TCP as previously described [5–7].

Results

The differences in the amount of [^{3}H]TCP binding at a single radioligand concentration and in saturation studies among control, suicide and schizophrenic groups were, for the most part, unremarkable and not specific to schizophrenia in the 7 brain regions examined. These data suggest that PCP receptors were not altered selectively in the brains of schizophrenics. A comparison between binding site characteristics in the suicide control and PCP addict populations also revealed no significant differences in the affinity or density of [^{3}H]TCP binding between the 2 clinical groups across 9 brain regions.

[^{3}H]Haloperidol-labelled *sigma* binding showed more consistent and specific alterations in several brain regions from schizophrenics. Binding (at 1 nM) was significantly lower in temporal cortex in the paranoid (49%) and in the undifferentiated (58%) schizophrenic groups and in the dentate nucleus for both the schizophrenic groups (paranoid, 25% and undifferentiated, 34%) and schizoaffectives (43%) when compared to normal controls. [^{3}H]Haloperidol binding was also lower in the paranoid schizophrenic group in the parietal cortex (20%) and in the schizoaffective group in the temporal cortex (24%); however, these differences were not statistically significant. In addition, no significant differences in *sigma* binding were seen in the suicides as compared to the normal controls in any of the brain regions examined.

Saturation studies in parietal and temporal cortex of schizophrenics showed lower maximal densities of *sigma* binding sites (i.e. B_{max}). No significant differences were seen in the affinity (K_d) for *sigma* binding in any of the groups examined. In temporal cortex, significantly lower B_{max} values in the paranoid schizophrenics (49%) and schizoaffectives (51%) were seen when compared to neurologically normal and to suicide groups. There were no significant differences in the affinity or density of [^{3}H]haloperidol-labelled *sigma* binding between the PCP addict and suicide groups in eight of the same brain regions examined in the schizophrenic population.

Discussion

These studies suggest an alteration in *sigma*, but not PCP binding sites in schizophrenia. The specificity of the reduction in *sigma* binding in the brains of schizophrenics is supported by several observations. First, no significant change in *sigma* binding was seen in the brains of suicide victims as compared to controls in any of the brain regions examined. Second, the decrease in *sigma* binding appeared to be confined to discrete brain regions, a finding which argues against a general neurochemical derangement or a global pathology in schizophrenia.

Several mechanisms can be proposed for the regional decreases in *sigma* binding in schizophrenics. One possibility is an alteration in the level of a putative endogenous ligand(s) for the *sigma* binding site. Alternatively, a focal lesion of neurons bearing *sigma* binding sites may occur in the disorder. In this regard, decreases in neuronal density have been observed in several regions, including the temporal cortex, of brains from schizophrenics [8]. The loss of *sigma* binding in the dentate nucleus of the cerebellum may be related to cerebellar structural abnormalities and dysfunction that has been previously reported in approximately 10% of schizophrenic patients [9]. However, in view of preclinical data, the long-term role of neuroleptics in reducing *sigma* binding sites cannot be ruled out, and it will be important to validate our findings in a drug-naive population. One possibility is that the changes in *sigma* sites are an integral part of the therapeutic actions of the neuroleptics. The present demonstration of specific regional decreases in *sigma* binding in postmortem schizophrenic brains, the high affinity of neuroleptics for this site, and the psychotomimetic activity and/or antipsychotic activity of *sigma* ligands, suggest the utility of pursuing the link between schizophrenia and the *sigma* system further.

Acknowledgements

The studies described were carried out in collaboration with Drs. Manual Casanova and Joel Kleinman of NIMH and Dr. Edythe London of NIDA.

References

1. Luisada PV and Brown BI (1976) Clin. Toxicol. 9: 539–554.
2. Luby ED, Cohen BD, Rosenbaum G, Gottlieb JS and Kelley R (1959) Arch. Neurol. Psychiatry 81: 363–366.
3. Largent BL, Wikstrom H, Snowman AM and Snyder SH (1988) Eur. J. Pharmacol. 155: 345–347.
4. Sircar R and Zukin SR (1983) Life Sci. 33: 259–262.
5. Weissman AD, Su T-P, Hedreen JC and London ED (1988) J. Pharmacol. Exp. Ther. 247: 29–33.
6. Weissman AD, Casanova MF, Kleinman JE, London ED and De Souza EB (1991) Biol. Psychiatry 29: 41–54.
7. Weissman AD, Casanova MF, Kleinman JE, London ED and De Souza EB (1991) Neuropsychopharmacology 4: 95–102.
8. Brown R, Colter N, Corsellis JAW, Crow TJ, Frith DC, Jogoe R, Johnstone EC and Marsh L (1986) Arch. Gen. Psychiatry 43: 36–42.
9. Heath R, Franklin D and Shraberg D (1979) J. Nerv. Ment. Dis. 16: 585–592.

Biological Psychiatry, Volume 1. G. Racagni et al., editors.

Dopaminergic and glutamatergic abnormalities in postmortem schizophrenic brain

Michio Toru[1], Akeo Kuramaji[1], Shin Kumashiro[1], Masahiko Ishimaru[1], Ichiro Suga[2] and Toru Nishikawa[3]

[1]Department of Neuropsychiatry, Tokyo Medical and Dental University, Yushima, Bunkyo-ku, Tokyo; [2]Tokyo Metropolitan Matsuzawa Hospital; and [3]National Institute of Neuroscience, NCNP, Tokyo, Japan

The treatment of the chronic schizophrenia is an unsolved problem. Most of the chronic patients are hospitalized without expectation of discharge. Antipsychotic drugs are effective in treating acute symptoms of this disease but not effective for chronic patients. We analyzed the postmortem brain of chronic schizophrenics to reveal neurotransmitter abnormalities which might be responsible to the chronicity of the disease.

Material and Methods [1]

Subjects

The brain samples were from 14 chronic schizophrenic patients whose diagnosis was ascertained by the catamnesis, and the type and course were categorized according to DSM III and 10 controls. Brain was dissected into 35 areas, homogenized in 3 vol of chilled 0.32 M sucrose and dispensed into small tubes to be stored at −80°C until analysis.

Biochemical measurements

Amines and metabolites were measured by the high performance liquid chromatography with electrochemical detection. Tyrosine hydroxylase (TH) was measured by a $^{14}CO_2$-trapping method with a two-step procedure. Dopamine D_2 receptors were measured by using ^{3}H-spiperone and (±) sulpiride, kainic acid receptors were measured by ^{3}H-kainic acid and L-glutamic acid, N-methyl-D-aspartate (NMDA) receptors by ^{3}H-MK801 and L-glutamic acid, and quisqualic acid receptors by ^{3}H-N-methyl-isoxazole-4-propionic acid (AMPA) and L-glutamic acid. Glutamic acid and aspartic acid were measured by spectrometry.

Results

Dopamine (DA)-related substances

No significant changes were found in DA concentration in the caudate, putamen and n. accumbens. We found a significant increase in homovanillic acid (HVA) values in the putamen and substantia nigra, but no change in the caudate. The change was marked in on-drug cases. TH was significantly increased in the caudate, putamen, n. accumbens, substantia nigra, n. ruber and n. subthalamicus. A significant positive correlation was found between TH activity in the caudate and HVA contents in the putamen ($P < 0.005$), substantia nigra ($P < 0.005$) or n. subthalamicus ($P < 0.005$). The mean B_{max} value of ^{3}H-spiperone binding labelling D_2 receptors to the putamen for 10 schizophrenics was 2.2 times higher than the controls ($P < 0.002$) without changes in KD. The B_{max} value of 5 on-drug cases was 2.8 times higher ($P < 0.002$), and that of 5 off-drug cases was 1.6 times higher than the controls ($P < 0.02$).

Excitatory amino acidergic neurons

Glutamic acid was measured in 35 brain areas. In only 2 areas (superior temporal gyrus and angular gyrus), significantly reduced levels were found. The contents of aspartic acid were significantly increased in 5 of 11 brain areas measured. The specific ^{3}H-kainic acid binding in schizophrenics was greater than the controls in the medial frontal cortex and eye-movement area. The values were significantly increased both in off-drug and on-drug cases in both areas. ^{3}H-Kainic acid binding to the angular gyrus was significantly elevated in schizophrenics. The specific ^{3}H-801 binding was significantly increased in the superior temporal gyrus, superior parietal cortex and supra-marginal cortex. No significant changes were found in ^{3}H-AMPA binding in 22 brain areas measured. A significant negative correlation was found between specific ^{3}H-kainic acid binding/^{3}H-MK801 binding values and glutamic acid contents in various brain areas.

Discussion

Our postmortem biochemical analysis revealed that a hyperdopaminergic state coexisted with a hypoglutamatergic state in the chronic schizophrenic brain [2]. Our findings on kainic acid receptors were recently confirmed by Deakin et al. [3] and we confirmed the increase in NMDA receptors reported by Kornhuber et al. [4].

The increase in glutamic acid receptors might result from a hypoactivity in glutamatergic neurons in the brain, because there exists a clear negative correlation between kainic acid receptors/NMDA receptors and glutamic acid contents. Another reason for this is the observation that phencyclidine, a strong schizophrenomimetic drug, is a non-competitive antagonist of NMDA receptors. DA was reported to exert an inhibitory influence on glutamic acid release from nerve terminals of corticostriatal glutamatergic neurons [5]. The hyperdopaminergic state found in the nigrostriatal tract of the same postmortem brain might induce hypoglutamatergic state resulting in an increase in glutamic acid receptors. A significant positive correlation between specific ^{3}H-kainic acid binding in the medial frontal cortex and TH activity in 5 brain areas supports this inference.

An activation of glutamatergic neurons in the chronic schizophrenic brain constitutes a hopeful attempt to treat these patients.

References

1. Toru M, Watanabe S, Shibuya H, Nishikawa T, Noda K, Mitsushio H, Ichikawa H, Kurumaji A, Takashima M, Mataga N and Ogawa A (1988) Acta. Psychiatr. Scand. 78: 121–137.
2. Toru M, Takashima M, Mataga N, Noda K, Mitsushio H and Nishikawa T (1987) In: Cazzullo CL, Invernizzi G and Bressi C (eds.) Schizophrenia: An Integrative View, 2. Ghedini Editore, Milan, pp. 207–211.
3. Deakin JFW, Slater P, Simpson MDC, Gilchrist AC, Skan WJ, Royston MC, Reynolds GP and Cross AJ (1989) J. Neurochem. 52: 1781–1786.
4. Kornhuber J, Mack-Burkhardt F. Riederer P, Hebenstreit GF, Reynolds GP, Andrews HB and Beckman H (1989) J. Neural Transm. 77: 231–236.
5. Rowlands GJ and Roberts PJ (1980) Eur. J. Pharmacol. 62: 2073–2081.

Biological Psychiatry, Volume 1. G. Racagni et al., editors.

Entorhinal cortex pathology in schizophrenia and affective disorders

Manuel Casanova, Richard Saunders, Lori Altshuler, Terry Goldberg, Este Armstrong, Daniel Weinberger and Joel Kleinman

Clinical Brain Disorders Branch, National Institute of Mental Health, Neurosciences Center at St. Elizabeths, 2700 Martin Luther King Jr. Ave., Washington, D.C., U.S.A.

Introduction

Previous studies support the idea that temporal lobe pathology may, in part, be involved in the pathogenesis of schizophrenia. The initial report of parahippocampal thinning by Bogerts et al. [1] was soon corroborated by Brown et al. [2] and provided impetus for future research. Soon afterwards, planimetric analysis of the parahippocampal cortex revealed that the area of maximal gray matter reduction was located at the crest of the gyri as opposed to the walls of the collateral sulcus, while microscopic examination of the entorhinal cortex (rostral parahippocampal gyrus) has provided evidence of neuronal loss and heterotopic-like arrangements of cells in its more superficial layers [3,4]. This study attempts to corroborate the cytoarchitectural disruption of the entorhinal cortex of schizophrenic (SC) patients and also examines whether these abnormalities are present in other psychiatric conditions.

Materials and Methods

All of our patients were selected from the Yakovlev Brain Collection at the Armed Forces Institute of Pathology. Eight schizophrenic patients were selected for our study (mean age of 59.8 years). In only 6 of these patients was there sufficient documentation to establish a diagnosis based on DSM III-R criteria. In order to eliminate any confounding effects of the leukotomy, we compared our measurements to those made in 3 control groups. The first control group consisted of 5 patients leukotomized for reasons other than schizophrenia (i.e. intractable pain) (mean age of 53.6 years). There were 5 patients in our second control group of leukotomized affective disordered patients (mean age of 64.6 years). The last group consisted of 8 non-leukotomized patients without any history of neurologic or psychiatric impairment (mean age of 61.7 years). Photomicrographs of the stellate cells of layer II of the entorhinal cortex were taken at an initial magnification of 160×. Neuronal perikarya were measured from the corresponding negatives. Using the Loats computerized image analysis system, photomicrographs were magnified 13× with a final resolution of 1.25 μm.

Results

Areas of entorhinal cortex cells did not differ significantly among the groups in the left and right rostral and caudal levels. All group comparisons of harmonic amplitudes yielded non-significant results. For phase angle 2, a significant difference was noted on uniform scores in the right posterior section by Kruskal–Wallis analysis (Kruskal–Wallis = 7.96, $P = 0.05$). This reflected the low score of the leukotomized control patients (0.37); other groups had mean uniform scores between 8.8–14.9. Differences in phase angle were not significant in other regions of the entorhinal cortex (Kruskal–Wallis = 4.64, $P > 0.20$).

In the left entorhinal cortex cell counts among the groups differed significantly by ANOVA ($F = 3.31$, $P = 0.05$). Individual *t*-test indicated the presence of significant differences ($P < 0.05$) between the SC patients and both control (leukotomized and non-leukotomized) groups. Significant differences by ANOVA were also noted in the cell counts of the right entorhinal cortex ($F = 4.39$, $P = 0.02$). Schizophrenic and affective disordered patients differed significantly from non-leukotomized control patients by *t*-test; in addition SC patients differed from the leukotomized for pain subjects ($P < 0.05$).

Discussion

Results from the present study indicate marked reductions in neuronal numbers in the entorhinal cortex of SC and affective patients as compared to non-psychiatric controls. No significant differences between groups was detected for any other morphometric parameter examined. Cell loss occurred within a pathological spectrum of severity spanning from a complete absence of layer II to normal cell numbers. Neuronal counts indicated the greatest reduction in the schizophrenic group; however, no significant difference in cell numbers was observed between the schizophrenic and manic depressive groups. Severely affected cases exhibiting total lack of glomerulation in layer II also manifested marked cytoarchitectural disruption of other layers. Most strikingly these cases showed blurring of the cytological characteristics defining each cortical layer and an overall reduction in width of the parahippocampal gyrus. In a few cases, the deeply pigmented cells in layer II appeared displaced and intermingled with those of the third layer; however, no heterotopic-like glomeruli were observed.

Our study provides a microscopic correlate to previous reports of parahippocampal thinning in schizophrenia and simultaneously corroborates the initial microscopic findings of cytoarchitectural abnormalities in this region by Jakob and Beckman [3]. In the present study the microscopic findings proved non-specific for schizophrenia, as they were also observed in patients leukotomized for affective disorders but not in those individuals leukotomized for pain. The similarity in pathological findings (i.e. neuronal cell loss in the entorhinal cortex) between affective and schizophrenic patients is worth emphasizing. A recent neuroimaging study by Hauser et al. [5] suggested temporal lobe volume reduction in patients with primary affective disorders. According to Altshuler et al. [6] this volumetric abnormality may be explained, in part, by thinning of the parahippocampal gyrus. The results of their study indicated structural abnormalities in the parahippocampal gyrus of schizophrenic (bilateral) and depressive (right hemisphere) patients. This observation echoes the previous report by Brown et al. [2] of a difference in thickness between the left and right parahippocampal gyrus in patients with affective disorders.

In summary, our findings indicate neuronal cell loss in the entorhinal cortex of SC and affective patients. There was no additional evidence of cellular disarray, distortion or shrinkage. Previous studies suggest that the underlying lesion accounting for the neuronal loss has an onset during brain gestation. Although dysfunction of the entorhinal cortex may provide a physiological basis for some of the salient symptoms observed in these disorders, it is insufficient, by itself, to explain the whole spectrum of psychiatric manifestations characterizing both schizophrenia and affective disorders. The rich connections of this limbic region and the shared pathological vulnerability with other sites of the nervous system lead us to believe that instead of an isolated foci of cellular abnormality there is a neuroanatomically defined system whose degree of aberrant function provides a variable clinical expression spanning affective and schizophrenic disorders.

References

1. Bogerts B, Meertz E and Schonfeldt-Bausch R (1985) Arch. Gen. Psychiatry 42: 784–791.
2. Brown R, Colter N, Crow TJ et al. (1986) Arch. Gen. Psychiatry 43: 36–42.
3. Jakob H and Beckman H (1986) J. Neural Transm. 65: 303–326.
4. Falkai P, Bogerts B and Rozumek M (1988) Biol. Psychiatry 24: 515–521.
5. Hauser P, Altshuler LL, Berritini W, Dauphanis D, Gelertner J and Post RM (1989) J. Neuropsychiatry Clin. Neurosci. 1: 128–134.
6. Altshuler LL, Casanova MF, Goldberg TE et al. (1990) Arch. Gen. Psychiatry 47(11): 1029–1034.

Biological Psychiatry, Volume 1. G. Racagni et al., editors.

Postmortem brain morphology in schizophrenia: Studies from the new Düsseldorf brain collection

Peter Falkai, Bernhard Bogerts, Sabine David and Benno Greve
Department of Psychiatry, University of Düsseldorf, Bergische Landstraße 2, 4000 Düsseldorf 12, Germany

Introduction

Since 1972, 32 post-mortem brain studies on schizophrenia have been published [1]. With the exception of 3, all of these studies found structural differences between controls and schizophrenics. Most of them focused on limbic system structures. Fourteen studies found changes consistent with a disorder in brain development, 6 reported findings consistent with an inflammatory process, whereas in 12 there was no comment on the possible etiology.

To further clarify the pathomorphology of schizophrenia, the volumes of the cingulate gyrus, stria terminalis, basal limbic forebrain, amygdala, hippocampal formation, septum, fornix, third ventricle, basal ganglia (caudate, putamen, accumbens, external and internal pallidum), thalamus and hypothalamus were determined in the brains of 19 schizophrenic patients and 21 control subjects. In addition, astrocyte densities were counted in 11 brain regions in each hemisphere and the occurrence of heterotopias in the entorhinal cortex was assessed in the same sample.

Patients and controls

Postmortem brains of 19 schizophrenic patients (9 males, 10 females; age: mean/range 51.4/27–72 years) were obtained postmortem between the years 1985–1988. Time between first hospital admission and death was 18 years (males: 20 years, range 10–26; females: 16 years, range 2–27). Clinical records were reviewed retrospectively; all patients fulfilled ICD 9 and DSM III-R criteria for schizophrenia. Fifteen patients had a predominant paranoid-hallucinatory symptomatology, 4 patients had prevailing negative symptoms. Further details of clinical symptoms, disease duration and cause of death of the patients have been published recently [2].

Ten patients had their first hospital admission before age 25 years, 7 patients had their first admission after age 25 years. Four patients had a documented family history of psychiatric illness, whereas for 12 patients no family history of psychiatric disease was reported.

Twenty-one control brains from individuals without history of neuropsychiatric disorders (13 males, 8 females; age: mean/range 53.3/33–72) were obtained from the same pathological or forensic institutes during the same time period. Information on age and cause of death of the control cases has been published recently [2].

Methods

Morphometry

The volumes of the cingulate gyrus, stria terminalis, basal limbic forebrain, amygdala, hippocampal formation, septum, fornix, third ventricle, basal ganglia (caudate, putamen, accumbens, external and internal pallidum), thalamus and hypothalamus were measured by planimetry of myelin-stained 20 micron whole brain serial coronal sections.

Immunhistochemistry

From each brain section were chosen at the level of the anterior commissure, mammillary bodies and posterior commissure which were stained with the PAP-(peroxidase-antiperoxidase) method for GFAP-(Glia Fibrillary Protein). Using a light microscope at a magnification of × 200, GFAP-positive astrocytes were counted with a grid. The density of GFAP-positive astrocytes was counted manually in the following areas separately for each hemisphere: periventricular grey matter, hippocampus CA4 region, amygdala, substantia innominate, mammillary bodies, anterior thalamic nucleus, entorhinal cortex and periaqueductal region.

Rating of heterotopias

On 10–15 subsequent myelin and Nissl sections the amount of heterotopic pre-α-cell clusters in the entorhinal cortex was assessed qualitatively using a scale from +1 to +3 (+1 = one heterotopic cluster, + = two heterotopic clusters, +3 = three heterotopic clusters) by two independent raters separately for each hemisphere.

Results

Morphometry

The volume of the hippocampal formation (left: – 15%, $P < 0.02$, right: – 15%, $P <$ 0.019) was significantly reduced in the right and left hemisphere; male patients were more affected than female patients. Patients with their first hospital admission before age 25 years had significantly smaller hippocampi compared to patients with their first admission after age 25 years (controls vs. hospital admission before age 25 years: – 20%, $P < 0.0009$, controls vs. hospital admission after age 25 years: – 11%, $P < 0.24$).

There was a non-significant trend towards an enlargement of the third ventricle (+26, $P < 0.07$). All other structures showed no difference between schizophrenic patients and controls.

Astrocyte counts

The schizophrenic group revealed a moderate but significant increase in GFAP positive cell densities in the periventricular grey matter around the third ventricle (left: +57%, $P < 0.01$, right: +44%, $P < 0.05$), the left periaqueductal area (+61, $P < 0.03$) and the left anterior thalamic nucleus (+63, $P < 0.05$). There was a tendency towards gliosis in the right amygdala and an insignificant trend towards increased glial cell densities in the entorhinal cortex. No significant gliosis could be observed in the mamillary bodies, hippocampus CA4 region and the substantia nigra.

Rating of heterotopias

Schizophrenic patients showed significantly more heterotopic pre-α-cell clusters in the left entorhinal cortex compared to the control group (+43%, $P < 0.032$). Late onset cases compared to healthy controls had significantly more heterotopias in the left entorhinal cortex than early onset patients (+58%, $P < 0.03$). Patients with a family history of psychiatric illness compared to patients lacking a family lacking a family history of psychiatric illness had an excess of heterotopias in both hemispheres of about 100% (patients with a family history vs. control subjects: left + 62%, $P < 0.03$; right +77%, $P < 0.04$).

Discussion

This study demonstrates hippocampal pathology in schizophrenia already shown in other post-mortem and recent MRI studies [1]. In addition, it shows a subtle but significant increase in astrocyte densities mainly around the third ventricle in brains of patients with schizophrenia. With the exception of the amygdala there is a lack of significant gliosis in temporal lobe structures, but an increase of heterotopias in the left entorhinal cortex in schizophrenics.

Although these data can only be regarded as preliminary, they suggest that there are several disease processes causing different pathologies in the brains of schizophrenic patients. Periventricular gliosis suggests a disease process starting after the 17–18th week of gestation [3], possibly due to birth complications (Dr. Norman, personal communication). Lack of gliosis and an excess of heterotopias in the temporal lobe, on the other hand, would point to a defect of cellular migration in the second trimester of gestation [4]. This idea is supported by a recent paper, suggesting that cerebral morphological abnormalities studied in schizophrenia may be classified into medial fronto-limbic system defects, periventricular damage and cerebral specialization abnormalities [5]. Each abnormality occurs independently, has its specific cause and is followed by a defined course of the disease. More work has to be done to support this tempting notion, which accounts well for the clinical heterogeneity of schizophrenic symptoms.

Acknowledgements

These studies were kindly supported by Deutsche Forschungsgemeinschaft (Bo 799/1–3) and the Alfried Krupp von Bohlen und Halback Stiftung.

References

1. Bogerts B (1991) In: Mednick SA, Cannon TD and Barr CE (eds.) Fetal Neural Development and Adult Schizophrenia. Cambridge University Press, pp. 153–173.
2. Bogerts B, Falkai P, Haupts M, Greve B, Ernst S, Tapernon-Franz U and Heinzmann U (1990) Schizophr. Res. 3: 295–301.
3. Norman MG and Ludwin SK (1990) In: Davis RL and Robertson DM (eds.) Textbook of Neuropathology. 2nd Edn., Williams and Wilkins, Baltimore, 1991, Chapter 7, p. 207.
4. Williams RS (1989) In: Evrard P and Minkowski A (eds.) Developmental Neurobiology. Nestle Nutrition Workshop Series, Vol. 12, Raven Press, N.Y., 1989, pp. 11–20.
5. Bilder RM and Degreef G (1991) Morphologic markers of neurodevelopmental paths to schizophrenia. In: Mednick SA et al. (eds.) Neurodevelopmental Pathology of Schizophrenia. Plenum Press, N.Y. (in press).

Biological Psychiatry, Volume 1. G. Racagni et al., editors.

Brain changes in schizophrenia and their meaning

T.J. Crow
Division of Psychiatry, Northwick Park Hospital, Harrow HA1 3UJ, U.K.

In his work on dementia praecox and paraphrenia [1], Kraepelin wrote that in dementia praecox "perception.....is not usually lessened" (p. 5), "orientation is not usually disordered" and "memory is comparatively little disordered. The patients are able, when they like, to give a correct detailed account of their past life and often know accurately to a day how long they have been in hospital".

These views are challenged by the phenomenon of "age disorientation". Approximately 25% of long-stay patients with a diagnosis of schizophrenia believe themselves to be 5 or more years younger than they really are [2]. Such patients make errors with respect to the present year and the duration of their hospital stay that are consistent with their concept of their own age. Thus age disorientation is part of a constellation of deficits of temporal orientation – for these patients "time stands still". Such intellectual deficits cannot be attributed to past physical treatments. The pattern is difficult to distinguish from that seen in Alzheimer's disease. Patients with age disorientation (defined as a 5-year discrepancy between subjective and true age) are younger at first admission than age-matched patients without age disorientation; age disorientation may thus be a feature of a type of schizophrenic illness with early onset and poor outcome [3].

These deficits were part of the background to the first CT scan study of schizophrenia [4]. A group of long-stay patients with schizophrenia, some of whom had age disorientation and other cognitive impairments, were found to have larger cerebral ventricles than age-matched controls. This finding was subsequently extended to larger samples of patients with a wider age range [5]. An important but neglected finding of these early studies was that the distribution of ventricular size in the patient group was shifted relative to that in the comparison groups. Harvey et al. [6] have recently confirmed that the ventricle-to-brain ratio distribution in schizophrenia is unimodal not bimodal. The conclusion to be drawn is that morphological alterations are intrinsic to the disease process in schizophrenia and are therefore an important clue to its nature.

Two syndromes

The concept of 2 syndromes [7] attempted to explain some of the variability associated with the disease on the basis that there are separate neuroleptic sensitive (and potentially reversible) and irreversible components, the former being particularly associated with positive and the latter with negative symptoms. Although cognitive impairments and negative symptoms may progress, it is not yet clear that the brain changes increase over time beyond what would be expected in the course of normal ageing. On the whole the evidence supports the contention that such brain changes are associated with the negative symptom component, although the relation is weak [8]. Dyskinesias appear to be more closely related to negative symptoms (the type II syndrome) than to exposure to neuroleptic medication.

The 2 syndromes represent "dimensions of pathology" and not separate disease processes; there is considerable overlap between them, and transitions occur over time, some patients losing and gaining positive symptoms, and some gaining, but less frequently losing, negative symptoms.

Asymmetry of brain changes

In a population of chronic patients we found that when other relevant variables (e.g. age and duration of illness) were controlled, age of onset predicted a number of aspects of outcome [9]. Thus patients who were first admitted to hospital at an age below the mode for the group as a whole (25 years for males and 28 years for females) were more likely than those who were first admitted at a later age to show negative symptoms, intellectual impairment (e.g. age disorientation) and behavioural deterioration.

One structural index, the difference between the widths of the 2 sides of the brain in the posterior segments (but not lateral or third ventricular size or brain area) distinguished age of onset groups. Patients with early onset had significant ($P < 0.01$) reductions in measures taken in the occipital and temporal regions in relative width of the left hemisphere [10]. Early onset of a schizophrenic illness apparently arrests the development of the normal asymmetries which are present in the posterior part of the brain. This finding may be a clue to the meaning of the structural changes in the brain – that these changes indicate that the core disturbance involves the mechanisms that control the development of asymmetry in the human brain.

Some other findings suggest that the structural changes in the brain in schizophrenia are lateralised. In a post-mortem study we [11] found a reduction in width of the parahippocampal gyrus in schizophrenic by comparison with affective patients and this change was significantly greater in the left hemisphere. In a further study [12] the area of the various components of the lateral ventricle was assessed radiologically after introduction of radio-opaque medium; enlargement was relatively selective to the temporal horn and highly ($P < 0.001$) selective to the left hemisphere. Although temporal horn enlargement was seen in Alzheimer-type dementia, this showed no predilection for the left side of the brain.

In an NMR study temporal lobe area was relatively reduced on the left side in patients with schizophrenia in comparison with those with affective disorder and age-matched controls [13]. These findings are in agreement with a number of other

CT scan and NMR studies that indicate that increases in ventricular size and reductions in mass in the temporal lobe are greater on the left than on the right side [14]. Such changes can be explained if in schizophrenia there is an arrest of asymmetry development that leads to a temporal lobe that is smaller and a temporal horn that is bigger than would otherwise be the case.

The asymmetries in the human brain are localized in the temporal lobe and include particularly the planum temporale [15]. They relate to handedness which itself could be determined by a simple mendelian gene [16]. Thus this gene may be the focus of the disturbance in schizophrenia.

Linguistic correlates of the disease process

If the primary change is in the genetic mechanisms of cerebral asymmetry, functional correlates in speech might be expected. Relative to patients with affective disorder and normal controls, patients with schizophrenia generate sentences of simpler structure [17,18]. Such deficits are associated with negative symptoms and may progress [19]. Of particular interest is the finding [17] that patients with an early onset are more likely to have reduced complexity of language structure.

Conclusions

1. Morphological changes in the brain in schizophrenia are consistent: they provide a clue to the nature of the disease process.
2. Such changes affect particularly the temporal lobe on the left side of the brain and can be understood as an arrest of development of cerebral asymmetry.
3. The psychosis gene may be the cerebral dominance gene, the genetic determinant of cerebral asymmetry.

References

1. Kraepelin E (1919) Dementia Praecox and Paraphrenia. Translated by RM Barclay and GM Robertson. RE Krieger, New York .
2. Crow TJ and Mitchell WS (1975) Br. J. Psychiatry 126: 360–363.
3. Crow TJ (1986) In: Kerr A and Snaith P (eds.) Contemporary Issues in Schizophrenia. Gaskell, London, pp. 168–174.
4. Johnstone EC, Crow TJ, Frith CD, Husband J and Kreel L (1976) Lancet ii: 924–926.
5. Weinberger DR, Torrey EF, Neophytides AN and Wyatt RH (1979) Arch. Gen. Psychiatry 36: 735–739.
6. Harvey I, McGuffin P, Williams M and Toone BK (1990) Psychiatr. Res. Neuroimag. 35: 61–69.
7. Crow TJ (1980) Br. Med. J. 280: 66–68.
8. Crow TJ (1985) Schizophr. Bull. 11: 471–486.

9. Johnstone EC, Owens DGC, Bydder GM, Colter N, Crow TJ and Frith CD (1989) Psychol. Med. 19: 91–103.
10. Crow TJ, Colter N, Frith CD, Johnstone EC, Owens DGC (1989) Psychiatr. Res. 29: 247–253.
11. Brown R, Colter N, Corsellis JAN, Crow TJ, Frith CD, Jagoe R, Johnstone EC and Marsh L (1986) Arch. Gen. Psychiatry 43: 36–42.
12. Crow TJ, Ball J, Bloom SR, Brown R, Bruton CJ, Colter N, Frith CD, Johnstone EC, Owens DGC and Roberts GW (1989b) Arch. Gen. Psychiatry 46: 1145–1150.
13. Johnstone EC, Owens DGC, Crow TJ, Frith CD, Alexandropolous K, Bydder GM and Colter N (1989) J. Neurol. Neurosurg. Psychiatry 52: 736–741.
14. Crow TJ (1990) Schizophr. Bull. 16: 433–443.
15. Geschwind N and Levitsky W (1968) Science 161: 186–187.
16. Annett M (1985) Left, Right, Hand and Brain: The Right Shift Theory. Erlbaum, London.
17. Morice RD and Ingram JCL (1983) Psychiatr. Res. 9: 233–242.
18. Thomas P, King K, Fraser WI and Kendell RE (1990) Br. J. Psychiatry 156: 204–210.
19. King K, Fraser WI, Thomas P and Kendell RE (1990) Br. J. Psychiatry 156: 211–215.

Biological Psychiatry, Volume 1. G. Racagni et al., editors.

The timing of morphological brain changes in schizophrenia: Do they progress?

Lynn E. DeLisi, Peter Strizke, Henry Riordan, Victor Holan, Maureen Kushner, Angela Boccio, Olga van Eyl and Azad Anand

Department of Psychiatry, HSC, T-10, SUNY Stony Brook, Stony Brook, NY 11794, U.S.A.

It is well established that subtle brain pathology, particularly ventricular enlargement and reduced temporal lobe size, exists in some chronic schizophrenic patients. However, whether these changes antedate the onset of psychosis, are a result of the psychotic process and/or progress with the chronic course in some patients, is unknown. If the latter is true, then brain morphology at the onset of illness may not be seen to differ from normal, or at least structural abnormalities would not be as pronounced as those found among chronic patients. An examination of the timing of morphological change could begin with studies of first episode psychotic patients when they are first identified at a clinical facility. Several attempts to study ventricular size in these patients have suggested that enlargement of the ventricles may be present early in the course of the illness, but these studies are not conclusive (see [1] for review). Of the reports on ventricular size in chronic patients, the majority do not find the size to be correlated with duration of illness (reviewed in [2]). Thus, either ventricular enlargement is an abnormality that is present in association with the initial acute illness process, or it does not increase linearly with time. The few studies of chronic patients studied twice over variable periods of time, each at different stages in their illness process, do not show definitive progressive change [3–5], but 2 [6,7] suggest that a subgroup of schizophrenic patients may have increasing ventricular size with time.

Several studies have been published of reduced whole temporal lobe size, as well as medial limbic structures, in chronic schizophrenic patients [8–12] and one study is reported of smaller hippocampal/amygdala volumes at the first episode of schizophrenia [13], but none have studied whether temporal lobe structures change with time.

In an initial report from our institution [1], 30 consecutive first admissions who had a schizophrenia-like episode had an MRI scan obtained and compared with controls (non-psychiatric patients referred for MRI scans to the same scanning facility). Nineteen of the patients were diagnosed DSM III-R schizophreniform and thus were less than 6 months ill; the rest were ill longer. Significant ventricular enlargement was present in these patients, greater on the left than on the right, but the total enlargement was not as great as that present in more chronic hospitalized schizophrenic patients. Ventricular enlargement was not correlated with the duration of illness, although the earlier the age of onset, the larger the ventricles.

Temporal lobe size, however, was not deviant in the 1st episode patients, although it was abnormal in chronic patients and weakly correlated with duration of illness.

Methods

The present report contains data from a 2-year follow-up examination of the above initial 30 patients. In addition, data from a new sample of schizophreniform patients is presented in order to further clarify the timing and prevalence of these changes.

Subject descriptions

Consecutive first hospital admissions for a schizophrenic-like psychosis were recruited for the present study from 2 area hospitals. Patients (n = 28; 15 males and 13 females; mean age 27.0 ± 7.1 years) who satisfied DSM III-R criteria for schizophreniform disorder or schizoaffective disorder of less than 6 months duration received MRI scans. These patients were compared with 33 controls (18 males and 15 females; mean age 28.0 ± 6.3 years) who were recruited from the same geographical area (20 of whom received MRI scans for minor medical reasons and were used in the previous study). Outcome at 2 years was measured by:

1. The total number of hospitalizations;
2. Total time (in months) spent in hospital;
3. The Global Assessment Scale ([14]; 100 = best, 0 = worst);
4. The Strauss/Carpenter Outcome Scale ([14]; 16 = best, 0 = worst);
5. Total Brief Psychiatric Rating Scale (BPRS) scores (18 items, scored as 1 = not present, 7 = worst).

Magnetic resonance imaging (MRI)

All scans were performed on a GE, 1.5 Tesla scanner. T1 weighted images with a spin echo pulse sequence (coronals: TR600 and TE 24 ms; axials: TR2000 and TE 80 ms) were used (slice thickness 5 mm with a 2-mm gap). The total volume for individual brain regions were computed by adding measured volumes of all slices containing these regions, multiplied by the slice thickness and the number of centimeters (cm^3) to a voxel ($0.93^2 \times 10^{-3}$). Regional measurements were adjusted for total brain size.

Results

Cerebral hemispheres

There were no differences between patients and controls. Females tended to have smaller right and left hemispheres than males; however there were no significant interactions between sex, diagnosis or laterality.

Lateral ventricles

The patients had a trend for larger ventricles than controls (MANCOVA, $F = 2.47$, $P < 0.12$), the left ventricle tended to be larger than the right ($F = 2.30$, $P < 0.14$) with a trend for a diagnosis by laterality interaction ($F = 2.60$, $P = 0.11$).

Temporal lobes

There were no overall temporal lobe volume differences between patients and controls. However the right temporal lobe was significantly larger than the left (MANCOVA, $F = 12.97$, $P = 0.0007$) and males had larger temporal lobes than females (MANCOVA, $F = 4.75$, $P < 0.04$); there was a trend for a sex by diagnosis interaction ($F = 2.92$, $P < 0.10$). In a post hoc analysis, however, neither male nor female schizophrenics tended to have smaller left or right temporal lobes than the same sex controls. On the left side only, the difference between male and female controls was greater than the difference between male and female patients, but this difference did not reach significance.

Twenty-nine of the 30 initial first episode patients [1] were available for follow-up, 4 patients recovered, 16 were diagnosed chronic schizophrenia (4 residual type, 6 undifferentiated, 6 paranoid types) and 9 chronic schizoaffective disorder. Their mean (±S.D.) scores for the BPRS were 26.41 ± 7.1, GAS: 63.79 ± 15.1 and Strauss/Carpenter Outcome Scale: 11.17 ± 3.1. Their mean number of hospitalizations was 1.8 ± 0.9 and months spent in hospital was 4.2 ± 3.0. The larger the ventricles at onset, the poorer the outcome as measured by the number of hospitalizations (left: Pearson $r = 0.53$, $P < 0.003$; right $r = 0.51$, $P < 0.005$), the amount of time in hospital (left: $r = 0.44$, $P < 0.02$; right: $r = -0.35$, $P = 0.057$) and the BPRS (left: $r = 0.18$, $P = 0.35$; right: $r = 0.39$, $P = 0.03$). Correlations of ventricular size with the GAS and Strauss/Carpenter Scales, however, were non-significant. Temporal lobe volume did not correlate with any measures of outcome.

Nineteen of the above 30 patients and 5 controls completed a 2-year follow up MRI scan. Among the 19 patients, a subgroup of patients had a substantial change in ventricular ($n = 5$) and temporal lobe ($n = 4$) measurements from the first to the second scan, although there were decreases as well as increases. Viewed as a group, there was no statistical evidence for an increase in total ventricular size with time, although there was a trend for a specific increase in left ventricular volume when compared with controls (MANOVA, $F = 2.78$, $P = 0.11$). Temporal lobe volumes tended to be smaller, with a greater difference on the right (paired t-test, $t = 2.23$, $P = 0.039$) than left ($t = 1.41$, $P = 0.176$) although no temporal lobe volume changes were significant when the change in patients was compared with the change in controls (MANOVA, left: $F = 1.059$, $P = 0.32$; right: $F = 0.17$, $P = 0.68$.

The change in ventricular volume was inversely correlated with the number of hospitalizations (Spearman r, left: -0.47, $P = 0.04$; right $r = -0.43$, $P = 0.6$) and months in hospital (left: $r = -0.45$, $P < 0.05$; right: $r = -0.53$, $P < 0.02$), while there were no significant correlations with BPRS, the GAS or Strauss/Carpenter Scores at outcome. Thus, the smaller the change in ventricular size, the greater the number and time spent in hospital. This may reflect a trend for greater change in size in those individuals with smaller ventricles on the initial scan. Changes in temporal lobe volume did not correlate with outcome.

Discussion

The timing of brain morphological change may be crucial to the understanding of the pathogenesis of schizophrenia. The present study of a large group of first episode psychotics, all less than 6 months ill, shows a trend for ventricular enlargement specific to the left side only, although this difference does not reach statistical significance. It is possible that the ventricular enlargement begins early in the illness process or even before clinical symptoms are evident and progresses slowly, but is only quantitatively distinguishable from controls several months to years later. Despite an overall lack of change in ventricular size within a 2-year period, there were a few patients in the group whose ventricles appeared to enlarge a substantial percent (greater than 20%). Whether this increase is related to the clinical course of illness in these patients remains to be seen in further follow-up.

We did not find a difference temporal lobe size between new onset patients and controls, although some suggestion of temporal lobe reduction 2 years later was present, which did not reach statistical significance when compared with controls. Since reduced temporal lobe size is present to a greater degree in some chronic patients it may be that this change occurs after the onset of illness in association with a deteriorating illness course.

The finding that ventricular enlargement may predict outcome at 2 years has some clinical utility. All first admissions for treatment of a psychotic episode might benefit from a MRI evaluation; however, further research into whether poor outcome can be prevented by specific treatment strategies and environmental manipulation in this subgroup of patients is needed.

In summary, these studies begin to address the issue of the timing of brain morphologic abnormalities in schizophrenia. Our data suggest that, while some subtle pathology can be seen at the onset of psychosis, it also could be progressing with time in a subgroup of individuals. The changes detected by brain imaging studies may be indications that an active degenerative brain process is occurring. What causes this process is unknown. It is hoped that further detailed evaluation of the present subjects over time will clarify whether brain morphologic abnormalities in schizophrenia are progressively degenerative and ultimately lead to its etiology.

Acknowledgements

This project was supported by The Scottish Rite Schizophrenia Research Foundation, The Stanley Foundation and NIMH RO1 44233-01A2.

References

1. DeLisi LE, Hoff AL, Schwartz JE et al. (1991) Biol. Psychiatry 29: 159–175.
2. Shelton RC and Weinberger DR (1986) In: Nasrallah HA and Weinberger DR (eds.) The Neurology of Schizophrenia. Elsevier, Amsterdam, pp. 207–250.
3. Nasrallah HA, Olson SC, McCalley-Whitters M et al. (1986) Arch. Gen. Psychiatry 43: 157–159.
4. Illowsky BP, Juliano DM, Bigelow LB and Weinberger DL (1988) J. Neurol. Neurosurg. Psychiatry 51: 209–213.
5. Kemali D, Maj S, Galderisi G et al. (1985) J. Psychiatr. Res. 19: 587–596.
6. Vita A, Sacchetti E, Valvoassori G and Cazzullo CL (1988) Acta Psychiatr. Scand. 78: 618–621.
7. Woods BT, Yurgeliun-Todd D, Benes FM et al. (1990) Biol. Psychiatry 26: 341–352.
8. DeLisi LE, Alexandropolous A, Colter N et al. (1988) Schizophr. Res. 1: 169–170.
9. DeLisi LE, Dauphinais ID and Gershon ES (1988) Schizophr. Bull. 14: 185–191.
10. Suddath RL, Casanova MD, Goldberg TE, Daniel DG, Kelsoe JR and Weinberger DR (1989) Am. J. Psychiatry 146: 464–472.
11. Rossi A, Stratta P, Dimichele V, Galluci M, Splendiani A and Cassacchia M (1990) American Psychiatric Association Annual Meeting, New York, New Research Abstracts, NR657, p. 302.
12. Dauphinais ID, DeLisi LE, Crow TJ et al. (1990) Psychiatr. Res. Neuroimag. 35: 137–147.
13. Bogerts B, Ashtari M, Degreef G et al. (1976) Psychiatr. Res. Neuroimag. 33: 1–13.
14. Endicott J, Spitzer RL, Fleiss JL et al. (1976) Arch. Gen. Psychiatry 33: 766–771.
15. Strauss JS and Carpenter WT, JR. (1974) Arch. Gen. Psychiatry 31: 37–42.

Biological Psychiatry, Volume 1. G. Racagni et al., editors.

Cholinergic activity and schizophrenic symptoms

Rajiv Tandon, John Greden, James Shipley, Nancy Mann and William Eisner
Schizophrenia Program, University of Michigan Medical Center, Ann Arbor, MI 48109-0120 U.S.A.

Introduction

Although historical pharmacological treatments of schizophrenia included anticholinergic agents or cholinergic stimulation, the cholinergic system is generally considered unimportant in the pathophysiology of schizophrenia. Evidence from several lines of research [1,2], however, suggests that the cholinergic system may differentially influence positive and negative symptoms in schizophrenia. The failure to assess separately the effects of cholinergic modulation on these distinct dimensions of schizophrenic psychopathology may account for some of the discrepant findings of previous years. Data from phenomenological, pharmacological, polysomnographic, substance abuse comorbidity, neuroendocrine and drive-reduction literature implicate muscarinic cholinergic hyperactivity in the pathogenesis of negative symptoms [1,2]. Another body of evidence suggests that an increase in positive symptoms may be associated with decreasing cholinergic activity in the acute phase of the illness [1,2]. Based on these data that suggest the involvement of cholinergic hyperactivity in the production of negative symptoms, the observed association between decreasing cholinergic activity and positive symptoms and the course of positive and negative symptoms during the acute phase of the illness [3], we proposed the following model of dopaminergic/cholinergic interactions in schizophrenia (Fig. 1). The model suggests that:

1. disruption of cholinergic/dopaminergic balance is of central importance in the expression of schizophrenic psychopathology;
2. as dopaminergic activity increases in the psychotic phase of the illness, cholinergic activity increases in a homeostatic response to restore balance;
3. the cholinergic system exerts a damping effect on the emergence of positive symptoms associated with dopaminergic hyperactivity; and
4. this compensatory increase in cholinergic activity is accompanied by an intensification of negative symptoms during the acute phase of the illness.

While unproven, it has heuristic merit and warrants testing in a more systematic fashion. Towards this end, we have conducted the following series of studies.

Series of studies

Although several factors influence sleep-EEG measures, certain sleep variables

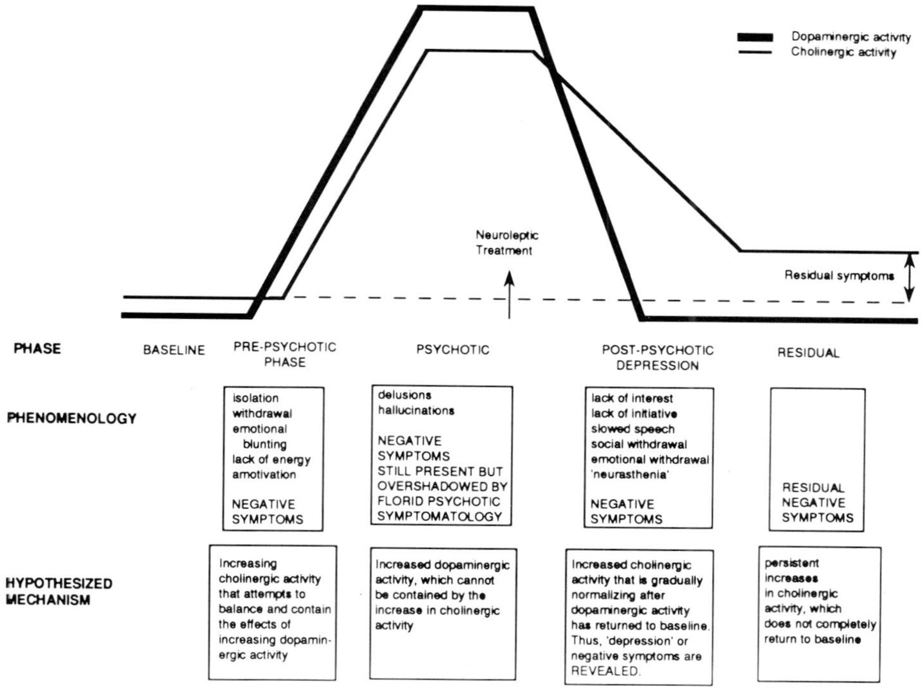

Fig. 1. Dopaminergic-cholinergic interactions and the phenomenology of an acute psychotic episode.

(such as REM latency) are strongly regulated by cholinergic neurotransmission and may provide an indirect measure of central cholinergic activity. To test the hypothesis that cholinergic activity is increased in the psychotic phase of the illness, we compared polysomnographic measures in 40 drug-free schizophrenic patients with those of 20 normal controls [4]. Schizophrenic patients showed significantly impaired sleep continuity and REM latency than controls; findings consistent with the hypothesized increase in cholinergic activity in schizophrenia.

We studied the effects of 6 mg biperiden on REM latency in 12 drug-free schizophrenic patients and matched normal controls [5]. We found that biperiden caused a smaller increase in REM latency in schizophrenic patients. We then studied the effects of 10 mg biperiden (an anticholinergic agent) on sleep measures in 15 otherwise drug-free schizophrenic patients and matched normal controls [6]. REM latency was significantly shorter in schizophrenic patients. These findings are consistent with the hypothesis of increased cholinergic activity.

We tested the prediction that an anticholinergic agent would increase positive and decrease negative symptoms by studying the effect of 8 mg biperiden/day for 2 days in 30 otherwise drug-free schizophrenic patients [5]. Biperiden produced a significant increase in positive symptoms ($t = 6.4$; $P < 0.01$) and reduction in negative symptoms ($t = 2.5$; $P < 0.05$).

Finally, we tested the prediction that positive and negative symptoms would covary in the psychotic phase of the illness by correlating changes in positive symptoms with changes in negative symptoms during 4 weeks of neuroleptic therapy in 40 schizophrenic patients [7]. We found that negative symptoms improved in tandem with positive symptoms ($r = 0.63$; $P < 0.01$).

Conclusions

These findings, overall, suggest that cholinergic activity may be increased in the psychotic phase of schizophrenia and may be relevant to the expression of positive and negative symptoms. It should be emphasized that the DA/ACh model is not intended as an exhaustive explanation of schizophrenia; other neurotransmitters and neurobiological abnormalities are undoubtedly important. The DA/ACh model is congruent with current knowledge about schizophrenia, is internally consistent, may explain some apparently discrepant findings in schizophrenia and is supported by the findings of our present series of studies. The hypothesis of DA/ACh interactions is testable using various strategies and is proposed as a heuristic formulation that may help to elucidate the role of cholinergic mechanisms in schizophrenia.

Acknowledgements

We gratefully acknowledge the support from the National Alliance for Research in Schizophrenia and Depression (NARSAD) and the Scottish Rite Schizophrenia Research Program in the conduction of these studies.

References

1. Tandon R and Greden JF (1989) Arch. Gen. Psychiatry 46: 745–753.
2. Tandon R and Greden JF (1990) In: Greden JF and Tandon R (eds.) Negative Schizophrenic Symptoms: Pathophysiology and Clinical Implications. American Psychiatric Press, Washington.
3. Docherty JP, van Kammen DP, Siris SG and Marder SR (1978) Am. J. Psychiatry 135: 420–426.
4. Tandon R, Shipley JE, Taylor S, Greden JF, Eiser A, DeQuardo JR and Goodson J (1991) Sleep electroencephalographic abnormalities in schizophrenia. Arch. Gen. Psychiatry (in press).
5. Tandon R, Shipley JE, Greden JF, Mann NA, Eisner WH and Goodson J (1991) Schizophr. Res. 4: 23–30.
6. Tandon R, Shipley JE, Taylor S, Eisner A and Goodson J (1991) Effect of biperiden on sleep-EEG measures in schizophrenia. Biol. Psychiatry (submitted).
7. Tandon R, Goldman R, Goodson J and Greden JF (1990) Biol. Psychiatry 27: 1323–1326.

Biological Psychiatry, Volume 1. G. Racagni et al., editors.

Experimental pharmacology in schizophrenia: Partial dopamine agonists

Carol A. Tamminga, Nicola G. Cascella and Robert R. Conley
Maryland Psychiatric Research Center, Department of Psychiatry, University of Maryland, Baltimore, MD 21228, U.S.A.

Introduction

Several kinds of evidence exist to understand the neurotransmitter systems involved in schizophrenia; these include clinical pharmacology, postmortem biochemical analysis, cerebrospinal fluid (CSF) measurements and now, results from brain imaging studies. Biochemical strategies, both postmortem and CSF, would be more powerful if the pathophysiologic site(s) of schizophrenia in CNS were clear. Imaging studies are now beginning to answer this pivotal localizing question. However, little is understood about the biologic status of the schizophrenic brain or of the type or localization of regional dysfunction in the illness. The target symptoms and the overall life course of schizophrenic symptoms have been described. But how to use these observations to be informative about brain biology is not clear. Perhaps the most salient biologic observation about the illness, is that dopamine (DA) receptor antagonists consistently reduce psychotic symptoms with a clinical potency which correlates with their D_2 receptor affinity. Moreover, other antidopaminergic strategies have been shown to be antipsychotic as well, like reserpine, tetrabenazine and apomorphine. These pharmacologic observations have been the most replicable and consistent pieces of biologic information about the illness.

The pharmacology of schizophrenia is simple: on one hand, several kinds of drugs produce psychotomimetic reactions which resemble schizophrenic psychosis to some variable degree. The dopamine (DA) agonists produce symptom exacerbation in patients with active symptoms (although not inevitably) and can induce paranoid delusions in normals. PCP induces a schizophrenia-like psychosis, with positive and negative symptoms and often delayed onset and offset of the syndrome. On the other hand, and more importantly, drugs which are antipsychotic in schizophrenia are all antidopaminergic. These antidopaminergic agents include: 1) DA-receptor blockers (e.g., haloperidol, chlorpromazine); 2) DA terminal transmitter depleters (e.g., reserpine, tetrabenazine); 3) atypical DA-receptor blockers (e.g., clozapine, remoxipride); and 4) autoreceptor agonists especially partial DA agonists.

Antidopaminergic strategies

Different mechanisms are available to diminish DA mediated neurotransmission in humans. The most widely applied is blockade of postsynaptic DA receptors. This strategy is potent, produces a broad blockade in all DA terminal areas and functionally affects all cerebral systems utilizing DA. But, while effective, it is a strategy which is non-selective and side-effect intensive. Therefore, other antidopaminergic strategies with more selective and milder actions have been sought. Several are currently being evaluated. One approach along this line is to use receptor blockers with low in vivo affinity, e.g., clozapine and remoxipride. Another approach is to decrease DA synthesis and release presynaptically with partial DA agonists. This latter technique will be discussed here.

Partial dopamine agonists

Partial agonists are drugs with full affinity, but limited intrinsic activity at a transmitter receptor [1]. Dependent on the intrinsic activity of the agonist and the usual state of the receptor, the partial agonist can be either an effective agonist or an antagonist. A partial DA agonist can simultaneously have different levels of intrinsic activity in different receptor populations, allowing a single drug to behave as a partial agonist in one area and an effective antagonist elsewhere. Partial DA agonists are preferentially active at autoreceptors compared with the postsynaptic receptors.

Positive results from several therapeutic trials of full DA agonists have been interpreted as drug actions at the DA autoreceptor [2]. Although no ergot or ergolines have had an antipsychotic action, the aporphine DA agonists have been tested and found to be antipsychotic. The purported mechanism of antipsychotic action of a partial agonist would be an inhibition of DA synthesis and release through DA autoreceptor stimulation, thus leading to a decrease in DA-mediated neurotransmission and a neuroleptic-like effect.

Results

–3PPP, the prototypal partial DA agonist

The levoenantiomer of 3PPP has relatively selective properties of a partial DA agonist. –3PPP decreases firing of DA neurons, reduces DA release in reserpinized rats, and reduces locomotor activity and stereotypies in rats [3]. Moreover, in the nucleus accumbens of the rat, –3PPP mimics the metabolic action of haloperidol on glucose utilization.

We have begun to study the action of –3PPP in man in preparation for efficacy studies of the drug in schizophrenia. –3PPP has an oral bioavailablity in man of approximately 4% (n = 1). A single 30 mg intramuscular administration produces plasma levels in the predicted behaviorally active range of 200–500 pmol/ml. Drug half-life in man is 2–2.5 h.

In the active plasma level range, –3PPP has certain biochemical and behavioral actions in man characteristic of a DA agonist. It increases plasma growth hormone (GH) concentrations in a dose-dependent manner up to 30 mg. Moreover, it causes yawning in test subjects, a common behavioral effect of apomorphine. However, the drug produces no nausea or any involuntary movements of any sort, either hypokinetic or hyperkinetic. Curiously, at the highest dose given to man (40 mg i.m.), the drug produced no effect on GH, perhaps representing a dose-dependent additional action of –3PPP on a new receptor population in brain.

The behavioral actions of –3PPP in schizophrenia were rated as a secondary outcome measure in this drug safety study. This study was conducted in a double-blind, placebo controlled manner, for the sake of mental status evaluation. Four schizophrenics, otherwise drug-free, received up to 40 mg i.m. of –3PPP in single daily doses. Psychosis was rated before and after drug administration by experienced research clinicians blind to drug or placebo using mental status assessment scales in a semistructured interview. All subjects reported a "calming" effect and often appeared more "relaxed". Two out of the four subjects had no measurable change at all in their psychosis, whereas, the other two subjects had some antipsychotic response, one mild, and the other, a pronounced antipsychotic action. The subject who had the most pronounced antipsychotic response to –3PPP was the most robust neuroleptic responder. This partially positive outcome with –3PPP in schizophrenia, taking into account the low patient number, suggests that further study of its action in schizophrenia may be warranted.

Conclusions

Several novel pharmacological strategies exist for treating schizophrenia. These have reasonably compelling rationales and, in some cases, preliminary data. Most often, although not inevitably, these strategies are antidopaminergic. As new tools and new knowledge become available these opportunities will broaden. It is timely to expect some new developments in antipsychotic treatments for schizophrenia.

References

1. Kenakin T (1990) The Pharmacologic Basis of Drug Action. Wiley, New York, U.S.A.
2. Tamminga CA, Gotts MD, Thaker GK, Alphs LD and Foster NL (1986) Arch. Gen. Psychiatry 43: 398–402.
3. Clark D, Hjorth S, Carlsson A (1985) J. Neural Transm. 62: 1–52.

Biological Psychiatry, Volume 1. G. Racagni et al., editors.

Clinical pharmacology of clozapine

George M. Simpson and Julie B. Kessel
Department of Psychiatry, Medical College of Pennsylvania/Eastern Pennsylvania Psychiatric Institute, 3200 Henry Avenue, Philadelphia, PA 19129, U.S.A.

Introduction

Clozapine, an atypical antipsychotic, was developed at the Wander pharmaceutical company in Berne, Switzerland in the early 1960s as a potential antidepressant compound, as it had a tricyclic core. By the early 1970s, however, in open and double-blind trials in Europe, clozaril had been clearly established as a potent antipsychotic compound with an unusual side-effect profile. It was noted to cause marked sedation and hypersalivation. Most importantly, clozaril demonstrated a striking absence of extrapyramidal symptoms such as rigidity, akinesia and akathisia. Early investigators also reported that it may have a beneficial effect on tardive dyskinesia [1]. The drug was soon noted to have the significant adverse effects of seizure induction and depression of bone marrow and in 1974, 16 cases of agranulocytosis (8 resulting in fatality) were reported in Finland. The search to find a similar agent that lacked the side-effect of agranulocytosis proved unsuccessful. It remained in use in some European countries which instituted more stringent blood monitoring practices and demonstrated that the drug was able to be used safely in this setting. Nevertheless, entry of the drug into the U.S. market was blocked until 1989 when double-blind, controlled studies were completed and clearly demonstrated its superiority over chlorpromazine in reducing both positive and negative symptoms in treatment-resistant schizophrenic patients [2].

Over the past thirty years, several classes of compounds with antipsychotic activity have been developed. Despite considerable differences in chemical structure, all of these agents appear to share an ability to bind to dopamine receptors. The role of this property in antipsychotic efficacy is supported by in vitro binding assays that demonstrate D_2 receptor antagonism and therapeutic efficacy to be highly correlated. These compounds also have "neuroleptic properties", meaning that they are associated with the propensity to induce extrapyramidal effects, including tardive conditions. Typical antipsychotics also produce catalepsy in animal models, block apomorphine or amphetamine-induced stereotypy, antagonize the conditioned avoidance response and cause an elevation in prolactin. The behavioural correlates are frequently used to screen potential antipsychotics.

Like the typical antipsychotic agents, clozapine does have central depressant properties and blocks the conditioned avoidance response in animals [3]. It also blocks muscarinic and adrenergic receptors [4,5]. However, clozaril does not produce catalepsy in animal models, does not block apomorphine- or amphetamine-induced stereotypy [3], is virtually devoid of extrapyramidal side-effects including tardive dyskinesia and is not believed to exert its antipsychotic action primarily via blockade of the D_2 receptor [6]. In marked contrast to the increase in prolactin levels in patients on typical antipsychotic drugs caused by D_2 blockade in the tuberoinfundibular neurons, clozapine only causes acute, brief and modest elevations with return to normal or below normal levels in 1–2 h [7]. There is also evidence that clozapine antagonizes D_2 receptors though it is not associated with the development of dopaminergic supersensitivity, unlike the typical antipsychotic drugs [8].

Some speculate that clozapine exerts its antipsychotic activity by preferentially blocking mesocorticolimbic dopamine neurons. The drug has been shown to cause selective depolarization inactivation of A10, but not A9 neurons with a suppressed release of dopamine from neurons in the accumbens but not from the striatum [9,10]. This, in addition to the profound anticholinergic effect of clozapine, has been postulated to account for the lack of extrapyramidal symptoms produced. However, addition of anticholinergic compounds to the typical neuroleptics does not produce the same effect [11].

Clozapine may also be distinguished from classical antipsychotic agents by its ability to antagonize D_1 receptors with nearly equal potency to its D_2 blocking effect [12]. The D_1/D_2 ratio for clozapine is, therefore, approximately 1.0. Additionally, clozapine is a very potent serotonin antagonist [13]. In fact, it is becoming increasingly attractive to postulate a role for serotonin in antipsychotic efficacy of the atypical antipsychotics, particularly clozapine [14,15]. It may be important to consider the relative contribution of D_1, D_2 and 5-HT in the etiology and treatment of these disorders. Atypical neuroleptic drugs, compared to typical neuroleptics, have a high ratio of ability to antagonize 5-HT and D_1, relative to D_2 receptors.

The claim has been made that certain atypical neuroleptics such as the benzamides may have a specific beneficial effect on negative symptoms. This has not, however, been definitively shown [16]. Kane et al. [2] did report that clozapine was superior to chlorpromazine, the reference antipsychotic, in the reduction of both positive and negative symptoms. Negative symptom scores have been shown to correlate positively with drug-induced parkinsonism [17]. Typical antipsychotics may then appear to cause or exacerbate negative symptoms. The collaborative study [2] may, therefore, be criticized. Since clozapine does not produce parkinsonism and chlorpromazine does, the apparent improvement in negative symptoms may, in part, be due to the lack of iatrogenic parkinsonism. In addition, since akathisia may appear to exacerbate positive symptoms, the decreased incidence of akathisia on clozapine may also lead to a diminished score on the positive subscales of the BPRS. Therefore, some of the beneficial effects of clozapine may relate to the absence of some of the negative effects of conventional neuroleptics.

Despite these criticisms, clozapine is the first antipsychotic to be demonstrated in clinical trials to be more efficacious than another antipsychotic. In clinical practice, the effect of clozapine on negative symptoms may be particularly important. Meltzer [15] suggests that if the ratio of serotonergic to dopaminergic activity is high, negative symptoms may predominate while, in the opposite case, positive symptoms may predominate. Clozapine has sparked a great interest in the role of serotonin antagonists in the treatment of the psychoses and in the interaction between the dopaminergic and serotonergic systems. A variety of drugs affecting serotonin are currently in clinical trials, e.g. risperidone. This drug is a potent antagonist at both dopamine D_2 and serotonin 5-HT_2 receptors [18].

Finally, clozapine is an atypical antipsychotic agent that has a marked therapeutic advantage over conventional antipsychotic agents in the treatment of a substantial number of schizophrenic patients. It does not lead to elevations in prolactin and does not appear to cause significant extrapyramidal effects or tardive conditions. It has pronounced D_1, D_2 and 5-HT_2 receptor antagonism and preferentially affects the dopamine neurons in the mesocorticolimbic areas, all of which may help to account for its mechanism of action. Its unique pharmacological profile has broadened the arena of investigation in this area. Clozapine provides an effective alternative to traditional antipsychotic treatment in the chronically psychotic patient.

References

1. Simpson GM, Lee JH and Shrivastava RK (1978) Psychopharmacology 56: 105–112.
2. Kane J, Honigfeld G, Singer J, Meltzer H and the Clozaril Collaborative Study Group (1988) Arch. Gen. Psychiatry 45: 789–796.
3. Stille G, Lauener H and Eichenberger E (1971) Pharmacology 26: 603–625.
4. Snyder S, Greenberg D and Yamamura H (1974) Arch. Gen. Psychiatry 31: 58–61.
5. Van Praag HM, Korf J and Dols LC (1976) Br. J. Psychiatry 129: 547–555.
6. Coward DN, Imperato A, Urwyler S and White TG (1989) Psychopharmacology 99: S6–S12.
7. Meltzer HY, Nash JF, Koenig JI and Gudelsky GA (1986) Clin. Neuropharmacol. 9 (Suppl. 4): 316–318.
8. Sayers AC, Burki HR, Ruch W and Asper H (1975) Psychopharmacologia 41(2): 97–104.
9. Chiodo LA and Bunney BS (1983) J. Neurosci. 3(8): 1607–1619.
10. Hand TH, Hu XT and Wang RY (1987) Brain Res. 415: 257–269.
11. Sayers AC, Beurki HR, Ruch W and Asper H (1976) Psychopharmacology 51: 15–22.
12. Farde L, Wiesel FA, Nordstrom AL and Sedvall G (1988) Psychopharmacology 96 (Suppl.): 79.
13. Fink H, Morgenstern R and Oelssner W (1984) Pharmacol. Biochem. Behav. 20(4): 513–517.
14. Lee T and Tang SW (1984) Psychiatr. Res. 12(4): 277–285.
15. Meltzer HY (1989) Psychopharmacology 99: S18–S27.
16. De Leon J and Simpson GM (1991) Integr. Psychiatry 7: 39–46.
17. Hoffman WF, Labs SM and Casey DE (1987) Biol. Psychiatry 22: 427–439.
18. Leysen JE, Gommeren W, Ens A et al.(1988) J. Pharmacol. Exp. Ther. 247(2): 661–670.
19. Anderson PH, Nielsen EB, Gronvald FC and Baestrup C (1986) Eur. J. Pharmacol. 120: 143–144.

Biological Psychiatry, Volume 1. G. Racagni et al., editors.

Serotonergic receptor subsystems and their functional significance

Ray W. Fuller
Lilly Research Laboratories, Eli Lilly and Company, Lilly Corporate Center, Indianapolis, IN 46285, U.S.A.

Introduction

Serotonin (5-hydroxytryptamine), discovered to be present in brain in 1953, is one of the most widely distributed, though not necessarily the most abundant, neurotransmitters in brain [1]. Serotonin neurons with cell bodies in midbrain-brain stem raphe areas project to many parts of the brain and thus can influence many things controlled by the brain, such as behavior, mood, appetite, temperature, sleep, pain and hormone secretion. Dysfunction of serotonin neurons might underlie some psychiatric and other disorders and drugs that modify serotonergic function might have therapeutic use in psychiatric and other illnesses. Dopamine is the monoamine most clearly implicated in schizophrenia, but there continues to emerge some evidence for serotonergic dysfunction in schizophrenia as well [2,3].

Serotonin receptor heterogeneity

One of the most important developments in serotonin pharmacology during the past decade has been the definition and characterization of multiple subtypes of serotonin receptors in brain [4]. Functional evidence for heterogeneity of brain serotonin receptors had existed earlier, but the introduction during the 1970s of radioligand-binding as a technique for studying brain serotonin receptors triggered the rapid progress in elucidating multiple receptors. Currently at least seven different serotonin receptors are defined in brain (Table 1). These receptors are widely but unevenly distributed among brain regions [5]. All are thought to occur postsynaptically and to receive neural signals transmitted by serotonin. Whether a single receptor or multiple receptors receive signals within a given neuroanatomical pathway or at a specific synapse remains unclear. In addition, the 5-HT_{1A} receptor occurs as an autoreceptor on cell bodies of serotonin neurons, where it modulates neuronal firing. The 5-HT_{1D} receptor apparently occurs presynaptically as a terminal autoreceptor on serotonin neurons and modulates serotonin release, except in rodents (where the 5-HT_{1B} receptor has this function).

All four of the brain serotonin receptor subtypes that have been cloned are monomeric G-protein-interacting receptors with seven transmembrane regions, similar to adrenergic and muscarinic receptors. Agonists and antagonists having some selectivity for these multiple receptor subtypes have been described. These

Table 1. Currently identified serotonin receptors in brain

Receptor	Cloned?	Species cloned
5-HT_{1A}	Yes	Human [6]; rat [7]
5-HT_{1B}	No	
5-HT_{1C}	Yes	Mouse [8]; rat [9]
5-HT_{1D}	Yes	Human [10]
5-HT_2	Yes	Rat [11]; mouse [12]; human [13]
5-HT_3	No	
5-HT_4	No	

agonists and antagonists are not only useful pharmacologic tools for investigating functional roles of the receptors, but in addition have potential therapeutic applications in psychiatric illnesses [14].

Serotonin receptors and schizophrenia

5-HT_2 and 5-HT_{1C} receptors

Abnormalities of brain 5-HT_2 receptors have been reported in schizophrenia and attributed to the disease process rather than to drug-induced changes [15,16]. Evidence has been presented that 5-HT_2 receptors are sites of action of hallucinogenic drugs such as phenylisopropylamines and LSD [17]. Antagonists at 5-HT_2 receptors have been postulated to have therapeutic potential in schizophrenia and some clinical data to support their utility has existed. Of wide interest has been the idea that simultaneous blockade of 5-HT_2 receptors and of dopamine D_2 receptors may result in the most satisfactory alleviation of positive and negative symptoms of schizophrenia while minimizing extrapyramidal side-effects [18]. The 5-HT_2 and 5-HT_{1C} receptors have considerable structural homology [19], reflected in their coupling to the same intracellular signaling system – activation of phospholipase C – and in marked pharmacological similarity [20]. Many antagonists of 5-HT_2 receptors are also potent antagonists of 5-HT_{1C} receptors. Clozapine, for example, whose antagonism of 5-HT_2 receptors has been postulated to be relevant to its usefulness in the treatment of schizophrenia [16], has even higher affinity for 5-HT_{1C} receptors [21]. The significance of clozapine's affinity at 5-HT_{1C} sites with regard to its desirable properties as an antipsychotic drug is still unknown.

5-HT_3 receptors

The 5-HT_3 receptors have recently been shown to exist in brain, their distribution has been mapped and considerable evidence has been presented to suggest that 5-HT_3 receptor antagonists might be useful in treating schizophrenia [22].

5-HT_{1A} receptors

Attention has been focused on 5-HT_{1A} receptors in relation to schizophrenia by recent findings of increased 5-HT_{1A} receptors in prefrontal and temporal cortices of patients with chronic schizophrenia [23] and by reports that 5-HT_{1A} receptor agonists antagonize neuroleptic-induced catalepsy in rats [24,25].

References

1. Tork I (1990) Ann. N.Y. Acad. Sci. 600: 9.
2. Bleich A, Brown SL, Kahn R and Van Praag HM (1988) Schizophr. Bull. 14: 297.
3. Lindstrom LH, Wieselgren IM, Klockhoff I and Svedberg A (1990) Biol. Psychiatry 28: 435.
4. Peroutka SJ (1990) Pharmacol. Toxicol. 67: 373.
5. Palacios JM, Waeber C, Hoyer D and Mengod G (1990) Ann N.Y. Acad. Sci. 600: 36.
6. Fargin A, Raymond JR, Lohse MJ, Kobilka BK, Caron MG and Lefkowitz RJ (1988) Nature 335: 358.
7. Albert PR, Zhou Q-Y, Van Tol HHM, Bunzow JR and Civelli O (1990) J. Biol. Chem. 265: 5825.
8. Lubbert H, Hoffman BJ, Snutch TP, van Dyke T, Levine AJ, Hartig PR, Lester HA and Davidson N (1987) Proc. Natl. Acad. Sci. U.S.A. 84: 4332.
9. Lubbert H, Snutch TP, Dascal N, Lester HA and Davidson N (1987) J. Neurosci. 7: 1159.
10. Branchek TA, Weinshank RL, Macchi MJ, Zgombick JM and Hartig PR (1990) Abstracts, Second IUPHAR Satellite Meeting on Serotonin. Basel, Switzerland, p. 35.
11. Pritchett DB, Bach AWJ, Wozny M, Taleb O, Dal Toso R, Shih JC and Seeburg PH (1988) EMBO J. 7: 4135.
12. Lan N, Yang W, Chen K, Wang K and Shih JC (1989) Soc. Neurosci. Abstr. 15: 673.
13. Kao H-T, Olsen MA and Hartig PR (1989) Soc. Neurosci. Abstr. 15: 486.
14. Murphy DL (1990) Neuropsychopharmacology 3: 457.
15. Bennett JP Jr, Enna S, Bylund DB, Gillin JC, Wyatt RJ and Snyder SH (1979) Arch. Gen. Psychiatry 36: 927.
16. Mita T, Hanada S, Nishina N, Kuno T, Nakai H, Yamadori T, Mizoi Y and Tanaka C (1986) Biol. Psychiatry 21: 1407.
17. Teitler M, Leonhardt S, Appel NM, DeSouza EB and Glennon RA (1990) Ann. N.Y. Acad. Sci. 600: 626.
18. Meltzer HY (1989) Psychopharmacology 99: 518.
19. Julius D, Huang KN, Livelli TJ, Axel R and Jessell TM (1990) Proc. Natl. Acad. Sci. U.S.A. 87: 928.
20. Hartig PR, Hoffman BJ, Kaufman MJ and Hirata F (1990) Ann. N.Y. Acad. Sci. 600: 149.
21. Canton H, Verriele L and Colpaert FC (1990) Eur. J. Pharmacol. 191: 93.
22. Costall B, Naylor RJ and Tyers MB (1990) Pharmacol. Ther. 47: 181.
23. Hashimoto T, Nishino N, Nakai H and Tanaka C (1991) Life Sci. 48: 355.
24. Invernizzi RW, Cervo L and Samanin R (1988) Neuropharmacology 27: 515.
25. Hicks PB (1990) Life Sci. 47: 1609.

Biological Psychiatry, Volume 1. G. Racagni et al., editors.

The MCPP challenge test in schizophrenia: Hormonal and behavioral responses

Naveed Iqbal, Gregory M. Asnis, Scott Wetzler, Rene S. Kahn, Stanley R. Kay and Herman M. van Praag

Albert Einstein College of Medicine/Montefiore Medical Center, Department of Psychiatry, New York, NY 10467, U.S.A.

The recent introduction of antipsychotic drugs that combine dopamine and serotonin (5-hydroxytryptamine) receptor antagonistic activity had revived the interest in the possible involvement of 5-HT dysfunctions in the pathogenesis of schizophrenia [1]. In the present study, we investigated 5-HT receptor sensitivity in schizophrenic patients using the m-chlorophenylpiperazine (MCPP) challenge paradigm. Based on the 5-HT_2 receptor hypersensitivity hypothesis [2] we made two predictions: 1) that the schizophrenic patients would have an augmented hormonal response to MCPP in comparison to normal subjects; and 2) that MCPP would cause an exacerbation of psychotic symptomatology in schizophrenic patients. A dose of 0.25 mg/kg MCPP p.o. was selected because it had previously been shown to identify patients with 5-HT receptor hypersensitivity in terms of their hormonal and behavioral responses [3,4].

Methods

Male schizophrenic patients were selected from the inpatient and outpatient services at Montefiore Medical Center (n = 7, mean age 32.7, S.D. 14.0 years; 2 outpatients and 5 inpatients). Normal male controls were paid volunteers recruited by advertisement in a community newspaper (n = 8, mean age 27.5, S.D. 6.8 years). The patients met Research Diagnostic Criteria (RDC) [5] for chronic schizophrenia of at least two years' duration (range: 2–35 years) and they had been medication-free for a two-week period prior to participation in the challenge tests. Five patients met RDC criteria for paranoid subtype and two patients met criteria for undifferentiated subtype.

The procedure of the MCPP test was as described in Kahn et al. [6]. A research psychiatrist used an abbreviated version of the Positive and Negative Syndrome Scale (PANSS) [7] to rate the behavior and mental status of the schizophrenic subjects during the challenge procedure at time 0, and at 60, 120, 180 and 210 min following administration of the tablets.

Hormonal release was calculated using placebo-corrected change-from-baseline scores. Accordingly, at each point in time, the subjects change-from-baseline value on placebo was subtracted from his change-from-baseline value on MCPP. Repeated measure MANOVAs were then conducted with one repeated measure (time: 0, 30, 60, 90, 120, 150, 180 and 210 min) and one group variable (schizophrenia vs. normal controls). For the schizophrenic subjects, behavioral response on the PANSS was calculated using δ (peak-minus baseline) values, and significance of the difference between MCPP and placebo response was analyzed by paired t-test.

Results

The schizophrenic patients had a peak MCPP blood level of 7.3 ng/dl (S.D. 10.0) as compared with 22.4 ng/dl (S.D. 24.1) for the normal subjects. Given the small number of subjects, this difference was not statistically significant ($t = 1.53$, $P = 0.15$). Using an area-under-curve analysis, there was not a significant group difference ($t = 1.47$, $P = 0.17$). Two of the schizophrenic patients had trace or nondetectable levels of MCPP. For both groups, peak blood levels were reached at 120 min after administration of MCPP.

The PANSS behavioral data for the schizophrenic subjects on placebo vs. MCPP, revealed a significant difference on total psychopathology ($df = 6$, $t = 2.71$, $P < 0.05$), indicating overall worsening of symptoms on MCPP. Both of the patients with trace or non-detectable levels of MCPP had a behavioral response to the drug. Predicated on this finding, we analyzed the component scores to clarify the nature of the drug-related changes. The results showed significant drug/placebo differences that were specific to the positive syndrome ($t = 3.29$, $df = 6$, $P < 0.02$) and activation ($t = 9.30$, $df = 6$, $P < 0.001$) components. In this abbreviated PANSS, the positive syndrome was composed of the symptoms of conceptual disorganization, hallucinatory behavior, excitement, suspiciousness/persecution, and hostility. Activation was composed of excitement, tension, and mannerisms and posturing.

There were no baseline differences between the groups (placebo: $t = 0.07$, $P = 0.95$; drug: $t = 0.93$, $P = 0.37$). The schizophrenic patients had lower placebo corrected change-from-baseline cortisol levels over time than did normal subjects. This was found to be statistically significant (group × time: $F = 4.96$, $df = 6,8$, $P < 0.05$).

There were no baseline differences between the groups (placebo: $t = 1.76$, $P = 0.10$; drug: $t = 1.45$, $P = 0.17$). The schizophrenic patients also had lower placebo-corrected change-from-baseline prolactin levels than did normal subjects. The main effect for the group difference was statistically significant ($F = 6.18$, $df = 1,13$, $P < 0.05$).

Discussion

MCPP induced a significant exacerbation of psychopathology in the schizophrenic subjects, which was characterized primarily by increased positive symptoms, specifically those associated with activation. We also found that the schizophrenic patients had statistically significant blunted cortisol and prolactin responses in comparison to the normal subjects. The schizophrenic patients had a low blood level of MCPP, but it was obviously sufficient to induce the behavioral response observed. Alternatively, it may have been an unmeasured metabolite of MCPP which induced the exacerbation of psychopathology.

The dissociation between behavioral and hormonal effects of MCPP in schizophrenic patients may be due to the drug's effects on multiple 5-HT receptor subtypes in various cortical and subcortical areas. For example, an upregulation of excitatory 5-HT receptors in the frontal cortex (i.e. 5-HT_2 and 5-HT_3 receptors) could be responsible for the exacerbated psychopathology; and an upregulation of inhibitory 5-HT autoreceptors in the subcortical region (i.e. 5-HT_1 receptors) could be related to the blunted hormonal release. Alternatively, certain postsynaptic 5-HT receptors in schizophrenic patients may be hyposensitive, thereby causing a blunted hormonal response.

An alternative explanation for the blunted hormonal response in the schizophrenic patients may be the unusually low MCPP blood level in these patients. The schizophrenic patients in this study had lower MCPP blood levels on 0.25 mg/kg than any other patient group we studied thus far [6,8,9]. This may be a result of pharmacokinetic differences in the schizophrenic subjects, such as absorption of MCPP or increased hepatic microsomal activity secondary to prior neuroleptic treatment [10].The residual effect of chronic neuroleptic use on hormonal or behavioral parameters is unclear [11]. However, the presence of a behavioral response to MCPP as well as low baseline levels of prolactin suggest that the effect of prior neuroleptic use on the findings presented was insignificant [12].

References

1. van Praag HM (1991) In: Lindenmayer JP and Kay SR (eds.) Positive and Negative Syndromes in Schizophrenia. Brunner Mazel, New York (in press).
2. Bleich A, Brown S, Kahn R and van Praag NM (1988) Schizophr. Bull. 14: 297–315.
3. Kahn R, Wetzler S, van Praag HM and Asnis GM (1988a) Psychiatr. Res. 25: 101–104.
4. Kahn R, Asnis G, Wetzler S and van Praag HM (1988b) Psychopharmacology 96: 360–364.
5. Spitzer R, Endicott J and Robins E (1978) Arch. Gen. Psychiatry 35: 773–782.
6. Kahn R, Wetzler S, Asnis G, King M, Suckow R and van Praag HM (1990) Psychopharmacology 100: 339–344.
7. Kay S, Fiszbein A and Opler L (1987) Schizophr. Bull. 13: 261–267.
8. Kahn R, Wetzler S, Asnis G, Papolos D and van Praag HM (1990) Biol. Psychiatry 28: 358–362.
9. Kahn R, Asnis G, Wetzler S and van Praag HM (1988) Psychopharmacology 98: 360–364.
10. Cooper T (1983) In: Lajpha A (ed.) Handbook of Neurochemistry. Plenum Press, New York.
11. Sramek J, Herrera J, Costa J and Heh C (1987) J. Clin. Psychiatry 7: 437.
12. Meltzer H, Matsurbara S and Lee J (1989) J. Pharmacol. Exp. Ther. 251: 238–246.

Biological Psychiatry, Volume 1. G. Racagni et al., editors.

5-HT_2 receptor antagonists in schizophrenia: Preclinical and clinical considerations

C.J.E. Niemegeers, F. Awouters, S.L.E. Heylen and Y.G. Gelders
Janssen Research Foundation, B-2340 Beerse, Belgium

Introduction

Central serotonin antagonism is long known to be an activity component of several classical neuroleptics. In recent years the interest in serotonin antagonism has greatly increased with the availability of potent and selective serotonin 5-HT_2 antagonists. A brief survey of the effects of 3 different serotonin 5-HT_2 antagonists, ritanserin, risperidone and ocaperidone is presented.

Ritanserin

Ritanserin is pharmacologically a potent and selective serotonin 5-HT_2 antagonist [1]. At low doses, ritanserin was found to possess disinhibitory properties in animals with induced anxiety-like behaviour, but in contrast to benzodiazepines it did not provoke indifference to punishment. Ritanserin increased the total amount of deep SWS, but it did not induce hypnosis, motor incoordination, sedation, or other abnormal behavioural effects up to very high doses. Ritanserin was found to be effective in several tests predictive for antidepressant activity and to possess anti-abuse potential against alcohol, cocaine and fentanyl, although it is not a substitute for any of these drugs.

Clinically ritanserin can be described as a thymosthenic agent [2] which restores energy and mood, reduces inhibition and anxiety and improves the quality of sleep, a clinical profile which is predictive for antidepressant activity.

In chronic schizophrenia, ritanserin at an average dose of 20 mg daily, associated with classical neuroleptic therapy, was reported to improve negative and affective symptoms, to favour the resocialization of the patients and to attenuate extrapyramidal side-effects.

In reducing EPS ritanserin was at least as effective as orphenadrine (Mindham total scores) [3]. Neuroleptic-induced akathisia considerably improved [4]. Based on single-dose administration, ritanserin was found to have a general-sleep promoting effect in schizophrenics [5]. Motor disturbances of Parkinson's disease, mainly tremor, were also found to respond [6]. New trials to study the effects of ritanserin in doses of 5–10 mg daily as add-on to neuroleptic treatment are in preparation.

Risperidone

Risperidone is a benzisoxazole derivative, with mixed serotonin 5-HT_2 and catecholamine (mainly dopamine D_2) antagonist properties, devoid of anticholinergic activity [7]. As a direct dopamine D_2 antagonist, risperidone is about 10 times less potent than as a serotonin 5-HT_2 antagonist.

Risperidone is also a potent and selective LSD antagonist, devoid of LSD-like agonist activity. In behavioural studies in rats, risperidone was found to possess disinhibitory properties, whereas dopaminergic overactivity was reduced in a dose-range overlapping the disinhibitory doses. With increasing doses blockade of the dopaminergic neurotransmission gradually became enhanced, to be complete at a very high dose only.

From the pharmacological studies, antipsychotic activity with a low propensity for induction of EPS was predicted.

In both open and double-blind phase II clinical studies in more than 500 chronic psychotic patients, risperidone was found to have a potent antipsychotic effect, to improve negative and affective symptoms of schizophrenia and to reduce pre-existing EPS [8,9].

Preliminary results of the first international multicentre dose-finding comparative trial indicate that the antipsychotic activity of ripseridone is superior to that of haloperidol. The evaluation of EPS, the associated consumption of antiparkinson medication together with the efficacy outcome, showed doses of 4–8 mg risperidone daily to be optimal.

Ocaperidone

The next compound is ocaperidone (R 79 598), a very potent neuroleptic, acting with the same intensity on both dopamine D_2 and serotonin 5-HT_2 receptors [10].

In the first open pilot clinical investigation on 81 schizophrenic patients with acute psychotic symptoms, ocaperidone was shown to be a very potent neuroleptic with a rapid onset of action and a mild EPS inducing potential at mean doses of 2.3 mg daily.

Based on pharmacological and clinical work with the 3 new serotonin antagonists ritanserin, risperidone and ocaperidone, it is suggested that in schizophrenia, 5-HT_2 antagonism, which is the common link between the 3 compounds presented, is likely to play an important role in the improvement of negative and affective symptoms and in the attenuation of EPS. Additional studies will have to define the precise role of 5-HT_2 antagonism on patient resocialization, compliance with medication and subjective improvement of sleep.

References

1. Awouters F, Niemegeers CJE, Megens AHP, Meert TF and Janssen PAJ (1988) Drug Dev. Res. 15: 61–73.
2. Reyntjens A, Gelders YG, Hoppenbrouwers MLJA and Vanden Bussche G (1986) Drug Dev. Res. 8: 205–211.
3. Bersani G, Grispini A, Marini S, Pasini A, Valducci M and Ciani N (1990) Clin. Neuropharmacol. 13: 500–506.
4. Miller CH, Fleischhacker WW, Ehrmann H and Kane JM (1990) Psychopharmacol. Bull. 26: 373–376.
5. Benson KL, Csernansky JG, Zarcone VP Jr (1991) Schizophr. Res. 4: 330.
6. Auff E, Birkmayer W, Deecke L et al. (1987) New Trends Clin. Neuropharmacol. 3: 140–158.
7. Janssen PAJ, Niemegeers CJE, Awouters F, Schellekens KHL, Megens AAHP and Meert TF (1988) J. Pharmacol. Exp. Ther. 244: 685–693.
8. Gelders YG, Heylen SLE, Vanden Bussche G, Reyntjens AJM and Janssen PAJ (1990) Pharmacopsychiatry 23: 206–211.
9. Borison RL, Pathiraja AP, Diamond BI and Meibach RC (1991) Schizophr. Res. 4: 314.
10. Megens AAHP, Awouters FHL, Meert TF, Schellekens KHL, Niemegeers CJE and Janssen PAJ (1991) J. Pharmacol. Exp. Ther. (submitted).

Biological Psychiatry, Volume 1. G. Racagni et al., editors.

$5\text{-}HT_3$ receptor antagonists: Preclinical and clinical considerations

B. Costall[1], A.M. Domeney[1], M.E. Kelly[1], R.J. Naylor[1], H.Y. Meltzer[2]

[1]Postgraduate Studies in Pharmacology, The School of Pharmacy, University of Bradford, Bradford, West Yorkshire, BD7 1DP, U.K.; and [2]Case Western Reserve University School of Medicine, Hanna Pavilion, 2040 Abington Road, Cleveland, OH 44106, U.S.A.

Introduction

Hypotheses of a raised mesolimbic dopamine function in schizophrenia have provided the rationale for treatment with dopamine receptor antagonists. The side-effects of neuroleptic treatment caused by a blockade of normal as well as abnormal dopamine function are well known and include extrapyramidal side-effects and endocrine disturbances. For over 30 years agents have been sought which selectively reduce a raised mesolimbic dopaminergic activity without affecting other brain dopamine systems. The $5\text{-}HT_3$ receptor antagonist ondansetron demonstrates such properties in animal models.

Preclinical studies

Animal models were developed in the rodent and primate to raise mesolimbic dopamine function by the injection of amphetamine or infusion of dopamine into limbic areas of the rat and marmoset brain. The effect of amphetamine to release endogenous dopamine or exogenously applied dopamine, was to produce the same behavioural response of increased locomotor activity. The increase in activity was inhibited by ondansetron and other $5\text{-}HT_3$ receptor antagonists. In contrast, the co-administration of amphetamine with the selective $5\text{-}HT_3$ receptor agonist 2-methyl-5-HT further enhanced the locomotor activity, a response again inhibited by ondansetron. The $5\text{-}HT_3$ agonist-antagonist effects to inhibit the dopamine response are most likely to be mediated via the $5\text{-}HT_3$ receptors which have been shown to be located in limbic brain areas of many species including man [1].

In further test procedures, a stimulation of dopamine cell bodies in the midbrain was achieved by local injection of the neurokinin receptor agonist DiMe-C7. The behavioural consequence is an increased activity and enhanced dopamine release in the forebrain; both the behavioural and biochemical responses were antagonized by ondansetron [2]. The data indicated that $5\text{-}HT_3$ receptors may normally act to facilitate dopamine function.

In all such manipulations there were important features to distinguish the actions of ondansetron compared with neuroleptic agents. Most striking was its ability to inhibit a raised dopamine function without affecting normal behaviour, the levels of activity simply returning to normal values. Ondansetron also failed to produce signs of extrapyramidal or endocrinological disturbance in animals, providing further evidence for the absence of dopamine receptor blockade. Furthermore, there were no changes in receptor sensitivity following withdrawal from ondansetron treatment, to contrast with the development of dopamine receptor supersensitivity following chronic neuroleptic-induced changes in dopamine receptor sensitivity. An intriguing finding was a lessened efficacy of ondansetron when using very high doses, although at these and lower doses animals retained an alert and normal appearance with no evidence of sedation.

The effectiveness of ondansetron to reduce a raised mesolimbic dopamine activity in the absence of effects to reduce normal behaviour provided the rationale for the clinical investigation of its effects in schizophrenia.

Open clinical studies in schizophrenia

Two open, uncontrolled multicentre studies were performed in the U.K. and the U.S.A. in hospitalized patients with a DSM III diagnosis of acute schizophrenia. One study employed doses of ondansetron of either 4 mg b.i.d. or 8 mg b.i.d. while the other study employed 2 flexible dosing regimens: a low dose regimen with a maximum possible dose of 8 mg b.i.d. and a high dose regimen with a maximum possible dose of 16 mg t.i.d. In these studies, ondansetron appeared to possess antipsychotic activity but, most interestingly, the drug's efficacy appeared to be inversely related to dose. For this reason, a double-blind placebo-controlled study was undertaken at a dose of 4 mg b.i.d.

A double-blind placebo-controlled study in acute schizophrenia

One hundred and fourteen DSM III schizophrenic patients from 13 participating centers in the U.K. were randomly assigned to ondansetron 4 mg b.i.d. or placebo, for a 4-week double-blind trial. Chlorpromazine (CPZ) in multiples of doses of 50–100 mg or diazepam were permitted for additional clinical management, if needed. The doses of CPZ were higher in the placebo-treated group but 45–50% of patients in both groups did receive some CPS. Thirty-eight of 55 (69.1%) ondansetron and 41 of 59 (69.5%) placebo patients completed the study. Analysis of the total BPRS, BPRS positive and negative symptoms and the clinical global impression (CGI) using the last value before chlorpromazine carried forward or the last value regardless of CPZ administration did not show a significant drug treatment effect or drug × CPZ interaction. There was also no difference in the proportions of the entire group of patients who responded to ondansetron (30.1%) or placebo (31.6%) with a decrease in BPRS score ≥ 50%. However, inspection of several measures suggested that the group of patients treated with ondansetron alone may have had a more favourable outcome than the other 3 groups, e.g. in final CGI scores and final BPRS positive and negative symptoms. Ondansetron produced no significant extrapyramidal or other side-effects and was well tolerated.

The use of CPZ and diazepam, which was requested by the review boards of the participating centers, clearly compromised the ability of this study to assess the antipsychotic effects of ondansetron. The antipsychotic effect of ondansetron observed in previous open trials could not be definitively confirmed or rejected. Further study of the antipsychotic efficacy of 5-HT_3 antagonists such as ondansetron, using more conventional research designs, is still warranted.

References

1. Costall A, Domeney AM, Naylor RJ and Tyers MS (1987) Br. J. Pharmacol. 92: 881–894.
2. Hagan RM, Butler A, Hill JM, Jordan CC, Ireland SJ and Tyers MB (1987) Eur. J. Pharmacol. 138: 303–305.

Biological Psychiatry, Volume 1. G. Racagni et al., editors.

Psychophysiological approaches to schizophrenia: Introduction and historical overview

Charles Shagass
Temple University and Philadelphia Psychiatric Center, Ford Road and Monument Ave, Philadelphia, PA 19131, U.S.A.

Psychophysiology is a vast domain, devoted to studying the relationships between physiological processes and behavior. While knowledge of such relationships may date back to antiquity, the pioneer of systematic studies in this area was probably Wilhelm Wundt. Credited with founding the first experimental psychology laboratory, he wrote a book on physiological psychology that guided the field for many years. During the early twentieth century, interest in recording and measuring physiological activities was encouraged by developments in instrumentation and introduction of concepts such as homeostasis. Measurements of autonomic nervous system activities offered a means of attempting to objectify emotional aspects of experience. From 1930 to 1960, the galvanic skin response (CSR) was perhaps the favorite tool of psychophysiological research, but other autonomic effector systems, e.g. cardiorespiratory, also received attention. Measures related more to central, rather than autonomic, nervous system activities, were also increasingly employed, e.g. electromyogram (EMC) and electroencephalogram (EEC). By 1955, the first scientific periodical devoted exclusively to psychophysiology was initiated; it became the journal Psychophysiology. The field has burgeoned ever since, with a remarkable growth spurt when computer techniques became available to relieve the drudgery of hand measurement of physiological records and of complex statistical calculations.

Most psychophysiological methods were applied to the study of psychiatric patients soon after their introduction, e.g. Hans Berger, discoverer of the human EEC, recorded the EEC of psychiatric patients early in his work. Schizophrenia has probably received more psychophysiologic study than any other psychiatric condition. Certainly, there is ample rationale for hoping that the manifold aberrations of perception, cognition and affect that are found in schizophrenia should be associated with deviant physiology. The results of these investigations have been generally positive, but disappointing. They have been positive in the sense that numerous statistical differences have been demonstrated between schizophrenics and comparison populations, most often nonpatient controls. They have been disappointing because the measurements of schizophrenics usually overlap substantially with those of other groups; also, differences from normal have generally not been unique to schizophrenics, often being found in other kinds of psychiatric patients. Apart from low diagnostic specificity, findings in schizophrenia have failed to identify convincingly specifically dysfunctional mechanisms. As peripheral findings have always been speculated about in terms of postulated CNS dysfunctions, newer methods to examine CNS function more directly in schizophrenia offer hope for more specificity in the future.

Many plausible reasons can be advanced for our failure to progress further toward identifying the nature of psychophysiological dysfunctions in schizophrenia (I must emphasize the plural). Here are a few:

1. heterogeneity of schizophrenic populations;
2. inadequate control over the state of the subject when recordings were made; this includes such difficult matters as level of alertness and degree of emotional arousal, as well as superficially simple factors like time of day, time since tobacco or alcohol use, and number of hours slept, etc.;
3. relative crudeness of available methods, e.g. scalp EEGs measure directly only surface cortical activities and these are attenuated and distorted by intervening tissues;
4. stimuli or tasks used in the laboratory situation do not tap adequately functions that are specifically deviant in schizophrenia;
5. more physiological systems need to be measured simultaneously in order to reveal patterns of dysfunction.

There are many other possible reasons for variable and nonspecific results. Awareness of such issues has led to more and more sophisticated methods of instrumentation, research design and data analysis.

One general conceptual problem may underlie much of the disappointment concerning the psychophysiology of schizophrenia. Psychophysiology is a correlational science, dealing with relationships and not with causes. This fact sets real limits on what can be expected and achieved. The approach can show that certain bodily processes, under particular circumstances, are associated with certain behaviors, or behavioral attributes. It can also show whether normal physiology/behavior relationships differ in schizophrenics; e.g. the task-related P300 wave, is of lower amplitude in schizophrenics even when task performance is correct. However, the cause of this altered normal relationship must be sought at some other level of observation. The experienced psychophysiologist may be content to demonstrate the P300/schizophrenia relationship and to do further experiments to define aspects of the P300 or the behavior involved in the correlation. However, others often want a causative explanation. They may say: "So what?" when informed that the cause of the altered relationship is not only unknown, but could not be revealed by the method. This kind of reluctance to understand and accept the limits of an approach is not unique to psychiatric psychophysiology. It has taken a long time for useful biological markers of clinical medicine, e.g., body temperature, arterial blood pressure, leukocyte count, blood glucose, etc., to be placed in perspective as possible correlates of disease processes, rather than the disease itself and certainly not its cause.

Another probable consequence of the correlational nature of psychophysiology is the paucity of useful theoretical concepts, without which the plethora of empirical observations is difficult to organize meaningfully. A.A. Alexander's [1] list of concepts employed to organize psychophysiological data in relation to psychopathology, include:

a) responsivity-reactivity;
b) activation/arousal;
c) defective physiological regulation;
d) physiological imbalance, including autonomic imbalance;
e) homeostasis.

Such concepts may be useful starting points for research, as they can be operationalized in many ways, but they hardly qualify as incisive theory. Findings showing, for example, that a particular kind of reactivity differs statistically from normal in schizophrenics can lead only to questions about what structures are working differently, the mechanisms involved, whether the dysfunction is transitory or permanent, etc.

Perhaps the main hope of theorists in this field lies in identifying brain structures that are specifically dysfunctional in at least a definable subgroup of schizophrenics. A localized specific dysfunction could point to pathology caused by an anatomical or neurochemical lesion. The newer brain imaging techniques, some of which will be discussed in the Symposium, have been received enthusiastically as possible avenues for identifying dysfunctional brain areas that may be specific for schizophrenia. This would have an enormous impact on theory, on organization of disparate psychophysiological observations, and on the focusing of research. Some indication of the power of a concept involving identification of a dysfunctional brain area can be gained from the impact of such a relatively non-specific theory as Flor-Henry's [2] proposal that schizophrenic disorders involve mainly the left brain hemisphere. This hypothesis has generated an enormous amount of productive research. The more focused concept of dorsolateral prefrontal lobe dysfunction in schizophrenia [3] may be having even more impact.

This Symposium is a very small sampling of approaches to psychophysiological investigation of schizophrenia, but it should convey an idea of the current status of some of the relevant research areas.

Acknowledgement

Author's research supported (in part) by USPHS Grant MH12507.

References

1. Alexander AA (1972) In: Greenfield MS and Sternbach RA (eds.) Handbook of Psychophysiology. Holt, Rinehart, Winston, New York, pp. 925–964.
2. Flor-Henry P (1969) Am. J. Psychiatry 126: 399–404.
3. Weinberger DR, Berman KF and Zec RF (1986) Arch. Gen. Psychiatry 43: 114–124.

Biological Psychiatry, Volume 1. G. Racagni et al., editors.

Computerized EEG in psychiatry

W. Günther, U. Klages, C. Haag, I. Bscheid and R. Riedel
Psychiatric University Hospital, Nussbaumstr. 7, D 8000 Munich 2, Germany

Introduction

Computerized EEG is increasingly used in the study of brain dysfunction in psychiatric patients [1]. Findings obtained so far can only be outlined. In *Alzheimer's patients*, the most widely accepted results concern increases in delta and theta power values along with a decreased (and slower) alpha activity [2–4].

Further fields of application of computerized EEG involve patients with various forms of *dependence* (e.g. increased absolute and relative alpha power in crack users [5], and neuropsychiatric manifestations of *HIV infection* [6].

Further widely-accepted findings have been reported for patients with *affective disorders*, namely increases of fast frequencies both over the non-dominant and dominant sides of the brain [7,8]. Additionally, in patients meeting RDC criteria for depression, Schatzberg et al. [9] found an increase in delta and theta in right posterior temporal regions and an increase in frontal beta activity bilaterally.

Findings in *schizophrenics* do not yield consistent results thus far. However, in several studies, an increase of delta and theta amplitudes is reported [10–13].

Additional information might be available using functional activation tasks, both to reduce the variability of "resting" conditions and to increase group differences by involving dysfunctional circuits.

Materials and Methods

We applied motor and music listening tasks as compared to resting conditions and used 16-channel EEG mapping to study 26 (13 male/13 female) untreated (1-week wash-out to drug-naive) schizophrenics and 34 matched controls. Experimental conditions were resting/eyes closed, fist opening and simple music listening conditions. Each activation was compared to an own preceding reference (resting/eyes closed) state in order to control for "sequential cerebral activation".

Results

In this mixed sample of predominantly "chronic" schizophrenic patients with distinct negative symptoms (total SANS averaging 36), we found increased delta power in resting conditions predominantly bifrontally.

However, additional results yielded a complete non-reactivity of EEG changes (as compared to resting EEG) in alpha and delta frequency bands in schizophrenic patients as compared to normals. This non-reactivity was detected both during motor and music listening tasks.

Interestingly, when the patients were subdivided according to this EEG reagibility to functional stimulation, two distinct subgroups were separated. One group of patients, reacting to stimulation almost like normals, was characterised by predominance of positive symptoms and absence of negative symptoms. The other subgroup, in contrast, showed in the EEG "inverse to normal" activation patterns and displayed markedly negative symptoms, with or without "overlaying" positive ones. Interestingly, such "inverse" patterns had been found in our former investigations exclusively in patients with Alzheimers disease [14].

For further details, we refer the interested reader to Günther [15] and Klages [16].

Comment

Computerized EEG in psychiatry has advanced scientific interest in investigating brain dysfunction in various psychiatric disorders. Studies using functional activation paradigms may additionally enhance the information that can be obtained by this method. Own investigations using 16-channel computerized EEG in a mixed sample of predominantly "chronic-negative" schizophrenic patients during motor and music listening tasks are examples of this approach.

Possible future developments may use a greater number of channels in an attempt to increase topographical resolution and the multimodal combination with other imaging methods like SPECT and PET, in order to improve the potential value of computerized EEG for use in clinical psychiatry.

References

1. Williamson PC and Kaye MD (1989) Can. J. Psychiatry 34: 680–686.
2. Busse EW (1983) In: Reisberg B (ed.) Alzheimer's Disease. Collier MacMillan, New York.
3. Saletu B, Paulus E, Anderer P et al. (1989) In: Saletu B, Biologische Psychiatrie. Thieme Verlag, Stuttgart, pp. 225–231.
4. Maurer K, Riederer P and Beckmann H (eds.) (1990) Alzheimer's Disease. Springer, Berlin.
5. Alper et al.
6. Riedel RR, Bader L, Naber D et al. (1991) Fortschr. Neurol. Psychiatr. Grenzgeb. 59: 69–80.
7. Flor-Henry P et al. (1975) IRCS Med. Sci. 3: 87.
8. Vacca L et al. (1980) Adv. Biol. Psychiatry 4: 111–118.
9. Schatzberg AF et al. (1986) In: Duffy FH (ed.) Topographic Mapping of Brain Electrical Activity. Butterworths, Boston.
10. Morihisa JM, Duffy FH and Wyatt RD (1983) Arch. Gen. Psychiatry 40: 719–728.

11. Buchsbaum MS, Guich SM, Burgwald L et al. (1989) Schizophr. Res. 2: 439–448.
12. Günther W and Breitling D (1985) Biol. Psychiatry 20: 515–532.
13. Günther W, Breitling D, Banquet JP et al. (1986) Biol. Psychiatry 21: 249–262.
14. Engel RR, Satzger W, Günther W et al. (1990) Abstr. ECNP Congr., Gothenburg.
15. Günther W (1990) In: Möller HJ and Pelzer E (eds.) Neuere Ansätze zur Diagnostik und Therapie schizophrener Minussymptomatik. Springer, Berlin, pp. 155–166.
16. Klages U (1991) Dissertation Med. Fakultät LMU München, Munich.

Biological Psychiatry, Volume 1. G. Racagni et al., editors.

Exploratory eye movements in schizophrenics: Comparison with temporal lobe epileptics and patients with frontal lobe lesions

Takuya Kojima, Eisuke Matsushima, Kazunori Nakajima, Shigeru Ohbayashi, Harunobu Ando, Katsumi Ando and Yasuo Shimazono

Department of Neuropsychiatry, Faculty of Medicine, Tokyo Medical and Dental University, 5-45 Yushima 1-chome, Bunkyo-ku, Tokyo 113, Japan

Introduction

In our previous studies it was reported that chronic schizophrenics and their relatives had less frequent eye fixations and a more limited area of inspection than normal controls [1]. Eye movements while responding to a question were scored to give the responsive search score (RSS) [2]. Schizophrenic patients had a significantly lower RSS than non-schizophrenic patients and in our other studies could be discriminated from non-schizophrenic patients with 75% sensitivity and 81% specificity [3]. Recently it was reported that schizophrenics were found to have areas of abnormal psychophysiological parameters or abnormal values of chemical neurotransmitters localized to the frontal or temporal lobes. The present study was conducted to compare the eye movements of schizophrenics with those of patients with localized brain dysfunction such as frontal lobe lesions and temporal lobe epilepsy.

Subjects

Nine patients with right frontal lobe lesions (RF group), 9 patients with left frontal lobe lesions (LF group), 12 temporal lobe epileptics with right-sided spike foci (EpR group), 21 temporal lobe epileptics with left-sided spike foci (EpL group), 50 schizophrenic patients (S group) and 50 normal controls (NC group) were tested. Mean ages and standard deviations for each of the groups were 38.8 ± 11.6, 40.6 ± 8.2, 35.9 ± 11.5, 36.1 ± 10.1, 38.2 ± 7.8 and 37.1 ± 7.2 years, respectively. Ages were matched for each group.

Method

Procedure

The subjects were asked to sit on a chair 1.5 m in front of a screen with an eye mark recorder on their heads. Three S-shaped figures were projected in turn on the screen for 15 s each. Each subject was shown an original S-shaped figure, followed by 2 figures slightly different from the original. The subjects were requested to look at the figures and compare each one with the original. Eye movements and fixation points during each viewing were recorded on videotape.

Measurement

The elementary components of eye movements (the number of eye fixations and the mean eye scanning length) were measured while the subject viewed the original figure. The **RSS** was calculated by scoring the eye movements made when the subjects were asked: "Are there any other differences?"

Results

Temporal lobe epileptics and schizophrenics

The elementary components of eye movements. The EpL group had significantly shorter mean eye-scanning length (MESL) than the EpR group and the NC group, although they had significantly longer MESL than the S group. On the other hand, there was no difference between the EpR group and the NC group.

RSS. Each epileptic patient group and the NC group had significantly higher RSS than the S group. No significant difference was found to exist between the epileptic groups and the NC group.

Patients with frontal lobe lesions and schizophrenics

The elementary components of eye movements. The RF group and the S group had less frequent eye fixations than the NC group. The TESL of the RF group was significantly shorter than that of the NC group. No significant difference in these components was found between the LF group and the NC group.

RSS. The RF, LF and NC groups had significantly higher RSSs than the S group.

Discussion

The similarities in the elementary components of eye movements between the EpL and S groups and between the RF and S groups suggest that dysfunction of the left temporal lobe and the right frontal lobe may exist in schizophrenia. These findings coincide with Flor-Henry's report [4] on temporal lobe epilepsy and our other

Table 1. Eye movements for each group

Group	Number of eye fixation (n)	Mean eye scanning length (MESL)	Total eye scanning length (TESL)	Responsive search score (RSS)
S group	29.6 ± 9.1[d,h]	13.9 ± 2.7[c,e,h]	415.7 ± 56.5[d,e,h]	6.6 ± 2.6[d,f,h]
EpL group	39.3 ± 6.4[b,e]	16.0 ± 3.1[a,g]	624.6 ± 156.8[b,g]	10.3 ± 2.2[b]
EpR group	43.8 ± 8.8[b,e]	19.8 ± 4.0[b,d]	870.1 ± 266.4[b,d,f]	11.3 ± 1.2[b]
RF group	34.0 ± 7.4[c,g]	16.8 ± 3.2[a]	575.3 ± 190.6[a,g]	10.6 ± 1.1[b]
LF group	37.8 ± 5.4[b]	19.1 ± 3.7[b]	721.9 ± 142.3[b]	11.0 ± 1.1[b]
NC group	40.0 ± 7.4[b,e]	18.2 ± 3.4[b,c]	710.3 ± 179.6[b,c,e]	10.6 ± 1.9[b]

[a]$P < 0.05$; [b]$P < 0.01$ vs. S; [c]$P < 0.05$; [d]$P < 0.01$ vs. EpL; [e] $P < 0.05$; [f]$P < 0.01$ vs. RF; [g]$P < 0.05$; [h]$P < 0.01$ vs. NC (Mann-Whitney U test).

report [5] on eye movements and neuropsychological tests for schizophrenia. The RSS is regarded as a parameter that is specific for schizophrenia. However, RSSs for the 2 patient groups (EpL and RF) were significantly different from those of the S group but were very similar to those of the NC group. These findings and the results described earlier suggest that schizophrenia is not produced by a frontal or temporal lobe lesion alone, but through disturbance of a neural system which may consist of both lobes, the basal ganglia, the thalamic nuclei and association areas.

References

1. Shimazono Y, Ando K, Moriya H, Kojima T, Ando H, Harada N and Iwama H (1983) Proc. WPA Regional Symposium. Kyoto, pp. 128–134.
2. Kojima T, Matsushima E, Iwama H, Ando H, Moriya H, Ando K, Takahashi R and Shimazono Y (1986) Psychopharmacol. Bull. 22: 768–777.
3. Ohta K, Kojima T, Matsushima E, Nakajima K, Kawashima M, Ohbayashi S, Matsuura M, Ando H, Ando K, Takahashi R and Shimazono Y (1988) Jpn. J. Psychiatry Neurol. 42: 677.
4. Flor-Henry P (1969) Epilepsy 10: 363–395.
5. Kojima T, Matsushima E, Ando K, Ando H, Sakurada M, Moriya H, Ohta K and Shimazono Y (1991) Schizophr. Bull. (in press).

Biological Psychiatry, Volume 1. G. Racagni et al., editors.

Slow response-related negativities in chronic schizophrenics

Rudolf Cohen, Patrick Berg and Gereon Hopmann
Fachgruppe Psychologie, Universität Konstanz, Postfach 5560, D-775 Konstanz, Germany

Event-related potentials (ERP) of schizophrenic and other psychotic patients have consistently [1] been found to show reduced amplitudes of the late endogenous components N1/PN, N2, P3, and the contingent negative variation (CNV). This attenuation does not seem to be a function of neuroleptic medication; it is related to a decreased signal-to-noise ratio and corresponds with a diminished responsiveness to experimental demands. There seems to be only one late component – rarely seen in normals – that has frequently been found to be enhanced in groups of psychotic patients during warned reaction time tasks: the post-imperative negative variation (PINV). This slow fronto-central negativity, extending far beyond the motor response, is frequently interpreted as a prolonged CNV (implying some sort of prolonged stimulus evaluation). Results from the following studies suggest that it might better be understood as a functionally distinct component possibly related to an appraisal of the immediately preceding response.

Material and Methods

Subjects and ERP analyses

In 4 studies medicated, chronic or subchronic inpatients with a schizophrenic disorder according to DSM III criteria were compared with healthy volunteers and alcoholic inpatients (≥6 weeks after withdrawal). Groups were matched for age (med. = 35 years, range: 18–55 years), sex and education. Alcoholics and healthy volunteers were combined in one "control group" whenever the groups did not differ ($P > 0.20$) in their respective averages. The EEG was recorded from Fz, Cz and Pz with Ag/AgCl electrodes referred to linked earlobes, the EOG from above and below the right eye. Amplifiers were set to a high frequency cut-off of 35 Hz and a time constant of 10 s. Trials with eye movements were rejected, trials with blink artifacts corrected by a linear regression approach [2].

Procedure

Study I (18 schizophrenics, 8 alcoholics, 10 normals)
In a warned reaction time task, both warning and imperative stimuli (ISI = 4 s) either consisted of arrows on a CRT, indicating whether to press the left or the right

hand button, or diamonds, requiring the subjects to choose which button to press. In blocks I and III (two-thirds of trials consisted of arrows) subjects had to press the button corresponding to the direction of the arrows; in block II (arrows only) the opposite button. Epoch: 8400 ms.

Study II (23 schizophrenics, 25 normals)
Blocks with compatible and incompatible trials as in Study I; in additional blocks, directional information was given only with the imperative stimulus. Epoch: 5800 ms.

Study III (24 schizophrenics, 12 alcoholics and 12 normals)
Different subjects were presented with different pairs of vowels (A,E,I,U) randomly delivered either acoustically through earphones or as letters on a CRT with intertrial intervals of 1200 ms. One of the 2 vowels was designated target (P = 0.33), requiring a fast button press.

Study IV (18 schizophrenics, 18 alcoholics, 18 normals)
Light and tone stimuli (800 Hz, 72 dB), matched for subjective intensity, were presented in random order with variable intervals (1.7 to 2.3 s); subjects were required to press the same button at every stimulus.

Results

In all 4 studies the ERPs of schizophrenic patients had a more pronounced slow fronto-central negativity to stimuli requiring a fast motor response than the ERPs of controls. In Study I (Fig. 1) the mean amplitude from 1300 to 4000 ms after the imperative stimulus was more negative at Fz and Cz in schizophrenics than in the control group ($F(1,34) \geq 7.46$, $P < 0.01$). Across groups this PINV was more pronounced at Fz, Cz and Pz ($F(2,68) \geq 12.60$, $P < 0.01$) if the subject had to choose which button to press. Whether or not the directional information of the arrows had to be reversed did not influence the PINV ($P > 0.20$). In Study II the PINV could only be determined from 800 to 1300 ms after the imperative stimulus; again, it was larger in schizophrenics than in controls ($F(1,46) = 17.51$, $P < 0.01$) independent of whether the directional information had to be reversed. If the directional information was given only with the imperative stimulus, the PINV at Cz was increased relative to the terminal CNV, particularly among schizophrenics ($F(1,46) = 20.79$, $P < 0.01$). Across these patients larger PINV amplitudes were associated with shorter reaction times in all experimental conditions ($0.18 \geq \text{rho}(20) \geq 0.61$).

Study III and Study IV [3] showed similar group differences (F(2,51 resp. 2,45) ≥ 8.72; $P < 0.01$) for auditory reaction time tasks without warning signals: in both studies the average factor scores for the frontal lead of the slow wave from principal component analyses of the ERPs to auditory stimuli were significantly

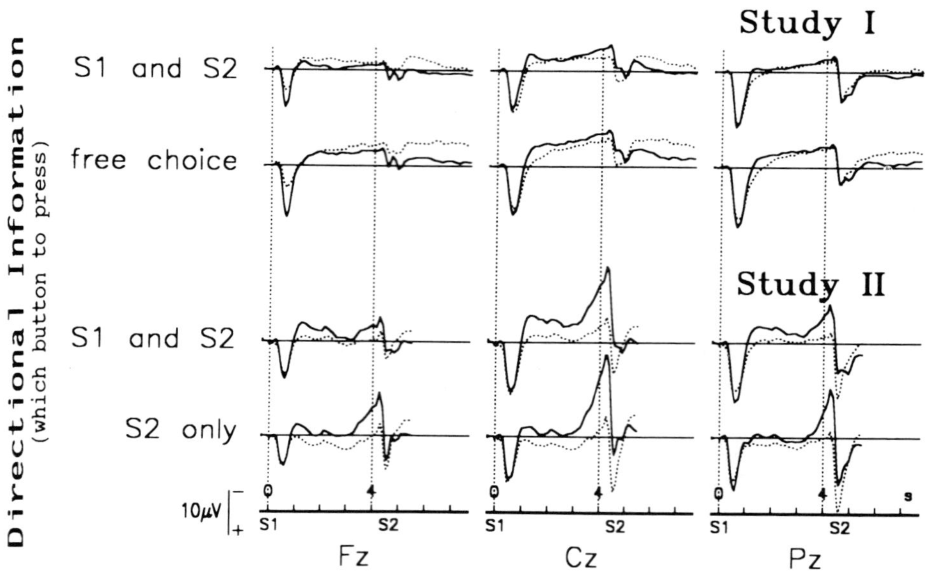

Fig. 1. Grand mean ERPs of schizophrenic inpatients (dotted lines) and control subjects (solid lines) from Studies I and II. (ERPs from compatible and incompatible blocks of trials combined.)

($P < 0.01$) more negative in schizophrenics than in alcoholic or in normal controls. No comparable group effects were found for visual stimuli, and in Study III the group effect was confined to auditory stimuli requiring a motor response. These slow negative waves appear somewhat more frontally distributed than those of the visual warned reaction time tasks.

We interpret these slow response-related negativities as variants of the PINV [4], which may reflect uncertainty about the appropriateness of the preceding response. The increased negativity following auditory target stimuli could be a function of the automatically alerting power of acoustic stimuli [5] which schizophrenics might have difficulty in discriminating from the irritation arising from failure in the monitoring and appraisal of their own actions [6].

References

1. Cohen R (1991) In: Häfner H and Gattaz WF (eds.) Search for the Causes of Schizophrenia, Vol. II. Springer-Verlag, Berlin, pp. 342–360.
2. Berg P (1986) Psychophysics 23: 354–364.
3. Cohen R, Rist F, Finger T and Mussgay L (1991) In: Brunia CHM, Gaillard AWK and Kok A (eds.) Psychophysiological Brain Research, Vol. II. Tilburg University Press, pp. 203–208.
4. Rockstroh B, Elbert T, Birbaumer N and Lutzenberger W (1990) Slow Brain Potentials and Behavior. Urban and Schwarzenberg, Baltimore.
5. Posner M (1978) Chronometric Explorations of Mind. Erlbaum, Hillsdale.
6. Frith CD and Done DJ (1988) Br. J. Psychiatry 153: 437–443.

Biological Psychiatry, Volume 1. G. Racagni et al., editors.

Sertindole: A new concept in neuroleptic research

John Hyttel
Pharmacological Research, H. Lundbeck A/S, Ottiliavej 9, DK-2500 Copenhagen-Valby, Denmark

Introduction

Classical neuroleptics (e.g. haloperidol) induce extrapyramidal side-effects (EPS) in addition to their antipsychotic activity. While EPS are believed to result from dopamine (DA) receptor blockade in the nigrostriatal system, the antipsychotic action involves inhibition of limbic DA systems. The first antipsychotic compound which did not induce EPS in man, clozapine, preferentially inhibits limbic DA function in animal experiments.

We have recently identified a new atypical neuroleptic, sertindole (1-[2-[4-[5-chloro-1-(4-fluorophenyl)-1H-indol-3-yl]-1-piperidinyl]ethyl]-2-imidazolidinone) [1,2]. The present study surveys its pharmacological profile in vitro and in vivo, and further shows its limbic selectivity after treatment for 3 weeks.

Pharmacology in vitro

Sertindole has high affinity (nmol range) for 5-HT_2 receptors, α-adrenoceptors and DA D_2 receptors. The affinity for D_1 receptors is lower but still in the nmol range. The affinity for α_2-adrenoceptors, histamine H receptors and sigma receptors is low and no affinity for 5-HT_{1A} receptors, muscarine cholinergic receptors and β-adrenoceptors is seen.

The receptor binding profile deviates from the profile of haloperidol which has higher affinity for DA D_2 receptors than for 5-HT_2 receptors and α_1-adrenoceptors. Haloperidol has relatively high affinity for sigma receptors. Sertindole also deviates from clozapine. Both compounds have high affinity for 5-HT_2 receptors and α_1-adrenoceptors, but clozapine also has high affinity for muscarine cholinergic receptors and low affinity for DA D_2 receptors.

Ex vivo binding confirms the profile shown above (effect on 5-$HT_2 > \alpha_1 > D_2$). Maximal inhibition is obtained within the first 48 h. Occupancy of 5-HT_2 receptors (^{3}H-ketanserin) is still observed 10 days after dosing. No binding to α_1-adrenoceptors and D_2 receptors is seen after 5–6 days and after 3 days, respectively.

Pharmacology in vivo

Sertindole has no DA antagonistic activity in classical tests for stereotypy (methylphenidate, amphetamine) and does not induce catalepsy. Sertindole has moderate antagonistic effect on central α_1-adrenoceptors, as measured by the discriminative stimulus induced by the α_1-agonist St 587.

Sertindole is a potent 5-HT_2 antagonist (quipazine induced head twitches, d-LSD cue) with a long duration of action and a high oral availability.

The effects on spontaneously active DA neurones in ventral tegmental area (VTA) and substantia nigra pars compacta (SNC) after repeated drug treatment was tested in rats. Inhibition of the number of spontaneously active DA neurones in VTA indicates an antipsychotic effect of a compound, while inhibition of the number of DA neurones in SNC might indicate the development of neurological side-effects [1,3].

Compared to both the classical (haloperidol) and the atypical (clozapine) neuroleptic, sertindole shows an extreme selectivity for DA neurones in VTA.

Sertindole selectivity inhibits the DA neurones in VTA with an ED_{50}-value (0.015 µmol/kg/day) more than 100 times lower than the ED_{50}-value (1.6 µmol/kg/day) for inhibition of DA neurones in SNC [2].

The antagonism of the hyperactivity response to continuous DA infusion into the rat nucleus accumbens was performed by Professor B. Costall and colleagues at the Neuropharmacology Research Group, University of Bradford, England [4].

Bilateral DA infusion into the nucleus accumbens of rats (25 µg/day) causes a hyperactivity response between days 2–6 and 9–12 [5,6]. This overstimulation of the mesolimbic DA system is sensitive to neuroleptic treatment. The effect of sertindole (s.c. once daily) on locomotor activity has been studied during the DA infusion (13 days) and during a 3-week post-infusion period without any treatment.

Sertindole antagonizes the hyperactivity response to DA infusion. The minimal effective doses of sertindole (MED 0.0057 µmol/kg, s.c.) are comparable to those used in the electrophysiological studies. However, the profile of sertindole does not resemble that of a typical neuroleptic agent since it fails to produce a rebound hyperactivity on withdrawal from treatment, and only reduces locomotor activity below normal control levels at a dose 500-fold higher than the minimal effective doses (i.e. 2.8 µmol/kg, s.c.). In contrast, this ratio is only 5 for fluphenazine which causes a marked rebound increase in activity after withdrawal of infusion and treatment.

In order to study the neurological side-effects, sertindole was injected s.c. to 3 green vervet monkeys, which were sensitized to neuroleptic treatment. After injection the monkeys were observed continuously for presence of neurological disturbances. Dose levels of 1.0, 2.1 and 4.2 µmol/kg were studied. At the 2 lower dosages only minimal side-effects were observed, consisting of slight sedation, hypokinesia and, in 1 monkey, slight restlessness. After 4.2 µmol/kg increasing sedation developed during the first 2 h after injection. At this time, marked dystonic reactions developed (retrocollis, catatonic postures) and, in one monkey, a full dystonic episode.

The potency of sertindole to induce neurological side-effects in green vervet monkeys is low. For comparison, the classical neuroleptic haloperidol induces neurological side-effects at doses as low as 0.067 and 0.13 μmol/kg, s.c. and clozapine induces marked sedation at doses between 3.1 and 15 μmol/kg.

Conclusion

In conclusion, sertindole has unique pharmacological properties. It clearly differs from classical neuroleptics, and has many similarities to clozapine. However, sertindole has higher potency in the tests predicting antipsychotic activity (effect on DA neurones in VTA, effect on DA infusion into nucleus accumbens), better oral activity, longer duration of action and has fewer risks for peripheral side-effects than clozapine.

References

1. Skarsfeldt T and Perregaard J (1990) Eur. J. Pharmacol. 182: 613–614.
2. Sánchez C, Arnt J, Dragsted N, Hyttel J, Lembøl HL, Meier E and Skarsfeldt T (1991) Drug Dev. Res. (in press).
3. Chiodo LA and Bunney BS (1983) J. Neurosci. 3: 1607–1619.
4. Domeney AM, Arnt J, Costall B, Naylor RJ, Sánchez C and Smith AG (1991) Br. Pharmacol. Soc. Joint Meeting, Lyon, April 25–27, France.
5. Costall B, Domeney AM and Naylor RJ (1982) Neuropharmacology 21: 327–335.
6. Costall B (1987) Br. J. Pharmacol. 92: 881–894.

Biological Psychiatry, Volume 1. G. Racagni et al., editors.

Depression in chronic schizophrenia

D.A.W. Johnson
University Hospital of South Manchester, Manchester, M20 8LR, U.K.

The presence of depressive mood disorders in schizophrenia has been recognized since the days of Kraepelin and Bleuler. Indeed, Bleuler declared it one of the most frequent acute disturbances in schizophrenia. More recent surveys suggest that 15–57% of schizophrenic outpatients will experience significant depression and it is the most frequent symptom described by schizophrenic patients living in the community. The exact prevalence is difficult to establish since the criteria for diagnosis often vary, but those studies using strict criteria taking care to isolate depression from negative symptoms confirm its frequency. Over the last 10–15 years there has been an increased interest in exploring the aetiology and significance of depression in schizophrenia.

Aetiology

The aetiology is complex and varied. It is most unlikely that a single cause is responsible for all depression even in an individual patient. The following possibilities should be considered.

Personality

The premorbid personality of the patient and his attitude towards his psychiatric illness and its consequences are important. Roy et al. [1] have suggested that depressed schizophrenic patients were more likely to be living alone, have suffered parental loss, have been treated for previous depression, have had previous attempts at self-harm, have had more undesirable life-events in the previous 6 months and have had more hospital admissions.

Genetic predispositions

A number of authors have suggested that relatives have suffered from depressive illness. Others have suggested that depression is a response to neuroleptic medication because of a genetic-based sensitivity. Both hypotheses lack adequate evaluation.

Postpsychotic depression

It is generally agreed that 6–12 months after recovery from an acute episode is a time of particular risk. Overall, 25% of patients experience depression within this interval and 50% of all suicides occur within 3 months of discharge.

There are 2 principal theories of aetiology: theories based on the psychological development of reaction to the experience of psychosis and the suggestion that depression identified at this time is an apparent phenomenon due to the differential response of existing symptoms ("revealed depression") [2,3]. It is important to note that both theories suggest that postpsychotic depression is part of the resolution of psychosis. The argument that postpsychotic depression has a different aetiology to depression at other times is supported by the failure to demonstrate any relationship to future relapse or prognosis in contrast to depression at other times.

Neuroleptic-induced depression

Neuroleptics may produce a true pharmacogenic depression, but this is likely to be relatively uncommon since depression was frequently reported before the introduction of these drugs. In recent research it has been reported as a prodrome to relapse in patients never prescribed drugs and also occurs as frequently in placebo-treated patients as those on active drugs in double-blind trials. It should also be noted that postpsychotic depression resolves on continuing medication.

A number of authors have identified "akinetic depression" which is a drug-induced neurological or psychological syndrome of extrapyramidal origin which responds rapidly to a challenge test with anticholinergic drugs.

Depression as a symptom of schizophrenia

The frequency of depressive symptoms and their presence in all phases of illness; the recognition of the "revealed depression" syndrome and the observation that it responds to continuing neuroleptic treatment; the report that new depressive symptoms in stable patients is related to relapse and natural history; the discovery that non-specific affective symptoms precede acute relapse often enough to be helpful in determining treatment must all suggest that at least some depression is part of the schizophrenic disorder.

Schizoaffective disorder

At the present time there is no consensus on the definition, natural history or prognosis of this condition. It remains a useful research hypothesis, but at the present time it is of unproven clinical value.

Treatment

Since there is no single aetiology there can be no single or "correct" treatment for all depression.

The first response to the development of depressive symptoms should be a full clinical review coupled with increased staff-patient contact and careful monitoring, rather than hastily added new treatments or a change of management. In the absence of any change of treatment or management, a significant proportion of depression resolves without any apparent adverse effect. During the postpsychotic phase (0–6 months) nearly 50% of depression settles within 2 months with the continuing improvement of the patient. However, in 10% of patients depression heralds an impending psychotic relapse. In depression which develops in stable patients who have lived in the community for 12 months or longer, the risk of an impending relapse is higher (over 20%). The association of other non-specific emotional changes coupled with a deterioration of social function again doubles the risk of relapse (30–40%). Although apparent spontaneous resolution is lower in this group than in the postpsychotic phase, some 20–30% have lost all depression within 2 months.

A full clinical review may reveal environmental changes or stress factors. Stress may result in a direct affective response or as a trigger for schizophrenic deterioration which includes affective changes. The presence of physical illness and drugs, both of prescription and abuse (including alcohol), must not be forgotten.

In the presence of schizophrenic deterioration, appropriate physical, social or psychological therapy is prescribed. In the presence of stress, physical illness and drugs without relapse the primary change is again addressed. It is only after these possibilities have been exhausted that other treatments are considered. The therapeutic concern in the long-term treatment of chronic schizophrenia is to minimize the dose and number of drugs prescribed.

The possibility of akinetic depression should be considered. Muscle sensations even in the absence of extrapyramidal symptoms are usually described. A challenge test of i.m. anticholinergic drugs is rapidly effective.

In the presence of long-lasting but mild depressions a change of neuroleptic should be considered. Flupenthixol has antidepressant properties in low doses and has been shown to influence mood in acute psychosis. Agitated or excited patients should not receive this drug but rather clopixol.

Surveys of drug prescriptions to schizophrenic patients reveal that 10–20% are likely to receive tricyclic drugs in any one year. The issues surrounding the prescription of these drugs are complex and the solutions far from clear. Schizophrenic deterioration can occur. Siris [4] has comprehensively reviewed the controlled trials. Research does not currently allow firm recommendations. In our present state of knowledge, antidepressants are probably overprescribed and any prescription should be in the nature of a carefully-monitored therapeutic trial.

Some studies report that recurrent mood disorders are reduced by the introduction of lithium. One view is that prescribing should be symptom-specific rather than syndrome-specific.

The use of ECT may rarely be required in severe or resistant depression. However, there is no evidence of a lasting-effect on the illness.

It should be noted that the lowest prevalence of depression is amongst well-controlled schizophrenic patients living in the community on long-term neuroleptics receiving modest doses. Maintenance therapy should always be a personalized flexible dose regime in which the majority of patients receive substantial reductions in dose, particularly over the 6–36 months after discharge. A proper regard for social and environmental factors must be included in the management programme.

References

1. Roy A et al. (1983) Br. J. Psychiatry 142: 465–470.
2. McGlashan TH (1976) Am. J. Psychiatry 133: 14–19.
3. Knights A and Hirsch SR (1981) Arch. Gen. Psychiatry 38: 806–811.
4. Siris SG (1989) Depression in Schizophrenics. Plenum Press, New York, pp. 215–232.

Biological Psychiatry, Volume 1. G. Racagni et al., editors.

Zuclopenthixol acetate and liquid oral haloperidol in the treatment of schizophrenic patients with acute exacerbation

Guy Chouinard[1,2], Gabriel Safadi[2] and Linda Beauclair[2]
[1]*Psychiatric Research Centre, Louis-H. Lafontaine, Hospital, University of Montreal, Montreal; and* [2]*Clinical Psychopharmacology Unit, Allan Memorial Institute, Montreal, Quebec, Canada*

Introduction

Clopenthixol, a neuroleptic of the thioxanthene group, has been available in Europe for many years. Recently, a preparation with a duration of action of 2 to 3 days, zuclopenthixol acetate in Viscoleo® has become available for clinical trials. To our knowledge, no controlled studies of a double-blind design have been reported for zuclopenthixol acetate. The present paper describes the first double-blind trial of intramuscular zuclopenthixol acetate in patients with acute schizophrenia (DSM III criteria) admitted to the emergency department, and compares its effect with those of liquid oral haloperidol.

Method

Study design

Forty schizophrenic patients satisfying the study criteria were selected for inclusion in the trial immediately after admittance to the emergency department of Louis-H. Lafontaine Hospital. Patients entered the study as they became available, and for each patient the trial was of nine days duration. Twenty patients were randomly assigned to each of 2 drug treatments: zuclopenthixol acetate or oral liquid haloperidol. After treatment with the research drug began, no other psychotropic medications including hypnotics were administered except for an antiparkinsonian drug whenever it was judged necessary.

All patients completed the clinical trial. Treatment groups did not differ with regard to age, sex, weight, height, age at manifestation of first symptoms of schizophrenia, course and duration of the illness (unpaired *t*-test or Fisher's exact test or Pearson's χ^2, as appropriate).

Medications

Zuclopenthixol acetate supplied in 1-ml vials containing 50 mg of zuclopenthixol acetate dissolved in a vegetable oil (Viscoleo®) was given intramuscularly every

3 days, and oral liquid haloperidol (2 mg/ml Haldol® supplied in 100-ml dropper bottles) was given 3 times a day in equally divided doses. To ensure double-blind conditions, patients treated with zuclopenthixol acetate also received identical haloperidol oral liquid-placebo 3 times a day, while those treated with haloperidol received identical zuclopenthixol acetate-placebo injections every 3 days. Initial dosages of zuclopenthixol were 50–150 mg every 3 days (maximum of 150 mg every 3 days), whereas dosage of liquid haloperidol was 10–30 mg 3 times a day (maximum of 60 mg/day).

Results

All 40 patients completed the study and were evaluated for both drug efficacy and safety.

Zuclopenthixol acetate and haloperidol dosages

For zuclopenthixol acetate, 18.9% of the total dose was given as PRN medication, whereas 10.9% of the total dose of liquid oral haloperidol was given as PRN (P = 0.03). Overall, the total mean daily dose was 18.9 mg (range: 9.2–34.4 mg) for haloperidol as compared to a mean dose per 3 days of 117.6 mg (range: 58.3–200 mg) of zuclopenthixol. Therefore, 1 mg of liquid oral haloperidol daily was equivalent to 6.2 mg every 3 days of intramuscular zuclopenthixol acetate.

Concomitant antiparkinsonian medication

Procyclidine, a central anticholinergic medication, was needed for control of parkinsonian reactions by all patients on at least 1 day during the course of the study. No statistically significant differences ($P < 0.05$) were found between the 2 groups for the total mean daily dose per 9 days. However, there was a trend for zuclopenthixol-treated patients to receive less procyclidine than haloperidol-treated patients.

Psychopathology

There was no evidence of statistically significant ($P < 0.05$) differences between the 2 drugs with respect to adjusted final mean BPRS total or factor scores or the CGI severity of illness score. For individual BPRS items, no statistical difference ($P < 0.05$) was found except for hostility ($P = 0.02$), with a better response in the haloperidol group; zuclopenthixol tended ($P < 0.10$) to have a better effect on guilt feelings ($P = 0.07$) and grandiosity ($P = 0.06$). Within treatment groups relative to baseline, most of the variables under investigation demonstrated significant improvement and both drugs seemed equally efficacious. Only in the zuclopenthixol group was there a statistically significant improvement from baseline on emotional withdrawal ($P < 0.01$) and on motor retardation ($P < 0.05$). For both treatment groups, 16 (80%) of the patients were classified by the physician as having moderately or markedly improved under treatment.

Extrapyramidal symptoms

On the Extrapyramidal Symptom Rating Scale (ESRS), no statistically significant differences were found for parkinsonism except for tremors ($P < 0.01$) and hyperkinesia (tremors + akathisia) ($P < 0.01$) which was more important in the zuclopenthixol group. However, both drugs were comparable in terms of other parkinsonian symptoms such as rigidity and akinetic symptoms. Tardive dyskinesia was also rated on the ESRS. There was a statistical trend for zuclopenthixol patients to have higher score on the "other involuntary movements" item (swallowing, irregular respiration, frowning, blinking, grimacing, sighing, etc.) for dyskinetic movements ($P = 0.08$) and on the extremities dyskinetic factor ($P = 0.08$). This would suggest that the drug had a lesser masking effect than haloperidol on dyskinetic movements. It is also possible that, since dyskinetic movements were rated on the ESRS at the end of the injection period, the masking effect of the medication was no longer present.

Sedation

At 3 h post-injection, a significantly higher degree of sedation was seen in the zuclopenthixol group ($P < 0.01$) where 15 (75%) of the 20 patients receiving the drug exhibited some form of sedation as compared to 7 (35%) of the patients in the haloperidol group.

Discussion

The results of this first double-blind study confirm previous reports from open labelled studies that zuclopenthixol acetate is an effective antipsychotic medication. Given every 3 days with supplementary doses as necessary, the drug brought schizophrenic symptoms under control at a rate similar to that of oral liquid haloperidol. Potential benefits from such a medication are its sedative effect, good tolerance at the injection site, rapid elimination in case of an adverse reaction as compared to parenteral neuroleptics of longer duration of action.

Biological Psychiatry, Volume 1. G. Racagni et al., editors.

Zuclopenthixol decanoate vs. haloperidol decanoate: A double-blind comparative study

T. Koskinen[1], B. Wistedt[2] and S. Thelander[3]
[1]*Kuopio Mental Health Centre, Finland;* [2]*Danderyd Hospital; and* [3]*Huddinge Hospital, Sweden*

Introduction

The long-acting depot formulations of zuclopenthixol and haloperidol have been developed for maintenance treatment of chronic psychoses. This study was undertaken to evaluate the clinical efficacy and unwanted effects of zuclopenthixol decanoate and haloperidol decanoate in maintenance treatment of chronic schizophrenic patients.

Materials and Methods

This double-blind, group comparative, multicentre study included patients from outpatient clinics in Finland and Sweden. Patients were randomly allocated to receive either zuclopenthixol decanoate or haloperidol decanoate at 4-week intervals for 9 months.

Outpatients of either sex between 25–60 years of age with the diagnosis "chronic schizophrenia" according to DSM III were selected for possible study entry.

Assessments were made at baseline and after 12, 24 and 36 weeks of treatment. The patients were rated according to the CGI [1] (by psychiatrists as well as nurses), the BPRS [2] and the MADRS [3]. Side-effects were assessed according to the UKU Scale [4] and the Simpson-Angus Scale [5]. A dose of 200 mg zuclopenthixol decanoate was considered to be equivalent to 50 mg haloperidol decanoate. Lorazepam or oxazepam could be given for restlessness and orphenadrine or biperiden for extrapyramidal symptoms.

Results

From the 64 patients entered into the study, 3 patients were withdrawn early and were only assessed at baseline. Statistical analyses were made on the 61 remaining patients. Four patients in the haloperidol group were withdrawn prematurely in period B because of deterioration, and 1 patient in the zuclopenthixol group terminated her life 3 months after entry into the study.

The doses of zuclopenthixol decanoate and haloperidol decanoate at week 36 were 284 mg (range 100–600 mg) and 92 mg (range 38–200 mg), respectively.

Antiparkinson drugs were given to 5 patients throughout the study period (3/34 zuclopenthixol, 2/27 haloperidol). About one-third of both treatment groups received oxazepam at some time during the study.

The results of the global assessment of severity of illness psychiatrists' assessment are shown in Fig. 1. At week 24 the difference between the groups was statistically in favour of zuclopentixol decanoate ($P = 0.02$). Figure 2 shows the BPRS total scores. There were no significant between-group differences. The MADRS total scores were very low throughout the trial period.

The global assessments of side-effects showed that the majority of patients in either group had no or only mild side-effects which had no adverse influence on the patients' functioning. The number of psychic symptoms (UKU Scale) decreased in both groups and there were very few neurological symptoms. The number of autonomic symptoms observed in the zuclopenthixol decanoate group clearly decreased during the study period, contrasting with increases noted in the patients treated with haloperidol decanoate.

Discussion

The results of this study reaffirm the efficacy of depot injections of zuclopenthixol decanoate or haloperidol decanoate in the maintenance treatment of chronic schizophrenia. Four patients receiving haloperidol decanoate deteriorated and had to be withdrawn. It is possible that these patients would have done better if higher doses had been given, or the injections had been given at shorter intervals.

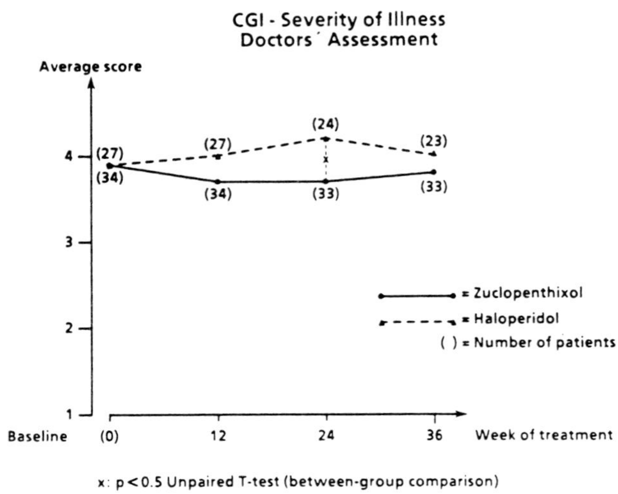

Fig. 1.

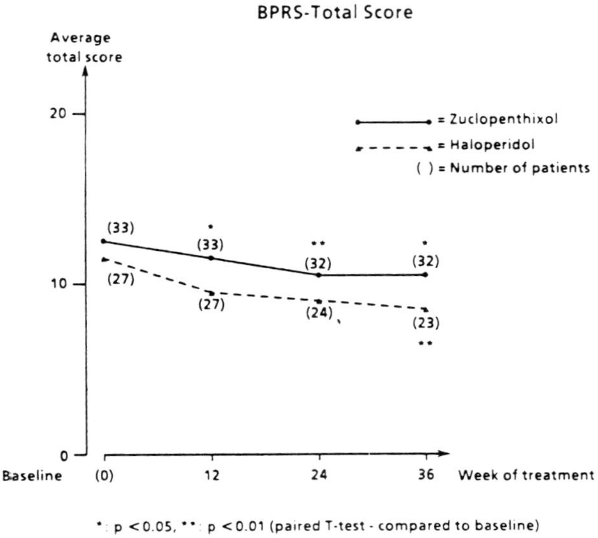

Fig. 2.

As the release half-lives of zuclopenthixol decanoate and haloperidol decanoate are very similar [6], it is not surprising that both depot neuroleptics in most patients may be given at comparable 4-week dosage intervals.

Conclusions

It was concluded that:

1. Zuclopenthixol decanoate and haloperidol decanoate are effective in maintenance treatment of chronic schizophrenia. Only 4 patients relapsed, all were receiving haloperidol.
2. Side-effects are few and usually mild.
3. Zuclopenthixol decanoate and haloperidol decanoate can be given at 4-week injection intervals.

References

1. Guy W (1976) In: Early Clinical Drug Evaluation (ECDEU) Assessment Manual for Psychopharmacology. Natl. Inst. of Mental Health, Publ. No. 76-338.
2. Bech P, Kastrup M and Rafaelsen OJ (1986) Acta Psychiatr. Scand. 73: S326.
3. Montgomery SA and Åsberg M (1979) Br. J. Psychiatry 134: 382–389.
4. Lingjærde O, Ahlfors UG, Bech P, Dencker SJ and Elgen K (1987) Acta Psychiatr. Scand. 76: S334.
5. Simpson GM and Angus JWS (1970) Acta Psychiatr. Scand. 212 (Suppl.): 11–19.
6. Jann MW, Ereshefsky L and Saklad SR (1985) Clin. Pharmacokinet. 10: 315–333.

Biological Psychiatry, Volume 1. G. Racagni et al., editors.

Dopamine modification and atypical neuroleptic properties

David M. Coward[1], Rudolf Markstein[2] and Assunta Imperato[3]
[1]Sandoz Research Institute Berne, P.O.Box, CH-3001 Berne; [2]Preclinical Research, Sandoz Ltd, Basle, Switzerland; and [3]Institute of Pharmacology, University "La Sapienza", Rome

Introduction

Antischizophrenic drugs are considered to owe both their antipsychotic activity and their undesirable propensity to induce extrapyramidal side-effects (EPS) to an ability to reduce central dopaminergic activity [1,2]. Moreover, attempts to move away from this principle have so far resulted in inadequate clinical efficacy. Two approaches have now emerged which might offer the possibility of retaining the principle of reducing dopaminergic tone whilst minimising EPS-liability. In addition, overall response rate and/or the reduction of negative symptoms might be improved in some cases.

Dopamine-based principles

Partial D_2 agonism

Interest in the principle of partial agonism at dopamine D_2 receptors stems from the hypothesis that compounds exhibiting high affinity and low intrinsic activity at the D_2 receptor might act as dopaminergic "buffers", reducing dopaminergic activity when it is excessive, but promoting it when it is reduced [3]. The former situation might be relevant to the reduction of positive symptoms, the latter to an improvement of negative symptoms [3–6]. A further advantage of partial D_2 agonists should be a failure to elevate serum prolactin levels, avoiding e.g. gynocomastia.

The ideal profile of a partial D_2 agonist should include an ability to potently and completely inhibit dopamine agonist-induced stereotypies in animal studies, while at the same time causing little or no catalepsy. In fact, studies with the prototypic agent terguride (trans-dihydrolisuride) confirmed that such a separation is possible and also showed that the compound's intrinsic agonism was reflected in a suppression of prolactin release and the induction of circling in rats with unilateral 6-hydroxydopamine (6-OHDA) lesions of the substantia nigra [7]. Since the limited clinical feedback available on terguride suggested a beneficial effect on negative symptoms, with only little improvement of positive symptomatology [8,9], we attempted to develop a range of partial D_2 agonists with differing degrees of intrinsic activity and, at the same time, greater potency than terguride with regard to apomorphine inhibition. Two ergoline-derived substances emerged from these endeavours – SDZ 208-911 and SDZ 208-912 – and their pharmacological properties have now been reported in detail [10].

In addition to showing high affinity for dopamine D_2 receptors in vitro, these agents are:

- equipotent to haloperidol as inhibitors of apomorphine- or amphetamine-induced stereotypies;
- weakly (208-912) or non-cataleptogenic (208-911);
- potent and selective inhibitors of conditioned avoidance;
- strong inhibitors of prolactin release;
- weak (208-912) or strong (208-911) inducers of contralateral circling behaviour in 6-OHDA-lesioned rats.

Confirmation that the low cataleptogenicity, prolactin suppression and circling induction shown by these agents stems from partial agonistic activity is provided by studies examining their ability to modify the effects of gamma-butyrolactone (GBL) on striatal L-dopa accumulation in the rat. Thus, in contrast to haloperidol, SDZ 208-912 only partially reverses the inhibition of GBL activity produced by apomorphine, whereas SDZ 208-911 itself reverses GBL's effects at low doses and partially reverses apomorphine's action at high doses [10].

D_1 and D_2 receptor blockade

While early studies suggested a primary role for D_2 receptor blockade in relation to the antipsychotic activity of both classical and non-classical neuroleptics [1], there has been a re-kindling of interest in the possible contribution of D_1 receptor blockade. This is attributable to the fact that compounds exhibiting selective D_1 blockade show preclinical profiles very similar to those of D_2 antagonists and, more interestingly, indications that some of the superior antischizophrenic activity of clozapine might stem from its concomitant blockade of both D_1 and D_2 receptors [11]. Thus, this atypical neuroleptic is known to be effective in a substantial proportion of otherwise therapy-resistant subjects and, as also shown in this population, to bring about a better improvement of negative symptoms that occurs with conventional drugs [12].

Indications from in vitro binding studies that this agent might show preferential affinity for D_1 as opposed to D_2 receptors [11] have now been extended and confirmed by in vivo investigations. For example, studies employing trans-striatal dialysis in the conscious rat indicate that low doses of clozapine cause selective blockade of D_1 receptors, whereas higher doses result in concomitant blockade of both receptor subtypes [11,13]. Following-up on these findings, Waddington and colleagues have now provided evidence for the expression of a similar phenom enon at the behavioural level [14]. The question as to whether similar effects occur in man is still open, but is being addressed by PET-scan studies examining the degree of D_1 and D_2 receptor occupancy to be found in the caudate nucleus of schizophrenics responding to various neuroleptics. The evidence available to date suggests that clozapine may be more active at D_2 than D_1 receptors in man, but that the D_2 occupancy is lower and the D_1 occupancy appreciably higher than that seen with classical neuroleptics [15].

Since there are good reasons for hypothesising that moderate, concomitant blockade of both D_1 and D_2 receptors might be relevant to both neurological side-effect liability and superior clinical efficacy [11], it would be worthwhile searching for new agents with similar properties.

D_1 blockade and partial D_2 agonism

In searching for a partial D_2 agonist exhibiting intrinsic activity intermediate between that of SDZ 208-911 and SDZ 208-912, a compound has been identified which may combine the attributes of partial D_2 agonism and moderate D_1 blockade. SDZ 212-327 ((−)-N-[(5R, 8S, 10R)-2-methyl-ergoline-8-yl]-2-ethyly-2-methyl-butanamide) is an ergoline showing high affinity for the spiperone-labelled D_2 receptor (pKi = 8.5) and moderate affinity for the SCH 23390-labelled D_1 receptor (pKi = 7.6). Studies in the rat show this agent to be equipotent to haloperidol as an apomorphine antagonist, but virtually non-cataleptogenic. Moreover, its agonistic activity in the 6-OHDA-lesioned rat is intermediate between that of SDZ 208-911 and SDZ 208-912, although its prolactin-suppressing action is weaker than both of these agents. Evidence for in vivo blockade of D_1 receptors by low doses of this compound stems from the finding that it shows a "dialysis profile" virtually identical to that of clozapine, the compound's normal elevation of striatal dopamine recovery in this test procedure being reduced in animals pretreated with the D_1 agonist CY 208-243.

Conclusions

There are good reasons for believing that partial D_2 agonism might be a viable principle for achieving broad-spectrum antischizophrenic activity in the absence of strong EPS and that concomitant D_1 and D_2 blockade contributes to the superior clinical qualities of clozapine. Clinical testing of the ergolines described in this report is expected to throw considerable light on both of these issues.

References

1. Creese I, Burt DR and Snyder SH (1976) Science 192: 481–483.
2. Tarsy D and Baldessarini RJ (1977) Biol. Psychiatry 12: 431–459.
3. Coward DM, Dixon K, Enz A, Shearman G, Urwyler S, White TG and Karobath M (1989) Psychopharmacol. Bull. 25: 393–397.
4. Gerlach J and Luehdorf K (1975) Psychopharmacologia 44: 105–110.
5. Angrist B, Peselow E, Rubinstein M, Corwin J and Rotrosen J (1982) Psychopharmacology 78: 128–130.

6. Van Kammen DP, Bunney WE, Docherty JP, Marder SR, Ebert MH, Rosenblatt JE and Rayner JN (1982) Am. J. Psychiatry 139: 991–997.
7. Wachtel H and Dorow R (1983) Life Sci. 32: 421–432.
8. Schanz H, Olbrich R and Aufdembrinke B (1988) Psychopharmacology 96: 239.
9. Filip V, Alda M, Filipova M, Hynek K and Posmurova M (1985) Abstracts, IVth World Congress of Biological Psychiatry, Philadelphia, p. 301.
10. Coward DM, Dixon K, Urwyler S, White G, Enz A, Karobath M and Shearman G (1989) J. Pharmacol. Exp. Ther. 252: 279–285.
11. Coward DM, Imperato A, Urwyler S and White TG (1989) Psychopharmacology 99: S6–S12.
12. Kane J, Honigfeld G, Singer J and Meltzer HY (1988) Arch. Gen. Psychiatry 45: 789–796.
13. Imperato A and Angelucci L (1988) Psychopharmacology 96: 79.
14. Murray AM and Waddington JL (1990) Eur. J. Pharmacol. 186: 79–86.
15. Farde L, Wiesel F-A, Nordstrom A-L and Sedvall G (1989) Psychopharmacology 99: S28–S31.

Biological Psychiatry, Volume 1. G. Racagni et al., editors.

$5\text{-}HT_2$, $5\text{-}HT_{1C}$ and DA_2 receptors in the action of clozapine and other atypical antipsychotic drugs

Herbert Y. Meltzer and Craig A. Stockmeier
Department of Psychiatry, Case Western Reserve University, Cleveland, OH 44106, U.S.A.

Introduction

Clozapine differs from typical antipsychotic drugs in being a more effective antipsychotic drug for both positive and negative symptoms in treatment-resistant schizophrenic patients [1]. Clozapine also produces fewer extrapyramidal symptoms and is not associated with tardive dyskinesia [2]. Understanding its mechanism of action is critical to developing more effective and safer antipsychotic drugs and may also provide insight into the etiology of schizophrenia.

There are numerous suggestions concerning the neuropharmacological basis of the action of clozapine which we have reviewed elsewhere [3,4]. This article will consider only the evidence for the role of serotonin (5-HT) and dopamine (DA) in the etiology of schizophrenia.

$5\text{-}HT_2$ antagonism

Clozapine has been shown to antagonize many effects of 5-HT including the plasma corticosterone and prolactin responses to MK-212, a $5\text{-}HT_2/5\text{-}HT_{1C}$ antagonist [5]. In man, clozapine also blocks the cortisol response to MK-212 [6]. Clozapine also downregulates $5\text{-}HT_2$ receptors in rat frontal cortex after a single dose [7]. $5\text{-}HT_2$ antagonism may be relevant because $5\text{-}HT_2$ receptors are abundant in the frontal cortex and are important to the action of hallucinogenic drugs [4]. It is of interest that $5\text{-}HT_2$ receptors are already decreased in density in the frontal cortex of deceased schizophrenics [8,9].

$5\text{-}HT_2/DA_2$ ratio: In vitro

The evidence that $5\text{-}HT_2$ antagonism is relevant to the action of atypical antipsychotic drugs comes from comparison of typical and atypical antipsychotic drugs [10,11]. Although the mean $5\text{-}HT_2$ affinities of 20 typical and 17 putative atypical antipsychotic drugs do not differ, the ratio and the affinities of the atypical antipsychotic drugs for $5\text{-}HT_2$ receptors compared to DA_2 receptors are highly significantly different [11]. Expressed as pK_i values (negative log of the k_i, the

$5\text{-}HT_2/DA_2$ pK_i values for the atypical drugs are significantly greater than for the typical drugs). Only loxapine, amoxapine and HP-370 have high ratios that would be more characteristic of atypical drugs [11]. It should be noted that it is the relative difference between $5\text{-}HT_2$ and DA_2 affinities of the two classes of drugs that is important. Some typical drugs are strong $5\text{-}HT_2$ antagonists but even stronger DA_2 antagonists, e.g., spiperone. These results suggest that in vivo atypical antipsychotic drugs produce relatively more occupancy of cortical $5\text{-}HT_2$ than DA_2 limbic or striatal DA_2 receptors.

$5\text{-}HT_2/DA_2$ ratio in vivo

We have determined in vivo binding of cortical $5\text{-}HT_2$, olfactory tubercle (limbic) and striatal DA_2 receptor occupancy following acute administration of typical and atypical antipsychotic drugs follow i.v. administration of ^3H-N-methyl-spiperone as ligand [12]. Table 1 provides the ED_{50} (negative log of the i.p. dose which produces 50% occupancy) of the striatal and olfactory tubercle (OT) DA_2 and cortical $5\text{-}HT_2$ binding sites.

The typical antipsychotic drugs have higher pED_{50} values for the OT and striatal DA_2 sites than the atypical antipsychotics but the two classes do not differ in pED_{50}

Table 1. pED_{50} of typical and atypical antipsychotic drugs for cortical $5\text{-}HT_2$ and striatal and olfactory tubercle DA_2 binding sites

Drugs	pED_{50}			$5\text{-}HT_2/DA_2$ ratio	
	Cortex	Striatum	OT	Striatum	OT
Typical					
Chlorpromazine	6.1	5.4	5.6	1.11	1.09
Fluphenazine	6.0	6.4	6.3	0.93	0.95
Haloperidol	5.4	6.5	6.4	0.84	0.84
Loxapine	7.1	7.8	6.7	1.03	1.06
Raclopride	4.3	5.2	5.2	0.82	0.83
Thioridazine	4.8	4.5	4.4	1.06	1.09
	5.6 ± 1.0	5.8 ± 0.89	5.8 ± 0.88	0.97 ± 0.12	0.98 ± 0.12
Atypical					
Amperozide	5.6	4.0	4.0	1.40	1.40
Clozapine	5.7	4.3	4.8	1.32	1.19
Fluperlapine	5.8	4.1	4.4	1.41	1.32
Melperone	5.2	4.9	5.0	1.06	1.04
Tiospirone	6.5	5.9	6.1	1.10	1.07
HP-370	5.7	4.3	4.2	1.33	1.36
Risperidone	6.7	6.1	6.1	1.10	1.10
	5.9 ± 0.49[b]	4.8 ± 0.81[a]	4.9 ± 0.80[a]	1.25 ± 0.14[a]	1.21 ± 0.14[a]

[a] $P < 0.05$ vs. typical antipsychotic drug; [b] S.D.

values for 5-HT_2 receptors. The in vivo ratios of the 5-HT_2/DA_2 (striatal) and 5-HT_2/DA_2 (OT) for the atypical antipsychotics were significantly greater than those of the typical drugs. These results confirm the previously reported in vitro data [11]. The in vivo data further illuminates some of the apparent discrepancies in the in vitro data. HP-370, which had a low 5-HT_2 ratio in vitro [11], has a high ratio in vivo. Loxapine, in vivo, has approximately equal ability to occupy 5-HT_2 and DA_2 receptors, whereas it was more potent at 5-HT_2 in vitro. Melperone and tiospirone, both of which are less effective than clozapine, have the lowest 5-HT_2/DA_2 pED_{50} ratios of any atypicals. HP-370, fluperlapine and amperozide, in this regard, have higher in vivo 5-HT_2/DA_2 ratios than clozapine. Clozapine appears more active in the OT than at striatal DA_2 receptors, which may contribute to its low EPS. These results suggest that in vivo binding may complement in vitro studies to identify candidate atypical antipsychotic drugs. Further studies of in vivo occupancy after chronic administration of atypical and typical antipsychotic drugs may be even more illuminating.

Conclusions

Atypical antipsychotic drugs may be distinguished from typical antipsychotic drugs by virtue of their relatively stronger 5-HT_2 than DA_2 receptor affinities in vitro and greater occupancy of 5-HT_2 receptors in vivo. This may be relevant to their clinical profile through 5-HT_2-mediated modulation of dopaminergic activity. Clozapine produces less interference with the availability action of DA in the limbic system [13], perhaps because of its 5-HT_2 antagonism.

Acknowledgements

The research reported was supported in part by USPHS MH 41684, GCRC MO1RR00080, the Department of Veterans Affairs and a grant from the Cleveland Foundation. H.Y.M. is the recipient of a USPHS Research Career Scientist Award MH 47808. The secretarial assistance of Ms. Lee Mason is appreciated.

References

1. Kane J, Honigfeld G, Singer J, Meltzer HY et al. (1988) Arch. Gen. Psychiatry 45: 789–796.
2. Casey DE (1989) Psychopharmacology 99S: S47–S53.
3. Meltzer HY (1989) Psychopharmacology 99S: S18–S27.
4. Meltzer HY (1990) In: Kales A, Stefanos GN and Talbott JA (eds.) Recent Advances in Schizophrenia. Springer-Verlag, Heidelberg, pp. 237–246.
5. Nash JF, Meltzer HY and Gudelsky GA (1988) Eur. J. Pharmacol. 151: 463–469.
6. Meltzer HY (1988) In: Schulz C and Tamminga C (eds.) Schizophrenia: A Scientific Focus, Int. Conf. on Schizophrenia. Oxford Press, New York, pp. 302–309.

7. Matsubara S and Meltzer HY (1989) Life Sci. 45: 1397–1406.
8. Mita T, Hanada S, Nishino N, Kuno T, Nakai, Yamadori T, Mizoi Y and Tanaka C (1986) Biol. Psychiatry 21: 1407–1414.
9. Matsubara S, Arora RC and Meltzer HY (1991) J. Neural Transm. (in press).
10. Altar CA, Wasley AM, Neale FF and Stone CA (1986) Brain Res. Bull. 16: 577–525.
11. Meltzer HY, Matsubara S and Lee J-C (1989) J. Pharmacol. Exp. Ther. 251: 238–246.
12. Frost JJ, Smith AC, Kuhar MJ, Dannals RF and Wagner HN (1987) Life Sci. 40: 987–995.
13. Ichikawa J and Meltzer HY (1990) Eur. J. Pharmacol. 176: 371–374.

Biological Psychiatry, Volume 1. G. Racagni et al., editors.

Can the unique effect of clozapine on the functioning of midbrain dopamine neurons explain any of its special clinical properties?

B.S. Bunney

Department of Psychiatry and Pharmacology, Yale University School of Medicine, New Haven, CT 06510, U.S.A.

Introduction

Clozapine's lack of many neurological side-effects, ability to treat negative symptoms and ability to produce significant improvement in one-third of psychotic patients unresponsive to other medications, clearly gives it highly desirable properties that classical antipsychotic drugs (ADs) lack [1]. How does clozapine act in the brain to produce its unique clinical profile? The answer is not yet known, but a great deal of information is now available about the chronic effects of clozapine on brain functioning. The following is a review of one small set of that data and is focused exclusively on clozapine's effects on the electrophysiological activity of midbrain dopaminergic (DA) neurons.

Materials and Methods

In these studies, extracellular single unit recording from chloral hydrate anesthetized or gallamine paralyzed rats was used to determine the number of spontaneously firing DA neurons in the zona compacta of the substantia nigra (A_9) and ventral tegmental area (A_{10}) in control animals and animals treated for 21 days with ADs [2–4]. A variety of ADs and control drugs were tested. All of the typical ADs produced similar results; therefore only the effects of haloperidol will be described. Haloperidol, whether administered 0.5 mg/kg/day s.c. or in the drinking water, produced the same effects. Clozapine was administered orally in doses of either 24.0 mg/kg/day or 10.0 mg/kg/day. There was no difference in the results obtained from the two doses. Spontaneously firing cells were counted in stereotaxically defined blocks of tissues in the A_9 and A_{10} areas by passing electrodes through them 12 times in a preset pattern, kept constant from animal to animal. The results are, therefore, expressed as number of cells per track.

Results

In both A_9 and A_{10} areas there were approximately 0.8 spontaneously active cells per track in non-treated animals and animals treated acutely or chronically with comparison control drugs. These included d-sulperide (the inactive isomer of sulperide), promethazine (a phenothiazine and close structural analog of chlorpromazine which lacks both antipsychotic efficacy and neurological side-effects) and the vehicles in which haloperidol and clozapine were dissolved [4]. Acute administration of both haloperidol and clozapine increased the number of spontaneously active cells in both the A_9 and A_{10} regions. Repeated treatment with haloperidol markedly decreased the number of spontaneously active cells in both areas (0.08 cells per track). Clozapine, on the other hand, although having an identical effect to that of haloperidol on A_{10} DA neurons, produced no diminution in the number of spontaneously active DA cells in the A_9 area compared to that found after acute administration. Intra- and extracellular studies of identified DA neurons have demonstrated that those DA cells inactive after chronic treatment with haloperidol and clozapine are inactive because they are in a state of depolarization block (DPB) [3–5].

Discussion

Can the difference between the effects of repeated clozapine and haloperidol treatment on the functioning of A_9 and A_{10} neurons explain their different clinical profiles in terms of the possession or lack of Parkinson-like side-effects and tardive dyskinesia? Autopsy studies of the brains of Parkinson patients and animal studies of postsynaptic DA receptor blockade both suggest that a 80–90% depletion of DA or blockade of receptor is required before any behavioral effects are observed. Extrapolating from these findings, one can hypothesize that an equally effective blockade of DA receptors is necessary before one can observe the therapeutic and neurological side-effects of ADs. If one could demonstrate that there is a difference in postsynaptic DA receptor blockade depending upon whether DA cells are in a state of DPB or not, one would have a possible explanation for the difference in neurological side-effect profiles between haloperidol and clozapine. On a theoretical basis, such a difference can be proposed. Since ADs are competitive DA receptor blockers, the increased release of DA demonstrated to occur after acute administration of either clozapine or haloperidol [6] might prevent effective postsynaptic receptor blockade by these agents. However, if over time something were to occur that would decrease DA release while AD administration continued, postsynaptic blockade might become more and more effective. A variety of studies now suggest that the induction of DPB on midbrain DA cells over a three-week period of repeated treatment with ADs may be such an event. However, since clozapine does not produce DPB block in the A_9 system, synaptic DA levels would not be expected to diminish in the striatum, and consequently effective blockade should not occur.

In summary, the inability of clozapine to produce DPB block in A_9 DA neurons is one possible explanation for its lack of Parkinson-like side-effects and tardive dyskinesia. This hypothesis should be testable by carrying out carefully designed positron emission tomography experiments in patients naive to ADs who are studied after acute treatment and then studied once more when maximum side-effects and/or therapeutic effects have been obtained. Such studies should be able to determine whether or not D_2 receptor occupancy changes with repeated administration of these agents.

Acknowledgements

This work was supported by U.S. PHS Grants, MH28849, MH25642 and the Abraham Ribicoff research facilities of the state of Connecticut.

References

1. Kane JM, Honigfeld G, Singer J, Meltzer H and the Clozaril Collaborative Study Group (1988) Arch. Gen. Psychiatry 45: 789–796.
2. Bunney BS, Walters JR, Roth RH and Aghajanian G (1973) J. Pharmacol. Exp. Ther. 185: 560–571.
3. Bunney BS and Grace AA (1978) Life Sci. 23: 1715–1728.
4. Chiodo LA and Bunney BS (1983) Neuroscience 3: 1607–1619.
5. Grace AA and Bunney BS (1986) J. Pharmacol. Exp. Term. 238: 1092–1100.
6. Moghaddam B and Bunney BS (1990) J. Neurochem. 54: 1755–1760.

Biological Psychiatry, Volume 1. G. Racagni et al., editors.

Amperozide, a putative antipsychotic drug with atypical properties

Erik Christensson

Department of CNS-Research, Kabi Pharmacia Therapeutics AB, P.O. Box 839, S-201 80 Malmö, Sweden

Chemically amperozide (FG5606) is related to several potentially psychotropic agents by its diphenylpiperazine moiety but differs in containing an 1-piperazine-carboxamide moiety. From a pharmacological point of view amperozide differs strongly from classical neuroleptics by lacking a high affinity for dopamine receptor binding sites and by its outstanding limbic mode of action. Yet it has similarities to some atypical neuroleptics in that it demonstrates a high affinity for 5-HT_2 receptor binding sites in brain.

The limbic selectivity of amperozide is obvious if its effect in a number of biochemical tests is compared with that of haloperidol [1]. In receptor binding studies carried out in vitro, amperozide was found to be a selective 5-HT_2 receptor blocker [2]. Its 5-HT_2 receptor blocking potency has been confirmed in behavioural tests by studying its effects on 5-HTP-induced head twitch behaviour [3], by its ability to block 5-HT-induced contractions in rat tail artery [4] and by its ability to antagonize inositol-1-phosphate formation in brain [2]. Also biochemical [5] and electrophysiological [6] studies confirm a limbic mode of action. The modification of the dopamine neuron activity in the midbrain seemed to be confined to the DA neurones of the ventral tegmental area (VTA) in 2 ways: 1) increasing firing rate and burst firing, i.e. an excitation; or 2) regularization of the firing pattern [6]. In unilaterally 6-OHDA lesioned animals amperozide antagonized only pergolide-induced turning behaviour while having a dualistic effect on apomorphine-induced turning behaviour, demonstrating both antagonistic and agonist potentiating effects [7]. Presynaptically amperozide interacted with the ability of amphetamine to induce turning behaviour in 6-OHDA lesioned rats [7] and by antagonizing amphetamine-induced locomotion [8]. In vitro tests showed that amperozide has the ability to interact with the DA carrier [9,10] and antagonizes the effect of amphetamine [9]. The antagonism of ketamine noticed in behavioural tests [11] and of glutamate-induced release of DA [12] suggests that amperozide also interacts with the presynaptic effects of glutamate. Like pimozide and other diphenyl derivates amperozide is characterized by a potent blocking effect of 5-HT reuptake but also to some extent of DA and NA [10].

The carboxamide moiety of amperozide on the other hand seems to be important for its interaction with the functional response in some receptor complexes. Obvious is its antagonistic effect on the α_2-adrenergic receptor message without having any affinity for the clonidine binding sites. The α_2-antagonistic effects of amperozide were noticed early during the documentation of the drug as a veterinary medical product for treating stress and maladaptation in pigs. The effect was observed by studying the antagonism of clonidine-induced motility in rat pups and by its effect of antagonizing the clonidine-induced flexor reflex in spinalectomized rats. But the effect was at that time difficult to explain, as amperozide had no affinity for the clonidine binding sites. Its interaction with the α_2-adrenergic receptor complex was obvious when comparing the effect of amperozide with that of cyproheptadine in wasting pigs suffering severely from chronic stress due to maladaptation. Cyproheptadine, which impairs the release of insulin, drastically increased the mortality in such pigs within 12 h after a dose of 1 mg/kg while amperozide decreased the mortality when given at a dose of 1 mg/kg. Preliminary studies of the ATP, UTP, CTP and GTP contents of cerebral cortex in brain from rats suggest that amperozide below 1 mg/kg had no significant effect on the levels, while 5 mg/kg significantly increased the levels after 1–2 h. In some cases a significant increase was also noticed after treatment with 1 mg/kg. Also the levels of NAD seemed to be increased. Apart from that, preliminary studies on the uptake of glucose in brain by the Sokoloff technique have given indications that a low dose of 0.5 mg/kg i.v. decreased the uptake while 5 mg/kg increased the uptake of glucose in most brain areas. All results are unanimous that amperozide has a strong influence on the adrenergic neuro-transmission in brain. Already a very low dose increases the firing of locus coeruleus [13], antagonizes the suppressive effects of clonidine on HA turnover [14] and increases the disappearance of HA in brain of α-MPT pre-treated animals [5,7]. At higher doses some affinity to α_1-receptor binding sites counteracts some of the noradrenergic effects, but the antagonism of the α_2-adrenergic message is obvious at all doses. The probability of increased release of insulin being induced by amperozide may be of importance in discussing an observed increase in the synthetic activity of DA and HA [5], as it has been reported that insulin activated the THase enzyme. The weak affinity by amperozide for the clonidine receptor binding sites in spite of a strong α_2-adrenergic property, suggest that the effect is due to an interaction with the transduction of the message from the receptor complex, as has been reported earlier for sulfonlyurea derivates and glibenclamide-like compounds. However, its interaction with other receptor complexes as well as its antiarrhythmic type III effect suggest blockade also of types of K^+ channels other than those associated to the α_2-adrenergic receptor complex. The occurrence of α_2 antagonistic and 5-HT_2 antagonistic properties in combination with the absence of DA receptor blocking potency point very strongly towards a drug with less anhedonic effects than earlier antipsychotics and without extrapyramidal side-effects. Amperozide has in ongoing clinical open phase 11 studies shown promising effects on both type 1 and type 2 schizophrenic symptoms [15,16].

References

1. Christensson E and Björk A (1990) Pharmacol. Toxicol. (Suppl. I): 5–7.
2. Svartengren J and Simonsson P (1990) Pharmacol. Toxicol. (Suppl. I): 8–11.

3. Gustafsson B and Christensson E (1990) Pharmacol. Toxicol. (Suppl. I): 34–39.
4. Christensson E (1991) (to be published).
5. Pettersson G, Johanessen K, Hulthe P and Engel JA (1990) Pharmacol. Toxicol. (Suppl. I): 40–44.
6. Grenhoff J, Tung Che-Se, Ugedo L and Svensson TH (1990) Pharmacol. Toxicol. (Suppl. I): 29–33.
7. Christensson E (1990) Pharmacol. Toxicol. (Suppl. I): 22–28.
8. Gustafsson B and Christensson E (1990) Pharmacol. Toxicol. (Suppl. I): 12–17.
9. Eriksson E and Christensson E (1990) Pharmacol. Toxicol. (Suppl. I): 45–48.
10. Eriksson E (1990) Life Sci. 47: 2111–2117.
11. Christensson E (1991) ACNP Meeting USA Satellite Symp., San Juan 1990.
12. Eriksson E (1991) (to be published).
13. Haskins JT, Muth BA and Andree TH (1987) Brain Res. Bull. 19: 465–471.
14. Waters N, Pettersson G, Carlsson A and Svensson K (1989) Naunyn-Schmideberg's Arch. Pharmacol. 340: 161–169.
15. Axelsson R, Nilsson A, Christensson E and Bergman I (1989) ECNP Abstr. 96.
16. Mertens C, DeWilde J, Dierick M, Bergman I and Gustavsson G (1989) In: CN Stefanis, CR Soldatos and AD Rabavilas (eds.) Excerpta Medica, Int. Congr. Series 899, p. 502.

Biological Psychiatry, Volume 1. G. Racagni et al., editors.

CSF peptides and long-term neuroleptic treatment in schizophrenia: Effects of haloperidol withdrawal and relapse

D.P. van Kammen, J.L. Peters, D.T. O'Connor, J. Gelernter, R. Ekman, E. Widerlöv, A. Guidotti, J. Perel, M.E. Kelley, M. Beuger and J. Gurklis
Highland Drive, VAMC, Pittsburgh, PA 15206 U.S.A.; and WPIC, University of Pittsburgh, Pennsilvania, U.S.A.

Introduction

The study of neuropeptides in the CSF is potentially of interest in schizophrenia, as they modulate monoamine transmission hypothesized to be involved in schizophrenia. We measured CSF neuropeptide Y (NPY-IR) [1], because NPY is coreleased with somatostatin, GABA and norepinephrine (NE), which we had found to be increased in drug-free relapsed patients [2,3]. Similarly, we measured: a) δ-sleep-inducing-peptide (DSIP), because of the reported decrease in δ sleep in schizophrenia [4]; b) diazepam-binding-inhibitor (DBI) (an endogenous allosteric ligand for the τ-aminobutyric $acid_A$ ($GABA_A$) receptor complex [5]), because of the proposed therapeutic effects of benzodiazepines and the potential relationship between GABA and schizophrenia; and c) CSF chromogranin A (CgA), because it is a secretory protein marker of the diffuse endocrine system while it is coreleased with monoamines [6].

Methods

Subjects: Fifty-three male chronic schizophrenic patients (DSM III-R) (age: 34.3 ± 7.2 years, range 20–50 years) participated in 2 lumbar punctures after informed consent, during chronic haloperidol treatment and following blind withdrawal on placebo for up to 6 weeks. Doses of haloperidol ranged from 2–40 mg/day (20.3 ± 17.9 mg/day). Psychosis severity was rated daily by the blind nursing staff [7]. Patients were considered to have relapsed if the 3 day psychosis ratings increased 3 points compared to the 7 day mean of these ratings prior to haloperidol withdrawal. Twenty-two patients met relapse criteria before the sixth week and 31 patients were considered to be clinically stable, having not shown signs of relapse before the end of the sixth week. NPY-IR (n = 31), DSIP-IR (n = 41), DBI-IR (n = 53) and CgA-IR (n = 33) were measured with a double antibody radioimmune assay (RIA) according to previously reported methodology [1,8–10]. We used paired T and Student's *t*-tests to examine the effect of withdrawal on the relapsers, non-relapsers and the total groups, because not all peptides were measured in all patients.

Results

As shown in Table 1, CSF NPY-IR, DBI-IR and CgA-IR increased significantly following haloperidol withdrawal, while CSF DSIP-IR did not increase significantly. In the relapsers only CSF DSIP-IR increased significantly (n = 21); the other 3 peptides did not increase significantly. In the non-relapsers, CSF NPY-IR (n = 18), DBI-IR (n = 31) and CgA-IR (n = 19) increased significantly, while CSF DSIP-IR (n = 20) did not change.

Discussion

Following withdrawal from haloperidol treatment CSF NPY-IR, DBI-IR and CgA-IR increased. Chronic dopamine receptor blockade may have led to decreases in CSF NPY-IR, CgA-IR, DBI-IR and DSIP-IR in our patients. We propose that the observed changes in the non-relapsers reflect a direct effect of the disappearance of DA receptor blockade, thus stable non-relapsers should be compared with normal controls. Changes associated with relapse could not be explained by the shorter duration of the drug-free time prior to the LP, therefore, they may have

Table 1.

		Total group		t	*P*
		Haloperidol	Drug-free		
NPY-IR	n = 31	139 ± 23.1	152 ± 25.6	−3.43	0.002
DSIP-IR	n = 41	374.8 ± 92.3	386.4 ± 88.4	−1.07	N.S.
DBI-IR	n = 53	0.83 ± 0.20	0.90 ± 0.24	−3.08	0.003
CgA-IR	n = 33	43.2 ± 21.1	53.4 ± 26.4	−2.29	0.029
		Relapsers		t	*P*
		Haloperidol	Drug-free		
NPY-IR	n = 13	143 ± 25.7	149 ± 24.9	−1.03	N.S.
DSIP-IR	n = 21	352.7 ± 66.2	380.3 ± 80.7	−2.54	0.02
DBI-IR	n = 22	0.79 ± 0.18	0.84 ± 0.26	−1.30	N.S.
CgA-IR	n = 14	41.2 ± 13.0	44.2 ± 15.8	−1.32	N.S.
		Non-relapsers		t	*P*
		Haloperidol	Drug-free		
NPY-IR	n = 18	135 ± 22.0	152 ± 24.9	−3.39	0.003
DSIP-IR	n = 20	398.1 ± 110.6	392.8 ± 97.5	0.28	N.S.
DBI-IR	n = 31	0.87 ± 0.21	0.95 ± 0.22	−3.01	0.005
CgA-IR	n = 19	45.3 ± 25.8	61.8 ± 29.7	−2.28	0.035

been mediated by the relapse process itself, either directly or as an epiphenomenon. Because none of these peptides correlated with psychosis ratings, we concluded that these peptides did not cause the psychotic decompensation, but could still be involved in the pathophysiology of schizophrenia. Because of the lack of change in DSIP-IR following haloperidol withdrawal in the clinically stable patients we propose that this peptide is less likely to have a primary involvement in schizophrenia. The difference in changes in the relapsers could be explained as being secondary to the biochemical changes associated with relapse. Relapsers differ mostly in schizophrenic symptoms from non-relapsers [2,3]. Peters et al. [3] found CSF NPY-IR to be decreased in chronic schizophrenic patients, to correlate significantly with CT scan measures and to be related to schizophrenic symptoms in relapsers and clinically stable patients. CSF DBI-IR and CgA-IR also relate to schizophrenic symptomatology, suggesting that further studies are needed to tell us more about their role in schizophrenic pathophysiology. CgA-IR is also involved in the immune system and could be a marker of an altered immune system in schizophrenia.

Acknowledgements

The authors are grateful to the patients and the nursing staff under Ms. D. McAdam, RM of the Schizophrenia Research Unit for their collaboration and cooperation.

References

1. Peters J, van Kammen DP, Gelernter J, Yao J and Shaw D (1990) Schizophr. Res. 3: 287–294.
2. van Kammen DP, Peters J, van Kammen WB, Nugent A, Goetz KL, Yao J and Linnoila M (1989) Biol. Psychiatry 26: 176–188.
3. van Kammen DP, Peters J, Yao J, van Kammen WB, Neylan T, Shaw D and Linnoila M (1990) Arch. Gen. Psychiatry 47: 161–168.
4. Feinberg I, Braun M, Koresko RL and Gottlieb F (1969) Arch. Gen. Psychiatry 21: 414–420.
5. Guidotti A, Forchetti CM, Corda MG, Konkel D, Bennett CD and Costa E (1983) Proc. Natl. Acad. Sci. U.S.A. 80: 3531–3535.
6. O'Connor DT and Frigon RP (1984) J. Biol. Chem. 259: 3237–3247.
7. Bunney WE Jr and Hamburg DA (1963) Arch. Gen. Psychiatry 9: 280–294.
8. van Kammen DP, Peters J, Yao J, Neylan T, Pontius E and O'Connor DT (1991) Haloperidol withdrawal increases CSF chromogranin A-like immunoreactivity (CgA-LI) in schizophrenic patients. Schizophr. Res. (in press).
9. van Kammen DP, Widerlöv E, Neylan T, Ekman R, Kelley ME, Mouton A and Peters JL (1991) Delta sleep-inducing-peptide-like immunoreactivity (DSIPLI) and delta sleep in schizophrenic volunteers (submitted).
10. van Kammen DP, Guidotti A, Kelley M, Gurklis J, Gilbertson M, Yao J, Peters J and Costa E (1991) Diazepam-binding inhibitor and schizophrenia: clinical and biochemical relationships on and off haloperidol (in preparation).

Biological Psychiatry, Volume 1. G. Racagni et al., editors.

Depressive symptoms in chronic schizophrenia: Clinical and pharmacological variables

Carlo A. Altamura, Massimo C. Mauri and Patrizia Leva
Department of Clinical Psychiatry, University of Milan, Policlinico-Guardia II, Via F. Sforza 35, 20122 Milan, Italy

Introduction

Schizophrenic patients have been reported to demonstrate a high prevalence of depressive symptoms and syndromes (25–80%) at various times and contexts during their illness [1].

Depression has been sustained to coexist with schizophrenia as an integral part of schizophrenic illness, commonly present during the acute phase when the florid psychosis is most evident and only noticed after the psychotic symptoms have been removed by treatment (*revealed depression*) [2,3].

The concept of *pharmacogenic depression* assumes that depressive symptoms may be induced by neuroleptic medication and "akinetic depression" may be considered a variation of the same concept [2,4].

The concept of *post psychotic depression* (PPD) refers to the possibility that depression may occur as a reaction to being ill as insight returns during the recovery from psychosis in some patients [5]. On the other hand, a clear overlap between PPD and negative symptoms, has been found [6].

A proportion of the schizophrenic patients have depressive symptoms that correspond to criteria for a diagnosis of depression in its own right, including endogenous features in some patients [7]. This is supported by suicide, the leading cause of premature death among schizophrenics [8].

The aim of the study was to assess: the frequency of depressive symptoms in chronic schizophrenic in-patients during an exacerbation phase. The possible relationship between age, sex, duration of illness, basal and post dexamethasone plasma levels, type of drug and dosage, extrapyramidal symptoms (EPS) and depressive features before and after 6 weeks of neuroleptic treatment.

Materials and Methods

One hundred and thirty-four chronic schizophrenic in-patients (45 disorganized, 25 paranoid, 1 catatonic, 63 undifferentiated) (DSM III-R), with acute exacerbation, 95 M and 39 F, age ranging from 17 to 73 years (mean 36.19 years ± 1.23 S.E.) and with a mean duration of illness of 10.31 years ± 0.92 S.E., were studied.

Prevalence and severity of depressive symptomatology were assessed by HRS-D and clustering three items of BPRS (guilt feeling, depressive mood, motor retardation) at admission (T_0) and after 3 weeks (T_6) of neuroleptic treatment.

Forty-three patients were treated with fluphenazine decanoate (FLD) (0.3 mg/kg ± 0.01 S.E. every two weeks), 68 patients with conventional haloperidol (HL) (0.14 mg/kg daily ± 0.01 S.E.) and 23 patients with haloperidol decanoate (HLD) (0.44 mg/kg daily ± 0.13 S.E. with an administration i.m. every four weeks).

EPS were evaluated by using the Simpson and Angus Rating Scale at T_6. Basal (at 8 a.m.) and post-dexamethasone cortisol levels (at 4 p.m.) (DST) were determined in 48 patients. Statistical analysis was made on the basis of ANOVA and regression analysis.

Results

At admission, the frequency of guilt feelings, rated according to severity (mild: scores 2–3; moderate: scores 4–5; severe: scores 6–7 at BPRS item) was 26% (mild), 12% (moderate) and 5% (severe). As regards depressive mood, the frequency was 35% (mild), 25% (moderate) and 5% (severe) while motor retardation showed a frequency of 23% (mild), 29% (moderate) and 13% (severe).

All patients showed a significant amelioration on BPRS total scores (mean values T_0: 58.11 ± 1.24 S.E. vs. T_6: 38.93 ± 1.27 S.E.; $P < 0.01$) and the BPRS depression "cluster" and HRS-D scores during the treatment period (mean values T_0: 782 ± 0.32 S.E., 21.22 ± 0.91 S.E. vs. T_6: 6.17 ± 0.27 S.E., 11.88 ± 1.03 S.E.; $P < 0.01$).

There was no relation between the duration of illness, sex, drug dosages and severity of depression at BPRS. There was a positive correlation between age ($r = 0.17$, $P < 0.05$, $r = 0.40$, $P < 0.01$), basal BPRS total scores ($r = 0.39$, $P < 0.01$, $r = 0.68$, $P < 0.01$) and depression scores evaluated at T_0 and T_6. There was no correlation between age and EPS, EPS and depression scores, in patients with EPS scores over 3 (Fig. 1).

No correlation was observed between drug dosages and EPS total scores. BPRS depression "cluster" scores and EPS total scores at the end of the study were significantly higher ($P < 0.01$) in patients treated with FLD (7.69 ± 0.58 S.E.; 1204 ± 1.44 S.E.) than in patients treated with HL (5.51 ± 0.32 S.E.; 3.44 ± 0.5 S.E.) or HLD (4.86 ± 0.50 S.E.; 2.7 ± 0.9 S.E.).

There was no correlation between basal, post DST cortisol levels and depression scores at T_0 and T_6. Non-suppressors to DST (NS) showed a higher variability of improvement in depression scores than suppressors (SS).

Conclusions

Our data confirm that a high prevalence of depressive symptoms occur throughout the course of schizophrenia, this symptomatology coexisting with schizophrenic

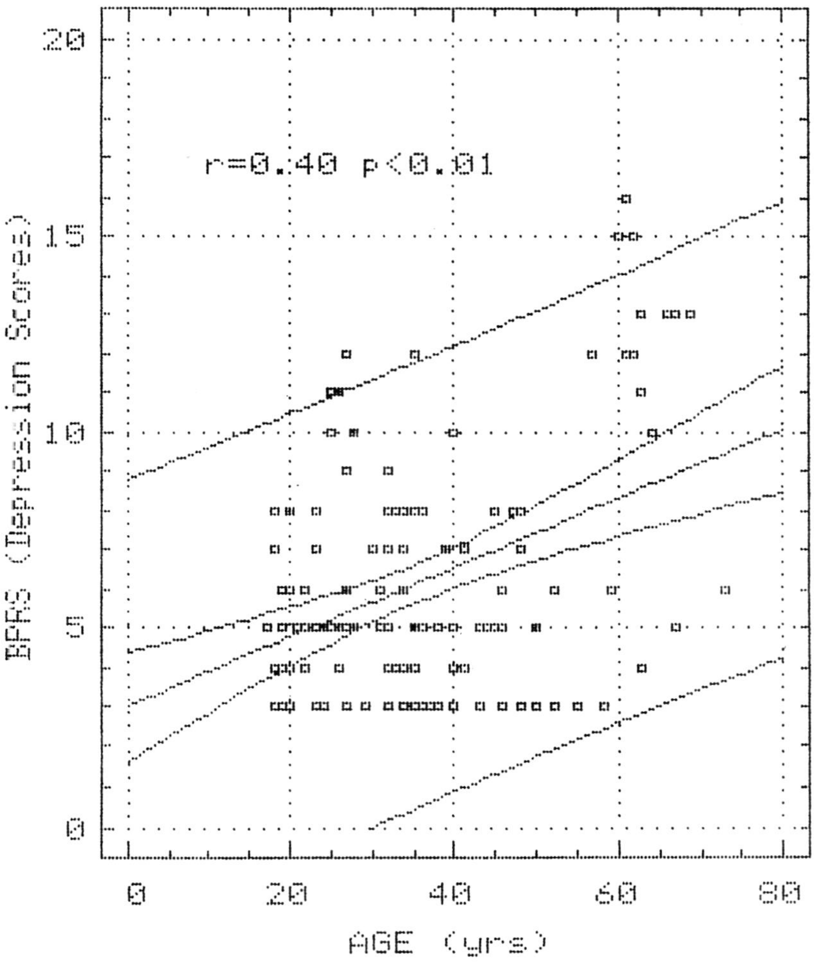

Fig. 1. A positive correlation between age and BPRS (depression scores) at the end of the study (Time 6).

illness. Depression seems to be related to age of patients, irrespective of sex, duration of illness, basal and post DST cortisol levels, drug dosage and EPS induced by neuroleptics. Patients treated with FLD showed a more pronounced depressive picture with higher EPS, without any relation between them, at the end of the study.

References

1. DeLisi LE (1990) In: DeLisi LE (ed.) Depression in Schizophrenia. Am. Psychiatric Press Inc., Washington.

2. Hirsch SR (1982) Br. J. Psychiatry 140: 421–424.
3. Green MF, Keith H and Ventura J (1990) Am. J. Psychiatry 147: 179–182.
4. VanPutten T and May PRA (1978) Arch. Gen. Psychiatry 35: 1101–1107.
5. Kramer MS, Wolfgang H and DiJohnson C (1989) Arch. Gen. Psychiatry 46: 922–928.
6. Siris SG, Adan MD and Cohen M (1988) Am. J. Psychiatry 145: 1532–1537.
7. Altamura AC, Mauri MC and De Novellis F (1989a) Pharmacopsychiatry 22: 246–249.
8. Cohen LJ, Test MA and Brown RL (1990) Am. J. Psychiatry 147: 602–607.

Biological Psychiatry, Volume 1. G. Racagni et al., editors.

Tardive dyskinesia: The long-term outcome

Daniel E. Casey
VA Medical Center, 3710 SW US Veterans Hospital Road, Portland, Oregon 97207 U.S.A.

Introduction

Tardive dyskinesia (TD) is a major problem for the long-term therapy of chronic psychoses with neuroleptic drugs [1]. It is widely believed that TD will inevitably worsen with continued neuroleptic treatment, since these drugs are the purported causative agents of TD. If this is true, a clinical dilemma inevitably develops. Without neuroleptic drugs TD will stay the same or improve, but there is a high risk of psychotic relapse. With continued neuroleptic treatment psychotic symptoms can be controlled, but there is the fear that TD will develop or that existing TD will be aggravated. However, results from many outcome studies challenge this concept. Most data suggest that TD gradually improves rather than worsens during continued neuroleptic treatment. These observations were even noted in the initial TD reports in either conditions of continued or discontinued neuroleptic therapy [2,3]. Though it is difficult to compare and contrast outcome studies because of their diverse data collection and analytical procedures [4], important features of the long-term outcome of TD will be reviewed.

Outcome

The range of TD improvement across studies varies widely from 0–92% [1,4]. Though a few patients have rapid resolution of TD [4,5], this is an uncommon course. In most patients, TD improves or resolves slowly over many months or years. Some patients do not improve at all, but only a few have symptoms increase with continued neuroleptic treatment [4].

Patient variables

Age is the factor most consistently correlated with TD outcome. Younger patients show much greater improvement than older patients. However, this is not predictable for each individual. Some younger patients show only mild or no improvement, whereas in some elderly patients, TD is completely resolved.

There are no data to clearly document whether gender influences outcome of TD. TD severity is negatively correlated with prognosis [6].

Drug factors

Discontinuing neuroleptic therapy is the preferred method for reducing the risks of aggravating or producing TD. Unfortunately, extended drug discontinuation is not usually a feasible option for the majority of patients with chronic psychosis. The alternate strategy of continued neuroleptic treatment with the lowest effective dose in psychotic patients who benefit from these drugs is the more practical approach.

Most studies evaluating continued neuroleptic treatment report that TD either improves or stabilizes [4,6]. The relative risk of this treatment approach is that the resolution of TD may be impaired due to the presence of neuroleptic drugs, whereas improvement may be more rapid without drug therapy. However, the difference in improvement rates in those patients continuing or discontinuing neuroleptics is only modest [4].

Interrupted or periodic neuroleptic treatment has sometimes been proposed as a method of drug holidays to reduce the risk of TD. A mandatory one day per week or one month per year off neuroleptics is not feasible in most cases. Rather, it is preferred to continuously use the lowest effective dose. There are some possible undesirable effects of interrupted drug therapy, though the data are somewhat conflicting. One retrospective study found a significantly higher rate of irreversible TD in patients who received intermittent neuroleptic treatment [7], though others have found the opposite [6].

Total neuroleptic exposure after TD diagnosis is negatively associated with a good outcome. The greater the exposure to neuroleptic drug, the less likely a favorable prognosis will be.

Temporal aspects

Time may be the most important factor in the outcome of TD. Length of follow-up is positively correlated with increasing improvement and resolution of TD. Studies evaluating TD outcome over more than 5 years have substantially more favorable results than short-term follow-up studies. Symptom resolution over a 5- to 10-year period shows that approximately 50% of patients will have at least 50% improvement in TD, independent of whether neuroleptic drugs have been continued or discontinued [4]. Just as it may take several years for TD to develop, so it may also take many years for TD to resolve or stabilize. Early detection of TD is also associated with a favorable outcome. However, this is not the course for all cases of TD detected early, since in some patients TD may have existed for a long period of time before it broke through current neuroleptic treatment or was unmasked by decreasing neuroleptic doses.

Conclusion and Summary

The outcome data for TD is more favorable than is commonly recognized. Most cases improve or stabilize, while only a minority increase over time. The outcome results are highly dependent on patient factors (age, symptom severity), drug factors (continued vs. discontinued treatment, dose) and temporal aspects (length of follow-up, duration of TD). These data give reason for cautious optimism that the course of TD, especially with continued neuroleptic treatment that is needed by most chronically psychotic patients, is favorable. However, much additional research is needed to clarify the important characteristics for identifying prognosis once TD has been established. In the meantime, it is possible to achieve a desirable clinical tradeoff of controlling the psychosis with the lowest effective neuroleptic dose in patients who benefit from these valuable drug treatments.

References

1. Casey DE (1987) In: Meltzer HY (ed.) Psychopharmacology: The Third Generation of Progress. Raven Press, New York, pp. 1411–1419.
2. Schönecker M (1957) Nervenarzt 28: 35.
3. Uhrbrand L and Faurbye A (1960) Psychopharmacologia 1: 408–418.
4. Casey DE and Gerlach J (1986) In: Casey DE and Gardos G (eds.) Tardive Dyskinesia and Neuroleptics: From Dogma to Reason. American Psychiatric Press, Washington DC, pp. 76–97.
5. Gardos G and Cole JO (1980) Am. J. Psychiatry 137: 776–781.
6. Gardos G, Cole JO, Salomon M and Schniebolk S (1987) Am. J. Psychiatry 144 (7): 895–902.
7. Jeste DV, Potkin SG, Sinha S et al. (1979) Arch. Gen. Psychiatry 36: 585–590.

Biological Psychiatry, Volume 1. G. Racagni et al., editors.

Subjective experiences of extrapyramidal side-effects in schizophrenia

S.R. Marder, T. van Putten, W.C. Wirshing, M. Aravagiri and T. Hicks-Gray
West Los Angeles Veteran Affairs Medical Center, Brentwood Division and Department of Psychiatry, University of California, Los Angeles, California, U.S.A.

Extrapyramidal side-effects (EPS) of neuroleptic medications – particularly akathisia and akinesia – may be experienced as anxiety, irritability, or depression. This presentation will focus on a number of factors associated with subjective experiences of distress from neuroleptic medications. We studied this issue by using dosage comparison studies. In separate inpatient and outpatient studies, patients were assigned to different doses of potent neuroleptics and side-effects as well as subjective experiences were measured.

Studies in acute schizophrenia

Dose comparison with haloperidol

Eighty patients with schizophrenia diagnosed by DSM III from the Brentwood Veterans Affairs Medical Center were assigned to receive 5, 10, or 20 mg daily of haloperidol for 4 weeks for an acute exacerbation of their illness [1].

Patients who received the 20-mg dose did better in some respects and worse in others. On the Clinical Global Impression Scale (CGI) the patients on the highest dose were significantly better than those on the lower 2 doses ($P = 0.024$). On the thought disturbance factor of the Brief Psychiatric Rating Scale (BPRS), the 20-mg dose was superior to the 5-mg dose ($P = 0.02$), but not to the 10-mg dose. On the other hand, patients assigned to 20 mg were significantly worse than the other 2 dosage groups on the withdrawal-retardation factor of the BPRS ($P < 0.001$). In addition, the high-dose patients experienced higher scores for akinesia ($P < 0.001$) and akathisia ($P = 0.07$). The discomfort experienced by these patients may have been the cause of the significantly greater likelihood that the 20-mg patients would leave the hospital "against medical advice" ($P < 0.0001$). Moreover, individuals who left the study showed a trend toward increased depression ($P = 0.08$), more akathisia ($P = 0.002$), and more withdrawal-retardation ($P = 0.007$), but not more psychosis.

We interpret these findings as indicating that a 20 mg per day dose of haloperidol can be psychotoxic for some patients and lead to dysphoric symptoms characterized by anxiety, depression, withdrawal and non-compliance. These problems are probably secondary to akathisia and akinesia.

Dose comparison with fluphenazine

In a later study [2], 72 newly readmitted schizophrenic men were randomly assigned to receive 5, 10, or 20 mg of fluphenazine daily for 4 weeks. Outcome was measured in a manner that was similar to the haloperidol study. Plasma concentrations of fluphenazine were measured using a highly specific and sensitive radioimmunoassay [3]. In this study we focused on the relationship between plasma fluphenazine concentrations and both clinical improvement and side-effects. Patients were evaluated as to whether or not they demonstrated "global improvement", which was defined as either marked or moderate improvement on the CGI. They were also rated as to whether they experienced "disabling side-effects" which were defined as side-effects that significantly interfered with the patient's functioning or side-effects that outweighed the drug's therapeutic benefit. It should be noted that in this study, these side-effect ratings were based upon the patient's own interpretation of side-effect severity.

Using logistic regression with the above variables as the outcome and the log of plasma fluphenazine concentration as the independent variable, we found significant relationships between fluphenazine level and both global improvement ($P = 0.015$) and disabling side-effects ($P = 0.0008$). Higher fluphenazine levels up to 4.23 ng/ml were associated with greater improvement. However, nearly 90% of patients had disabling side-effects at plasma levels above 2.7 ng/ml. These findings confirmed our impression that at therapeutic levels of a neuroleptic, patients may experience subjective side-effects that can severely compromise a drug's effectiveness.

Side-effects in maintenance therapy

Dosage comparison with fluphenazine decanoate

Our maintenance study [4] was a double-blind trial of either 5 mg or 25 mg of fluphenazine decanoate administered every 2 weeks for 2 years. The subjects were 66 male veterans referred to a research clinic at a large, urban V.A. hospital. All were candidates for maintenance neuroleptic treatment who fulfilled DSM III criteria for schizophrenic disorder. Prior to study entry, subjects were stabilized for 2 months or more on fluphenazine decanoate. Those who required more than 25 mg every 14 days were dropped from this study. Patients were maintained on the fixed dose of 5 or 25 mg for as long as they did well. When subjects demonstrated an increase of 3 or more points on BPRS cluster scores for thought disturbance or paranoia, they were considered to have had a "psychotic exacerbation".

Using survival analysis, we found that patients assigned to the higher dose had significantly better survival rates without psychotic exacerbations ($P < 0.05$). However, when we evaluated the subjective state of patients using the SCL-90, we found differences between the 2 groups. All of the factor scores from this scale were higher in the 25-mg group. These differences were statistically significant for depression and phobic anxiety. These findings indicate that even though the higher dose provides somewhat more protection, it is at a price. Individuals receiving 25 mg appeared to feel more uncomfortable, as indicated by their higher SCL-90 ratings at 1 and 3 months. Significant correlations of the elevated SCL-90 factors with the various side-effect factors – including akathisia and retardation – indicate that this discomfort was probably extrapyramidally-based. There may have also been a more tangible effect. Eight patients dropped out of the study during the first 6 months. Six of these individuals had been receiving the higher dose. We looked carefully at these patients to determine whether dropping out may have been related to the dose they were receiving. At 1 month, the patients who eventually dropped out on the higher dose during the first 6 months were experiencing more internal distress, as indicated by higher SCL-90 ratings for all of the subscales. The differences were statistically significant for the obsessive-compulsive ($P = 0.03$) and depression ($P = 0.02$) subscales. This suggests that a number of patients receiving 25 mg experience drug-induced discomfort which resulted in their abandoning treatment.

Summary

The above studies, taken together, indicate that akathisia and akinesia can be experienced as vague dysphorias that can have serious effects on a patient's subjective experiences and on their cooperation with treatment.

References

1. Van Putten T, Marder SR and Mintz J (1990) Arch. Gen. Psychiatry 47: 754–758.
2. Van Putten T, Marder SR, Wirshing WC, Aravagiri M and Chabert N (1991) Schizophr. Bull. (in press).
3. Midha KK, Cooper JK and Hubbard JW (1980) Commun. Psychopharmacol. 4: 107–114.
4. Marder SR, Van Putten T, Mintz J, Lebell M, McKenzie J and May PRA (1987) Arch. Gen. Psychiatry 44: 518–521.

Biological Psychiatry, Volume 1. G. Racagni et al., editors.

Side-effect profiles of atypical versus classical neuroleptics

Jes Gerlach
Sct Hans Hospital, Department P, Roskilde, Denmark

Introduction

The side-effect profiles of neuroleptic drugs are determined by the compounds' receptor affinities: high dose neuroleptics (which induce a wide spectrum of side-effects) bind to a variety of brain receptors including dopamine (DA), norepinephrine (α_1), serotonin (5-HT) and acetylcholine receptors, while low dose neuroleptics (which cause mainly extrapyramidal side-effects (EPS)) are relatively selective in binding to D_2 DA receptors.

Mental side-effects can also be related to receptor affinities. Thus DA receptor blockade produces emotional indifference, akathisia (which may aggravate psychotic symptoms) and during long-term treatment, lethargy and sometimes depression. Blockade of α_1 receptors causes sedation and blockade of muscarinic acetylcholine receptors may lead to confusion. It is still unknown whether 5-HT_2 antagonism has any effect in schizophrenia, beneficial or detrimental.

A whole range of new antipsychotics have been making their appearance [1]. No common pharmacological feature unites these new antipsychotic drugs, but they all induce a relatively low level of EPS (due to a low or atypical blockade of DA receptors). In the following the side-effect profiles of 4 groups of new, atypical neuroleptics shall be discussed with special focus on EPS and mental aspects.

Selective antagonism of dopamine receptors

$D_{2/3/4/5}$ *DA receptor blockers*

Recent molecular and receptor binding studies indicate that a variety of different DA receptors exist, including the newly discovered $D_{3/4/5}$ receptors [2]. It appears that some substituted benzamides such as sulpiride and remoxipride have a selective affinity to subgroups of such receptors [3]. This may explain why these antipsychotics induce few side-effects, not only few autonomic, cardiovascular and sedative side-effects, but also few EPS. Furthermore, these drugs may have a slightly deviant EPS profile in that they produce a relatively low level of bradykinesia compared to tremor and akathisia [1]. By means of such drugs it may also be possible to limit or avoid some of the mental side-effects associated with a traditional D_2 antagonist treatment. In this connection it should be mentioned that sulpiride exhibits a special activating, antiautistic potential [4].

D_1 DA receptor blockers

These are potential antipsychotics. They are cataleptogenic and react positively in other antipsychotic models. However, the side-effect profile of D_1 antagonists seem to differ from the side-effect profile of traditional D_2 blockers. Thus D_1 antagonists do not produce dystonia or akathisia in drug-naive monkeys, only bradykinesia and tremor (parkinsonism). Only when given following a D_2 antagonist treatment do D_1 antagonists produce dystonia, and even then, some tolerance to the dystonia develops during long-term treatment. Furthermore, D_1 antagonists appear to induce less dyskinesia than D_2 antagonists during as well as following long-term treatment (acute and tardive dyskinesia). This suggests a relatively benign side-effect profile of D_1 antagonists, also with respect to mental side-effects. D_1 antagonists have not yet been tested in the clinic.

Partial D_2 dopamine agonists

Partial D_2 agonists are an interesting new group of antipsychotic drugs that act both as agonists and antagonists at the D_2 receptors, dependent upon their intrinsic activity and the basal endogenous DA activity. The hypothesis is that the antagonistic activity might moderate the DA hyperactive brain regions responsible for the positive symptoms, while the agonistic effect might normalize DA hypoactive regions connected with negative symptoms, and at the same time prevent EPS and mental side-effects related to D_2 receptor blockade [5].

A drug with low intrinsic activity (SDZ HDZ 912) is effective upon positive and negative symptoms, but also produces EPS (D_2 antagonism) and tachycardia (D_2 agonism). Drugs with higher intrinsic activity (e.g. terguride) may improve negative symptoms, but have no or limited effect upon positive symptoms [1]. Further studies are warranted to evaluate whether partial D_2 agonists represent a useful treatment principle in schizophrenia.

Drugs with low binding to D_2 receptors and additional binding to other receptors

Clozapine is the well-established representative of this group, with a well-documented therapeutic effect in therapy resistent schizophrenic patients. Clozapine blocks D_1 and D_2 receptors (both with 40–50% occupancy), α_1, muscarinic and 5-HT_2 receptors. This leads to induction of a number of side-effects including autonomic and cardiovascular reactions, sedation and sometimes confusion. On the other hand, clozapine rarely induces EPS, tardive dyskinesia and D_2 related mental side-effects such as akathisia.

No other drug with an equal combination of D_1 and D_2 receptor blockade has yet been developed to replace clozapine. However, several potential antipsychotics with low D_2 blocking effect and additional blocking of 5-HT_2 receptors have been developed (e.g. amperozide and ICI 204.636), although there is still no significant clinical documentation for a beneficial effect of 5-HT_2 blockers in schizophrenia. Further clinical testing will clarify the crucial question of whether such drugs may have antipsychotic effect comparable to traditional neuroleptics or clozapine.

Non-dopaminergic antipsychotics

Different non-dopaminergic transmitter systems are under evaluation in the search for new antipsychotic drugs including the 5-HT, the GABA-A/benzodiazepine, the glutamate and peptidergic systems (for review, see [1]). If it can be proved that significant antipsychotic effects and not just mild modulatory effects can be obtained through one of these transmitters, it will open up a new era in the pharmacotherapy of schizophrenia – hopefully with fewer side-effects. Clinical results are still inconclusive.

References

1. Gerlach J (1991) Schizophr. Bull. 17:
2. Tol HHMV, Bunzow JR, Guan H-C, Sunahara RK, Seeman P, Niznik HB and Civelli O (1991) Nature 350: 610–619.
3. Ogren S-O, Florvall L, Hall H, Magnusson O, Ängeby-Möller K (1990) Acta Psychiatr. Scand. 82 (Suppl. 358): 21–26.
4. Härnryd C, Bjerkenstedt L, Bjork K, Gullberg B, Oxenstierna G and Sedvall G (1984) Acta Psychiatr. Scand. (Suppl. 311) 69: 75–92.
5. Coward DM (1991) In: Tamminga CA and Schulz SC (eds.) Advances in Neuropsychiatry and Psychopharmacology: Schizophrenia Research. Raven Press Ltd., New York, pp. 297–305.

Biological Psychiatry, Volume 1. G. Racagni et al., editors.

Differential plasticity of dopamine receptors after pharmacological or functional deafferentation

P.F. Spano, M. Pizzi, A. Valerio, C. Missale and M. Memo

Department of Biomedical Sciences and Biotechnology, Section of Pharmacology, Toxicology and Experimental Therapeutics, University of Brescia, Via Valsabbina 19, 25124 Brescia, Italy

Heterogeneity of dopamine receptors

In 1978 we first proposed to classify dopamine (DA) receptors into D_1 and D_2 subtypes on the basis of their pharmacological properties and the intracellular responses they mediate. In recent years we have accumulated biochemical evidence on the existence of at least two pharmacologically and functionally distinguishable D_2 receptor subtypes which we proposed to designate as D_{2A} and D_{2B} [1,2]. Functional evidence for the existence of different subtypes of D_1 receptors has also been provided recently [3]. The DNA cloning methodology has allowed knowledge to be obtained of the molecular basis of DA receptor heterogeneity [3]. Two forms of the D_2 DA receptor were identified by gene cloning and shown to be derived from alternative splicing of a common gene. More recently, novel dopamine receptors, termed D_3 and D_4 [4] were discovered, which display similar but not identical pharmacological properties when compared to the D_2 receptor subtypes. DA D_1 receptors were also cloned from both rat and human brain. In the last few months, data have been reported on the cloning of D_5 receptors, which present a pharmacological profile related to that of D_1 receptors [5].

Supersensitivity of dopamine receptors

We studied the possible functional modifications of both D_1 and D_2 receptor subtypes following repeated administration to rats of DA antagonists that act selectively on a single class of DA receptors. We found that persistent blockade of D_1 receptors induces a selective upregulation of D_1 receptors while persistent blockade of D_2 receptors results in an upregulation of D_2 receptors in the mesostriatal areas [6]. The supersensitivity of the distinct DA receptors was apparent in both number and function. On the other hand, the repeated administration of D_2 selective agonists down-regulated DA D_2 receptor function in both mesostriatal and in mesolimbocortical rat brain regions [7]. Treatment of rats with reserpine, which depletes the intracellular stores of DA and putative cotransmitters, causes the target neurons to increase the functional response of the receptors to DA due to an increase in the G protein activity without changing the number of receptor proteins [8]. This implies that the number of receptors does not always reflect the functional state of the transduction machinery.

Expression of dopamine receptors

The changes in functional activity of DA receptors may thus stem from a modification in the availability of specific component of the multiprotein receptor complex. To evaluate this hypothesis, we measured the relative abundance of the mRNAs encoding the two isoforms of D_2 receptors and various G protein α-subunits in the striata of rats chemically denervated by unilateral injection with 6-hydroxydopamine (6-OHDA) in the substantia nigra. The steady state levels of the mRNAs encoding the two isoforms of the D_2 receptors were similar in the 6-OHDA lesioned and in the control striatum. On the contrary, we found a different pattern of expression in the mRNAs specific for the α-subunits of the G_i and G_o proteins in the 6-OHDA lesioned striatum as compared with controls. The calculated amount of $G\alpha i_1$ and $G\alpha_o$ mRNAs was significantly higher in the striatum from the lesioned side, the steady state of $G\alpha i_2$ mRNA appeared to be unchanged while that of $G\alpha i_3$ was slightly decreased. The increase in the mRNA levels of Gi_1 and G_o α-subunits may be related to the functional supersensitivity of DA D_2 receptors. Our results suggest that the expression of the genes encoding the different components of the DA D_2 receptor complex is regulated by specific and unidentified factors originating from afferent fibers. An alteration in this very balanced input results in a change of signal processing.

References

1. Castelletti L, Memo M, Missale C, Spano PF and Valerio A (1989) J. Physiol. 410: 251–265.
2. Pizzi M, Valerio A, Benarese M, Missale C, Carruba MO, Memo M and Spano PF (1990) Mol. Neuropharmacol. 1: 37–42.
3. Strange PG (1991) Trends Neurosci. 14: 43–45.
4. Van Tol HHM, Bunzow JR, Guan HC, Sunahara RK, Seeman P, Niznik HB and Civelli O (1991) Nature 350: 610–614.
5. Sunahara RK, Guan HG, O'Dowd BF, Seeman P, Laurier LG, Ng G, George SR, Torchia J, Van Tol HHM and Niznik HB (1991) Nature 350: 614–619.
6. Memo M, Pizzi M, Nisoli E, Missale C, Carruba MO and Spano PF (1987) Eur. J. Pharmacol. 138: 45–51.
7. Nisoli E, Memo M, Missale C, Carruba MO and Spano PF (1990) Eur. J. Pharmacol. 176: 85–90.
8. Missale C, Nisoli E, Liberini P, Rizzonelli P, Memo M, Buonamici M, Rossi A and Spano PF (1989) Brain Res. 483: 117–122.

Biological Psychiatry, Volume 1. G. Racagni et al., editors.

Rodent models of tardive dyskinesia: Methodological considerations

Gaylord Ellison
Department of Psychology, UCLA, 405 Hilgard Ave, Los Angeles, CA 90024, U.S.A.

In spite of considerable efforts to develop annual models of tardive dyskinesia (TD), this has remained a controversial field. Rodent models of TD, which principally rely upon counts of vacuous oral movements (OMs) have been recently reviewed by Waddington [1]. Different laboratories report quite diverse results and few general inferences are possible, even including whether what is being demonstrated when rodents given neuroleptics exhibit increased OMs models TD or acute dystonia.

While the sources for these discrepancies remain largely unknown, methodological differences probably contribute to this problem. In most rodent studies, rats are administered neuroleptics and tested in an "open cage test", where some investigators find gradually increasing OMs in drugged animals and conclude that this models TD, but others report that "vacuous OMs" occur as soon as 24 h after drug administration and conclude [2] that the OMs observed represent acute dystonic reactions in rats. An alternative testing procedure, the "tube-test", leads to different results. Here the rat rests within a loosely-fitting tube to which it has been well habituated, with the head protruding through a large hole made in the end of the tube. OMs, as well as head movements, are monitored via a TV camera focussed on the oral region by an operator in an adjacent room pressing computer-linked keys. These are not simply 2 different measures of the same behavior, for neuroleptics induce a different pattern of results in the 2 tests. When rats were administered chronic neuroleptics and repeatedly observed in both tests [3–5], observers in the tube-test reported no or very small increases in OMs in the chronic neuroleptic animals compared to controls. Yet when these animals were tested in the cage test, much larger differences were observed, often with strikingly increased OMs in the drug-treated groups. Other results further indicated profound discrepancies between these tests. Rats given acute HAL immediately showed increased OMs (a "dystonia-like result") in the cage test, but not in the tube test. When the drug was withdrawn after chronic administration there were immediate increases in OMs in the tube test (a "TD-like result"), whereas in the cage test OMs rapidly returned to control levels [5]. It was concluded that there is an artifact related to activity levels in the cage test [6]. Oral activity of rats is dramatically inhibited during bouts of exploratory behavior, when the animals are rearing and sniffing. If all that is measured is number of OMs, misleading results can be obtained as rats which have been injected with neuroleptics show inflated OM scores simply because they are less exploratory.

But the assumption behind both tests – that counting OMs in rodents can model TD – may not be valid. The Abnormal Involuntary Movements Scale (AIMS) is a composite of 10 ratings, 4 of which focus on the oral region, 3 on the arms, legs and trunk, and 3 of which consist of ratings of the severity, degree of incapacitation and patient's awareness of the abnormal movements. Attempts to simplify it by only counting oral movements in humans with TD yielded data which correlated very poorly with all other ID scales, including the AIMS Scale [7]. It seems likely that simple counting of oral activity will not develop into a non-controversial model of TD, a disorder which is fundamentally a dyskinesia.

A less controversial model of rodent TD may be possible when the form of oral movements is actually quantified. In the tube test experiments reviewed above, simultaneous with the reports of the human observer a computerized system precisely recorded the rat's oral movements using a video analysis system [8],and with 2 small UV-sensitive spots painted on the upper and lower jaws of the rat. A TV close-up of the muzzle was fed to a computer which determined the distance between the 2 spots, stored this and converted the data into unidirectional individual openings or closings of the mouth. The detailed analysis of these data using fast-Fourier (FFT) analysis revealed a phenomenon in the rats which clearly also develops in humans. It was found that when the animals were first started on the neuroleptics, during the initial period of sedation, energy was decreased at all frequencies [9]. This indicates that the OMs at this time were fewer, but had a relatively normal form. But then the rats administered chronic HAL or fluphenazine (and especially the latter animals) began to show oral movements which had an altered energy spectrum compared to controls, with relatively increased energy at 1–3 Hz together with decreased energy at higher frequencies (5–7 Hz). This was not just a tranquilization effect, for upon drug withdrawal, when the animals showed a dramatic increase in the total number and average amplitude of oral movements, this shift in the energy spectrum also increased substantially.

This is an important finding because it means that rodents given chronic neuroleptics do not necessarily develop more OMs per se, but that the pattern generator underlying their movements is gradually altered, giving rise to movements of a new typography. Even more striking is that this implies that a direct link to human tardive dyskinesia is apparently possible, for this is the same altered energy spectrum which has been repeatedly reported in humans with TD [10–12] and confirmed in 3 studies in humans using FFT analyses. Wirshing et al. [13], recording from 50 patients with TD, analyzed the data with FFT and concluded that TD was characterized by increased energy in the 1–2 Hz frequency band. Wirshing and Cummings [14] recorded from another set of patients and again found that TD has a characteristic signal at 1–2 Hz. Caligiuri et al. [15], recording tongue movements, found that the spectrum from 0–3 Hz best characterized TD.

This close agreement between the altered form of the movements recorded in rats administered chronic neuroleptics and those of humans with TD would appear to indicate that these alterations in the actual form of OMs are a highly promising animal model of TD. Precisely measuring the form of OMs in rodents may clarify some other controversies in this field, such as the "primed dystonia" vs "tardive dyskinesia" controversy. We have compared [5] the progressive effects of chronic HAL when administered in 2 quite different drug regimens: either continuously (similar to the way it is given to human patients) or, at the same overall dosage, intermittently (1 large dose weekly, as in the primate "primed dystonia" drug regimen). Strikingly different forms of oral syndromes developed in the 2 groups. The rats administered continuous HAL developed the TD-like syndrome, with increased energy at 1–3 Hz, an effect which increased upon drug withdrawal. However, the rats administered intermittent HAL began to show large, jerky OMs, reflected in the computerized files by large amplitude OMs with steep slopes and a peak FFT energy at 5–7 Hz. Thus, entirely different types of abnormally-formed oral movements progressively develop when HAL is given in different regimens. Perhaps "primed dystonia" occurs in rodents as well as primates.

This rodent model of TD may also offer some new tests of potential antipsychotic drugs. When chronic effects of the atypical neuroleptics clozapine and raclopride were compared with those of HAL [16], the rats chronically treated with either atypical neuroleptic did not show increased OMs in either the cage or the tube test. However, a highly unusual syndrome of oral behavior was induced by chronic clozapine, for the longer the rats were on the drug the more OMs were inhibited or suppressed, falling to levels well below those of the controls. Because so few OMs occur, FFT indicated energy well below control levels at all frequencies, including 1–3 Hz. However, progressive changes in OM form did occur with clozapine (but not raclopride), for the relative energy distribution shown by clozapine animals, even though well beneath controls, did have increased energy at 1–2 Hz relative to that at 5–8 Hz. Although clozapine was clearly not inducing TD in this model, there were progressive changes developing in the pattern generator underlying OM form which only could be revealed by sensitive analyses. I conclude that when the form of OMs are actually measured, both in rats and humans, considerably more promising rodent models of TD appear possible than when rating scales and simple counting of OMs are employed.

References

1. Waddington JL (1990) Psychopharmacology 101: 431–447.
2. Rupniak N, Jenner P and Marsden C (1986) Psychopharmacology 88: 403–419.
3. Ellison G and See R (1990) A computerized methodology for the study of neuroleptic-induced oral dyskinesias. Neuromethods 20.
4. See RE, Levin E and Ellison GD (1988) Psychopharmacology 94: 421–427.
5. See RE and Ellison GD (1990a) Psychopharmacology 100: 404–412.
6. Levy AD, See R, Levin E and Ellison G (1987) Life Sci. 41: 1499–1506.
7. Chien C, Jung K and Ross-Townsend A (1980) In: Fann W, Smith R, Davis J and Domino E (eds.) Tardive Dyskinesia: Research and Treatment. Spectrum Publications, New York, pp. 233–241.

8. Ellison G, See R, Levin E and Kinney J (1987) Psychopharmacology 92: 122–126.
9. Ellison G and See R (1989) Psychopharmacology 98: 564–566.
10. Alpert M, Diamond F and Friedhoff AJ (1976) Psychopharmacol. Bull 12(2): 5–7.
11. Sprague R, van Emmerik R and Newell K (1990) Movement Disord. 5: 57
12. Rondot P and Bathien N (1986) Adv. Neurol. 45: 361–366.
13. Wirshing WC, Cummings J, Dencker S and May P (1991) J. Neuropsychiatr. Clin. Neurosci. 3: 10–17.
14. Wirshing WC and Cummings JL (1990) Neuropsychiatry, Neuropsychol. Behav. Neurol. 3: 23–35.
15. Caligiuri M, Jeste D and Harris M (1989) Neuropsychopharmacology 2: 309–312.
16. See RE and Ellison GD (1990b) Eur. J. Pharmacol. 181: 175–186.
17. Tyron W and Pologe B (1987) Am. J. Psychiatry 144: 1584–1587.

Biological Psychiatry, Volume 1. G. Racagni et al., editors.

Continuous versus discontinuous neuroleptic treatment in an animal model of tardive dyskinesia

Birte Glenthøj[1], Tom G. Bolwig[1] and Ralf Hemmingsen[2]
[1]Department of Psychiatry, Rigshospitalet, 2100 Copenhagen; and [2]Department of Psychiatry, Bispebjerg Hospital, 2400 Copenhagen, Denmark

The kindling phenomenon represents an example of neuronal plasticity in the nervous system. According to the original description [1], kindling is the development of permanent excitability changes in the brain produced by spaced electrical stimulations of specific brain sites with an initially subthreshold current. Altered neuronal plasticity caused by intermittent electrical stimulations bears resemblance to pharmacological sensitization, where a discontinuous regimen likewise is essential for a progressive augmentation of the behavioural response. Electrical or pharmacological sensitization has been connected with the development of pathological behaviour in a group of neuropsychiatric conditions including development of tardive dyskinesia [2–7].

Several studies have demonstrated increases in oral activities such as vacuous chewing movements (VCM) and tongue protrusion in rodents in connection with neuroleptic treatment. This syndrome might according to Casey [8] qualify for an analogous animal model of tardive dyskinesia. The outcome of studies of oral activity in rats following chronic treatment with antipsychiatric drugs has varied considerably. Hence increased oral activity, in agreement with development of tardive dyskinesia in humans, has been reported to develop slowly and to persist after discontinuation of neuroleptic treatment [9–12]. Other authors have concluded that development of VCM is a model for acute dystonia, as it appears shortly after initiation of neuroleptic treatment and disappears soon after withdrawal [13].

According to the hypothesis that a pharmacological sensitization is relevant to the development of tardive dyskinesia, we have in a number of studies observed the effect of discontinuous and continuous treatment of rats with dopamine D_1 and dopamine D_2 blocking agents. All experiments were carried out with male Wistar rats.

In one study [7] rats were randomly assigned to five groups receiving haloperidol (HAL) and zuclopenthixol (ZU) discontinuously (HAL = 1 mg/kg/day, 48 h weekly; ZU = 2 mg/kg/day, 48 h weekly) or continuously (HAL = 1 mg/kg/day; ZU = 2 mg/kg/day). Drug was added to the drinking water. All animals were treated for 15 weeks. They were observed during treatment and following termination of medication both in their home cages and in restraining plexiglass tubes in which they were videotaped. Two weeks after withdrawal, ZU-treated rats were tested for their reactivity to the D_1 receptor agonist SK&F 38 393. HAL-treated rats were operated and electrically kindled in the nucleus amygdala until generalized seizures developed.

Both discontinuously- and continuously-treated rats developed a significant increase in VCM compared to controls within the first week of treatment. Differences were most pronounced in home cages. Haloperidol-treated rats had more mouth movements than zuclopenthixol-treated rats during most of the study.

It was remarkable that the abnormal rise in VCM disappeared a few days after withdrawal in continuously-treated rats both in tubes and in home cages. The change persisted in animals treated discontinuously with HAL throughout the 11-weeks observation period after treatment had been terminated.

When ZU-treated rats were challenged with SK&F 38 393 the increase in tongue protrusions was only significant in treated rats, implicating behavioural D_1 receptor supersensitivity [14]. This supersensitivity was not connected with the spontaneous rise in oral activity seen only in discontinuously-treated rats. Thus, our results do not indicate that increased D_1 receptor responsiveness is significant for the increases in oral activity found after neuroleptic withdrawal.

Another observation of interest was that intermittently-treated rats during amygdala kindling demonstrated seizures earlier than continuously-treated rats and control animals. This difference points to cross-sensitivity between discontinuous neuroleptic treatment and electical amygdala-kindling ([5]; Glenthøj et al., in preparation).

To determine whether longer-lasting continuous neuroleptic treatment would result in persist increases in VCM, in another study we treated rats intermittently and continuously with haloperidol for 27 weeks. Rats were observed until 13 weeks after termination of medication. The results confirm findings of persisting rises in oral activity only following discontinuous treatment (Glenthøj et al., in preparation). We also treated rats continuously (subcutaneous osmotic minipumps) and discontinuously (injections once weekly) with the selective D_1 antagonist NO 756 for 15 weeks. Neither treatment regimen resulted in lasting changes in oral activity (Glenthøj and Hemmingsen, in preparation).

The outcome of studies of oral activity has been contradictory as to the onset and persistance of VCM in connection with neuroleptic treatment. Our results point to the treatment regimen as an important factor in rodent models of neuroleptic induced extrapyramidal side-effects (EPS). In studies using different treatment regimens, we found observable long-lasting changes only following withdrawal from intermittent treatment, whereas all treated groups demonstated elevations in VCM after a few days of treatment.

The increase in mouth movements seen from the beginning of medication might be a result of D_1 receptor preponderance (see [15,16]). The observation that the combined dopamine D_1 and D_2 receptor antagonist zuclopenthixol provoked fewer VCM than the predominantly D_2 receptor blocker haloperidol throughout the medication period is consistent with this hypothesis. The proposed mechanism of a prompt relative D_1 receptor preponderance during neuroleptic treatment could represent a rodent model of acute dyskinesia. The long-lasting changes seen after intermittent treatment might be the result of pharmacological sensitization. We consider this syndrome of sensitization to be an animal model of tardive dyskinesia. Our results are in agreement with clinical studies suggesting that persistent tardive dyskinesia is associated with a greater number of interruptions in drug therapy [17–20]. The exact pathogenetic mechanisms of both electrical kindling and pharmacological sensitization are still unknown, but the finding of cross-sensitivity is of interest, especially when compared with the reported supersensitivity to apomorphine following extensive amygdala kindling [21]. Also remarkable are the studies of Czernansky et al. [22], demonstrating sensitization to the acute effect of HAL on dopamine turnover in intermittently treated rats opposed to tolerance in continuously-treated animals.

References

1. Goddard GV, McIntyre DC and Leech CK (1969) Exp. Neurol. 25: 295.
2. Post RM (1980) Life Sci. 26: 1275.
3. Post RM and Ballenger JC (1981) In: Van Praag HM, Lader MH, Rafaelsen OJ and Sachar EJ (eds.), Handbook of Biological Psychiatry, Part IV. Marcel Dekker Inc., New York, p. 609.
4. Glenthøj B, Hemmingsen R and Bolwig TG (1988) Behav. Neurol. 1: 29.
5. Glenthøj B and Hemmingsen R (1989) Eur. J. Pharmacol. 164: 393.
6. Glenthøj B and Hemmingsen R (1991) Life Sci. 48: 2137.
7. Glenthøj B, Hemmingsen R, Allerup P and Bolwig TG (1990) Eur. J. Pharmacol. 190, 275.
8. Casey DE (1984) Psychopharmacol. Bull. 20: 376.
9. Waddington JL, Cross AJ, Gamble SJ and Bourne RC (1983) Science 220: 530.
10. Waddington IL, Molloy AG, O'Boyle KM and Youssef HA (1985) In: Shagass C et al. (eds.), Proc. IVth World Congr. Biol. Psychiatry, Sept. 1985, Philadelphia, U.S.A. Elsevier, New York, pp. 1151.
11. Levy AD, Sea RE, Levin ED and Ellison GD (1987) Life Sci. 41: 1499.
12. See RE and Ellison G (1990) Psychopharmacology 100: 404.
13. Rupniak NMJ, Jenner P and Marsden CD (1985) Psychopharmacology 85: 71.
14. Glenthøj B, Arnt J and Hyttel J (1990) 47: 1339.
15. Rosengarten H, Schweitzer JW and Friedhoff AJ (1983) Life Sci. 33: 2479.
16. Rosengarten H, Schweitzer JW and Friedhoff AJ (1986) Life Sci. 39: 29.
17. Jeste DV, Potkin SG, Sinha S, Feder S and Wyatt RJ (1979) Arch. Gen. Psychiatry 36, 585.
18. Branchey M and Branchey L (1984) J. Clin. Psychopharmacol. 4: 41.
19. Yassa R, Ghadirian AM and Schwartz G (1985) Can. J. Psychiatry 30: 344.
20. Gerlach J, Ahlfors UG, Amthor KF, Dencker SJ, Graven A, Gunby B, Hagert U, Korsgaard S, Lunding L, Noring U, Ojannen K, Pitkonen T, Povlsen UJ, Rossel T, Tolvanen E and Wæhrens J (1986) Psychopharmacology 90: 423.
21. Czernansky JG, Mellenun J, Beauclair L and Lombrozo L (1988) Psychopharmacology 92: 122.
22. Czernansky JG, Bellows EP, Barnes DE and Lombrozo L (1990) Psychopharmacology 101: 519.

Biological Psychiatry, Volume 1. G. Racagni et al., editors.

Ultrastructural changes in rat CNS with typical and atypical neuroleptics

Charles K. Meshul[1,2] and Daniel E. Casey[3]
[1]Research; [2]Laboratory; and [3]Psychiatry Services, V.A. Medical Center, Portland, OR 97201, U.S.A.

Introduction

Classical neuroleptic drugs, like haloperidol, may exert their therapeutic effect by blocking dopamine (DA) D_2 receptors [1]. Long-term blockade of such receptors within the caudate nucleus results in an increase in their numbers [2,3]. Prolonged treatment with the typical neuroleptic, haloperidol, results in a high incidence of extrapyramidal side-effects (EPS) and tardive dyskinesia (TD) [4,5] while treatment with the atypical neuroleptic, clozapine, is associated with a much lower incidence of EPS and TD [6].

As a possible correlate to the neuroleptic drug-induced changes in receptor density, we have focused on haloperidol-induced ultrastructural changes in a particular type of synaptic contact ("perforated" synapse, Fig. 1) made in the striatum that could correlate with the increase in DA D_2 receptors [7]. Fourteen-day administration of haloperidol to rats caused a significant increase in the number of perforated synapses within the dorsolateral caudate but not the nucleus accumbens. This effect reversed if the animals were subsequently taken off the drug for an additional 2 weeks. To further characterize the effects of neuroleptic drugs on rat brain, we examined the regional specificity of clozapine, an atypical neuroleptic, and haloperidol on the appearance of perforated synapses within the caudate nucleus, nucleus accumbens, and medial prefrontal cortex (MPCx).

Materials and Methods

Male Sprague-Dawley rats (180–200 g) (n=5 for each group) were injected with either haloperidol (0.5 mg/kg/day, s.c.), clozapine (35 mg/kg/day, s.c.), or normal saline for 14 days. Twenty-four hours following the final injection, the animals were anesthetized and perfused with fixative and the caudate nucleus, nucleus accumbens and medial prefrontal cortex (MPCx) were cut and processed for electron microscopic analysis as previously described [8]. All photographs (final mag. = × 42,000) were randomly taken throughout the section in the region of the neuropil, an area containing the greatest concentration of synapses. The number of synapses with and without perforations was determined and mean percentages between groups were statistically analyzed [7].

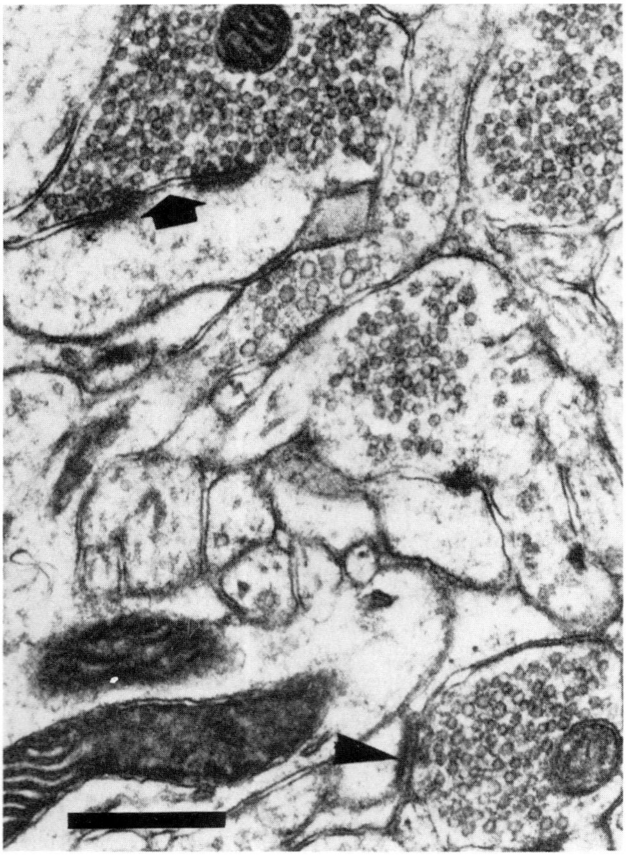

Fig. 1. Electron micrograph from the neurophil of the caudate nucleus of a rat treated with haloperidol for 14 days. A non-perforated (arrowhead) and perforated (arrow) synapse make an asymmetric contact with a dendritic spine. Calibration bar: 0.5 μm.

Results

The neurophil of the caudate nucleus is illustrated in Fig. 1. The majority of synapses within the caudate contain a postsynaptic density in which the post-synaptic density is continuous along the entire length of contact with the nerve terminal. The perforated synapse contains a break in the continuity of the post-synaptic density or specialization. Treatment with haloperidol for 14 days resulted in a statistically significant increase in the mean percentage of perforated synapses within the caudate as compared to either clozapine or saline ($P < 0.05$) (Table 1). There was no change within the nucleus accumbens or MPCx following either clozapine or haloperidol. The total number of synapses for each of the treatment groups did not differ (data not shown), meaning that the percent increase in perforated synapses within the caudate nucleus was due to an actual increase in the

Table 1. Effect of haloperidol and clozapine on perforated synapses

Treatment groups	Caudate[a]	Nucleus accumbens[a]	Medial prefrontal cortex[a]
Saline	8.8 ± 0.8	8.5 ± 0.6	10.4 ± 0.9
Clozapine	8.6 ± 0.7	8.9 ± 0.8	10.4 ± 0.8
Haloperidol	14.2 ± 0.8[b]	9.7 ± 0.6	10.1 ± 0.9

[a]Values are mean percentage of perforated synapses per 22 μm^2 ± S.E.M.
[b]Statistically significant versus saline or clozapine by Peritz' F-test ($P < 0.05$).

number of such synapses and was not due to a decrease in the total number of synapses.

Discussion

The dorsolateral caudate nucleus receives afferents from areas associated with motor functions [8], while the afferents to nucleus accumbens originate mainly from limbic structures [8]. This differential innervation pattern may lend support to the concept that the nucleus accumbens may be the site of antipsychotic action, whereas the more dorsal and lateral striatum may be involved in neuroleptic-induced EPS/TD [9].

We hypothesized that the perforated synapse was not of dopamine origin but was glutamatergic and was associated with the corticostriatal pathway [6,7]. Injection of a tracer (WGA-HRP) into a rat motor cortex labelled perforated synapses within the striatum [10]. We also speculated that the increased numbers of perforated synapses within the caudate may be dependent on increased activity of the corticostriatal pathway [6,7]. Kainate lesion of the thalamus, thereby decreasing activity of the thalamocortical and corticostriatal pathways, prevented the haloperidol-induced increase in perforated synapses [10].

Electrophysiological studies from midbrain DA neurons have shown that subchronic administration of haloperidol causes depolarization blockade of the neurons that project both to the caudate and nucleus accumbens [11]. Subchronic clozapine treatment results in depolarization blockade of only the DA neurons projecting to the nucleus accumbens and not the caudate nucleus [11]. We find that haloperidol but not clozapine treatment causes an increase in perforated synapses in the area of the caudate associated with motor function. However, clozapine blocks and down-regulates other receptors, such as serotonin ($5\text{-}HT_2$) [12] and the very low incidence of EPS/TD associated with clozapine may also be related to blockade of non-DA receptors. Future studies will focus on co-administration of haloperidol and a $5\text{-}HT_2$ antagonist in an attempt to mimic the effects of clozapine.

Acknowledgements

We thank Regina Stallbaumer for technical assistance. This work was supported by the Department of Veterans Affairs and U.S. Public Health Service Grant, MH 36657.

References

1. Seeman P and Grigoriadis D (1987) Neurochem. Int. 10: 1–25.
2. Burt D, Creese I and Snyder S (1977) Science 196: 326–328.
3. Baldessarini RJ and Tarsy D (1980) Adv. Biochem. Psyopharmacol. 24: 451–455.
4. Casey DE (1987) In: Meltzer HY (ed.) Psychopharmacology: The Third Generation of Progress. Raven Press, New York, pp. 1411–1419.
5. Casey DE (1989) Psychopharmacology 199: S47–S53.
6. Meshul CK and Casey DE (1989) Brain Res. 489: 338–346.
7. Meshul CK, Janowsky A, Casey DE, Stallbaumer RK and Taylor B (1991) (submitted).
8. Beckstead RM, Domesick VB and Nauta WJH (1979) Brain Res. 175: 191–217.
9. Stevens JR (1973) Arch. Gen. Psychiatry 29: 177–189.
10. Meshul CK, Janowsky A, Casey DE and Stallbaumer RK (1990) Soc. Neurosci. Abstr. 16: 419.
11. Chiodo LA and Bunney BS (1983) J. Neurosci. 3: 1607–1619.
12. Wilmot CA and Szczepanik AM (1989) Brain Res. 487: 288–298.

Biological Psychiatry, Volume 1. G. Racagni et al., editors.

D_1 dopamine hypothesis in tardive dyskinesia

Jes Gerlach, Lars Hansen and Linda Peacock
Sct Hans Hospital, Department P, Roskilde, Denmark

Introduction

Several hypotheses have been proposed to explain the pathophysiology of tardive dyskinesia (TD), e.g. dopamine (DA) supersensitivity, GABA hypofunction and a neurotoxic defect [1]. In this paper we shall discuss the potential role of DA, especially a D_1 hyperfunction in the pathophysiology of TD, mainly on the basis of recent studies in monkeys. First, however, a few clinical TD features will be mentioned as it is essential that a hypothesis of pathophysiology is anchored in clinical reality.

Acute and tardive dyskinesia

Neuroleptic-induced dyskinesia is and heterogeneous syndrome [2]. Typical TD is seen in elderly patients during or following long-term treatment, most often as oral dyskinesia. The syndrome may persist after withdrawal and be irreversible.

Paradoxical TD or acute dyskinesia occurs mainly in younger patients treated for a shorter period of time with relatively high doses. This syndrome is often more universal in its localization and accompanied by akathisia or dystonic features. Usually, it disappears following withdrawal.

It is likely, but not clinically proven, that there is a pathophysiological link between acute dyskinesia and typical TD.

Can D_1 receptors be involved in acute and tardive dyskinesia?

Effect of D_1 and D_2 agonists in Cebus monkeys

In Cebus monkeys (drug-naive or previously neuroleptic-treated) D_1 agonists induce oral dyskinesia (chewing and tongue protrusions) which strongly resembles human TD. The effect is especially pronounced in monkeys with pre-existing spontaneous or neuroleptic-induced dyskinesia (TD) and the oral movements are of essentially the same quality as the pre-existing dyskinesia. A few monkeys show only few or no movements, while others demonstrate a pronounced syndrome, sometimes with 60–120 tongue protrusions per min. Two features are unlike human TD: a) a few monkeys present their oral dyskinesia in the form of licking, e.g. licking the cage or their paws (especially with high doses of D_1 agonist); and b) some monkeys present their dyskinesia together with an atypical grooming, i.e. simple purposeless, repetitive acts such as examining, licking or biting the fur, the nails or the cage, the act being specific for each individual monkey. This behaviour is especially pronounced following a long-term D_1 antagonistic pretreatment (see later).

The D_1 agonist dyskinesia syndrome is induced in a weak form (together with sedation) by partial D_1 agonists such as SKF 38393 (10 mg/kg) and SKF 75670 (0.1–0.3 mg/kg). A D_1 agonist with higher intrinsic activity, SKF 81297 (0.3–0.9 mg/kg) has a much stronger dyskinesia effect, which in some cases is associated with mild activation and the repetitive "grooming" behaviour described above [3,4]. Also the mixed D_1/D_2 agonist apomorphine may induce oral dyskinesia which may be aggravated by concomitant blockade of the D_2 receptors [5].

In contrast, D_2 agonists induce no significant oral dyskinesia, but decreased locomotion at low doses, and increased arousal, psychosis-like behaviour and repetitive head and body movements at higher doses. In some cases, a weak suppression of oral dyskinesia may be seen, probably because the activation extinguishes other types of behaviour including the oral dyskinesia.

These observations of TD-like oral movements in Cebus monkeys induced by different D_1 agonists support the idea from rat studies [7] that a D_1 hyperactivity may be involved in TD.

Effect of D_1 and D_2 antagonists

Acute treatment with D_2 antagonists in relatively low doses, especially after a "priming" period with repeated drug exposure, can produce mild oral dyskinesia (most pronounced in monkeys with preexisting dyskinesia) reminiscent of acute dyskinesia seen in patients [3–5]. In contrast, D_1 antagonists induce only mild dyskinesia (and no dystonia) in drug-naive monkeys (and rats [6]), but in D_2 primed monkeys they produce dyskinesia and dystonia similar to D_2 antagonists [3,4]. This indicates that acute dyskinesia is related to the blockade of DA receptors, primarily the D_2 receptors and to processes beyond these receptors. D_1 stimulation may play a modulatory additive role.

Following chronic antagonist administration, oral dyskinesia is seen more frequently after D_2 than after D_1 antagonists, while "grooming" is significantly increased only after the D_1 antagonist treatment. D_1 agonist-induced dyskinesia is increased after both D_1 and D_2 blockade (although it is partly suppressed by "grooming" after the D_1 antagonist), while D_1 agonist-induced "grooming" is markedly more pronounced after the D_1 antagonist than after the D_2 antagonist. It should be added that some intensive, prolonged SKF-induced mouth openings and tongue protrusions are seen in some monkeys after the prolonged D_1 antagonist exposure, suggesting that the D_1 receptor may be especially dyskinesia-sensitized by the prolonged D_1 antagonist treatment.

Conclusion

In most but not all Cebus monkeys, D_1 agonists induce/aggravate oral dyskinesia which closely resembles human TD. A long-term pretreatment with D_1 antagonist aggravates some essential aspect of the D_1 agonist-induced dyskinesia, although atypical grooming hides some of the movements. This suggests that a D_1 hyperfunction may be involved in the pathophysiology of oral dyskinesia.

Acute dyskinesia can be induced by blockade of D_2 receptors, but also by D_1 receptors in the case of previous priming with D_2 antagonists. This suggests that acute dyskinesia primarily depends on processes beyond the D_1/D_2 receptors (e.g. in subgroups of GABA neurons), although some modulation may come from D_1 receptor stimulation.

TD (which appears to be "in family with" acute dyskinesia) may be related to similar postsynaptic processes, though in a more persisting form (and usually without akathisia and dystonic features). In TD a relative D_1 hyperfunction (compared to D_2 functions) may facilitate/modulate the syndrome. The observation of an increased D_1 receptor density and a decreased D_2 receptor density in human brains from elderly people supports this view.

References

1. Waddington JL (1989) Int. Rev. Neurobiol. 31: 297–353.
2. Gerlach J and Casey DE (1988) Acta Psychiatr. Scand. 77: 369–378.
3. Gerlach J, Casey DE and Kistrup K (1986) Clin. Neuropharmacol. (Suppl. 4) 9: 131–133.
4. Peacock L, Lublin H and Gerlach J (1990) Eur. J. Pharmacol. 186: 49–59.
5. Gerlach J and Casey DE (1990) Prog. Neuro-Psychopharmacol. Biol. Psychiatry 14: 103–112.
6. Collins P, Broekkamp CLE, Jenner P and Marsden CD (1991) Psychopharmacology 103: 503–512.
7. Rosengarten H, Schweitzer JW and Friedhoff AJ (1983) Life Sci. 33: 2479–2482.

Biological Psychiatry, Volume 1. G. Racagni et al., editors.

Ageing and other determinants of baseline levels of spontaneous orofacial movement in rodents during long-term neuroleptic treatment

John L. Waddington

Department of Clinical Pharmacology, Royal College of Surgeons in Ireland, St. Stephen's Green, Dublin 2, Ireland

Introduction

When tardive dyskinesia emerges in patients with long-term exposure to neuroleptic drugs, it is recognized by clinical observation; indeed, in some patients it can assume prominent and problematic proportions [1,2]. Thus, the long-standing difficulty in identifying readily an isomorphic model of this movement disorder in rodents remains enigmatic. Over the past decade, a number of studies have treated rodents with neuroleptic drugs for extremely prolonged periods, constituting considerable proportions of their adult lifespan. Review [3] of these searches for spontaneous orofacial movements, as the most likely putative counterpart of the typical buccal-lingual-masticatory movements of tardive dyskinesia, indicates a number of provocative findings but much inconsistency. This area is thwart not only with methodological difficulties [3] but also with conceptual problems relating to our perspectives of the clinical disorder we are seeking to model [2].

Baseline issues

The majority of rodent studies reporting the emergence of late-onset orofacial movements during long-term neuroleptic treatment, most commonly vacuous chewing, note such movements to be exacerbations in frequency and/or severity of those that are already present to at least some extent under baseline conditions in untreated control groups [3–6]; this might parallel an increasing appreciation that the baseline extent of buccal-lingual-masticatory movements in untreated non-human primates [7] and patients, particularly in older patient populations with more serious neuropsychiatric disorders [2], may have been seriously underestimated.

Such data support the notion that in both animal and clinical populations, long-term neuroleptic treatment may not so much "cause" tardive dyskinesia de novo but rather exacerbate the appearance of an idiopathic motor syndrome; tardive dyskinesia may reflect at least in part an inappropriate and over-elaborated manifestation of innate, fundamental motor patterns [2]. Baseline levels of orofacial movement appear to differ between rodent strains [5], and this may indicate genetic regulation thereof; similarly, there is evidence that during long-term neuroleptic treatment, vulnerability to the emergence of an excess of orofacial movements in rodents [5] and of tardive dyskinesia in patients [8–10] may include some element of genetic predisposition.

Ageing

Several long-term neuroleptic studies in rodents have reported the baseline level of orofacial movements in untreated animals to increase with ageing; this does not appear to be an artefact of observer sensitization over longitudinal assessment, as it is evident on cross-sectional examination of young vs. aged animals [3]. It has been suggested [11] that it may be an artefact of response incompatibility between oral movements and other more gross motor activities, with a perhaps lower level of such activities in aged animals favouring the manifestation of oral movements. Our own data (Molloy and Waddington, unpublished observations) do not support such an explanation; we could find no significant reduction in the prevalence of sniffing or locomotion, some reduction in rearing and some excess of grooming in aged animals who showed overall a highly significant increase in the prevalence and severity of oral movements in comparison with their young counterparts. Recent studies in young animals have also failed to confirm any reciprocal relationship between orofacial movements and other motor activities [6].

It thus appears that, in general, spontaneous orofacial movements in rodents become more prominent with ageing. While such a phenomenon may not be evident in purified samples of the "normal'" human elderly who are without significant medical or neuropsychiatric disorders, it is certainly apparent in populations that include those who are neuroleptic-naive but suffer from the common physical and mental frailties of old age [2]. In rodents, longitudinal studies suggest that long-term neuroleptic treatment may in fact act to precipitate/hasten the emergence of orofacial movements that have a generally high likelihood of emerging spontaneously with advancing age; indeed, in senescence the extent of age-related orofacial movements may be so prominent as to give a ceiling effect, such that late initiation of neuroleptic treatment has little action to elevate further so high a baseline [3]. Several clinical studies comparing untreated with treated populations of elderly patients are consistent with such a process [2].

Organic brain dysfunction

One of the most widely entertained vulnerability factors for tardive dyskinesia is pre-existing organic brain dysfunction [1,2].

Two studies in rodents have demonstrated that lesions of the frontal cortex result in an elevated baseline level of spontaneous orofacial movements; also, there was a yet greater increase in such movements during or after withdrawal from subsequent long-term neuroleptic treatment [3]. In a recent study [12], methylazoxymethanol-induced cortical brain lesions also resulted in a substantially elevated level of spontaneous orofacial movements; on long-term neuroleptic drug administration, little further increase in orofacial movements was evident, perhaps suggesting the operation of a ceiling effect similar to that considered above in senescence.

Several clinical studies [2] are consistent with the notion that organic brain dysfunction can result in prominent, involuntary buccal-lingual-masticatory movements indistinguishable from the typical tardive dyskinesia evident in comparable patient populations who have received long-term exposure to neuroleptics. Baseline issues are fundamental to our concept of tardive dyskinesia, and appear to influence critically how we interpret the effects of long-term neuroleptic treatment in putative animal models.

References

1. Kane JM and Smith JM (1982) Arch. Gen. Psychiatry 39: 473–481.
2. Waddington JL (1989) Int. Rev. Neurobiol. 31: 297–353.
3. Waddington JL (1990) Psychopharmacology 101: 431–447.
4. Stoessl AJ, Dourish CT and Iversen SD (1989) Psychopharmacology 98: 372–379.
5. Tamminga CA, Dole JM, Goodman L, Kaneda H and Kaneda N (1990) Psychopharmacology 102: 474–478.
6. Glenthoj B, Hemmingsen R, Allerup P and Bolwig TG (1990) Eur. J. Pharmacol. 190: 275–286.
7. Rupniak NMJ, Tye SJ, Steventon MJ, Boyce S and Iversen SD (1990) Mov. Disord. 5: 314–318.
8. Waddington JL and Youssef HA (1988) Br. J. Psychiatry 153: 376–381.
9. Ko GN, Zhang LD, Yan WW et al. (1989) Am. J. Psychiatry 146: 387–389.
10. Waddington JL, Youssef HA and Kinsella A (1990) Psychol. Med. 20: 835–842.
11. Levy AD, See RD, Levin ED and Ellison GD (1987) Life Sci. 41: 1499–1506.
12. Johansson P (1990) Psychopharmacology 100: 72–76.

Biological Psychiatry, Volume 1. G. Racagni et al., editors.

The reliability and significance of cognitive dysfunction in tardive dyskinesia

John L. Waddington

Department of Clinical Pharmacology, Royal College of Surgeons in Ireland, St. Stephen's Green, Dublin 2, Ireland

Introduction

Perhaps the most consistent finding in research on tardive dyskinesia is a general association with increasing age and the most widely considered individual vulnerability factor is pre-existing organic brain dysfunction [1]. Organicity is a heterogeneous concept. The classical literature on organicity in patients with vs. without tardive dyskinesia is inconclusive, but involves multifarious indices in often diagnostically-heterogeneous groups; though systematic studies, often utilizing selected indices in more homogeneous and predominantly schizophrenic populations, are provocative, they remain far from definitive on the issue [1,2]. However, on review [3], the putative index of organicity that has been reported most consistently (but by no means invariably) to distinguish populations of schizophrenic patients with tardive dyskinesia from those without such movement disorder is cognitive dysfunction; of the more recent studies, most [4–7] but not all [8] continue to report similar findings, although no specific or localizing cognitive deficit is apparent. Indeed, this association with tardive dyskinesia is perhaps most evident in older, chronically-ill schizophrenic inpatients whose cognitive function has been evaluated using unsophisticated procedures appropriate for their generally poor level of functioning [3].

Reliability

As not all studies have noted such a relationship, factors which might influence its reliability are of some interest. Most body regions are presumed to be potentially at risk for tardive dyskinesia, but some weight of evidence now suggests that orofacial (i.e. buccal-lingual-masticatory) movements may constitute a "core" syndrome that is pathophysiologically distinct from involuntary movements with other topographies [3]; indeed, 2 studies [9,10] have now indicated that the association between tardive dyskinesia and cognitive dysfunction in schizophrenia may be most evident for, if not exclusive to, involuntary movements with an orificial topography. Thus, including involuntary movements of other body areas in the diagnosis of tardive dyskinesia may obscure what appears to be a specific association with those of the orofacial region.

A further issue is whether such an association is apparent across other diagnostic groups. Though the majority of studies have involved patients with schizophrenia, some similar findings have been reported in those with affective illnesses, particularly bipolar affective disorder, and mental handicap who have been treated with neuroleptics [3]. However, systematic studies in such populations with non-schizophrenic diagnoses are as yet relatively few, and further work is clearly necessary.

Significance

It must be emphasized that studies of these phenomena do not utilize diagnostic instruments, and hence they cannot distinguish per se between neuroleptic-associated tardive dyskinesia and similar involuntary movement disorder(s) with other origins. There is increasing evidence [3] that the baseline level/prevalence of involuntary movements unrelated to neuroleptic exposure may have been underestimated; thus, there remains the possibility that neuroleptics may not so much "cause" tardive dyskinesia as precipitate the emergence of involuntary movements associated with the pathophysiology of the disorder for which neuroleptic treatment was prescribed. If tardive dyskinesia is indeed a neuroleptic-precipitated variant of a covert or overt disease-related movement disorder [3], is there any evidence that such spontaneous dyskinesia may also be associated with cognitive dysfunction? There are few systematic studies on this issue, but compatible data have been reported in neuroleptic-naive patients with chronic schizophrenia [11], Alzheimer's disease [12] and mental handicap [13].

Perhaps the most critical issue is the nature of the putative association between tardive dyskinesia and cognitive dysfunction. Does cognitive impairment imply organic brain changes that might be expected to have arisen before initiation of neuroleptic therapy, and which might therefore constitute a pre-existing vulnerability factor for this disorder on subsequent neuroleptic treatment? The vast majority of studies are cross-sectional in nature, comparing populations of affected with unaffected patients, and little is available in the way of prospective or longitudinal data. In one prospective study of younger, mixed affective and schizophrenic outpatients without involuntary movements [14], poor initial cognitive function was indeed found to be predictive of the subsequent emergence of tardive dyskinesia. In another longitudinal study of older, chronically-ill schizophrenic inpatients without such movement disorder [15], poor initial cognitive dysfunction was not predictive of the subsequent emergence of tardive dyskinesia; however, those patients who went on to develop tardive dyskinesia were distinguished by a selective deterioration in their cognitive function over the same time frame in which their movement disorder emerged, suggesting some close temporal relationship between these two phenomena. It cannot yet be excluded that such cognitive dysfunction is another manifestation, or an epiphenomenon, of the pathophysiological process(es) that underlay tardive dyskinesia, rather than a vulnerability factor for and the harbinger of its later emergence.

Acknowledgement

The author was supported by the Health Research Board of Ireland.

References

1. Kane JM and Smith JM (1982) Arch. Gen. Psychiatry 39: 473–481.
2. Waddington JL (1987) Hum. Psychopharmacol. 2: 11–22.
3. Waddington JL (1989) Int. Rev. Neurobiol. 31: 297–353.
4. Tegeler J, Strauss WH, Luthcke H and Bertling R (1988) Pharmacopsychiatry 21: 308–309.
5. Manschreck TC, Keuthen NJ, Schneyer ML, Celada MT, Laughery J and Collins P (1990) Biol. Psychiatry 27: 150–158.
6. O'Callaghan E, Larkin C, Kinsella A and Waddington JL (1990) Br. J. Psychiatry 157: 578–584.
7. Karson CN, Bracha S, Powell A and Adams A (1990) Am. J. Psychiatry 147: 1646–1649.
8. Gureje O (1988) J. Neurol. Neurosurg. Psychiatry 51: 1525–1530.
9. Waddington JL, Youssef HA, Dolphin C and Kinsella A (1987) Arch. Gen. Psychiatry 44: 907–912.
10. De Wolfe AS, Ryan JJ and Wolf ME (1988) J. Nerv. Ment. Dis. 176: 270–274.
11. Waddington JL and Youssef HA (1990) Br. J. Psychiatry 156: 106–108.
12. Molsa PK, Marttila RJ and Rinne UK (1984) Neurology 34: 1114–1116.
13. Dinan TG and Golden T (1990) Br. J. Psychiatry 157: 131–132.
14. Wegner JT, Kane JM, Weinhold P, Woerner M, Kinon B and Lieberman J (1985) Psychiatr. Res. 16: 331–337.
15. Waddington JL, Youssef HA and Kinsella A (1990) Psychol. Med. 20: 835–842.

Biological Psychiatry, Volume 1. G. Racagni et al., editors.

Essential fatty acids and α-tocopherol supplementation in tardive dyskinesia

K.S. Vaddadi
Larundel Hospital, Plenty Road, Bundoora, Victoria 3083, Melbourne, Australia

Introduction

The prevalence of tardive dyskinesia (TD) in neuroleptic exposed psychiatric population has varied between 5% to 50% [1]. Essential fatty acids (EFAs) which the body cannot make have many important functions such as:
1. maintaining cell membrane structure;
2. being precursors of prostaglandins (PGs) that have neuromodulatory functions;
3. confer on membranes properties like modulating the behaviour of membrane-bound proteins such as receptors, 80 ATPases and ion channels [2].

Due to some of their actions EFAs and PCs have been implicated in the causation of schizophrenia [3]. Open clinical trials and animal model studies have demonstrated the efficacy of EFAs in reducing involuntary movements [4,5].

Clinical studies

A double-blind placebo controlled trial of Efamol (each capsule contains linoleic acid 360 mg, γ-linolenic acid 45 mg, and vitamin E 10 IU) was undertaken in a group of 48 psychiatric patients [6]. There were 81.3% schizophrenic, 5 with bipolar affective disorder and four with personality disorders according to DSM III criteria. These patients had well established tardive dyskinesia. There were 17 diagnostically-matched psychiatric controls without TD and 20 age-matched non-psychiatric controls without abnormal involuntary movements. Regular blood samples were collected to estimate red blood cell (RBC) membrane EFA levels. Patients were rated at regular intervals on Abnormal Involuntary Movements Rating Scale (AIMS) and Comprehensive Psychopathological Rating Scale (CPRS) [7,8]. Patients were given up to 12 capsules of Efamol daily for a period of 16 weeks, following which there was a cross-over to a placebo group. In summary, this trial demonstrated that:

a) patients with severe TD (total AIMS > 12) had lowest levels of RBC membrane N-6 and N-3 series EFAs, when compared with psychiatric controls and normals. Since 81.3% had schizophrenia, the results suggested a close association between low membrane EFA levels, tardive dyskinesia and schizophrenia. The results could not be attributed to dietary factors;

b) Efamol supplementation had significant effect in lowering CPRS scores, thus reflecting a state of clinical improvement;
c) There was no improvement in TD scores;
d) Efamol elevated RBC membrane fatty acid levels.

During the last phase of the trial (4 weeks) after the completion of the double-blind period, that was open, all the patients received active Efamol and two active Efavit tablets (contains ascorbic acid 125 mg, pyridoxine hydrochloride 25 mg, nicotinic acid 7.5 mg and zinc sulphate 4.4 mg). These micronutrients are known co-factors in the metabolism of EFAs to prostaglandin E. The combination of Efamol and Efavit produced significant improvement in TD and in CPRS scores with elevations of both N-6 and N-3 series RBC membrane fatty acids. In another study conducted in Australia, we analysed RBC membrane fatty acids in a younger schizophrenic population with TD. The results were compared with age-matched group of normal controls. Patients were rated on TD Rating Scale [9] and psychiatric status recorded on BPRS (Brief Psychiatric Rating Scale) [10]. Examination of individual EFA levels showed no association with BPRS scores. Within a schizophrenic sample, movement disorder, rather than psychiatric state seemed most related to RBC membrane EFA levels. Subjects were grouped according to their TD status (no TD, mild TD, severe TD). Multivariate analysis of the data showed that age had no significant multivariate effect of EFA levels; however, multivariate tests of significance for the effect of TD status revealed highly significant results. Separate univariate analysis was then performed for each of the nine RBC membrane fatty acids examined, which revealed significant effects of clinical status on γ-linolenic acid (18:3 N-6) and marginally significant effects on α-linolenic acid (18:3 N-3) and arachidonic acid (20:4 N-6). Discriminant function analysis of the complete data for 85 subjects showed that 3 discriminate functions emerged; only one function was significant. This function ordered the groups along a continuum from normal to schizophrenics without TD, schizophrenics with mild TD and schizophrenics with severe TD. This function identified a group with severe TD who had low levels of γ-linolenic acid and elevated levels of 22:5 N-3 and 22:6 N-3 EFAs as most abnormal, and the control group as least abnormal, with high levels of N-6 series (18:3 N-6) and lower levels of N-3 series EFAs (22:5 N-3 and 22:6 N-3).

This study agrees with our previous work showing lower levels of N-6 series EFAs in schizophrenics with TD compared to schizophrenics without TD and normal controls. We also found increased metabolites of N-3 series EFAs in the most disabled group.

α-Tocopherol in tardive dyskinesia

Increased products of lipid peroxidation have been found in the cerebrospinal fluid of patients treated with phenothiazines [11]. Raised catecholamine turnover by neuroleptics may cause increased production of free radicals. These free radicals may destabilise cell membrane and cause structural damage and this may lead to persistent TD [12]. α-Tocopherol (vitamin E) is a membrane soluble antioxidant and protects biological membranes against peroxidation [13].

Due to these properties it has been tried in the treatment of movement disorders such as tardive dyskinesia. In a placebo-controlled study Lohr et al. [12] have shown a mean reduction in the AIMS score of 43% in TD patients when treated with α-tocopherol. Reduction in AIMS score in a smaller sample of TD patients has been reported with the use of α-tocopherol [14].

Discussion

These clinical studies using EFAs and α-tocopherol are very encouraging, and these studies need to be undertaken on larger samples and the duration of treatment period needs to be longer due to the fluctuating nature of TD. In addition, fluctuations in the mental state affect TD ratings. EFAs by getting incorporated into membranes and α-tocopherol with its antioxidant action may have an important preventive role in patients receiving neuroleptics. Prospective clinical trials using both EFA and α-tocopherol in patients receiving neuroleptics need to be undertaken to study their preventive role in TD development.

References

1. Johnson DAW (1988) In: Bebbington P and McGuffin P (eds.) Schizophrenia: The Major Issues. Heinemann Professional Publishing, Oxford pp. 158–171.
2. Horrobin DF and Manku MS (1990) In: Horrobin DF (ed.) Omega-6 Essential Fatty Acids: Pathophysiology and Roles in Clinical Medicine. A.R. Liss, New York, pp. 21–23.
3. Horrobin DF, Ally AI, Karmal RA and Manku MS (1978) Psychol. Med. 8: 43–8.
4. Vaddadi KS (1984) IRCS Med. Sci. 12: 678.
5. Costall B, Kelly E and Naylor RJ (1984) Br. J. Pharmacol. 83: 733–740.
6. Vaddadi KS, Courtney P, Gilleard CJ, Manku MS and Horrobin DF (1989) 27: 313–323.
7. Guy W (ed.) (1976) ECDEU Assesment Manual For Psychopharmacology. Publication ADM 76-338 Washington D.C., U.S. Dept. of Health, Education, and Welfare, pp. 534–537.
8. Asberg M, Montgomery S, Perris C, Schalling D and Sedvall G (1978) Acta Psychiatr. Scand. (Suppl.) 271: 5–27.
9. Simpson GM, Lee JH, Zoubok B and Gardos G (1979) Psychopharmacology 64: 171–179.
10. Overall JE and Gorham DR (1962) Psychol. Rep. 10: 799–812.
11. Pall HS, Williams AC, Blake DR and Lunec J (1987) 1: 596–599.
12. Lohr JB, Cadet JL, Lohr MA, Larson L, Wasli E, Wade L, Hylton R, Vidoni C, Jeste D and Wyatt RJ (1988) Schizophr. Bull. 14(2): 291–296.
13. Van Gossum A, Kurian R, Whitwell J and Jeejeebhoy KN (1988) Clin. Nutr. 7: 53–57.
14. Elkashef AM, Ruskin PE, Bacher N and Barrett D (1990) Am. J. Psychiatry 147: 4, 505–506.

Biological Psychiatry, Volume 1. G. Racagni et al., editors.

Nicotine and tardive dyskinesia

Darrell G. Kirch, Lauren L. Wing, Rena Li and Richard Jed Wyatt
Schizophrenia Research Branch and Neuropsychiatry Branch, National Institute of Mental Health, 5600 Fishers Lane, Room 10-105, Rockville, MD 20857, U.S.A.

Introduction

While there has been long-standing research interest in the psychophysiologic effects of nicotine and their relationship to smoking behavior, only recently has attention turned toward possible associations between smoking and psychiatric disorders. In one of the first studies to examine the prevalence of smoking among psychiatric patients, schizophrenic patients were noted to have a prevalence of smoking nearly 3 times that observed in the general adult population [1]. Among patients with schizophrenia, moreover, there appears to be a higher prevalence of smoking among patients with tardive dyskinesia (TD) than those who do not have TD [2–4]. This finding is of neurochemical significance because TD is hypothesized to involve nigrostriatal dopamine (DA) hyperactivity. In contrast, Parkinson's disease, a disorder associated with hypofunction of striatal DA neurotransmission, has been observed to be less likely to occur among smokers [5]. While a direct causal link between smoking status and TD or Parkinson's disease has not been established, these observations do present compelling reasons to study further the effects of nicotine on brain DA function.

Nicotine and central nervous system dopamine

Nicotine is a drug with complex pharmacologic properties that acts on multiple neurotransmitter systems in the brain [6]. While studies have indicated that acute doses of nicotine stimulate the release of DA, our own data in rats administered nicotine over 3 weeks using osmotic mini-pumps showed nicotine at a dose of 12 mg/kg/day to decrease striatal DA turnover [7]. Other studies of chronic administration reported a similar decrease in DA turnover in contrast to the acute effect of increased DA release [8].

Studies of post-synaptic effects of nicotine have yielded conflicting results. We found no effect of chronic nicotine (again at 12 mg/kg/day) on either D_1 or D_2 DA receptors in rat striatum [9]. Other investigators noted an apparent super-sensitivity of DA receptors after chronic nicotine administration [8], while one group reported that chronic nicotine, when combined with haloperidol, blocked the development of haloperidol-induced supersensitivity among DA receptors [10]. Therefore, while it is clear that nicotine interacts significantly with the DA system, it is not possible at this point to state conclusively how chronic nicotine exposure might affect DA function in order to be positively associated with TD. Neither of the most obvious possibilities, an increase in DA release or an increase in DA receptor supersensitivity, has been conclusively proven to occur with chronic nicotine administration.

Possible role of other neurotransmitters

It is important to note that nicotine affects multiple other central neurotransmitters in a fashion which might be relevant to the association between smoking and TD. For example, nicotine has been shown to have effects on norepinephrine, serotonin and various peptides [6,7]. It also is possible that the association between smoking and TD relates to other compounds. Smokers have higher blood levels of carbon monoxide, a substance that might alter oxidative mechanisms in the brain and be relevant to the progression of neurotoxic damage. We have preliminary data (unpublished) which indicates that schizophrenic patients who consume larger amounts of nicotine are also prone to consume greater amounts of caffeine. In a study of chronic caffeine administration we found that caffeine caused a decrease in rat striatal DA metabolites [11]. Caffeine, an adenosine antagonist, also affects the gamma-aminobutyric acid system (GABA). GABA is a neurotransmitter which some observers have thought might be involved in the development of TD.

Conclusions

This is an area of research characterized by preliminary findings. It is important that larger epidemiologic studies be done in order to confirm not only whether there is indeed a positive association between smoking and TD, but also whether specific clinical subtypes of patients are involved in this association. More research is needed regarding the interactions between nicotine and brain neurotransmitters, not only DA, but also norepinephrine, serotonin and GABA. This research will require the development of animal models which more closely parallel nicotine consumption in humans who smoke, i.e, frequent acute doses of nicotine in the context of chronic administration and tolerance. Such studies not only have the prospect of better defining the relationship between smoking and abnormal movements, but also may provide clues to the biological basis for nicotine dependence.

References

1. Hughes JR, Hatsukami DK, Mitchell JE and Dahlgren LA (1986) Am. J. Psychiatry 143: 993–997.
2. Yassa R, Lal S, Korpassy A and Ally J (1987) Biol. Psychiatry 22: 67–72.
3. Binder RL, Kazamatsuri H, Nishimura T and McNeil DE (1987) Biol. Psychiatry 22: 1280–1282.

4. Kirch DG, Alho A and Wyatt RJ (1988) Cell. Molecular Neurobiol. 3: 285–291.
5. Baron JA (1986) Neurology 36: 1490–1496.
6. Benowitz NL (1986) Ann. Rev. Med. 37: 21–32.
7. Kirch DG, Gerhardt GA, Shelton RC, Freedman R and Wyatt RJ (1987) Clin. Neuropharmacol. 10: 376–383.
8. Fung YK and Lau YS (1989) Pharmacol. Biochem. Behav. 32: 221–226.
9. Kirch D, Taylor T, Creese I, Xu S-X and Wyatt R (1991) (submitted).
10. Prasad C, Spahn SA and Ikegami H (1989) Biochem. Biophys. Res. Commun. 159: 48–52.
11. Kirch D, Taylor T, Gerhardt G, Benowitz N, Stephen C and Wyatt R (1990) Neuropharmacology 29: 599–602.

Biological Psychiatry, Volume 1. G. Racagni et al., editors.

Diabetes mellitus and tardive dyskinesia

Sukdeb Mukherjee, Ravinder Reddy and David B. Schnur
Department of Clinical Neuropsychiatry, The New York State Psychiatric Institute, 722 West 168th Street, Box 72, New York, NY 10032, U.S.A.

Although numerous studies across decades have found increased rates of impaired glucose tolerance and diabetes mellitus in patients with various neuropsychiatric disorders (see [1] for a review), the implications of this association for an understanding of neuropsychiatric disease processes or their complications has remained unclear. Following reports of high rates of impaired glucose tolerance in patients with Parkinson's disease, therapeutic trials were initiated with hypoglycemic agents. These did not yield consistent results and interest in this issue was lost because of the lack of ideas as to what implication it might have for an understanding of the neurological disease process.

In 1985 we proposed that abnormal glucose metabolism may be associated with an increased risk of tardive dyskinesia (TD) in neuroleptic-treated psychiatric patients [2]. This view was based on a series of incidental findings during our investigations of TD:

1. In two separate study populations, the proportion of TD patients who also had been diagnosed as having non-insulin-dependent diabetes mellitus (NIDDM) was greater than that expected from known rates in the general population.
2. A disproportionately large number of TD patients also had a positive family history of NIDDM.
3. On the average, fasting blood glucose level was significantly higher among TD patients than in non-TD patients, a difference that remained significant even after controlling for the variance due to age and sex.
4. Additionally, we found 15 (75%) of 20 diabetic neuroleptic-treated patients to manifest TD [3], a rate that is considerably higher than that reported previously in any group.

Using a within-subject, repeated measures, on-off haloperidol design we examined the effects of haloperidol on glucose tolerance in 15 chronic schizophrenic patients. There was no main effect of either TD or time (on or off haloperidol), but there was a significant TD × time interaction effect on post-load glucose level, with decreased glucose tolerance in TD patients, but improved glucose tolerance in non-TD patients [4]. A positive family history of NIDDM also predicted the presence of TD independent of neuroleptic effects on glucose tolerance. This was particularly intriguing since all patients in this study were younger than 45 years of age and none was diabetic.

Our initial finding of a relation between diabetes mellitus and TD [2–4] was recently replicated in a controlled study by an independent group, who found 79%

of elderly diabetic neuroleptic-treated patients to have TD, in contrast to 53% of non-diabetic patients who were matched with the former group on age, sex and neuroleptic exposure; the difference was statistically highly significant [5]. Surprisingly, they also found a high rate of dyskinesias (21%) in diabetic subjects who had never received neuroleptics, thereby raising the possibility that diabetes may be associated with an elevated rate of spontaneous dyskinesia, and thus contribute to high rates of TD by an additive effect.

In chronic schizophrenic patients it is difficult to determine whether impaired glucose tolerance is due to the coincident presence of NIDDM, or a consequence of the psychotic disease process and its treatment (e.g., with neuroleptics), or sedentary life style and institutional diet with attendant obesity. Since NIDDM is known to be influenced strongly by genetic factors, we undertook a systematic investigation of family history of NIDDM in these schizophrenic patients. The findings have been reported previously [6]. The patients were all younger than 45 years of age and none were diabetic. Of the 140 parents of 70 patients in the study, 20 were excluded for not having reached or having died before the age of 50 years. Fourteen (12%) of the 120 parents were diagnosed as having NIDDM, a rate higher than that expected from known rates in the population. In only one instance were both parents affected. Of the 57 patients who did not have an affected parent, 9 had a grandparent diagnosed as having NIDDM. Thus, across 2 generations, 22 (31%) of the 70 patients had a positive family history of NIDDM and could be assumed to be at risk for developing NIDDM.

It deserves reiteration that in two independent samples we found evidence of a relation between TD and family history of NIDDM in young subjects who themselves were not diabetic. This raises the fundamental question: is the increased risk of TD due to metabolic consequences of the diabetic state, or an effect of underlying genetic factors that antedate and may even be independent of the development of clinical diabetes? Our findings suggest the latter as the more likely explanation. It is noteworthy that, in the study by Ganzini et al. [5], in which a robust association between TD and diabetes was noted, all the neuroleptic-treated diabetic patients had NIDDM and could therefore be presumed to be insulin-resistant. Incidentally, the rate of depression in NIDDM patients has been found to be several-fold higher than in the general population and a high rate of insulin resistance has been found in non-diabetic patients with major depression, who are also more likely than others to develop TD if treated for long periods of time with neuroleptics.

Emerging evidence on the pathogenesis of NIDDM suggests that, early in the course of the disease, there is insulin resistance with peripheral glucose disposal maintained in the normal range by compensatory hyperinsulinemia, the failure of which results in the diabetic state with its characteristic hyperglycemia. Insulin sensitivity is, to a large degree, determined genetically, although it can also be influenced by other factors, such as obesity. Considering our finding of a relation between family history of NIDDM and TD, it is likely that this effect is mediated by insulin resistance. The emerging evidence indicates that some conditions, such as hypertension and coronary artery disease, that traditionally were regarded as complications of diabetes are, in fact, consequences of insulin resistance, rather than due to hyperglycemia. We add to the list a lowered threshold for developing specific neurological disorders.

Insulin resistance in most cases is due to postreceptor binding defects that result in defective intracellular signal transmission. Although most studies have focused on the effect of this defect on glucoregulatory processes, there is considerable evidence that, particularly in nerve cells, insulin is involved in a variety of actions that are unrelated to glucoregulation. These involve activation of immediate early genes (e.g., c-fos), activation of enzymes of intermediary metabolism (e.g., pyruvate dehydrogenase) and other specific enzymes, such as choline acetyltransferase, promoting neurite outgrowth and survival and maintaining the Na^+/K^+ pump, to mention but a few. At this early stage of the investigation it is difficult even to speculate on a particular cascade of insulin-dependent metabolic events the deregulation of which could lower the threshold for the development and expression of disorders as apparently disparate as parkinsonism, tardive dyskinesia, depression, Huntington's chorea, or schizophrenia. It has recently been proposed that a primary defect of brain insulin action may be involved in the pathology of Alzheimer's disease.

We hypothesize that insulin resistance with consequent inefficiency of insulin action results in the deregulation of normal physiological defensive and compensatory mechanisms and thereby has a permissive effect on the development of neurological and psychiatric syndromes. The nature of the clinical syndrome is determined by other factors that are independent of insulin actions. The high concentration of insulin receptors in the limbic and striatal regions of the brain may offer a clue as to why insulin resistance is associated with certain neurological disorders, but not others.

In 1899 Sir Henry Maudsley in "The Pathology of Mind" wrote that "Diabetes is a disease which often shows itself in families in which insanity prevails." Our studies indicate that the observations of this astute clinician, which have been virtually ignored during almost 100 years of research, may indeed be valid and worthy of systematic investigation. The marked advances from diabetes research and studies of the molecular basis of insulin actions now offer concepts and tools with which to attack this problem and it would be a detriment to our patients should we continue to ignore this phenomenon. In reviewing the evidence, Adamo et al. [7] noted: "In summary, insulin affects metabolism in the brain by stimulating glucose uptake into glial cells, activating pyruvate dehydrogenase, as well as stimulating protein and lipid synthesis. These effects are seen with nanomolar concentrations of insulin and thus, are probably mediated by insulin receptors. In addition to these metabolic effects, insulin may play an important role as a neuromodulator or neurotransmitter in the central nervous system. Finally, a role of insulin in brain growth and development is suggested by the effects of insulin on synaptogenesis and neurite formation." We would encourage active pursuit of research on the role of brain insulin actions in health, as well as in the development of neuropsychiatric disorders.

References

1. Wilkinson DG (1981) Br. J. Psychiatry 138: 1–9.
2. Mukherjee S et al. (1985) Arch. Gen. Psychiatry 42: 205.
3. Mukherjee S et al. (1986) Arch. Gen. Psychiatry 43: 193.
4. Mukherjee S et al. (1989) Psychiatr. Res. 29: 17–27.
5. Ganzini L et al.(1991) Arch. Gen. Psychiatry 48: 259–263.
6. Mukherjee S et al. (1989) Lancet i: 495.
7. Adamo M et al. (1989) Mol. Neurobiol. 3: 72–100.

Biological Psychiatry, Volume 1. G. Racagni et al., editors.

The subjective awareness of movement disorders

Pierluigi Scapicchio, Paolo Decina and Giovanni Caracci
S.M. Immacolata Hospital, Guidonia, Italy and the Research Division at door Psychiatric Center, Queens Village, New York, New York, U.S.A.

Introduction

The well established finding that a majority of chronic schizophrenics with tardive dyskinesia (TD) are often not aware of their abnormal movements has received little research attention despite its intrinsic interest and possible importance [1–5]. A basic issue is whether the unawareness of motor defect is specific to the TD symptom complex and should be regarded as an anosognosia. Relevant clinical questions are how firm and stable this unawareness is and whether it is responsive to clinical intervention. The studies reported here address these issues by examining the relations of unawareness with type of movement disorders (i.e. TD and tremor) and with the affective and cognitive statuses of the individuals affected, and by testing the temporal stability of unawareness in relation to enhancement by advisement procedures.

Study 1 – Differential lack of awareness of movement disorders

The main aims of this study [6] were: a) to determine whether the lack of awareness of movement disorders is limited to dyskinesia, or includes also neuroleptic-induced parkinsonian (NIP) tremor; and b) to examine the relation of unawareness to cognitive impairment.

Methods

The study group comprised 18 chronic schizophrenic inpatients with TD according to research criteria (RD-TD) [4] and 17 with NIP tremor, i.e. tremor and one or more cardinal signs of parkinsonism. After an initial interview to evaluate insight of patients into their illness, standardized examinations [7,8] were conducted to assess type and severity of involuntary movements, as well as cognitive function with a 10-question mental test evaluating the basic functions of orientation and immediate memory [9]. Two raters blind to the study hypothesis attended the procedure and independently rated each subject's awareness of both psychiatric illness and abnormal movements. The former was rated as being present or absent, and the latter was evaluated using a three-point scale, with three indicating full awareness of the presence and bodily distribution of movements, two indicating incomplete or inconsistent awareness, and one indicating a complete lack of awareness.

Results

Patients presenting with NIP tremor were significantly more aware of their motor defect than patients with TD. Only 24% of patients with tremor were completely unaware of their movements, compared to 78% of patients with dyskinesia. Lack of awareness of involuntary movements was not related to cognitive impairment, severity scores of motor deficits (tremor and global TD), or insight into psychiatric disorders.

Study 2 – Awareness among manic and schizophrenic patients

The aims of the study were: a) to examine whether schizophrenic patients are more aware than bipolars; and b) whether this may be attributable to a greater severity of affective blunting.

Methods

The sample comprised 57 schizophrenic and 18 manic patients with RD-TD who were admitted to a research unit for participation in discrete and largely unrelated protocols. While raters were not blind to diagnosis at the time of the clinical assessments, there was no a priori objective to compare the diagnostic group on awareness of involuntary movements or affective blunting. Clinical assessments were completed during routine baseline data collection, and these included standardized neurological examinations [7,8] and psychiatric assessments [10] from which the measure of affective blunting was extracted.

Results

Schizophrenic patients were significantly less aware of their dyskinetic movements than bipolars (79% vs. 44%). Among those variables differentiating the two diagnostic groups, only affective blunting was significantly associated with lack of awareness.

Study 3 – Stability of unawareness and effects of advisement procedures

The aims of the study were: a) to determine whether schizophrenic patients are able to understand and retain information relevant to the risk of developing TD; and b) to establish whether verbal or visual feedback to patients would enhance their subjective awareness and, if so, whether the improved awareness would be maintained at follow-up.

Methods

The sample comprised 20 chronic schizophrenic inpatients with RD-TD who, just before the study, had been previously briefed on the risk of TD and their involuntary movement status. Upon initiating the study, the patients were first asked if they had ever heard of TD. They were then subjected to a standardized neurological examination [7,8]. After that, the patients were interviewed to assess their awareness of movements. When a patient denied awareness of, or incompletely described, the involuntary movements, these were described to the patient (verbal feedback) and awareness was reassessed. If lack of awareness persisted, the patient was asked to stand in front of a mirror, the movements were pointed out (visual feedback), and awareness was again reassessed. At each step, two raters independently rated awareness using the same three-point scale described in study 1. Awareness of the presence and localization of movements was reassessed two weeks after the initial evaluation. All patients were in a stable clinical state across the two evaluations.

At initial evaluation only 25% of the patients knew about TD and were fully aware of their movement disorder. Both verbal and visual feedback resulted in significant immediate enhancement of awareness. Although patients were able to learn about their involuntary movements, there was impaired retention and recall of the learned information after 2 weeks, with a return to prefeedback baseline levels.

Discussion

Taken together, the findings of these three studies suggest that unawareness of the motor manifestations of TD is a relatively stable, partially improvable condition that, rather than being secondary to an impairment of cognition, is a specific correlate of the TD symptom complex associated with emotional blunting. Thus, unawareness of TD may be properly regarded as an anosognosia. The findings also underscore the need for developing methods that will enhance the insight of patients into their disabilities and allow them to participate more meaningfully in their own treatment.

References

1. Alexopoulos GS (1979) J. Nerv. Ment. Dis. 167: 125–127.
2. Caracci G, Mukherjee S, Roth SD and Decina P (1990) Am. J. Psychiatry 147: 295–298.

3. Myslobodsky MS, Tomer R, Holden NT, Kempler S and Sigal M (1985) J. Nerv. Ment. Dis. 173: 156–160.
4. Rosen AM, Mukherjee S, Olarte S, Varia V and Cardenas CC (1982) Am. J. Psychiatry 139: 372–373.
5. Smith JM, Kucharski LT, Oswald WT and Waterman LJ (1979) Am. J. Psychiatry 136: 918–922.
6. Decina P, De Bonis C, Saraceni F, Scapicchio P and Mukherjee S (1991) Differential lack of awareness of involuntary movements in chronic schizophrenic patients. Biol. Psychiatry (submitted).
7. Guy W (1976) ECDEU Assessment Manual for Psychopharmacology. U.S. Public Health Service, U.S. Government Printing Office, Wahington D.C., pp. 534–537.
8. Simpson G, Lee J, Zoubok B, Cole JO and Gardos G (1979) Psychopharmacology 64: 171–179.
9. Waddington JL and Youssef HA (1986) Am. J. Psychiatry 143: 1162–1165.
10. Andreasen NC (1982) The scale for assessment of negative symptoms. University of Iowa, Iowa City.
11. Schooler N and Kane JM (1982) Arch. Gen. Psychiatry 39: 486–487.

Stress, anxiety and personality disorders: Pathophysiology, biology and treatment issues

Biological Psychiatry, Volume 1. G. Racagni et al., editors.

A disorder of selective attention in post-traumatic stress disorder

A.C. McFarlane and C.R. Clark

University of Adelaide, Department of Psychiatry, Hillcrest Hospital, P.O. Box 233, Greenacres, SA 5086, Australia

Introduction

There has only been relatively recent interest in the nature of the disordered arousal that makes up the Group D diagnostic criteria of post-traumatic stress disorder (PTSD) [1]. Most of this work focused on the pattern of arousal in response to stimuli resembling the original traumatic experience. However, clinical experience dictates that sufferers have a disordered pattern of arousal in many non-specific situations.

In particular, disturbed concentration 8 months after a disaster was the one symptom that predicted the continued presence of PTSD 3 years later in a group of high risk firefighters [2].

The role of these attention-related phenomena was specifically investigated in this group by a series of questions focusing on distractibility. Factor analysis was used to characterize the pattern or grouping of phenomena incorporated in the existing diagnostic criteria. The first factor was characterized by a disturbance of attention suggesting that these impairments best distinguish people with PTSD from those who do not have the disorder. The findings from this study are supported by several other factor analytical studies [3,4].

This phenomenological observation may provide some insight into some of the proposed neurobiological abnormalities in PTSD, particularly in relation to the role of noradrenaline, which is the focus of this presentation and dopamine.

There is a growing body of work that has examined the psychobiology of the trauma response and PTSD which has focused on the biological substrates of arousal and, in particular, the locus caeruleus with its widespread cortical projections [1]. It has been proposed that much of the phenomenology of PTSD can be explained by a loss of the modulatory role of this system [1]. Both MAO inhibitors and tricylic antidepressants which affect locus caeruleus activity have been found to decrease the effects of unavoidable shock in animals [5], an experimental paradigm for PTSD.

An important omission from much of the discussion about the neurobiology of PTSD has been a corresponding examination of the role of noradrenaline in attention. A sizeable body of work accumulated during the 1980s provides evidence for a crucial role of central noradrenaline (NA) in attention [6]. Electrophysiological studies on the activity of cells of the locus caeruleus have indicated a role in the orienting of attention.

Against this background, there is a convergence of interest arising from phenomenological observations about a disturbance of attention as being the primary abnormality in PTSD, from the role of noradrenaline as a central neurotransmitter in the process of selective attention and from disturbances of noradrenergic functioning in PTSD.

In summary, the sorts of attentional problems which seem to be implicit in PTSD are an impairment in discrimination of relevant from irrelevant information and increased distractibility. The methodology of event-related potentials provides a means of examining these issues. This study aimed to investigate the attentional process in patients with PTSD by examining their responses to neutral stimuli, i.e. stimuli not reminiscent of the primary trauma.

Methodology and Results

A three-tone, auditory discrimination task was chosen [7]. This task tested both the subjects' ability to discriminate an infrequent target stimulus and to avoid being distracted by the other stimuli that were irrelevant, one of which occurred frequently and the other infrequently.

Nine outpatients diagnosed under the DSM III criteria as having PTSD using a standardized interview were included in the study. Ten control subjects were matched for age, a premorbid intelligence quotient and years of education. Subjects were also matched for the time of day of testing and sex.

The subjects were tested on two occasions approximately one month apart. The timing of the PTSD groups second testing was determined by their clinical response to the tricylic antidepressant, dothiepin.

Analysis of these 4 components from the PTSD group pretreatment, showed no abnormality in either the N_1 or N_2 component relative to controls. There was, however, a significant lack of a clear parietal focus to the target tone ($F[1,17] = 4.43$, $P < 0.05$), with P_3 amplitude depressed at Pz relative to controls (Tukey, $P < 0.05$). In addition, P_3 latency was abnormally long ($F[1,17] = 5.70$, $P < 0.05$), particularly to the distractor tone (Tukey, $P < 0.05$). Following treatment these effects diminished, with the PTSD group showing a close to normal profile for P_3 amplitude and latency. A pretreatment abnormality in the topography in the slope of the slow wave, however, persisted following treatment ($F[1,17] = 4.22$, $P < 0.05$).

A cross-correlation of ERP and behavioural measurements with clinical scale scores for the PTSD group revealed three significant relationships, all post-treatment: a negative correlation between P_3 amplitude to the distractor tone at the Pz site and the Intrusion Subscale of the Impact of Events Scale [8] ($r(7) = 0.88$, $P < 0.01$); a positive correlation between N_2 amplitude to the distractor tone at Fz and the measure of anxiety state ($r(7) = 0.85$, $P < 0.01$); and a positive correlation between reaction time to targets and avoidance ($r(7) = 0.85$, $P < 0.01$). There was no difference between groups, on either testing occasion, in either speed or accuracy of target detection.

Discussion and Conclusion

These data should be recognised as preliminary findings of a small pilot study on the disturbances of cognitive processing in PTSD traumatic stress disorder. These early data suggest that there is a change in the scalp topography of a number of cognitive components (P_3, slow wave) of the ERP in PTSD. This may indicate an abnormality in the coordination or timing of component generator activity within the neocortex.

The finding that P_3 latency was abnormally long to distractors in the PTSD subjects prior to treatment indicates that in PTSD the sufferers are taking longer than normal to evaluate the significance of irrelevant, distracting stimuli [9]. In the same vein, the reduced amplitude in the P_3 to targets indicates a less efficient or diminished allocation of processing resources to significant stimuli. Following treatment, however, these abnormalities appear to have been largely overcome. The significance of the slow wave component of the ERP is less certain. It has been suggested [10] that it may reflect a late, perhaps final, stage of evaluation associated with the cognitive processing of incoming information.

The use of the ERPs to investigate the attentional processes in PTSD would appear to be a promising technique. The unusual wave form patterns observed in these patients suggested that there was a significant information processing problem in these people even to affectively neutral tones. In this regard, it was of particular interest that in these patients the P_3 amplitude was inversely correlated with the intrusions score of the Impact of Events Scale. This suggested that intrusion may be associated with an increased sensitivity to the rapid evaluation of the significance of stimuli. In contrast, avoidance was correlated with reaction time, suggesting a tendency to shut out incoming stimuli. Thus, there was a preliminary suggestion that intrusion and avoidance may be reflective of response pattern characteristics other than phenomena specifically related to the trauma. The fact that the abnormalities in P_3 amplitude and latency were no longer present following treatment of PTSD sufferers with prothiaden, suggests that this drug may have some effect on correcting this information processing problem in PTSD.

References

1. Kolb LC (1989) Physiologic. Med. 19: 821–824.
2. McFarlane AC (1988) J. Nerv. Ment. Dis. 176: 22–29.
3. Silver SM and Iacono CU (1984) J. Clin. Psychol. 40: 5–14.
4. Pynoos RS, Frederick C, Nader K, Arroyo W, Steinberg A, Eth S, Nunez F and Fairbanks L (1987) Arch. Gen. Psychiatry 44: 1057–1063.

5. Martin P, Soubrie P and Simon P (1987) Prog. Neuro-Psychopharmacol. Biol. Psychiatry 11: 1–11.
6. Clark CR, Geffen GM and Geffen LB (1989) Neuropsychologia 27(2): 131–139.
7. Pfefferbaum A, Ford JM, Winegrat BG, Roth WT and Kopell BS (1984) Electroencephalogr. Clin. Neurophysiol. 59: 85–103.
8. Horowitz M, Wilner M and Alverez W (1979) Psychosom. Med. 41: 209–218.
9. Hillyard SA and Kutas M (1983) Ann. Rev. Neurosci. 34: 33–61.
10. Ruchkin DS, Sutton S, Kietzman ML and Silver K (1983) Electroencephalogr. Clin. Neurophysiol. 50: 35–47.

Biological Psychiatry, Volume 1. G. Racagni et al., editors.

Specific psychophysiological diagnosis in post-traumatic stress disorder

B. Raphael and D. Cumes-Rayner

Interest in, and understanding of PTSD has expanded rapidly in the past decade, with studies covering a wide range of traumatically stressful circumstances, from combat, to major disasters, rape to armed hold-up [1]. Questions have arisen about diagnosis and the role of the stressor event in the development of the disorder. These queries and their answers may have wide implications for prevention, treatment and even for litigation.

Diagnoses are made in terms of clinical judgement – whether or not the phenomena described by the patient, and observed by the clinician, meet diagnostic criteria, for instance as per DSM III-R [2].

Recently Watson [3] reviewed psychometric measurement techniques that could be used to assist diagnosis or quantify symptoms. He concluded that, of the 12 measures he considered, few had comprehensive reliability assessments, or establishment of concurrent validity, especially for non-clinic populations. Keane's Mississipi Scale for Combat-Related PTSD [4], Spitzer and Williams Structured Clinical Interview for DSM IV PTSD [5] and his own PTSD Interview (I) [6] were the measures of choice in terms of current developments.

Clearly difficulties arise because many measures and studies have related to combat induced PTSD and studies with Vietnam veterans and their degree of generalisability to other situations may not be established. Degrees of symptomatology present and effects on function are relevant to diagnosis. Post-traumatic phenomena such as intrusive memories and even some nightmares may occur occasionally for many years after an event, but their occurrence does not necessarily indicate disorder. McFarlane's studies of such phenomena in volunteer fire fighters illustrates the ubiquity of many intrusive memories which may only lead to, or be associated with, disorder in a relatively small proportion of those who experience them [7]. Early after a traumatic experience many, if not most of those exposed will experience some such phenomena but they will settle within a relatively short period of time and hence not reach criteria of deviation for diagnosis of disorder (1 month [2]).

A number of recent publications have looked at biological approaches to the diagnosis of PTSD. Petman et al. [8] studied psychophysiological assessment of Vietnam veterans using visual imagery associated with an individualised autobiographical traumatic anecdote. Blanchard et al. [9] studied psychophysiological arousal after exposure to audiotapes of combat sounds. More recently they have shown that five heart rate parameters can correctly discriminate 75% of a sample of

Vietnam veterans into those with and without PTSD and that adding 10 blood pressure parameters, increased discrimination to 80% [10]. Other parameters did not increase discrimination. Cross-validation in a new sample showed 83% correct discrimination [10] during the audiotape procedure which involved gunfire, helicopter and screams. Visual stimuli have also been used in such studies, for instance, footage from the movie "Platoon" [11].

Friedman's valuable 1991 review [11] has summarised the biological factors found to be relevant for diagnosis after surveying a number of different studies in the field. He discusses groupings of: sympathetic nervous system hyper-arousal; hypofunction of the hypothalamic – pituitary – chronocortial axis; abnormality of the endogenous opiate system; sleep abnormalities. He concludes that, in terms of the current state of knowledge, "*the best and most specific biological diagnostic test for PTSD is psychophysiological assessment*" [11] (p. 74). The techniques which use traumatogenic stimuli are sensitive and powerful, and are likely to be more so, the more specific and individualised the stimulus (e.g. specific experiences of the individual such as used by Pitman [3]).

Specific diagnosis in PTSD

While the above studies are helpful in establishing a diagnostic framework it is important to realise that they have, for the most part, derived from veteran (Vietnam) populations and their generalisability to other PTSDs is yet to be determined. Furthermore, whether or not psychophysiological measures can be used to validate a "real" as opposed to fictitious illness (malingering) is by no means clear and may have relevance not only for the patient's care, but for the legal consequences (e.g. possibilities for litigation).

Another related issue of great importance is whether, when a number of stressors have been experienced, it can be determined if one or other of these is responsible for the development of disorder. Such traumata may have occurred multiply, at the one time, or sequentially, or even over a relatively long period. While the clinical picture (e.g. the specific intrusive memories or nightmares) may indicate the likely aetiological agent, it seems psychophysiological responsiveness patterns could add further in identifying which elements are most significant. This may be particularly relevant to Vietnam veterans, who are for instance, subsequently exposed to other traumatogenic stimuli – to name one group.

A further consideration is as to whether or not psychophysiological measures could help to identify the stress or experience and its consequences when denial and avoidance predominate. Traumatic amnesia, repression and dissociation may all cloud this picture and psychophysiological responsiveness suspected traumatogenic material might be a valuable indicator. Effects of disclosure [12] are also relevant and whether or not they are associated with diminished arousal, or arousal during disclosure, may be important diagnostically as well as providing guidance for therapy.

The relationship between such overwhelmingly stressful experiences and physical morbidity is also relevant. This suggests pathways to adverse health outcomes ranging from sudden death through to cardiovascular and cerebrovascular episodes, hypertension and so forth. Attempts to dampen arousal may also be associated with substance abuse that is a frequent co-morbidity pattern and other adverse health practices contributing to somatic co-morbidity [13].

Finally, the legal implications of identifying the specific stressor must be considered. This might facilitate conclusions as to the relative contribution of a specific stressor effect. However the validity of this approach requires much further development and research study [11].

Psychophysiological reactivity and specific stimuli in post-traumatic stress disorder

Cumes-Rayner [14,15] has evolved techniques for measuring blood pressure reactivity in relation to disclosure and to other circumstances including perceived stressful life experiences. She uses a Dinamap 845 vital signs monitor which provides readings of systolic, diastolic, mean arterial pressure and pulse measurements which have been shown to be reliable [16] and correlate highly (0.8) with intra-arterial measures [17]. Testing takes place with measures across one hour. These include:

a) familiarisation with machine and test situation;
b) relaxed casual measurement (no vocalisation);
c) emotive events recall (one or more readings), including the perceived traumatic events and other situations (these may be either vocalised or visualised);
d) comparative stressor response: an *unrelated* event remembered as having been emotive;
e) control for vocalisation: reading aloud of non-emotive material (and some pressure of speech as emotive events recall);
f) final measurement with or without relaxation instructions.

The instructions are presented hypnoidally to enhance focus on recall. The measurement should occur 40–60 s into the reporting or visualisation process [15]. The use of this procedure in PTSD is also supported by Ramsay [18]. Elevations of 10–20 mmHg are considered to be indicative of reactivity to a stressor. The differential meaning of systolic, diastolic and mean arterial pressure changes is currently being investigated [14,15].

Clinical and psychophysiological diagnosis exploring specific aetiological factors is presented in 2 case studies.

Case 1 – Mr. A.

Mr. A. was in his early 40s. He had had a relatively happy childhood, although a somewhat critical father. There was no personal or family history of psychiatric disorder. He had seen active service including combat in Vietnam, when he entered the army at about the age of 19 years. Although he had had a number of life-threatening experiences in combat, he denied that these had had any long-term effects on him and he viewed his experience generally as positive and maturing. After leaving the army he applied for training as an air traffic controller. He had been successful and had worked happily in his chosen profession until 10 months prior to his presentation. He was happily married with 2 young children.

Approximately 10 months earlier he had witnessed a mid-air collision of 2 small planes. He had been on duty at the time, but had just left the tower briefly, with one of his colleagues in charge, to carry out other legitimate and required activities. As he returned he saw the collision and tried to stop it, but was too late. All the men were immediately taken off duty as was practice, and a full review occurred. He was fully exonerated in this. However, with his return to work in the weeks that followed, he experienced increasing difficulties.

He had to keep checking to make sure everything was safe. His concentration was poor. He was increasingly anxious every time he went to his work situation, although he felt alright away from it (i.e. non-anxious). He felt his work-mates blamed him for what had happened and became oversensitive to any of their comments. He had increasing difficulties sleeping, with some non-specific nightmares filled with threat and fear. He had lost interest in his usual activities and withdrawn not only from friends, but also from his wife and children. He was drinking heavily to try to deal with his distress. His work situation deteriorated, and even despite several periods of time off, he felt he was unable to continue. He was irritable and jumpy and constantly fearful that more terrible things would happen.

Clinical assessment

Clinical assessment indicated a considerable level of denial, despite the above symptoms. He said he had always coped in the past and couldn't see how this episode could have really affected him, although he recognised his increasing difficulties in his work and family life. He showed some re-experiencing phenomena in his dreams and in the triggering of distress in his work situation where all reminders of what had occurred brought intense experience of anxiety, almost to the level of panic. His avoidant phenomena and withdrawal were profound. He showed heightened arousal, irritability and poor concentration and persistent sleep difficulties. A clinical diagnosis of PTSD was made. Substance abuse disorder was not diagnosed as he had stopped his alcohol intake on the advice of his local doctor. His wife and the counsellor from his workplace confirmed his history and his previous high level of work and personal functioning.

Psychophysiological assessment: (summary of 8 reads)

	Systolic	Diastolic	M.A.P.	H.R.
Base rate:				
Matched for vocals	136	90	103	53
Talking about:				
1. Crash	154	108	*121*	72
2. Interpersonal work discomfort	*164*	105	119	72
3. Final read (nonrelaxed)	141	90	116	56

Case 2 – Mr. B.

Mr. B. was in his late 40s. He was a police officer and had been an extremely fit man and was very physically strong, devoting much of his spare time to body-building and exercise. He had had a reasonable childhood, but some difficulties in relationships with his parents. He had had no past personal or family history and psychiatric disorder. His marriage had broken up some years before because of his wife's disturbance and they had seen a counsellor at his insistence, but to no effect. He had the custody of his two teenage daughters and got on very well with them according to his report.

He presented for assessment approximately 8 months after an episode which "changed his life". He had been off duty and had gone into a night club where some disturbance occurred and was violently assaulted by a number of men. He was kicked and beaten and crawled out onto the pavement to escape. He remembers thinking that he was going to die before he lost consciousness from head injuries. He was taken to hospital and spent several days there and was finally discharged and returned to work. Some uncertainties occurred about the assault, for the assailant claimed that the injuries were the result of the patient's head-butting, not the attack. Support from within the force was variable.

Mr. B. tried to actively involve himself in work as these matters were clarified. However, he found his concentration was impaired and he had marked difficulty in interpersonal situations with increasing withdrawal he was also subject to bouts of irritability and at times rage, and had "overdone" his response to some domestic violence situations. He was increasingly afraid he would lose control and would even shut himself inside a wardrobe at times to deal with his tension. He experienced difficulties with his girlfriend and had lost interest in sex. He also lost interest in exercise and body-building and wanted to have nothing to do with people. He would have intrusive memories of the event and his terror, but also images of decaying bodies and other horrific scenes from his earlier police work. These had never troubled him before. Nightmares involved similar themes and he had great difficulty sleeping. He had voluntarily left the police force, although it was work that he loved, so that he could be sure he did not do "something that he would regret". He had received counselling and antidepressant treatment from his local doctor, who was skilled in dealing with police officers.

He had been reassessed recently by the neurologist who had cared for him in hospital and had had neuropsychological testing. This had shown no abnormalities on cerebral scan, but some suggestion of impaired frontal lobe function complicated by PTSD (poor concentration, impulsivity and poor emotional control). He was referred for assessment and court report.

Clinical Assessment

Clinical assessment indicated the presence of re-experiencing phenomena of both the event and earlier traumatogenic stimuli (e.g. decaying bodies). Avoidance and withdrawal were profound and were seriously interfering with his functioning. Heightened arousal with irritability, poor concentration and sleep disturbance as well as his rage reactions, constituted further evidence of disorder. The patient had previously met diagnostic criteria for major depressive disorder. His current diagnosis was considered to be post-traumatic stress disorder.

Psychophysiological assessment: (summary of 8 reads)

	Systolic	Diastolic	M.A.P.	H.R.
Base rate:	133	85	92	68
Visual imagery recall:				
1. Unrelated – decaying body	136	80	106	68
2. Attack	144	*100*	89	68
3. Current loss of function	151	*104*	*114*	67
4. Final relaxation	134	87	94	63

Discussion and Conclusions

These reports indicate the specific physiological responses that occurred for 2 men in regard to visualisation of a traumatic experience and/or talking about it. The second case clearly indicates the differential response for one traumatic stimulus (the assault and its effects) compared to other potentially traumatic episodes which had appeared in the intrusive images. In both instances reactions to the experience also contributed to psychophysiological responsiveness. These findings indicate the potential utility of such measures in defining a stressor and its contribution to the individual's distress. Further work is necessary to clarify these observations on large samples and to establish the validity of such measures in consolidating not only diagnosis but aetiological formulation in post-traumatic stress disorder in non-combat situations. Such measures have the advantage of immediate reactivity, easy use and can be developed in association with other clinical and biological assessments, and can provide models for meaningful interpretation of multiple tasks, and across individuals [20].

References

1. Wilson J and Raphael B (1991) International Handbook of Traumatic Stress Studies. Plenum, New York, U.S.A.
2. DSM III-R (1987) Diagnostic and Statistical Manual of the American Psychiatric Association. APA Press.
3. Watson C (1991) J. Consult. Clin. Psychol. 2(4): 460–469.
4. Keane TM, Caddell JM and Taylor KL (1988) J. Consult. Clin. Psychol. 56: 85–90.
5. Spitzer RL and Williams JW (1986) Structured Clinical Interview for DSM III-R. N.Y. Biometrics Res. Dept., N.Y. State Psychiatric Institute.
6. Watson C et al. (1991) J. Consult. Clin. Psychol. (in press).
7. McFarlane AC (1990) Post-Traumatic Stress Disorder. Doctoral Thesis (MD), University of Adelaide.
8. Pitman RK and Orr SP et al. (1987) Arch. Gen. Psychiatry 44: 970–975.
9. Blanchard E, Kolb L et al. (1982) Psychiatr. Q. 54: 220–229.
10. Blanchard E, Kolb L and Prins A (1991) J. Nerv. Ment. Dis. 179: 97–101.
11. Friedman M (1991) J. Traum. Stress 4: 67–91.
12. Pennebaker JW and Susman JR (1988) Soc. Sci. Med. 26: 327–332.
13. Shalev A et al. (1990) Psychosomatics 31: 197.
14. Cumes-Rayner D and Price J (1990) J. Psychosom. Res. 32: 181–190.
15. Cumes-Rayner D (1990) Applying Psychophysiology: The Clinical Measurement of Disparity Between Reported Affect and Arousal (Roneoed paper).
16. Silas JH et al (1980) Br. Heart J. 43: 202–205.
17. Ramsey M (1979) Med. Biol. Eng. Comput. 17: 11–18.
18. Ramsay R (1990) J. Psychosom. Res. 34: 355–365.
19. Dimsdale JE, Stern MJ and Dillon E (1988) Psychosom. Med. 50: 64–71.
20. Dimsdale JE, Berry C and Mills P (1990) Psychosom. Med. 52: 435–444.

Biological Psychiatry, Volume 1. G. Racagni et al., editors.

Panic disorder: Diagnosis and course

Robert M.A. Hirschfeld

Department of Psychiatry and Behavioral Sciences, University of Texas Medical Branch, 1.200 Graves Building, Galveston, TX 77550, U.S.A.

History

Although there were lucid descriptions of the phenomena of panic attacks in the mid-nineteenth century [1,2], panic disorder as a distinct clinical syndrome was largely ignored until the 1900s when American and European investigators published a number of studies on it. Panic disorder was first included in an official nomenclature, the Diagnostic and Statistical Manual of the American Psychiatric Association, in its third revision published in 1980 [3]. It has never been included in the International Classification of Diseases of the World Health Organization, but it is proposed for inclusion in the tenth revision.

Diagnosis

The world's two major nomenclatures, the ICD 10 and the DSM IV, are similar in that they both include the category of panic disorder which is defined similarly in both. However, the two nomenclatures regard panic disorder very differently, reflecting differences in European and American nosologic tradition. In Europe, panic is conceptualized as an extreme form of generalized anxiety, whereas agoraphobia is regarded as the most severe variant of phobia. In the United States, agoraphobia is viewed as a consequence of repeated panic attacks, based upon the work of Donald Klein and others in the 1960s and 1970s. Therefore, in DSM agoraphobia is secondary to panic disorder.

Clinical course

Much less research has been conducted on the clinical course of anxiety and panic disorders than on depressive disorders. However, eight medium to long-term follow-up studies have been completed in the last decade, which show fairly good convergence of findings. These studies were all naturalistic in that treatment was uncontrolled following, at most, the first several months.

In general, over half the patients have substantial improvement in panic attacks and agoraphobia at the follow-up point and perhaps 10–20% are fully recovered. Nevertheless, relatively few are symptom-free and up to 20% are still severely ill

[4–7]. Predictors of a worse long-term course include: severity of both anxiety [8] and phobic avoidant symptoms, presence of a personality disorder and current or past major depression [7].

With regard to long-term psychosocial outcome, significant persistent, social [7,9,10], familial, and occupational deficits remain [7,9]. In addition, there is significant illness-related disability, especially in patients with agoraphobia. As with symptomatic outcome, predictors of worse long-term psychosocial outcome include: severity of presenting features, especially anxiety and agoraphobia, the presence of a personality disorder, the presence or history of major depression, and poor social adaptation at the time of index assessment [7].

In conclusion, the clear inference that we can draw from the data at this point is that panic disorder is a prevalent long-term illness with lingering social and occupational disabilities. Major questions remain, however, about the relationship between panic disorder and agoraphobia.

References

1. Moral BA (1866) Arch. Gen. Med. 7: 385–402, 530–551, 700–707.
2. Westphal C (1871–1872) Arch. Psychiatr. Nervenkr. 2–3: 138–161.
3. American Psychiatric Association (1980) Diagnostic and Statistical Manual of Mental Disorders (3rd Edition) (DSM III). Am. Psychiatr. Assoc., Washington, D.C.
4. Coryell W, Noyes R and Clancy J (1983) J. Affective Disord. 5: 311–317.
5. Maier W and Buller R (1988) Eur. Arch. Psychiatr. Neurol. Sci. 238: 105–109.
6. Noyes R, Garvey MJ and Cook BL (1989) J. Affective Disord. 16: 249–257.
7. Noyes R, Reich J, Christiansen J, Suelzer M, Pfohl B and Coryell WA (1990) Arch. Gen. Psychiatry 47: 809–818.
8. Faravelli C and Albanesi G (1987) Compr. Psychiatry 28(6): 481–487.
9. Katsnig H, Stolk JM, Klerman GL, Ballenger JC, Amering M, Briggs A, Buller R, Cassano G, Garvey M, Roth M and Solyom C (unpublished).
10. Kreig JC, Bronisch T, Wittchen HU and von Zerssen D (1987) Acta Psychiatr. Scand. 76: 36–47.

Biological Psychiatry, Volume 1. G. Racagni et al., editors.

The place of pharmacotherapy in the management of panic disorder

Sir Martin Roth
Trinity College, University of Cambridge, U.K.

Introduction

This paper is mainly devoted to the use of pharmacological treatment in the clinical management of the panic agoraphobic group of disorders. To set the contribution of drug treatment in perspective, their efficacy will be briefly compared with the results recorded in recent years in relation to psychological therapies.

Controlled therapeutic trials serve to define the value and limitations of drugs in precise terms. However, the application of such findings in clinical practice requires strategies that differ from those which must be applied in the experimental evaluation of the efficacy of drugs. In the last section of the paper, drug treatments are set in the context of the general management of patients with panic-agoraphobic disorder.

MAO inhibitors were the first drugs to be employed in the treatment of disorders in which panic attacks and phobic symptoms were leading features [1,2]. It was Klein who first established the value of imipramine in panic disorders. But he reported benzodiazepine to be ineffective in this condition [3]. With the emergence of the triazolo benzodiazepines, favourable results began to be recorded in panic disorder [4]. The Cross-National Collaborative Panic Study initiated in 1982 was to provide the most comprehensive body of data regarding the efficacy of alprazolam in panic disorder. In phase I alprazolam proved to be superior in efficacy to placebo [5,6]. In phase II the effects of alprazolam were compared with placebo and with the tricyclic drug imipramine, for whose efficacy a considerable amount of literature had accumulated. The full data are in press [7]. The account given here will be confined to a brief summary of the main results.

The Cross-National Collaborative Panic Study: Second phase investigation

After evaluation and assessment during the first 1–2 weeks and a similar washout period, patients were randomly assigned to alprazolam, imipramine or placebo in a double-blind therapeutic regime that lasted 8 weeks. Assessments were carried out on admission to the study, at the point of randomization following the washout period and at weeks 1–4, 6 and 8 following the randomization of patients.

To qualify for admission to the study patients had to satisfy modified DSM III criteria for a lifetime diagnosis of panic disorder. They must also have experienced at least 1 panic attack with 3 or more symptoms per week for the previous 3 weeks. There was a set of other clinical criteria for inclusion. Patients had to be able to take oral medication and to participate voluntarily. Exclusion criteria comprised a range of medical conditions including epilepsy, systemic disease, suicidal tendencies, other psychiatric disorders and abnormal laboratory findings. Those with a recent history of alcoholism or drug abuse were also excluded. Full details are published in the definitive report.

The enquiry was conducted at 12 study centres. At each of these, patients were blindly assigned to 1 of the 3 modalities of treatment. Unit dosage was 25 mg imipramine or 1 mg of alprazolam. Dosage was increased according to a set schedule which specified dosage of 6 mg of alprazolam, 150 mg of imipramine or 6 placebo tablets by the nineteenth day. In the subsequent period a more flexible regime was permitted, the participant investigator being enabled to vary the dose according to the patient's clinical condition.

Patients were evaluated with the aid of the structured clinical interview for DSM III diagnosis, Upjohn (SCID-UP; [8]) which had been found to have a high interrelator reliability ($\kappa = 0.86$) for diagnosis of panic disorder.

Assessment of efficacy was undertaken by a number of measures including the Physicians Global Improvement Scale, the Panic Attack Scale of Sheehan and Sheehan [9], a modified version of the Overall Phobia Scale [10], Hamilton Anxiety Rating Scale [11,12] and the Hopkins SCL-90 Patient's Self-Rating Scale [13]. Anticipatory anxiety was assessed on the percentage of time spent in anticipation of episodes of panic. Overall impairment in work, social and leisure time activities and family life were rated on 5-point scales.

All serious adverse effects were noted. The weekly rating for adverse effects was recorded with the aid of a scale developed at the psychopharmacology research branch of the NIMH [14]. The scientific quality of the study at each centre was assessed by special teams containing independent assessors who made biannual visits.

One thousand one hundred and sixty-eight patients were randomized. Sixty-two percent of the sample was female with a mean age at entry of 34 years. Symptoms of panic disorder had been present for an average of 5 years. Fifty percent had uncomplicated panic and 76% panic with limited or extensive phobic avoidance. Of the 1168 patients 1010 were "evaluable", having completed 3 weeks of medication.

Every attempt was made to limit to a minimum the extent to which patients received any form of psychotherapy or behavioural treatment during the 8-week treatment phase.

Summary of results

The alprazolam group exhibited improvement at an earlier stage in respect of most variables than the imipramine group or the placebo group. By week 8 with alprazolam and imipramine group had improved to a closely similar extent, both drugs having proved significantly more potent in relieving symptoms than placebo.

In respect of panic attacks alprazolam patients showed improvement after week 1, the imipramine group by week 6. By week 8 both drugs had shown a significantly greater reduction in panic attacks than placebo both in the completer analysis and the end-point analysis. In the latter, 70% of alprazolam and imipramine patients had zero panic attacks compared with 50% of those on placebo.

On measures of anxiety, alprazolam showed improvement within the first 2 weeks but improvement was deferred until the fourth week in the case of imipramine. Both active compounds exerted a significantly greater effect than placebo on the Hamilton Anxiety Scale [11,12]. Fear and avoidance in respect of the patient's central phobia improved early in the trial in the alprazolam group; symptom relief occurred later in the case of imipramine.

Both end-point and completer analyses of ratings for phobias showed greater improvement with the 2 active drugs than with placebo except at week 8. Patient's self-report in the SCL-90 total score showed imipramine to be significantly more effective than both alprazolam and placebo at week 8 by completer and end-point analysis. But alprazolam proved more effective than placebo in the end-point analysis.

On the 4 measures of social functioning utilized, the pattern of drug effects was similar to that recorded in respect of symptoms. Improvement of those on alprazolam surfaced at an early stage, imipramine later. In the end-point analysis, both 2 active drugs were found to be better than placebo.

Discontinuation of drug

It proved possible to discontinue medication in the great majority of patients. A substantial proportion of those on alprazolam experienced some increase in anxiety, arising probably in part from a recrudescence of the original anxiety symptoms and withdrawal. In no case were serious complications such as convulsion, clouding or delirium recorded.

Completion and drop-out rate

Among those randomized, 83% of patients on alprazolam completed the trial compared with 70% of those on imipramine and 56% of those on placebo. The significantly higher drop-out rate in the placebo group owing to deterioration or failure of improvement provides an indirect measure of efficacy of the active compound. The highest rate of withdrawal on account of adverse side-effects was recorded in the imipramine group.

The high drop-out rate in the placebo group has a significant bearing upon the results of the completer analysis in particular. As only the best placebo responders would have remained in the trial until termination, the results of the completer analysis will have reflected bias in favour of the placebo.

As all 3 groups in the trial (including placebo) showed striking improvement during the 8-week trial period, the efficacy of the active drug was exposed to particularly stringent tests. Although attempts were made to minimize formal psychotherapy, the placebo patients are likely to have received considerable support from frequent visits, comprehensive assessment lasting an hour or more on each occasion, knowledge gained about their disorder and the reassurance to raise morale that will have resulted from interactions with the therapist. These non-specific psychological influences in the placebo group carry implications for ordinary clinical practice which are discussed in the final section of this paper.

The use of alprazolam and imipramine in clinical practice

The benzodiazepine most extensively studied in panic disorder is alprazolam. As noted, alprazolam has an efficacy equal to that of antidepressants, but it has a much more rapid onset of action. In severely distressed patients it is, therefore, the drug of first choice.

Alprazolam, because of its relatively short half-life, should be given in divided doses. A starting dose of approximately 0.5 mg is taken 2 or 3 times daily after meals to permit slow absorption; the final dose is variable. The dose should then be increased by 0.5 mg every 2–3 days depending on progress until a satisfactory measure of stable relief has been achieved.

Subsequent fixed dose studies have shown that about 60% of patients respond to 2 mg of alprazolam and 75% respond to 6 mg (Lydiard RB, Lesser IM et al., unpublished data). Many patients therefore respond to lower doses, but higher doses may be necessary to treat a proportion of them. Tolerance to the drug calling for or causing escalation of doses is very rare. The term dependence has been used to explain the withdrawal effects. This is questionable in the case of a chronic disorder liable to frequent relapse, with reappearance of the symptoms held in check by alprazolam, once medication ceases.

To avoid severe withdrawal symptoms discontinuation should always be undertaken slowly. For a high-potency agent like alprazolam, guidelines should include decreasing by no more than 0.5 mg per week when the patient is at the higher doses, slowing to 0.25 mg per week or less when dosage has reached approximately 2 mg. Even at this low rate, patients may experience return of the original symptoms.

Imipramine and MAOI's typically exert their therapeutic effects after 3 or 4 weeks. As there is commonly an early stage jitteriness or increased panic, an initial dose of 10–25 mg is prudent. After a few days at this low dose, the dose can be titrated upward.

The ultimate effective dose is variable; some patients may respond at doses lower than considered necessary for an antidepressant response. In a chronic disease often complicated by severe depression, account must be taken of the irreversible effects of overdoses; and panic disorder has its own suicidal risk.

Behavioural and cognitive treatments

A large body of evidence has been presented in recent years to suggest that behavioural treatments [15] and cognitive therapy (Beck, 1988) achieve results comparable with or superior to those obtained by drug treatment. Andrews and Moran [16], who employ a range of these and other psychological therapies have asked "are drugs essential in the treatment of agoraphobia with panic attacks?". They answer this question firmly in the negative. The technique used by this team in panic-agoraphobia (but also social phobic and obsessive-compulsive neurosis) entails 40–80 h of intensive therapy in a setting of small groups of patients. It includes education about the disorder, training in muscular relaxation and in "slow breathing", in vivo exposure and cognitive methods aimed at restructuring the attitudes and personality of the individual. The published results are impressive, and changes in basic personality are claimed as well as significant relief of symptoms.

These are interesting investigations and deserve replication by other centres in the near future. But there is need for further controlled investigation of behavioural and cognitive treatments and comparative studies of their effects as against those of drug treatment.

Aspects of management in clinical practice

The objectives and the approaches to management in clinical practice differ from those appropriate for controlled clinical trials. In the latter, all influences other than those that emanate from the specific treatment under trial have to be minimized or eliminated. In clinical practice on the other hand, every form of intervention that might contribute to the alleviation of the suffering needs to be utilized in management.

Those with agoraphobic and related disorders fear that they are losing their reason and may be at any moment plunged into insanity and suffer public humiliation. They may be reluctant to describe such symptoms lest such communications should elicit confirmation from the psychiatrist that their fears are indeed justified. The exploration that brings such fears to light, the reassurance that they are groundless and which reveals that the psychiatrist is familiar with the patient's inner experiences relieves anxiety and improves rapport. It is a powerful factor in securing compliance in any further measures adopted in treatment.

The present mental state has to be set in the context of the patient's past and recent history, the record of his development in childhood and adolescence, his adaptation to stresses and challenges and the character and quality of his interpersonal relations.

The personality problems of those with panic-agoraphobic and related disorders comprise emotional dependence on others, low self-esteem, impaired coping mechanisms and difficulties in handling anxiety. The dependance is manifest in a parodied form in their illness. For there is virtually nowhere these patients cannot go in tranquillity when accompanied by mother, husband, adult offspring or close friend. The resulting demoralization is commonly manifest as an associated depressive disorder. Treatment should be informed by knowledge of such vulnerable spots in the individual defences and aimed at improving patients' coping mechanism. Some evidence has been cited that such measures can accelerate and stabilize progress in the control and elimination of symptoms.

Analysis of the results of controlled double-blind trials of drug treatments and in particular the large placebo effects reportedly recorded [17] have directed attention to the fact that the care of those with the disabling symptoms of phobic and related disorders needs to be many-sided if it is to achieve optimal results.

References

1. Sargant W and Dally PJ (1962) Br. Med. J. 1: 6–9.
2. Kelly DGW, Frommer E, Mitchell-Hoggs N et al. (1970) Br. J. Psychiatry 116: 387–398.
3. Klein DF (1964) Psychopharmacologia 53: 397–408.
4. Chouinard G, Annable L, Fontaine R et al. (1982) Psychopharmacology 77: 229–233.
5. Ballenger JC, Burrows G, DuPont R et al. (1988) Arch. Gen. Psychiatry 45: 413–422.
6. Noyes R, DuPont RL and Pecknold JC (1988) Arch. Gen. Psychiatry 45: 423–428.
7. Klerman GL et al. (1991) Drug treatment of panic disorder: comparative efficacy of alprazolam, imipramine and placebo. Br. J. Psychiatry (in press).
8. Spitzer RL and Williams JBW (1988) J. Psychiatr. Res. 22 (Suppl. 1): 55–86.
9. Sheehan DV and Sheehan KE (1982) J. Clin. Psychopharmacol. 2: 235–243.
10. Marks IM and Matthews AM (1979) Behav. Res. Ther. 17: 263–267.
11. Hamilton M (1959) Br. J. Med. Psychology 32: 50–55.
12. Hamilton M (1960) J. Neurol. Neurosurg. Psychiatry 23: 56–62.
13. Derogatis LR, Lipman RS and Covi L (1973) Psychopharmacol. Bull. 9: 13–28.
14. Levine J and Schooler NR (1986) Psychopharmacol. Bull. 22: 343–381.
15. Marks IM (1987) Fears, Phobias and Rituals. Oxford University Press, New York.
16. Andrews G and Moran C (1988) In: Hand I and Wittchen HU (eds.) Panic and Phobias I. Treatments and Variables Affecting Course and Outcome. Springer-Verlag, Heidelberg.
17. Roth M (1991) Clinical and scientific implications of recent progress in the treatment of phobic disorders. Psychiatr. Ann. (in press).

Biological Psychiatry, Volume 1. G. Racagni et al., editors.

Cognitive therapy for panic disorder

M.G. Gelder, D.M. Clark and P. Anastasiades
Department of Psychiatry, University of Oxford, Warneford Hospital, Oxford, U.K.

There is substantial evidence for biological abnormalities in patients with panic disorder, affecting both the noradrenergic [1] and the serotonergic [2] systems. However, it is not certain whether these abnormalities reflect the primary disorder or are secondary to a more basic mechanism of another kind. In recent years, evidence has accumulated indicating that the basic aetiological mechanism may be psychological and take the form of a specific kind of fear concerning physical symptoms of anxiety [3]. The fear is that these symptoms are the forerunner of an immediate medical emergency such as a heart attack or a stroke. Such fears have been shown to characterize patients with panic disorder but not patients with other kinds of anxiety disorder and they have been demonstrated by several objective methods [4]. These fears are capable of setting up a vicious circle in which anxiety leads to physical symptoms and fear of the consequences of these symptoms generates more anxiety – until a panic attack results.

This hypothesis could explain the power of chemical agents to evoke panic attacks because such agents produce somatic symptoms which could activate the vicious circle of panic. If this view is correct, the effects of biochemical challenges should be reduced by a psychological intervention that reduces the specific fears. Since sodium lactate infusions regularly provoke panic attacks in panic disorder patients, a convincing test of the hypothesis would be to demonstrate that the sodium lactate response can be reduced by psychological means.

The sodium lactate response has been modified in two studies. In the first [5] with normal subjects, anxiety response to lactate was significantly reduced when the subjects were told that the infusion would produce pleasant excitement, rather than anxiety. In the second, by our group, the response of panic disorder patients to sodium lactate infusion was significantly reduced when it was preceded by specific reassurances directed to the fears of physical symptoms that characterise panic disorder patients. These experiments strongly suggest that there is an important psychological component to both normal subjects' and panic disorder patients' response to sodium lactate infusion.

The treatment of panic disorder

If psychological factors are as important in spontaneous panics as in lactate-induced ones, psychological treatment should be effective in panic disorder. The appropriate treatment is a specific kind of cognitive therapy which has three stages. Firstly, the patient is helped to identify fearful cognitions; secondly, the therapist identifies the patient's reasons for continuing to believe in the cognitions; thirdly, steps are taken to undermine these beliefs and help patients think of the symptoms in a more rational way.

Five uncontrolled studies have shown that cognitive therapy can diminish the frequency and intensity of panic attacks [6–10]. In three controlled studies, cognitive therapy has been shown to be more effective than supportive therapy [10] or relaxation training [11], and as effective as alprazolam [12].

A clinical trial in Oxford with panic disorder patients has compared cognitive therapy with imipramine, with intensive relaxation and with a waiting list group. Both psychological treatments were given for three months and this was the period spent on the waiting list. Imipramine treatment lasted for 6 months, with a starting dose of 10 mg a day (to avoid unpleasant side-effects) increasing to a maximum average dose of 225 mg per day. Assessments were made 3, 6 and 15 months after the beginning of treatment. After 3 months, cognitions had changed more in the cognitive therapy group than in the other three, showing that cognitive therapy has the required specific effect. Improvement in panic attacks was also greater in this cognitive therapy group than in those receiving imipramine or relaxation (which changed equally). The wait-list group did not change significantly, showing that the changes in the treatment groups were not simply due to spontaneous improvement. At this assessment point, the two psychological treatments had been completed but the imipramine treatment continued at maximum dose for a further 3 months became gradual withdrawal.

Fifteen months after the start of treatment – 12 months after the end of cognitive and relaxation treatment and 9 months after the end of imipramine – the cognitive therapy group was still more improved than the others. In the cognitive therapy group 80% of patients were free from panic attacks and had not had further treatment, while the corresponding figure in the imipramine and relaxation groups were 50% and 47% respectively.

These findings suggest strongly that psychological factors play an important part in maintaining panic disorder and that cognitive therapy which changes these cognitions has substantial therapeutic effects. The findings do not rule out biological causes of panic disorder which, indeed, play a part in all anxiety disorders. However, the results indicate that panic disorder is no different from other anxiety disorders in being caused by a combination of biological predisposition and psychological maintaining factors.

References

1. Charney DS and Heninger GR (1986) Arch. Gen. Psychiatry 43: 1042–1054.
2. Den Boer J, Westenberg HGM and Verhoeven WMA (1990) Psychiatr. Ann. 20: 494–499.

3. Clarke DM (1986) Behav. Res. Ther. 24: 461–470.
4. Clark DM, Salkovskis PM, Gelder MG, Koehler C, Martin M, Anastasiades P, Hackman A, Middleton H and Jeavons A (1988) In: Hand I and Wittchen HU (eds.) Panic and Phobias II. Springer-Verlag, New York.
5. van der Molen GM, van den Hout MA, Vroemen J, Lousberg H and Griez E (1986) Behav. Res. Ther. 24: 677–680.
6. Clark DM, Salkovskis PM and Chalkley AJ (1985) J. Behav. Ther. Exp. Psychiatry 16: 23–30.
7. Kopp M, Milhaly K and Vadasz P (1986) Ideggyogyaszati Szemle 39: 185–196.
8. Michelson L, Marchione K, Greenwald M, Glanz L, Testa S and Marchione N (1990) Behav. Res. Ther. 28: 141–153.
9. Salkovskis PM, Jones DRO and Clark DM (1986) Br. J. Psychiatry 148: 526–532.
10. Sokol L, Beck AT, Greenberg RL, Wright FD and Berchick RJ (1989) J. Nerv. Mental Dis. 177: 711–716.
11. Barlow DH, Craske MG, Cerny JA and Klosko JS (1989) Behav. Ther. 20: 261–282.
12. Klosko JS, Barlow DH, Tassinari R and Cerny JA (1990) J. Consult. Clin. Psychol. 58: 77–84.

Biological Psychiatry, Volume 1. G. Racagni et al., editors.

Discontinuation and long-term follow-up of participants in a clinical drug trial for panic disorder

Heinz Katschnig, John M. Stolk, Gerald L. Klerman, James C. Ballenger, Michaela Amering, Andrew Briggs, Raimund Buller, Giovanni Cassano, Michael Garvey, Martin Roth and Carol Solyom

Psychiatric Clinic, University of Vienna, Währinger Gürtel 18–20, A-1090 Vienna, Austria

Introduction

Conventional wisdom has been that panic disorder is a disabling and chronic disorder. While the natural history of untreated panic disorder remains to be clarified, data are now forthcoming about the naturalistic course of the disorder in patients who have participated in clinical drug trials [1,2]. These data do not unequivocally confirm the gloomy picture held hitherto. The present paper is intended to shed light on this question in documenting the 4-year outcome of panic disorder in patients who had participated in a large international multicenter clinical drug trial. In addition, the immediate effect of drug discontinuation is analyzed.

The original patient population had taken part either in the Cross-National Collaborative Panic Study Phase I (alprazolam vs. placebo) or Phase II (alprazolam vs. imipramine vs. placebo) and consisted of 1,647 panic disorder patients (defined according to a modified version of DSM III) from 15 countries in Europe, North and Latin America. Most patients had completed an 8-week trial protocol; in some centres the study was extended to 8 months. After 8 weeks, alprazolam and imipramine proved to be equally efficient and superior to placebo [3,4]. In two different studies on different samples the questions of: a) discontinuation problems (Rosenberg et al., forthcoming); and b) of the long-term outcome (Katschnig et al., forthcoming) were addressed.

Discontinuation study

Patients and Methods

Rosenberg et al. (forthcoming) analysed the effect of discontinuation of drug treatment in 289 patients of the 8-week trial and in 154 patients of the 8-month trial. Since attrition rates during the drug trial varied widely between treatment groups, the samples studied for discontinuation effects were no longer random. So far only results for relapse and rebound are available and not for withdrawal symptomatology.

Results

A symptomatic course after discontinuation was found – depending on the variables chosen – in 41–64% of alprazolam, in 29–34% of imipramine and in 4–19% of placebo patients. A relapse was observed in 26–42% of alprazolam, 2–15% of imipramine and 10–19% of placebo patients. A rebound of symptoms above pre-study levels was found in 8–18% of alprazolam, in 0–9% of imipramine and 0–15% of placebo patients. The peak incidence of symptom worsening and rebound generally occurred during the midpoint of rather fast alprazolam dose reduction (1 mg every 3–4 days), which was usually reached within 1–2 weeks after treatment termination. No systematic relationship between alprazolam dosage at the start of discontinuation and symptom reoccurrence was found, nor were there any differences in incidence of discontinuation symptoms between short-term and long-term treatment with alprazolam.

Long-term follow-up study

Patients and methods

Seven selected sites from North America and Europe with a total of 423 patients (= roughly one quarter of the original sample) were to be followed-up 2–6 years after leaving the protocol. A special follow-up interview was constructed, focusing among other issues on: a) symptom and disability comparisons between the post-study year and the year before the interview (called here the "current year"); and b) current medication use. Three hundred and sixty-seven patients (86.8%) could be re-interviewed. For a subsample of 220 patients the patterns of course could be established.

Results

Patients experiencing no panic attacks
Only 23.6% of all patients reported having experienced no panic attack during the post-study year. There was some but not a very dramatic increase in the population of patients experiencing no panic attack between the post-study year and the current year (29%).

Global phobic fear and avoidance
Global phobic fear and avoidance was measured on an 11-point scale (0 = no phobic avoidance, 10 = maximum phobic avoidance). During the post-study year 38.4% of all patients reported no or only mild phobic avoidance (0–4), with a substantial increase to 59.5% during the current year.

Disabilities
For work, family life/home and social life/leisure disability the same pattern could be found as for phobic avoidance, with, however, a much larger improvement for most disabilities (e.g. no or only mild work disability increased from 48% to 82.4%).

Outcome in relation to original study medication
None of the above variables (symptoms, disabilities and current medication use) showed differences in outcome in relation to type of study medication.

Deaths
Three patients developed malignant neoplasms and subsequently died. There was no suicide.

Current use of psychotropic medication
Forty-five percent of all patients were not taking any psychotropic medication at the time of the follow-up interview. Twenty-three percent were taking benzodiazepines alone, 12% antidepressants and 9% both. Eleven percent were using other psychotropic drugs.

Patterns of course
Thirty-one percent of 220 patients for whom these data were obtained recovered and stayed well, but 18.6% showed a severe chronic course. The rest (50.4%) showed intermediate patterns.

Discussion

The results show that both advocates of a poor and of a good outcome in panic disorder are right. Not all panic disorder patients have a bad outcome, some even do excellently; but there is a substantial amount of chronic or recurrent yet mild symptomatology, although not necessarily linked to disability.

Four explanations are possible for the relatively good outcome in a large subgroup of patients (Katschnig et al., forthcoming): a) a favourable natural history of the disorder in this subgroup; b) a statistical "regression to the mean" effect; c) the effect of treatments received during follow-up; and d) a "sleeper" effect of non-pharmacological factors operating during the original treatment study (e.g. self-monitoring of symptoms in a diary; inadvertent exposure in vivo).

The outcome of panic disorder does not seem as gloomy as once thought. It is the same question of perspective as regarding a glass of water as being half full or half empty – both statements are true and both should be accepted. One is reminded here of Kraepelin's dementia praecox, which, as Eugen Bleuler pointed out, is only one of several possible subtypes of "the schizophrenias". It seems that such a differentiated view is also necessary for panic disorder.

References

1. Noyes R, Garvey MJ and Cook BL (1989) J. Affective Disord. 16: 249–257.
2. Nagy LM, Krystal JH, Woods SW and Charney DS (1989) Arch. Gen. Psychiatry 46: 993–999.
3. Ballenger JC, Burrows GD, DuPont RL, Lesser IM, Noyes R, Pecknold JC, Rifkin A and Swinson RP (1988) Arch. Gen. Psychiatry 45: 413–421.
4. Cross-National Collaborative Panic Study Second Phase Investigators: Drug Treatment of Panic Disorder: Comparative Efficacy of Alprazolam, Imipramine and Placebo.

Biological Psychiatry, Volume 1. G. Racagni et al., editors.

What is obsessive-compulsive disorder: A review of the clinical syndrome

Christopher P. Freeman

Department of Psychiatry, Edinburgh University, Royal Edinburgh Hospital, Morningside Terrace, Edinburgh EH10 5HF, U.K.

Introduction

Obsessive compulsive disorder (OCD) is a fascinating but complex condition which has a long history in both literature and psychiatry. We are all familiar with Lady Macbeth's obsessions and ritual hand-washing driven by guilt and Freud's descriptions of the "rat man" and Wolfman [1] linking obsessional thoughts and compulsive actions with unconscious conflicts. Despite these insights psycho-analysis has not been helpful in the management or treatment of OCD. In recent years there has been a resurgence of interest in the condition driven by a number of important findings concerning the biology of the disorder and by the development of drugs that appear to have specific anti-obsessional properties. At the same time it has become clear that what was once thought to be an uncommon psychiatric disorder may in fact afflict not 0.05% of the population but between 2% and 3%.

The clinical picture

The central feature of the disorder are obsessions and compulsions. These are comprehensively defined in DSM III-R [2] and the elements of the definition include: a repetitive act or thought which is recognised by the individual, which they feel compelled to carry out and which they would like to resist but cannot. The compulsions must be purposive actions, performed in accordance with certain rules; usually not an end in themselves, they are designed to bring about some future state of affairs or magically prevent some future event occurring. Although cleansing and checking rituals are the most common, a wide range of obsessional behaviours occur and it has become increasingly recognised that a significant group of patients (between a quarter and a third) have only obsessional thoughts and no observable rituals. Primary obsessional slowness is an interesting variant where the patient does not repeat behaviour but does everything very slowly and meticulously, often becoming "stuck" at certain points for long periods of time, unable to go on or go back.

The disorder begins in adolescence or early adulthood but has been described in young children and occasionally begins for the first time in the elderly. Nevertheless, 65% of cases have their onset under the age of 25 years. Most studies have shown the male:female ratio to be equal, but the ECA study [3] showed a male:female ratio of 2:3. Once established, the disorder appears to run a chronic course with fluctuations in symptomatology. It was originally thought to be an uncommon disorder with a prevalence in the general population of 0.05%. The ECA study [3,4] has shown lifetime prevalence rates varying from 1.9% in St. Louis to 3.1% in Baltimore and other sites that have used the Diagnostic Interview Schedule (DIS) have shown similar high rates (Edmonton 3%, Puerto Rico 3.2%). Only the studies in Taiwan again using the DIS showed rates of under 1% lifetime prevalence.

Boundaries of the disorder

In both DSM III and DSM III-R OCD is grouped with the anxiety disorders partly because anxiety is an almost universal symptom in OCD but mainly because of the theoretical assumption that it is anxiety that drives the obsessional and compulsive behaviour. Hopefully this will not be the case in DSM IV or in ICD 10. The symptom pattern of OCD, the stability of the symptoms and lifelong pattern are all quite different to many anxiety disorders and the response to treatment and low placebo response rate are both specific to OCD. There is some overlap with phobic disorders though usually the distinction is clear. Although the phobic will go to great lengths to avoid contact with the feared object, most can more or less switch off their fear when the feared object is not there. In contrast, the OCD patient remains constantly vigilant, scanning their environment for the thing that they are afraid of and ruminating on the consequences of contact. For example, the dog phobic can usually relax if they are reassured that there are no dogs in their immediate environment. Someone with an obsessional fear of dogs will be afraid of any contact and will be constantly scanning their environment for signs or residues of dogs. Sometimes the two symptoms' patterns do merge and Marks has used the term "obsessive phobia" to describe these.

There does seem to be marked overlap of OCD and depressive disorders, the two symptoms' patterns commonly occurring together. In the ECA study 1/3 of OCD patients had had an episode of major depressive illness and obsessional patients frequently get milder episodes of depression. It is also clear that some patients with a primary depressive disorder develop obsessional symptoms when they are depressed and these disappear when their depression is treated. In contrast, the symptom pattern of the two disorders differs, major depressive illness runs an episodic course and has a different sex ratio. This has led to attempts to decide which disorder is primary by describing which had the earlier onset. If depressive illness occurred first, then OCD is not diagnosed as a primary disorder; however, the evidence from treatment studies suggests that OCD should be regarded as a distinct illness and that the symptoms of depression and anxiety should be seen as associated symptoms.

Gilles de la Tourette syndrome (GTS) is a movement disorder characterised by both multiple motor and one or more vocal tics which usually occur many times a day in bouts. Gilles de la Tourette himself [5] in 1889 noted the association between GTS and OCD. A range of studies has shown that between 11% and 80% of GTS patients have obsessional symptoms and pedigree studies have shown an excess of GTS and OCD in families. Twenty percent of OCD patients appear to have tics, and neuroanatomical studies suggest that both disorders may involve the frontal lobes, corpus striatum and basal ganglia. This has led to the suggestion that some forms of OCD may be a phenotype of GTS. Although the aetiology of GTS is not known, it may be inherited as an autosomal dominant disorder with incomplete penetrance [6]. Despite these findings, it is clear that the majority of OCD patients do not have tics and that there is little or no crossover in treatment effectiveness between the 2 disorders.

Finally, there are a wide range of other "compulsive" or "driven" behaviours such as compulsive stealing, fire-setting, hair pulling, shopping, eating, gambling, self-mutilation and water drinking, most of which have little in common with obsessive-compulsive disorder except for the adjective compulsive. All these tend to be repetitive behaviour but most lack the qualities of clear-cut OCD, and in particular they lack the magical quality of thinking that characterises OCD. When someone steals, gambles or sets fires compulsively, it is the direct act itself which provides the stimulation, relief of anxiety or change in mood rather than the act being used to magically bring about or prevent some future state of affairs.

References

1. Freud S and Rieff P (1973) In: Three Case Histories. Macmillan Publishing Co., New York, pp. 15–102.
2. Diagnostic and Statistical Manual of Mental Disorders Edn. 3 (Revised) (1987) Am. Psychiatr. Assoc., Washington D.C., pp. 245–247.
3. Robins LN, Melzer JE, Weissman MM et al. (1984) Arch. Gen. Psychiatry 41: 949–958.
4. Burnham MA, Hough RL, Escaber JI et al. (1987) Arch. Gen. Psychiatry 44: 687–694.
5. Gilles de la Tourette G. Semin. Med. 19: 15–156.
6. Robertson MM and Gourdie A (1990) Br. J. Psychiatry 156: 515–521.

Biological Psychiatry, Volume 1. G. Racagni et al., editors.

Neurobiology of obsessive-compulsive disorder: A review

Thomas R. Insel and James T. Winslow
Laboratory of Clinical Science, NIMH, P.O. Box 289, Poolesville, MD 20837, U.S.A.

The search for a neurobiological basis for obsessive-compulsive disorder (OCD) has included genetic, neuroanatomic and neuropharmacologic studies. Although the etiology of this disorder (or group of disorders) remains unclear, several interesting leads have emerged from each of these areas of study.

For instance, a genetic factor has been suggested from various reports of twins concordant for OCD, but it is not yet clear if the genetic factor in question codes for OCD or some character trait which may predispose to the development of the syndrome. In any case, these sorts of report are difficult to interpret. They are clearly subject to a reporting bias – discordant twins are less likely to be reported in the literature – and even the presence of a very high rate of concordance does not exclude epigenetic factors. Perhaps the most important report in this general area was the recent family study describing a high incidence of Tourette's syndrome in the family members of OCD probands, suggesting a genetic link between these two disorders [1].

There has long been a belief in the neurologic basis of OCD – partly because the symptoms seem so contrary to the conscious will of the patient and partly because some OCD patients often have subtle motor tics or clumsiness which might belie some neurologic disorder. Several frank neurologic disorders have been associated with the symptoms of OCD. Perhaps the best known example is the sequelae to the von Economo's influenza epidemic of 1919, but other neurologic disorders associated with OCD include Sydenham's chorea [2], bilateral necrosis of the globus pallidus [3] and Tourette's syndrome [1]. It is unlikely that any of these syndromes represents an etiology for very many of the psychiatric patients presenting with OCD, but the apparent association between disorders of striatal pathology and OCD symptoms may serve as a marker for an anatomic site in which to seek physiologic, if not pathologic changes in OCD.

Historically, another suggestion for neurological involvement in this disorder came from the relative success of psychosurgery. Specifically, two interventions appeared especially useful: cingulectomy and "stereotaxic leukotomy" (i.e. transection of the tracts from frontal cortex to subcortical sites such as striatum and thalamus). Indeed, using modern neurosurgical techniques with stereotaxic placement of both of these lesions, Kelly has reported about 80% success in OCD patients refractory to behavior therapy and pharmacotherapy [4]. These methods have not undergone rigorous double-blind testing with sham surgery, but even as extensive case reports, the results are impressive not only for their rate of improvement but also for the low frequency of reported adverse effects.

The most exciting development towards a neuroanatomic model of OCD is certainly the advent of new imaging techniques. Four studies have used PET scans with ^{18}F-2 deoxyglucose to localize regions of abnormal metabolic activity in the brains of OCD patients [5–8]. The studies vary with respect to conditions – in some, the patient's eyes were open [5,6], in others they were closed [8]; one study used a cognitive task to focus attention [7] and scanners of different resolution were used. However, results across studies describe two areas of abnormally high activity: the orbital region of frontal cortex and the caudate (one of the major nuclei of the striatum). In one study, cingulate cortex was also significantly more active in OCD patients [8]. The changes reported in orbital cortex and cingulate are perhaps most remarkable in view of the many regions such as hippocampus and temporal cortex, previously described as active in anxiety states, which appear normal in OCD. As the striatum was previously implicated by neurologic disorders associated with OCD, and surgically transecting the tracts projecting from orbital cortex to striatum appears to decrease obsessional symptoms, a circuit connecting orbital cortex to the basal ganglia may be "over-active" in OCD. Indeed, metabolic activity in this circuit appears to decrease following successful pharmacologic treatment of OCD patients [9].

From a neuropharmacologic perspective, the most remarkable aspect of OCD is its high selectivity for drug response. Most drugs that reduce anxiety, depression, or psychosis are not effective against obsessions. While individual OCD patients may respond to antidepressants such as the tricyclic imipramine or the monoamine oxidase inhibitor tranylcypromine, thus far the only medications that appear effective in studies of OCD are clomipramine, fluvoxamine and fluoxetine [10]. These three compounds are all antidepressants and yet they reduce obsessional symptoms in nondepressed OCD patients. For this reason, they have been described as antiobsessional drugs, in addition to being antidepressants. What is surprising is that so many other excellent antidepressants, many of which are structurally related to these anti-obsessional drugs, appear ineffective for the symptoms of OCD. The distinctive feature of these anti-obsessional agents appears to be their potency for inhibiting serotonin uptake. Although most antidepressants, including imipramine and amitriptyline, inhibit the synaptic uptake of serotonin, none are quite as potent as clomipramine (or its metabolite desmethylclomipramine), fluvoxamine and fluoxetine [11].

Beyond this unique selectivity of serotonin uptake inhibitors for reducing OCD symptoms, the following results from clinical studies support a role for serotonin in the mediation of antiobsessional drug effects. In some studies, but not others, the improvement in obsessional symptoms correlates with the plasma level of clomipramine and not its less selective metabolite desmethylclomipramine [12]. With clomipramine treatment, the decrease in obsessional symptoms correlates ($r = 0.75$) with the decrease in the concentration of the serotonin metabolite 5-HIAA in cerebrospinal fluid – implicating the inhibition of reuptake in the antiobsessional effect [13]. A similar result obtains with serotonin content in blood platelets [14]. Finally, in a study of changes after chronic treatment, a serotonergic antagonist, metergoline, was found to induce a partial relapse of symptoms in OCD patients who had improved on clomipramine [15].

Is serotonin involved in the pathophysiology of OCD? There are three kinds of study that have searched for an abnormality of serotonergic function in untreated OCD patients. Studies of blood serotonin have been inconsistent, with one early investigation reporting a decrease in whole blood serotonin concentration [16] and a more recent study in OCD children failing to find an abnormality [14]. Platelets, which are the major reservoir of serotonin in blood, show normal uptake of serotonin, although one study found a decrease in the number of platelet serotonin uptake sites in untreated OCD patients [17]. This latter finding might seem paradoxical. Since OCD patients improve with serotonin uptake blockade, one might expect an increase rather than a decrease in the number of sites available for uptake. The explanation might ultimately relate to the chronic versus acute effects of drugs that block serotonin uptake, but currently we are left with two observations that are not easily reconciled. In a second approach to assessing serotonergic functioning, we found an increase in CSF 5-HIAA in nine OCD patients compared to age-matched healthy volunteers [18]. This preliminary result suggests increased turnover of serotonin in the central nervous system, possibly reflecting increased synthesis, increased reuptake, or increased intraneuronal metabolism. Finally, the challenge strategy has been used to assess serotonergic responsiveness in OCD patients. Here, the main finding is that m-CPP, a mixed serotonin receptor agonist, can induce obsessional symptoms in OCD patients but is largely without effects in healthy controls [11]. Their responsiveness to the symptom-inducing effects of the drug suggests an increase in the sensitivity of that population of 5-HT receptors subserving behavioral effects. These effects are blocked by pretreatment with the nonselective serotonin antagonist metergoline and they are blunted by chronic treatment with clomipramine [19]. The exact subtype of receptor and the precise location of m-CPPs effects remains unknown.

In summary, we know more about the treatment than the cause of OCD. Genetic factors may have some role, but the genotype may be expressed across a broad range of diagnostic categories – not simply OCD. Increased activity in the orbital-frontal cortex appears with PET imaging, but this may be an associated rather than etiologic feature. And finally, some abnormality of brain serotonergic pathways seems likely based on pharmacologic responsiveness, but additional research will be necessary to define a pathophysiologic role for serotonin in OCD.

References

1. Pauls DL, Towbin KE, Leckman JF et al. (1986) Arch. Gen. Psychiatry 43: 1180–1182.
2. Swedo SE et al. (1989) Am. J. Psychiatry 146: 246–249.
3. Laplane D, Baulac M, Widlocher D et al. (1984) J. Neurol. Neurosurg. Psychiatry 47.

4. Kelly D (1980) Anxiety and Emotions. Charles C Thomas.
5. Baxter L, Phelps M, Mazziotta J, Guze B and Schuartz J (1987) Arch. Gen. Psychiatry 44: 211–218.
6. Baxter L, Schwartz J, Mazziotta J et al. (1988) Am. J. Psychiatry 145: 1560–1563.
7. Nordahl TE, Benkelfat C, Semple W et al. (1989) Neuropsychopharmacology 2: 23–28.
8. Swedo SE et al. (1989) Arch. Gen. Psychiatry 46: 518–523.
9. Benkelfat C, Nordahl TE, Semple WE, King AC, Murphy, DL and Cohen RM (1990) Arch. Gen. Psychiatry 47: 840–848.
10. Murphy D, Zohar J, Benkelfat C, Pato M, Pigott T and Insel T (1989) Br. J. Psychiatry 155: 15–24.
11. Zohar J and Insel TR (1987) Biol. Psychiatry 22: 667–687.
12. Insel T, Murphy D, Cohen R, Alterman I, Kilts C and Linnoila M (1983) Arch. Gen. Psychiatry 40: 605–612.
13. Thoren P, Asberg M, Bertilsson L, Mellstrom B, Sjoqvist F and Traskman L (1980) Arch. Gen. Psychiatry 37: 1289–1294.
14. Flament M, Rapoport J, Murphy D, Berg C and Lake C (1987) Arch. Gen. Psychiatry 44: 219–225.
15. Benkelfat C, Murphy DL, Zohar J, Hill JL, Grover G and Insel TR (1989) Arch. Gen. Psychiatry 46: 23–28.
16. Yaryura-Tobias J and Bhagavan H (1977) Am. J. Psychiatry 134: 1298–1299.
17. Weizman A et al. (1986) Am. J. Psychiatry 143: 335–339.
18. Insel T, Mueller E, Alterman I, Linnoila M and Murphy D (1985) Biol. Psychiatry 20: 1174–1189.
19. Zohar J, Insel TR, Zohar KR, Hill JL and Murphy DL (1988) Arch. Gen. Psychiatry 45: 167–172.

Biological Psychiatry, Volume 1. G. Racagni et al., editors.

Animal models of obsessive-compulsive disorder

Berend Olivier, Marianne Houben-Gelissen, Jan Mos and Guus van der Poel
CNS-Pharmacology, DUPHAR B.V., P.O.Box 900, 1380 DA Weesp, The Netherlands

Introduction

Obsessive-Compulsive Disorder (OCD) is clinically classified under the anxiety disorders in DSM III-R, although some doubts exist about its classification as an anxiety disorder [1], OCD is characterized by obsessions and compulsions in about 85% of patients, while the remainder have only obsessions. It is fairly common in the general population (1–3% lifetime prevalence). There is clear evidence for a biological basis of OCD, coming from different sources, viz. genetic studies, studies of neuroanatomical, neurophysiological and endocrinological deviations (basal state differences and biological markers), studies of pharmacological challenges provoking or exacerbating obsessive-compulsive symptoms and clinical pharmacology.

Although there are many case records and small uncontrolled studies indicating effects of a variety of psychoactive drugs in OCD, there seems to be only one group of compounds with proven efficacy, viz. the serotonin reuptake inhibitors (chlorimipramine, fluvoxamine, fluoxetine). These clinical findings can be used to steer animal research into preclinical models of OCD, because until now such models have been clearly lacking and no animal data are available to predict putative anti-OCD activity of new drugs.

The present paper outlines several possibilities to develop animal models of OCD and surveys data obtained in various anxiety paradigms in order to predict such anti-OCD potency.

Pharmacological models

Owing to the anti-obsessional qualities (and specificity) of the 5-HT reuptake blockers, a fruitful approach to find an animal OCD-model seems to be to sort out whether a certain (anxiety) model can distinguish specific 5-HT reuptake blockers from other anxiolytics, like the benzodiazepines, which are not active in OCD.

The ultrasonic distress vocalization paradigm in rat pups seems to offer such qualities [2,3]. Using a low-stress (37°C) and a high-stress (18°C) condition, 5-HT reuptake blockers inhibit vocalizations under high stress, but not under low stress conditions. Benzodiazepines reduce vocalizations under both conditions, but only partly under high-stress conditions. 5-HT_{1A}-agonists (ipsapirone, buspirone, flesinoxan) strongly reduce vocalizations under both stress situations, whereas mixed 5-HT_1-agonists (eltoprazine, RU 24969, TFMPP) mildly reduce vocalizations only under high-stress conditions. 5-HT_3 antagonists have no effect under these conditions. These data indicate that 5-HT reuptake blockers can be differentiated from other serotonergic ligands and from BDZ-agonists. Drugs with a similar profile in this paradigm could be predicted to have anti-OCD potency, although much more data have to be gathered to exclude false positives (and negatives) in this model.

Another approach to study OCD comes from clinical evidence demonstrating that pharmacological interventions can reduce as well as exacerbate obsessive-compulsive symptoms. The latter has been shown after application of the serotonergic agonist mCPP in OCD-patients. mCPP did not induce anxiety or obsessions in normal healthy volunteers, but exacerbated symptoms in OCD-patients. Metergoline reduced symptoms in OCD-patients. Moreover, the beneficial effects of clomipramine could be antagonized by the (nonspecific) 5-HT antagonist metergoline [4,5]. Since mCPP is primarily a 5-HT_{1C}-agonist (although it has various other activities) it could be hypothesized that 5-HT_{1C} receptors in the CNS are somehow involved in the emergence of obsessive and compulsive behaviours. It is noteworthy that mCPP, when given to rats induces "purposeless chewing", which could perhaps model compulsive behaviour in the rat. Theoretically, drugs which are able to antagonize this behaviour (e.g. 5-HT_{1C}-antagonists) could be considered as potential anti-OCD drugs.

Neuroanatomical models

Psychosurgical interventions (e.g. cingulectomy) have been applied successfully in severe OCD, suggestive for frontal lobe dysfunction in OCD. Moreover, co-morbidity with neurological disorders involving dysfunctions of the basal ganglia (e.g. Gilles de la Tourette syndrome) has frequently been described, pointing to an involvement of the basal ganglia in OCD too [6,7]. There is evidence that the orbitofrontal loop, including the orbitofrontal cortex, the caudate nucleus, the globus pallidus and part of the substantia nigra is malfunctioning, possibly leading to disinhibition of "innate motor programmes". It is worth remarking that part of these structures have high densities of serotonin receptors, viz. 5-HT_{1B}-receptors in rodents and their counterpart, 5-HT_{1D}-receptors in non-rodents, including humans [8]. An attractive hypothesis could be that modulation of these serotonergic receptors in the basal ganglia with specific ligands (or for some reason with 5-HT reuptake blockers) could lead to anti-OCD effects. There are suggestions [6] that OCD patients have a modified regulation of aggression. These authors suggest that "an increase in responsiveness at some cohort of serotonergic sites might lead to altered modulation of aggression, with OCD patients experiencing worry and guilt over aggressive acts not committed". Since serotonin is heavily involved in the regulation of impulsivity and aggression and OCD can be regarded as a disease with impulsive discontrol, it could be argued that certain anti-aggressive drugs, acting via 5-$HT_{1B/1D}$ receptors, could display anti-OCD efficacy. Therefore determination of the anti-aggressive potency of drugs in animal models of aggressive behaviour could be of help to find anti-OCD therapeutics.

Miscellaneous models

Various other animal models of OCD have been proposed, including ethologically derived models based on displacement behaviour, like ritualistic grooming, stereotypy or adjunctive behaviour. In this context, it is interesting to note that excessive hair-pulling (trichotillomania), a certain form of compulsive behaviour, seems to have an animal analogue, acral lick dermatitis in certain dogs [7]. CMI is able to antagonize this hair-pulling both in humans and in dogs, and therefore the "dog"-model seems to have attractive "face" and "predictive" validity.

Conclusions

Although OCD seems to be a "serotonergic" disease, it is highly unlikely that other neurotransmitter systems are not involved in such a complex disorder. Animal models of OCD therefore should not be based purely on a "one neurotransmitter hypothesis". Increasing knowledge on OCD in humans will lead to new approaches in the preclinical studies of OCD models and its neuropharmacology.

References

1. Montgomery SA (1990) In: Montgomery SA, Goodman WA and Goeting N (eds.) Obsessive-Compulsive Disorder. Duphar Medical Relations, pp. 1–6.
2. Mos J and Olivier B (1988) In: Olivier B and Mos I (eds.) Depression, Anxiety and Aggression. Preclinical and Clinical Interfaces. Medidact, Houten, pp. 85–93.
3. Mos J and Olivier B (1989) In: Bevan P, Cools AR and Archer T (eds.) Behavioural Pharmacology of 5-HT. Lawrence Erlbaum Ass., New Jersey, pp. 361–366.
4. Zohar J and Insel TR (1987) Biol. Psychiatry 22: 667–687.
5. Benkelfat C, Murphy DL, Zohar J, Hill JL, Grover G and Insel TR (1989) Arch. Gen. Psychiatry 46: 23–28.
6. Insel TR and Winslow JT (1990) In: Jenike MA, Baer L and Minichiello WE (eds.) Obsessive-Compulsive Disorders: Theory and Management. Year Book Medical Publishers Inc., Chicago, pp. 118–131.
7. Rapoport JL (1990) Psychol. Med. 20: 465–469.
8. Waeber C, Schoeffter P, Palacios JM and Hoyer D (1988) Naunyn-Schmiedeberg's Arch. Pharmacol. 337: 595–601.

Biological Psychiatry, Volume 1. G. Racagni et al., editors.

Studies of fluvoxamine in OCD

Christopher J. McDougle and Wayne K. Goodman
Yale University Department of Psychiatry, 34 Park Street, New Haven, CT 06519, U.S.A.

The past decade has witnessed significant advances in the pharmacotherapy of obsessive compulsive disorder (OCD). In particular, the clear efficacy of serotonin (5-HT) reuptake inhibitors (RUIs), such as fluvoxamine, clomipramine and fluoxetine, has been established in controlled studies in OCD patients. Consistent with these drug response data are the hypotheses that changes in 5-HT function are critical to the treatment of OCD and perhaps involved in the pathophysiology of at least some patients with the disorder.

Fluvoxamine is a unicyclic drug that possesses selective and potent effects on 5-HT reuptake inhibition. In addition to being an effective antidepressant medication, fluvoxamine has been demonstrated to significantly reduce obsessive-compulsive symptoms in patients with OCD. In a preliminary report by Price et al. [1], ten OCD patients received single-blind treatment with fluvoxamine (mean daily dose ± SD = 274 ± 30 mg/day) for at least 4 weeks (5.9 ± 2.0 weeks) following at least 2 weeks of placebo (3.4 ± 0.8 weeks). For the entire sample, fluvoxamine caused highly significant decreases in scores on the Yale-Brown Obsessive Compulsive Scale (Y-BOCS), the Hamilton Depression Scale and the Hamilton Anxiety Scale. On the basis of Clinical Global Impression Scale criteria, six patients were judged to be responders and four nonresponders.

A subsequent 6- to 8-week double-blind placebo-controlled trial of fluvoxamine was conducted in 42 patients with primary OCD [2]. Approximately one-half of the patients also had symptoms of major depression. Fluvoxamine (255 ± 60 mg/day) was significantly better than placebo on all measures of obsessive-compulsive symptoms including the Y-BOCS. Nine of 21 patients were responders with fluvoxamine compared with no responders with placebo. Fluvoxamine was effective in patients with OCD both with and without secondary depression. The anti-obsessive-compulsive efficacy of fluvoxamine demonstrated in this controlled study of OCD patients lends partial support to the 5-HT hypothesis of OCD. Although fluvoxamine is clearly superior to placebo in treating the target symptoms of OCD, it is also evident that it is not curative. Thus, although fluvoxamine-responsive OCD patients may be suffering from a dysregulation in 5-HT function, this leaves a substantial group of patients who may have OCD on the basis of some other neurochemical abnormality.

A recently published study by Goodman et al. [3] was conducted to evaluate whether 5-HT reuptake inhibition is critical to the treatment of OCD. Forty outpatients with a principal diagnosis of OCD were randomized in a double-blind fashion to 8 weeks of treatment with either fluvoxamine (213 ± 55 mg/day) (n = 21) or the norepinephrine reuptake inhibitor, desipramine hydrochloride (188 ± 68 mg/day) (n = 19). Fluvoxamine was significantly better than desipramine in reducing the severity of obsessive-compulsive symptoms as measured by the Y-BOCS and by the global response rate. Eleven of 21 patients were responders with fluvoxamine compared to 2 of 19 patients with desipramine. Fluvoxamine, but not desipramine, was also effective in reducing the severity of secondary depression. Fluvoxamine-induced improvement in symptoms of OCD was not correlated with the severity of baseline depressive symptoms. The finding that the selective and potent 5-HT reuptake inhibitor fluvoxamine was significantly better than the selective norepinephrine reuptake inhibitor desipramine strengthens the hypothesis that inhibition of 5-HT neuronal transport is relevant to anti-obsessive-compulsive efficacy. Furthermore, the selective efficacy of 5-HT reuptake inhibitors in OCD differentiates this condition from depression and panic disorder, two disorders in which drugs with variable effects on acute monoamine reuptake are roughly equal in efficacy.

Despite success with potent inhibitors of 5-HT reuptake, however, as many as 50% of OCD patients are clinically unchanged after an adequate trial with these agents. It is conceivable that this subgroup of treatment-resistant patients has OCD as a result of abnormalities in neurochemical systems (e.g. dopamine) different from or in addition to those involving 5-HT [4]. Alternatively, these refractory patients may have alterations in 5-HT neurotransmission different from those in patients who are responsive to 5-HT reuptake inhibitors. One approach to this treatment-resistant group has been to add agents such as tryptophan, buspirone, fenfluramine and lithium, which may act by enhancing 5-HT function, to ongoing treatment with antidepressants. In order to objectively evaluate this combination treatment approach in OCD patients, McDougle et al. [5] conducted 2- and 4-week double-blind placebo-controlled studies of lithium augmentation in 20 and 10 OCD patients, respectively, who had failed to respond to fluvoxamine alone. Although 2 weeks of double-blind lithium augmentation produced a small but statistically significant reduction in obsessive-compulsive symptoms, most patients did not have a clinically meaningful response. Furthermore, there was no statistical or clinical improvement in obsessive-compulsive symptoms during the subsequent 4-week double-blind place-controlled trial of lithium augmentation. On the basis of treatment response criteria, only 18% and 0% of the patients responded to lithium augmentation of fluvoxamine during the 2- and 4-week treatment trials, respectively. These data suggest that lithium augmentation of potent 5-HT reuptake inhibitors is not an effective treatment strategy in most patients with OCD who are refractory to 5-HT reuptake inhibition alone. Preliminary results from an ongoing 6-week double-blind placebo-controlled investigation of buspirone addition to the treatment of fluvoxamine-refractory OCD patients indicate that this treatment combination may be effective in a subgroup of OCD patients [6]. Taken together, however, these findings suggest that it is unlikely that a solitary disturbance in 5-HT function can fully account for the pathophysiology of OCD.

To date, the role of the brain dopamine (DA) system in the pathophysiology of OCD has not been carefully studied, despite preclinical and clinical evidence implicating it in the mediation of some obsessive-compulsive behaviors. For example, recent studies indicate that 45% to 90% of patients with the chronic tic disorder, Tourette's syndrome (TS), display obsessive-compulsive symptoms. That DA is involved in TS is based in part on the well-documented effectiveness of haloperidol and other DA antagonists in suppressing tics in the majority of TS patients. These pharmacologic data, taken together with reports of lower baseline and postprobenecid mean cerebrospinal fluid levels of the DA metabolite homovanillic acid in TS patients compared with available comparison groups, have led several groups of investigators to suggest that TS is a disorder in which postsynaptic DA receptors are supersensitive.

In a recent open case series by McDougle et al. [7], neuroleptic was added to ongoing treatment in 17 non-psychotic OCD patients unresponsive to fluvoxamine with or without lithium. These cases were then reviewed by a rater blind to treatment outcome to determine whether co-morbid tic-spectrum disorders or schizotypal personality disorder (SPD) were associated with a positive response to neuroleptic addition. According to conservative criteria, 9 out of 17 (53%) patients were judged responders to this combination treatment strategy. A concurrent diagnosis of chronic tics or SPD was associated with a positive response to addition of neuroleptic. Seven of 8 (88%) patients with comorbid chronic tic disorders or SPD were responders, whereas only 2 of 9 (22%) patients without these co-morbid diagnoses were responders. Preliminary results from a 4-week double-blind placebo-controlled study of haloperidol addition to fluvoxamine-refractory patients with OCD support the efficacy of this combination treatment strategy and suggest that OCD patients with a co-morbid chronic tic disorder may have a preferential response to this approach [8].

In summary, potent inhibitors of 5-HT reuptake, such as fluvoxamine, have clearly been established as the first-line pharmacologic treatment for patients with OCD. The controlled addition of agents which affect 5-HT function in ongoing treatment in 5-HT RUI-refractory OCD patients has not, to date, yielded robust clinical results. The addition of low-dose DA antagonists to ongoing 5-HT RUI treatment in refractory OCD patients has produced encouraging findings. In particular, OCD patients with a co-morbid chronic tic disorder such as TS may have a preferential response to conjoint 5-HT RUI-DA antagonist treatment. These drug response data suggest that the 5-HT systems and the DA systems may contribute to the pharmacotherapy, and possibly the mediation, of obsessive-compulsive symptoms in some patients with OCD.

References

1. Price LH, Goodman WK, Charney DS, Rasmussen SA and Heninger GR (1987) Am. J. Psychiatry 144: 1059–1061.

2. Goodman WK, Price LH, Rasmussen SA, Delgado PL, Heninger GR and Charney DS (1989) Arch. Gen. Psychiatry 46: 36–44.
3. Goodman WK, Price LH, Delgado PL, Palumbo J, Krystal JH, Heninger GR and Charney DS (1990) Arch. Gen. Psychiatry 47: 577–585.
4. Goodman WK, McDougle CJ, Price LH, Riddle MA, Pauls DL and Leckman JF (1990) J. Clin. Psychiatry 51(8S): 36–43.
5. McDougle CJ, Price LH, Goodman WK, Charney DS and Heninger GR (1991) J. Clin. Psychopharmacol. (in press).
6. McDougle CJ, Goodman WK, Price LH, Holzer IC, McCance-Katz EF and Heninger GR (1991) Am. Psychiat. Assoc. New Research Abstract No. 328.
7. McDougle CJ, Goodman WK, Price LH, Delgado PL, Krystal JH, Charney DS and Heninger GR (1990) Am. J. Psychiatry 147: 652–654.
8. McDougle CJ, Goodman WK, Price LH, Lee NC and Heninger GR (1991) (unpublished data).

Biological Psychiatry, Volume 1. G. Racagni et al., editors.

How then should we treat OCD?

N. Fineberg, D.B. Montgomery and S.A. Montgomery
Department of Psychiatry, St Mary's Hospital Medical School, London, U.K.

So far there have been 9 double-blind placebo-controlled studies of clomipramine (CMI) in OCD, reviewed by Montgomery [1] and in each case CMI has emerged as significantly superior to placebo, in some cases in spite of only small numbers of patients in the treatment groups.

Clomipramine was shown to have a direct antiobsessional effect in a study which excluded concomitant depression, so that the effect could not be secondary to effects on depression. This result was later confirmed in 2 large multi-centre studies [2,3].

Three studies have reported a weekly analysis of data and in these studies a significant advantage for CMI over placebo was seen as early as 1 or 2 weeks following the start of treatment. In addition, the studies show a low rate of placebo response at around 5%, which is unusual in treatment studies in psychiatry and might explain the ability of small studies to show significant results so early in treatment.

The strong evidence of efficacy for CMI can be contrasted with the lack of evidence of efficacy for tricyclic antidepressants, lithium, benzodiazepines and neuroleptics. CMI has been directly compared with a wide range of conventional antidepressants, including nortriptyline, amitriptyline, clorgyline, desipramine, and imipramine. The consistent demonstration of antiobsessional superiority for CMI in studies that tended to include quite small numbers of patients argues strongly for the efficacy of CMI and the lack of efficacy of the comparative drug.

Clomipramine is associated with a number of unpleasant and potentially dangerous side effects. Attention has turned, therefore, to the investigation of the newer, more selective 5-HT reuptake inhibitors. The results for fluvoxamine are convincing. So far there have been 4 placebo-controlled studies of fluvoxamine in OCD [1] and each study has demonstrated a significant advantage for fluvoxamine over placebo. Two studies reported data sequentially over the course of treatment, one found early onset of efficacy and one did not. A further direct comparison of fluvoxamine with the noradrenergic antidepressant desipramine demonstrated a significant superiority for fluvoxamine and supports the data suggesting efficacy for fluvoxamine in OCD.

There has been a single multi-centre study examining the effects of sertraline in non-depressed obsessional patients and the results show a significant advantage for sertraline over placebo at the 8-week end-point of the study. A separate report of data on what appears to be a small subgroup of these patients failed to show evidence of efficacy for sertraline.

From these results, it appears that CMI and the newer more highly selective 5-HT reuptake inhibitors are effective treatments for OCD, whereas conventional antidepressants without potent serotonergic effects are not.

These findings have led to the hypothesis that the biological abnormality underlying OCD principally involve serotonergic mechanisms. Demonstration of the nature of this serotonergic abnormality might direct future treatment for OCD.

We have applied the L-tryptophan (LTP) test to 16 untreated non-depressed obsessional patients and 16 matched controls and found a significant difference in endocrine response, with a significantly elevated growth hormone and a less markedly elevated prolactin response in the obsessional group, indicating a possible abnormality in $5\text{-HT}_1/5\text{-HT}_{1A}$ mechanisms which are thought to be involved in mediating the LTP-induced endocrine response. An LTP challenge study by Charney et al. [1] produced broadly similar results which lend support to these findings.

The evidence points, therefore, toward a serotonergic abnormality underlying OCD. The exact receptor mechanism associated with the abnormality remains unclear; however the development and investigation of drugs that are specific for different 5-HT receptor subtypes is likely to clarify the situation in the future.

References

1. Montgomery SA, Fineberg N and Montgomery DB (1990). In: Montgomery SA, Goodman WK and Goeting N (eds.) Obsessive Compulsive Disorders: Current Approaches. Pub. Duphar Med. Relations, pp. 54–63.
2. Chouinard G, Goodman, Griest J et al. (1990) Psychopharmacol. Bull. (Suppl. 3) 26: 279–284.
3. Fineberg N and Montgomery S (1990) In: Montgomery SA, Goodman WK and Goeting N (eds.) Obsessive Compulsive Disorders: Current Approaches. Pub. Duphar Med. Relations, pp. 19–25.
4. Charney DS, Goodman WC, Price LH et al. (1988) Arch. Gen. Psychiatry 45: 177–185.

Biological Psychiatry, Volume 1. G. Racagni et al., editors.

Obsessive-compulsive disorder in different cultures: An Egyptian perspective

A. Okasha
Department of Psychiatry, Ain Shams University, Cairo, Egypt

The material for this investigation was drawn from those patients suffering from obsessional disorders who had attended the University Department of Psychiatry of Ain Shams, Cairo and from those seen in private practice between the years 1968–1975. Those were followed-up for a period ranging up to 5 years and all were examined personally. Eighty-four cases, 54 males and 30 females were studied.

The majority of patients were between 20–30 years. All of them had religious ruminations and sexual impulses. The onset was sudden in 67% of cases but followed a gradual progressive course in the remainder.

The marital status was of no significant importance as regards obsessional illness. Ideas and ruminations were more common among the university educated patients, while rituals and impulses prevailed among those of low education.

Positive family history of obsessional illness in near relatives was observed in 26% (approximately 31%).

The main presenting symptoms in our study were anxiety in 71 patients, obsessional symptoms in 25, depression in 8 and social incapacity in 12. Precipitating factors, whether psychological or physical, were noted in about 69% of the cases. Most of the patients were neurotic as children, 78% with fears, anxiety, enuresis, irritability, shyness, sleep disturbances, etc. Actual compulsive personality was noticed in 22%, anxious, dependent and histrionic personalities in 39% and the others showed mixed types with no specificity.

The most common presentation was ruminations, then fears and rituals. The prevalent fears were those connected with diseases, death, madness, germs and extra-terrestrial powers.

The religious nature of upbringing and education, the emphasis on religious rituals, the warding off of blasphemous thoughts through the phrase "I seek refuge with the Lord from the accursed satan" can explain much of the phenomenology of the obsessive-compulsive moslem, even if he is not practising his religious duties. The emphasis on cleanliness (in Arabic, Tahara; in Hebrew, Taharat) or ritual purity is the cornerstone of most compulsive rituals. The number of prayers, the verbal content can be subject of scrupulousness, checking and repetition. A bath is necessary after ejaculation, whatever its nature and after menstruation.

The lines of management given to our patients were non-specific, namely sup-

Table 1. Form and content of obsessions (% in Egypt and India)

	Doubts	Thoughts	Fears	Urges	Images	Convictions	Egypt (%)	India (%)
Dirt	2	0	5	0	–	1	5	18
Religion	1	8	0	8	0	3	12.6	4.5
Sex	0	8	0	7	2	0	10.7	12.5
Death	0	6	8	3	0	0	10.7	6
Illness	1	3	15	0	1	0	12.6	8.2
Aggression	0	1	0	3	0	0	2.7	5.2
Harm	0	2	7	1	0	2	7.5	10.3
Past	0	7	0	1	3	1	7.5	9.3
Daily activities	13	3	0	2	0	5	14.6	14.2
Inanimate, impersonal	0	2	0	1	0	7	6.5	4.7
Others	2	4	1	8	0	0	9.1	6.5

portive psychotherapy, imipramine, amitriptyline and small doses of neuroleptics. Few cases received gradual desensitization and ECT and 2 had leucotomy.

The outcome after 5 years was 15% symptom-free, 56% improved with interrupted exacerbation and 29% unchanged. This may reflect to some extent the natural history of the disorder as the specific 5-HT re-uptake inhibitors and exposure prevention claimed to be of specific value were not used. Probably the outcome would have been different but this is left for the future follow-up studies on the advanced management of OCN.

We remain profoundly ignorant of the biological, psychological and social variables which influence the onset and outcome of various kinds of neurotic disorders. Retrospective follow-up studies such as reviewed here, cannot be expected to provide definitive answers concerning the efficacy of treatment and the outcome of the illness, but they can provide a framework for understanding the problems connected with such disorders.

Presentation of obsessional illness in Egypt varied according to culture. Rituals and impulses were common in patients from rural areas, while ideas and ruminations predominated in the educated.

Table 2. Common obsessional themes in Egypt, India, England and Jerusalem

	No.	Filth (%)	Harm (%)	Order (%)	Sex (%)	Religion
Egypt [1]	84	43	22	12	18	56
India [2]	82	46	29	27	10	11
England [3]	45	38	23	11	9	–
Jerusalem [4]	10	40	20	10	10	50

References

1. Okasha A (1973) Ain Shams Med. J. 21(4): 367–374.
2. Akhtar S, Wig N et al. (1975) Br. J. Psychiatry 127: 342–348.
3. Stern RS and Cobbs JP (1978) Br. J. Psychiatry 132: 233–239.
4. Greenberg D (1984) Am. J. Psychother. 38: 4.
5. Khanna S and Channabasavanna SM (1988) Psychopathology 21: 12–18.

Biological Psychiatry, Volume 1. G. Racagni et al., editors.

Obsessive-compulsive related disorders

Eric Hollander, Dan Stein, Concetta M. Decaria, Maxim Frenkel, Sari Trungold and Michael R. Liebowitz

OCD Biological Studies Program, Department of Psychiatry, Columbia University College of Physicians and Surgeons, 722 West 168th Street, New York, NY 10032, U.S.A.

Introduction

Current diagnostic classification systems are struggling with a possible overlap of obsessive-compulsive disorder (OCD) with several related spectrums, including specific somatoform, impulse control, eating, delusional and tic disorders. Based on clinical symptoms, associated features, family history, presumed etiology, and response to serotonin-reuptake inhibitors and behavior therapy, there appears to be a group of disorders which we might call obsessive-compulsive related disorders.

These include body dysmorphic disorder and hypochondriasis (somatoform disorders); trichotillomania, onychophagia, pathological gambling and sexual compulsions (disorders of impulse control and pathological grooming behaviors); depersonalization (dissociative disorders); anorexia nervosa and bulimia (eating disorders); Tourette's syndrome (tic-related disorders of childhood/adolescent onset); delusional disorders (monosymptomatic delusional hypochondriasis, delusional disorder somatic subtype and pathological jealousy); and personality disorders characterized by impulsivity (borderline personality).

The serotonergic system may be involved in risk aversiveness, estimation of future harm and impulsivity. A dimensional approach to the study of risk aversiveness vs. impulsivity may help describe where various disorders mentioned above lie on this serotonergic/risk aversive/impulsive spectrum.

Biological challenge studies with serotonergic agents such as m-CPP may assess sensitivity of 5-HT systems in the OCD-related disorders.

The use of serotonin reuptake blockers for the treatment of obsessive-compulsive related disorders will be described. Pharmacological dissection with 5-HT reuptake blockers may also help define the OCD-related disorders.

Methods

Biological challenge studies

Patients with obsessive-compulsive disorder, Tourette's syndrome, anorexia nervosa and borderline personality disorder underwent biological challenges with oral m-CPP (0.5 mg/kg) and placebo under double-blind, randomized conditions.

Subjects had clinician ratings of obsessive-compulsive symptoms using the Clinician Challenge OC Scale. Prolactin measurements over time prior to and following, m-CPP administration were collected.

Serotonin reuptake blocker treatment

Patients with obsessive-compulsive disorder, body dysmorphic disorder, depersonalization, sexual compulsions, hypochondriasis and trichotillomania underwent open treatment studies with serotonin reuptake blockers, including fluoxetine, clomipramine and fluvoxamine. A literature review of treatment studies with 5-HT reuptake blockers in the above disorders, as well as in eating disorders, Tourette's syndrome, onychophagia will be presented.

Results

Patients with obsessive-compulsive disorder, Tourette's syndrome and eating disorders may be particularly sensitive to the obsessogenic effects of the 5-HT agonist m-CPP. In contrast, patients with borderline personality disorder do not have a dysphoric response, but rather feel "high" in response to m-CPP.

5-HT reuptake inhibitors such as fluoxetine, clomipramine and fluvoxamine are highly effective in obsessive-compulsive disorder. Preliminary trials with these agents also appear promising in the treatment of body dysmorphic disorder, depersonalization disorder, trichotillomania, hypochondriasis, anorexia nervosa, bulimia nervosa, onychophagia and Tourette's syndrome. More work is needed, or findings are not yet promising, in the treatment of sexual compulsions, pathological gambling, pathological jealousy, borderline personality disorder and some delusional disorders. Further controlled trials are required for all of the OCD-related disorders. Response to serotonin reuptake blockers may have psychopathological significance in differentiating compulsive disorders from disorders of impulse control.

Acknowledgments

Supported in part by Research Scientist Development Award MH-00750 (Dr. Hollander) from the National Institute of Mental Health, Bethesda, Maryland.

References

1. Hollander E (1991) In: Pato M and Zohar J (eds.) Current Treatments of Obsessive-Compulsive Disorder. American Psychiatric Press Inc., Washington, D.C., pp. 173–191.
2. Hollander E, Liebowitz MR, Fallon B et al. (1990) J. Clin. Psychopharmacol. 10: 200–203.

3. Hollander E, Liebowitz MR, Winchel RW et al. (1989) Am. J. Psychiatry 146: 768–770.
4. Hollander E, Liebowitz MR and DeCaria C (1989) Psychiatr. Dev. 4: 267–296.
5. Hollander E, DeCaria C, Gulley R et al. (1991) Psychiatr. Res. 36: 1–17.

Biological Psychiatry, Volume 1. G. Racagni et al., editors.

Selectivity for ω-receptor subtypes as a strategy for a novel approach in the development of anxiolytic drugs

Salomon Z. Langer and Sonia Arbilla
Synthélabo Recherche (LERS), 31, avenue Paul Valiant Couturier, F-92220 Bagneux, France

Introduction

Despite their widespread use, the molecular mechanism by which benzodiazepines produce their anxiolytic actions remained speculative for several years. The recent development of drugs exhibiting only some of the pharmacological actions of benzodiazepines (hypnotic, anxiolytic) has reinforced the concept that different receptors or receptor subtypes exist, with which these drugs interact to exert their preferential pharmacological action [1–4]. This view is being confirmed by the recent advances in the field of molecular biology and the pharmacological characterization of transfected receptors [5,6].

It is well established that drugs which interact with ω (benzodiazepine) receptors possess different properties in relation to their intrinsic activity and their positive or negative allosteric modulation of the $GABA_A$-chloride channel macromolecular complex [7,8]. Thus, a drug with selectivity for an ω-receptor subtype [3,4,7,8] and varying degrees of intrinsic activity may produce a specific pharmacological action such as anxiolysis, sedation or myorelaxation [7,8].

Imidazopyridines as a new class of anxiolytics

In spite of previous controversy about the receptor subtype which is involved in the effect of anxiolytic drugs, it is now clear that sedative and hypnotic effects may result from the stimulation of ω_1-receptors by selective compounds possessing high intrinsic activity [1,9,10]. The imidazopyridine zolpidem is at present a typical representative of this type of drug. The low affinity and lack of intrinsic activity of zolpidem for ω_2-receptors may indicate that ω_2-receptors are involved in the mechanism of action of drugs possessing myorelaxant activity [9].

Alpidem is an imidazopyridine which possesses selective anxiolytic activity [9,10] as well as high selectivity for some ω-receptor subtypes. Due to its high affinity for ω_1-receptors, alpidem is as an excellent tool for assessing the receptor subtype as well as the allosteric interactions involved in the mechanism of action of anxiolytics.

The selectivity of alpidem for ω-receptor subtypes

The cerebellum, spinal cord and kidneys are typical examples of tissues that possess receptors of the ω_1-, ω_2- and ω_3-subtypes respectively [3,4]. It is now well established that the majority of benzodiazepines do not discriminate between ω_1- and ω_2-receptor subtypes: consequently, the selectivity of a compound for ω-receptor subtypes can be assessed by its relative potency to displace benzodiazepine binding to tissues differentially enriched in ω-receptor subtypes.

In receptor binding studies designed to evaluate the potency and selectivity of alpidem to displace either ^{3}H-diazepam binding to cerebellum and spinal cord, or ^{3}H-Ro 5-4864 binding to rat kidney, alpidem was found to possess higher affinity for ω_1-sites than for ω_2- sites [3,4,7]. In addition, these receptor binding studies have shown that alpidem has high affinity for ω_3-sites [7].

Confirming the ω_1-receptor selectivity of alpidem, the imidazopyridine displays preferential affinity for $GABA_A$ transfected receptors expressing the α_1 subunit variant when compared to those containing the α_3 variant. In addition, alpidem is devoid of significant affinity for $GABA_A$ receptors expressing the α_5 subunit variant (Pritchett, personal communication). A comparable selectivity for transfected $GABA_A$ receptors has been reported for zolpidem [6].

Characteristics of ^{3}H-alpidem binding to ω-receptor subtypes in human and rat brain

In human and rat brain, alpidem as a radioligand labels both ω_1- and ω_3-receptor subtypes. The affinity of ^{3}H-alpidem for ω_1-receptors is the same in the human parietal cortex and rat cerebral cortex [7], but there are marked differences in the affinity of ^{3}H-alpidem for ω_3-receptors. In fact, in the human brain, ω_3-receptors display an affinity for ^{3}H-alpidem which is 10 times lower than in the rat [7]. The affinity of alpidem for ω_3-receptors is one of the differences between this imidazopyridine and the benzodiazepines in relation to their pharmacological profile at ω-receptor subtypes. However, the involvement of ω_3-receptors in the anxiolytic effects of alpidem is unlikely, because the central pharmacological effects of alpidem in animal models are antagonized by flumazenil [7].

The allosteric interaction of alpidem with the $GABA_A$-ω site chloride channel macromolecular complex

The $GABA_A$-receptor that includes the chloride-ionophore and the picrotoxin-barbiturate site is known to be associated with ω-receptors on modulatory sites [7,8]. The GABA-mediated enhancement of the affinity of agonists for ω-receptors is considered as an index of the intrinsic activity of the compound at ω-receptors [14]. The binding of ^{3}H-alpidem occurs at an ω-site associated with the $GABA_A$-

receptor because it is increased in the presence of GABA. This confirms the agonist properties of alpidem at its recognition site. In contrast, alpidem does not interact directly with the chloride or the barbiturate modulatory site. In fact, neither the chloride ions nor pentobarbital allosterically modify the binding of ^{3}H-alpidem [7,8].

Conclusions

The concept that a receptor subtype-selective drug will offer a more specific therapeutic profile may be valid for the development of specific anxiolytic drugs. Alpidem is an imidazopyridine which represents a novel anxiolytic possessing considerable selectivity for the ω_1-receptor and very low affinity for the ω_2-site. Alpidem modulates the function of $GABA_A$ receptor by means of its positive allosteric interaction with the ω_1 modulatory site and it is likely that it does not modify in a direct manner the function of the barbiturate site and the chloride channel. The overall effect of alpidem at the macromolecular complex may be that of a partial agonist and this may account for its low sedative effects. The unique receptor profile and pharmacological spectrum of activity of this imidazopyridine may be relevant to its selective anxiolytic activity.

References

1. Arbilla S, Depoortere H, George P and Langer SZ (1985) Naunyn-Schmiedeberg's Arch. Pharmacol. 330: 248–251.
2. Braestrup C and Nielsen M (1981) J. Neurochem. 37: 333–341.
3. Langer SZ and Arbilla S (1988) Biochem. Behav. 29: 763–766.
4. Langer SZ and Arbilla S (1988) Fund. Clin. Pharmacol. 2: 159–170.
5. Pritchett DB, Lüddens H and Seeburg P (1989) Science 245: 1389–1392.
6. Pritchett DB and Seeburg P (1990) J. Neurochem. 54: 1802–1804.
7. Langer SZ, Arbilla S, Tan S, Lloyd KG, George P, Allen J and Wick A (1990) Pharmacopsychiatry 23: 106–107.
8. Langer SZ, Arbilla S, Benavides J and Scatton B (1990) In: Biggio G and Costa E (eds.) GABA and Benzodiazepine Subtypes. Raven Press, New York, pp. 61–72.
9. Depoortere H, Zivkovic B, Lloyd KG, Sanger D, Perrault G, Langer SZ and Barthoiini G (1986) J. Pharmacol. Exp. Ther. 237: 649–658.
10. Nicholson AN and Pascoe DA (1986) Br. J. Pharmacol. 21: 205–211.
11. More E, Perrault G and Zivkovic B (1987) Br. J. Pharmacol. 92 (Suppl.): 669P.
12. Perrault G, Morel E, Sanger DJ, Joly D, Zivkovic B and Lloyd KG (1988) Psychopharmacology 96 (Suppl.) Abstr. 33.03.17.
13. Zivkovic B, Arbilla S, Sanger DJ, Depoortere H, Scatton B and Langer SZ (1991) This volume.
14. Möhler H and Richards JG (1981) Nature 294: 763–765.

Biological Psychiatry, Volume 1. G. Racagni et al., editors.

Pharmacological and behavioural profile of alpidem as an anxiolytic

B. Zivkovic, G. Perrault and D.J. Sanger
Synthélabo Recherche (LERS), 31 Av. P.V. Couturier, 92220 Bagneux, France

Introduction

Benzodiazepines are undoubtedly efficacious drugs in the treatment of various forms of anxiety, but are still far from being specific anxiolytics. In addition to their anxiolytic action, they also induce anticonvulsant, myorelaxant, sedative and amnesic effects. A particularly difficult problem with benzodiazepines is the development of dependence which may lead to medically unjustified prolonged administration of these drugs.

It is now well established that benzodiazepines act at specific recognition sites within the $GABA_A$ receptor complex and enhance the efficacy of GABA in opening the associated chloride ion channel. These recognition sites, known as benzodiazepine receptors and recently classified as ω receptors, do not represent a uniform population, and at least 2 receptor subtypes, ω_1 and ω_2 can be differentiated pharmacologically [1]. While benzodiazepines are non-selective for the 2 receptor subtypes, several novel compounds structurally non-related to benzodiazepines display selectivity for the ω_1 receptor subtype. Among these ω_1 selective compounds, particular attention is given to the imidazopyridine, alpidem, which has been shown in clinical studies to be an anxioselective agent [2,3].

Anxiolytic activity of alpidem

In various animal tests, which were developed to evaluate the anxiolytic potential of benzodiazepines, alpidem showed an atypical pharmacological profile [4]. In mice, alpidem induced an increase in food consumption when the animals were placed in a novel environment, and inhibited marble-burying behaviour with a potency similar to that of chlordiazepoxide. However, in contrast to the benzodiazepines, alpidem failed to antagonize shock-induced fighting and was inactive in the four-plate test. In rats, alpidem decreased the rearing activity monitored in an experimental chamber equipped with a staircase as did the benzodiazepines, but in contrast to these drugs, it failed to produce any increase in exploratory activity. In a conflict procedure using mild electric shocks to suppress drinking in thirsty rats alpidem antagonized the punishment-induced behavioural suppression with a potency similar to chlordiazepoxide. However, in another conflict procedure involving operant behaviour and which is very sensitive to the action of benzodiazepines, alpidem was inactive. In social competition experiments, in which a group of 3 rats established a hierarchy of access to sweetened milk, alpidem increased the drinking time of subordinate rats in a manner similar to other anxiolytics [5].

Taken together, these results demonstrate that alpidem possesses anxiolytic properties but its overall anxiolytic profile is different from that of the benzodiazepines. Moreover, as the effects of alpidem in these tests were antagonized by the benzodiazepine antagonist flumazenil, it is clear that the action of alpidem involves omega receptors. In view of alpidem's selectivity for the ω_1 receptor subtype, it is tempting to hypothesize that this receptor subtype is essential for the anxiolytic action of benzodiazepines.

Central depressant effects of alpidem

In contrast to the central depressant effects of benzodiazepines, which are induced by doses within the anxiolytic range, the doses of alpidem active in tests predictive of anxiolytic activity are at least 10 times lower than the doses inducing sedative effects. Moreover, alpidem is devoid of myorelaxant activity and thus can be distinguished from benzodiazepines not only on quantitative but also on qualitative grounds.

Another striking difference between alpidem and benzodiazepines is related to the effects of these drugs on cognitive functions. It is well known that benzodiazepines produce anterograde amnesia and that this may occur not only when these drugs are given at sedative and hypnotic doses but also within the dose range recommended for the treatment of anxiety. In the test of acquisition of conditioned fear in mice, alpidem produced effects on learning with doses which exceeded by a factor of 4 the doses affecting exploratory activity, whereas the benzodiazepines, diazepam and chlordiazepoxide, produced a cognitive deficit with doses which were equal to or lower than doses inducing other behavioural effects. Therefore, it is likely that alpidem will have a lower potential than benzodiazepines for inducing cognitive deficits in man [4]. Indeed, clinical studies with alpidem support this prediction [3].

Potential of alpidem for inducing tolerance and dependence

A particular problem with the use of benzodiazepines in the treatment of anxiety is the development of dependence which may lead to the prolonged administration of these drugs. As the development of tolerance and dependence seems to be related to the level of receptor occupancy as well as the intrinsic activity of a given compound, it may be assumed that drugs with low intrinsic activity which are

Table 1. Effect of repeated treatment (10 days) with alpidem or diazepam on the latency to convulsions induced by isoniazid in mice

Repeated treatment (10 days)	Daily dose (mg/kg, p.o.)	Acute flumazenil (mg/kg, i.p.)	Latency to convulsions (min)	
			6 h withdrawal	42 h withdrawal
Vehicle	–	0	19.5 ± 1.0	19.9 ± 0.6
Alpidem	200	0	24.4 ± 1.4[a]	20.3 ± 0.7
Alpidem	200	5	19.3 ± 0.9	20.5 ± 0.6
Diazepam	10	0	23.8 ± 0.7[a]	13.9 ± 0.5[b]
Diazepam	10	5	14.2 ± 0.6[b]	13.1 ± 0.9[b]

[a]$P < 0.05$; [b]$P < 0.01$ vs. repeated vehicle.

selective for a subpopulation of receptors would be less likely to induce this phenomenon. Alpidem meets these criteria [2,4] and indeed in animals failed to induce tolerance and dependence. Thus, after repeated administration of alpidem to mice for 10 consecutive days there was no change in its potency in antagonizing convulsions induced by different convulsive challenges. In contrast to alpidem, tolerance developed to the anticonvulsant activity of diazepam. Moreover, 42 h after the last administration of diazepam mice became more sensitive to convulsions induced by isoniazid, an effect shown in Table 1 as a decrease in the latency to convulsion. A decrease in latency, which clearly indicates the occurrence of withdrawal, could also be precipitated by the benzodiazepine antagonist, flumazenil. In contrast to diazepam, after repeated treatment with alpidem neither spontaneous nor flumazenil-induced withdrawal was observed (Table 1).

Conclusions

In various behavioural tests in animals alpidem displays anxiolytic-like activity in the virtual absence of central depressant effects. Moreover, repeated administration of alpidem was not associated with the development of tolerance and dependence. The original profile of alpidem may be related to its selectivity for the ω_1 receptor coupled to a low intrinsic activity.

References

1. Langer SZ and Arbilla S (1988) Fundam. Clin. Pharmacol. 2: 159–170.
2. Langer SZ, Arbilla S, Tan S et al. (1990) Pharmacopsychiatry 23: 103–107.
3. Morton S and Lader M (1990) Pharmacopsychiatry 23: 120–123.
4. Zivkovic B, More E, Joly D et al. (1990) Pharmacopsychiatry 23: 108–113.
5. Joly D and Sanger DJ (1991) Behav. Pharmacol. (in press).

Biological Psychiatry, Volume 1. G. Racagni et al., editors.

Therapeutic activity of alpidem in anxious patients: An overview of European studies

Massimo Casacchia
Ospedale S. Maria di Collemaggio, 67100 L'Alquila, Italy

As described by previous speakers, alpidem is a new anxiolytic agent which binds in a preferential manner to ω_1 binding sites within the GABA-chloride channel supra-molecular complex.

In man, alpidem is characterized by linear non-saturable kinetics. Peak levels are obtained within 1.5–2 h after oral administration, with a bioavailability of 32–35% [1]. Alpidem is highly bound to plasma proteins [2] and has a terminal half-life of 16 to 20 h in normal adults [1]. The compound undergoes extensive metabolic degradation resulting in 3 active circulating metabolites, with a kinetic profile similar to that of the parent compound.

Several pharmacodynamic studies run in healthy volunteers have shown that unitary doses of 25 mg, 50 mg and 75 mg or repeated doses of 50 mg b.i.d. and 75 mg b.i.d. are virtually devoid of negative effects on sensori-motor performances in the young and middle-aged adult subject. Furthermore, doses of 25 mg and 50 mg are without detrimental effects on mnesic performance. EEG data indicate that alpidem does not induce "spindles" and has only minimal influence on Δ waves [3], while like other anxiolytics it increases β-activity and decreases α-activity.

In this report we critically review the available information on the therapeutic activity of alpidem as observed in therapeutic trials carried out in Europe, in adult patients suffering from different types of anxiety. The population studied so far consists of more than 1300 patients suffering from either generalized anxiety or adjustment disorders with anxious mood. Other observations refer to situational anxiety ($n = 400$) and anxiety in psychotic patients ($n = 81$). The anxiolytic activity of alpidem in life stress events has been tested in 400 patients who had to undergo minor surgical intervention, or gastroscopy or cardiovascular characterization, by means of 5 double-blind placebo-controlled studies with randomization [4]. Alpidem doses of 50 and 75 mg induced an anxiolytic effect significantly greater ($P < 0.001$) to that of placebo within 90 to 120 min. A short-lasting slight sedative effect was observed in about 16% of the cases only with the 75 mg dose.

Considering the anxiolytic action of alpidem in chronic anxiety, 3 double-blind trials carried out on 222 patients according to a parallel group design with randomization against placebo at doses of 50 mg/day to 200 mg/day indicated that an anxiolytic effect was evident within 3 to 5 days [5–7]. At an overall analysis such an effect was significantly superior to that of placebo ($P < 0.01$).

Best results were obtained with 50 mg b.i.d. and 50 mg t.i.d. doses. At the end of the active treatment period (3 weeks), 52% of alpidem treated patients were rated as responders against 28% in the placebo group ($P < 0.01$). Dropouts for inefficacy were 13.5% in alpidem and 17% in placebo groups, while dropouts for adverse effects were 6% and 1% respectively.

In another set of 7 studies [8–10], the anxiolytic activity of alpidem was compared (according to a parallel group double-blind design with randomization) to that of reference anxiolytics such as diazepam, chlorazepate, lorazepam, alprazolam and buspirone in 617 anxious patients suffering from chronic anxiety disorders. The study period varied from 3 to 6 weeks. Alpidem doses varied from 50 mg b.i.d. to 50 mg t.i.d. in most patients. In all studies the anxiolytic activity of alpidem was manifest within 7 days and was comparable to that of reference benzodiazepines, while it was significantly superior to that of buspirone ($P < 0.05$) [10]. According to the CGI, 73.5% of the patients were rated as responders in the alpidem group and 72% in the reference drugs group. No effects on memory or daytime performances were observed. Dropouts for inefficacy were 2.9% and 2.6% in the 2 groups while dropouts for adverse events amounted to 2.3% and 6.1% respectively.

Furthermore, in one open-labelled long-term study (274 patients at 6 months, and 101 at 12 months) no tachyphylactic phenomena could be observed [11]. No rebound anxiety after treatment discontinuation or withdrawal signs were noted.

On the basis of the above-mentioned results, it may be concluded that alpidem has an evident anxiolytic action comparable to that of currently available anxiolytic agents.

Globally the drug was very well tolerated, with sedative effects observed in about 6–7% of the cases. Alterations in laboratory tests, aspecific in nature and of limited clinical significance, were observed in about 1% of the patients.

Alpidem appears to be a new interesting psychotropic agent effective in various types of anxiety disorders. Because of its good tolerance and safety profile and its lack of negative effects on memory and cognitive functions, it may represent an improvement in the treatment of anxiety disorders, with a better benefit/risk ratio.

References

1. Dimsdale M, Friedmann JC and Morselli PL (1988) Drugs Future 13: 106.
2. Pacifici GM, Bianchetti G, Viani A et al. (1989) Eur. J. Clin. Pharmacol. 37: 29.
3. Saletu B, Gründberger J and Linzmayer L (1986) Int. J. Clin. Psychopharmacol. 1: 145.
4. Musch B, Morselli PL and Priore P (1988) Pharmacol. Biochem. Behav. 29: 803.
5. Casacchia M, Farolfi A, Priore P et al. (1989) Acta Psychiatr. Scand. 80: 137.
6. Bassi S, Albizzati MG, Ferrarese C et al. (1989) Clin. Neuropsychopharmacol. 12: 67.
7. Régnier F, Chastel A, L'Héritier C et al. (1989) Thérapie 44: 279.
8. Ropert E et al. (1991) (in press).
9. Morselli PL (1990) Pharmacopsychiatry 23: 129.
10. Garreau M, Georges P and Boval P (1991) (in preparation).
11. Mendlewicz J and Coupez-Lopinot M (1991) (in preparation).

Biological Psychiatry, Volume 1. G. Racagni et al., editors.

Pharmacological treatment of anxiety in the elderly: New perspectives

Paolo Lucio Morselli
Clinical Research Department, Synthelabo Recherche (LERS), 75622 Paris, France

The pharmacological treatment of the elderly patient constitutes a problem which in recent years has attained an unexpected dimension with social, medical and economic implications [1,2]. The extended welfare and the prolongation of life-span has led to an increased drug consumption where cardiovascular and psychotropic drugs play a primary role. Anxiety syndromes or reactions linked to organic disabilities, separation from active life, withdrawal from the family and institutionalization have brought about a constant increase in the prescription of anxiolytic drugs in the elderly. Such an increased consumption by frequently polymedicated patients has been accompanied by an alarming rise of severe drug reactions [3,4].

Falls, confusion episodes, memory disturbances, perceptual troubles, slow thinking and impaired sensorimotor functions are the most common side-effects described in the literature [5–9]. This type of side-effects may condition a vicious circle where anxiety is sustained by the increasing disability and by the fear of a more difficult integration with the surrounding environment. Modified pharmacokinetics, changes in receptor sensitivity and poor compliance due to errors in understanding or remembering the drug regimen are among the main reasons for the increased incidence and severity of ADR in the elderly [2]. The necessity of an alternative to the presently used benzodiazepine anxiolytics has been stressed on several occasions [10,11].

Within this frame, the availability of a new anxiolytic agent acting on a specific receptor subtype and devoid of evident sedative and myorelaxant properties may contribute positively to the issue.

The pharmacodynamic profile of alpidem as well as its therapeutic action have been evaluated in a population of more than 400 elderly people. The elderly volunteers and anxious elderly in- and outpatients participating in this evaluation may be considered as highly representative of the possible users of the drug.

Four studies were conducted on 68 elderly volunteers (60 to 85 years) in controlled laboratory conditions to assess possible effects of alpidem on sensorimotor functions and cognitive processes. Doses of 25 and 50 mg administered as single or repeated (7 days) doses were without any effect on mnesic capabilities and did not alter sensorimotor performances [12–14]. On the contrary, as in adults, a detrimental effect was observed with the unitary dose of 100 mg. The apparent plasma half-life values (20–24 h) were similar to those observed in adults

(18–20 h); however, higher C_{max} and AUC values were constantly noted. The data suggest that no increased sensitivity to alpidem is present in the elderly. Three clinically controlled studies run against placebo in 250 anxious elderly in- and outpatients (60 to 84 years), frequently suffering from concomitant organic diseases and polymedicated (~80%), showed that alpidem at the doses of 25 mg t.i.d. or 50 mg b.i.d. administered over 2 to 4 weeks, has a significant ($P < 0.01$) anxiolytic effect devoid of disturbing side-effects without detrimental effects on cognitive and sensorimotor performances. As in adults, the anxiolytic action is evident within 3 to 5 days in 70–75% of the population [12,15,16]. The global incidence of side-effects was 7 to 8% with only 3.1% as dropouts for ADR.

Furthermore, no tachyphylaxis could be noted up to 12 months' treatment in a long-term study run on 96 patients (60 to 85 years old) [12]. No rebound anxiety and no withdrawal signs were observed in those cases where alpidem treatment had to be discontinued abruptly, after 3–4 months or more, for intercurrent diseases [12].

Globally the data obtained in a population of more than 400 elderly subjects, representative of possible future users, suffering from various anxiety disorders and concomitant pathologies indicate that the anxiolytic action of alpidem (at doses of 75–100 mg/day) is comparable to that observed in adult anxious patients, without any increase in the incidence or severity of adverse drug reactions. In particular, the lack of detrimental effect on mnesic function should be stressed.

Alpidem therefore appears to be an anxiolytic drug with very favourable benefit/risk ratio in the elderly, and a very promising alternative to the existing agents.

References

1. WHO Drugs (1981) 22: 279-294.
2. Morselli PL and Guillet PH (1988) In: Burley D et al. (eds.) The Focus for Pharmaceutical Knowledge. MacMillan Press Ltd, Houndmills U.K., pp. 208–221.
3. Pickels H (1986) Lancet 8497: 40–41.
4. Freer CB (1985) Br. Med. J. 292: 1113–1115.
5. Curran HV (1986) Biol. Psychol. 23: 179–213.
6. Lister RG (1985) Neurosci. Biobehav. Res. 9: 87–94.
7. Ashton N (1986) Adv. Drug React. Bull. 118: 440–443.
8. Foy A, Drinkwater V, March S et al. (1986) Br. Med. J. 293: 1072.
9. Golombo KS (1989) Hum. Psychopharmacol. 4: 15–22.
10. Lader MH and Pertusson H (1981) Biol. Psychiatry 16: 1195–1201.
11. Lader MH and Pertusson H (1983) Neuropharmacology 22: 527–533.
12. Morselli PL (1990) Pharmacopsychiatry 23(3): 129–134.
13. Satzger W, Engel RR et al. (1990) Pharmacopsychiatry 23(3): 114–119.
14. Hindmarch I (1990) Pharmacopsychiatry 23(3): 124–128.
15. Singer L (1991) (in preparation).
16. Frattola L (1991) (in preparation).

Biological Psychiatry, Volume 1. G. Racagni et al., editors.

Anxiolytics and withdrawal signs: Comparative studies of alpidem and benzodiazepines

M. Lader and S. Morton
Institute of Psychiatry, London SE5 8AF, U.K.

Over the past decade, numerous researchers have shown that the benzodiazepines have a clinically important propensity to induce physical dependence on long-term usage [1]. Furthermore, even short-term use for a month or so may be followed by rebound on discontinuation, particularly when stopping shorter-acting compounds [2]. The danger is that such rebound will be misinterpreted by patient and prescriber as a recrudescence of symptoms, with resumption of medication.

Inevitably, when new putative anxiolytics are developed, questions arise as to whether a physical dependence potential exists which will evidence itself eventually as unacceptably wide long-term use. Thus, extensive programmes of research are now devoted towards addressing this issue and the quality and quantity of such data required by regulatory authorities are constantly increasing.

Assessing dependence potential

Animal tests are helpful predictors [3] and include spontaneous or induced elicitation of a physical withdrawal syndrome, suppression of withdrawal to known dependence-inducing drugs and the detection of tolerance. In normal subjects, short-term administration of a compound may be followed by rebound, or one can attempt to suppress rebound to known rebound-inducing drugs. These tests differ entirely from tests believed predictive of abuse potential.

A range of studies is needed in patients. Short-term courses of an anxiolytic should always be followed by a placebo-controlled discontinuation phase in which careful scrutiny is made for evidence of rebound. The test drug can be administered after a month of a known rebound-inducing compound such as a shorter-acting benzodiazepine. Longer-term studies can also be designed to search for rebound and withdrawal on controlled discontinuation. Similarly, suppression of withdrawal to known withdrawal-inducing drugs can be sought.

In more extensive usage, case-reports need careful evaluation as do post-marketing surveillance data. Finally, epidemiological surveys may use prescription and usage data and may focus on groups especially at risk, such as alcoholics.

Studies with alpidem

Alpidem has been the subject of extensive evaluations for efficacy and safety. It differs from the benzodiazepines chemically, it is more selective at the receptor level, perhaps with lower intrinsic activity and it has an untypical profile of anxiolytic activity in animal models [4]. Tests of dependence potential predict a low liability in man, but direct testing is essential. To that end, many studies have been completed or are in progress.

Repeated dose studies in normal subjects have not detected any problems with rebound on discontinuation. Clinical studies have often incorporated the assessments postdiscontinuation which are necessary to detect rebound. One such study which we conducted involved the administration in flexible dosage of alpidem (average daily dose 112.5 mg) or lorazepam (3.5 mg/day) for 4 weeks to 24 patients with the diagnosis of GAD. Improvement was seen in both groups by the end of week 1 and there were no appreciable differences between the groups. However, lorazepam but not alpidem was associated with marked deficits in memory function [5].

The second part of this study – the discontinuation phase – found that abruptly stopping alpidem after 4 weeks' treatment produced no rebound, whereas a significant withdrawal syndrome was shown by the lorazepam group. Scores on all anxiety scales, as well as a Tranquilliser Withdrawal Scale, rose by 7 days after stopping lorazepam and then subsided. However, the severity of this reaction led us to discontinue the trial prematurely.

In a second clinical study, we assessed the usefulness of alpidem in helping dependent patients withdraw from their long-term benzodiazepine. In these patients, alpidem or placebo was added to the benzodiazepine regimen. Then, the benzodiazepine was tapered off and finally the alpidem or placebo was discontinued. Alpidem proved inefficacious in these severely dependent patients and may even have been counter-productive. Similarly, alpidem does not seem to improve the postwithdrawal syndrome, i.e. the constellation of symptoms persisting a month or more after discontinuation. These data suggest only limited cross-tolerance between alpidem and the benzodiazepines.

Other large-scale trials are addressing the issue of possible rebound and withdrawal after several months of treatment with alpidem or a benzodiazepine. Yet others examine the problems with may arise when switching from a benzodiazepine to alpidem. In this way, as complete a dossier as possible will accrue on the possible dependence potential of alpidem.

References

1. Task Force Report (1990) Benzodiazepine Dependence, Toxicity, and Abuse. American Psychiatric Association, Washington D.C.

2. Chouinard G, Anne L and Fountaine R (1983) Progr. Neuropsychopharmacol. Biol. Psychiatry 7: 669–673.
3. Hartnoll R (1991) In: Willner P (ed.) Behavioural Models in Psychopharmacology: Theoretical, Industrial and Clinical Perspectives. Cambridge University Press, Cambridge, pp. 503–519.
4. Dimsdale M, Friedman JC, Morselli PL and Zivkovic B (1988) Drugs Future 13: 106–109.
5. Morton S and Lader M (1990) Pharmacopsychiatry 23: 120–123S.

Biological Psychiatry, Volume 1. G. Racagni et al., editors.

Anxiolytic and dependence: Two double-blind studies of alpidem versus benzodiazepines

M. Garreau, J. de Wilde, L. Frattola, C. L'Heritier, P. Boval and P.L. Morselli
Synthelabo Recherche (LERS) 58, Rue de la Glacière, F-75013, Paris, France

Introduction

Since the initial use of benzodiazepine 30 years ago, more than 30 derivatives have been widely prescribed throughout the world. Nevertheless, this class of compounds, which are effective in the treatment of anxiety, has been shown to induce many adverse events that are potentially dangerous.

Although some side-effects are well known (such as sedation, impaired performance, amnesia) [1,2], some of them have been noticed more recently.

In the last 10 years, withdrawal symptoms and rebound anxiety have been reported following the abrupt discontinuation of treatment with benzodiazepines, leading patients to return to benzodiazepines even though they do not need them any longer [3–5].

The possibility to have new effective drugs, which differ from benzodiazepines and are devoid of their adverse effects, appears to be of a major interest.

Alpidem is a new anxiolytic, chemically and pharmacologically unrelated to benzodiazepines, which appeared to have a low dependence potential during initial clinical studies in more than 2000 patients.

Material and Methods

To confirm these preliminary data, two double-blind studies have been carried out in Europe, using the same protocol. The specific aim of these studies was to evaluate the potential withdrawal signs at the end of treatment with alpidem, in comparison with the benzodiazepines.

One study was performed in Italy, by Pr Frattola et al., comparing alpidem 50 mg t.i.d. with alprazolam 0.5 mg t.i.d., the other in Belgium by Dr de Wilde et al., comparing alpidem 50 mg b.i.d. or t.i.d. with lorazepam 2.5 mg b.i.d. or t.i.d. These 2 studies included 223 patients randomized to two parallel groups, i.e. 122 in the first study (61 patients in each group), 101 in the second study (51 in the alpidem group, 50 in the lorazepam group).

During the active treatment period, efficacy was assessed by means of the Hamilton Anxiety Rating Scale. Evaluation of withdrawal signs was made using a specific withdrawal rating scale (H. Ashton Scale), by an independent investigator on a blind basis.

In view of the lack of internationally recognized definition of the "withdrawal syndrome", the following criteria have been used.

Increase of at least 2 points for 2 or more items of the scale and onset of 2 new symptoms between the end of the active treatment and the end of the 2-week placebo periods, combined with the diagnostic criteria for sedative, hypnotic or anxiolytic withdrawal syndrome, according to DSM III.

It should be emphasized that the analysis was made subsequently on the basis of specific withdrawal scale and was not a description of spontaneous adverse events reported by the patients.

Results

At the end of the active treatment period, the efficacy of alpidem and alprazolam was found to be equivalent, as well as that alpidem and lorazepam.

According to the selected criteria:

- In the first study, 26 of the 54 patients present at the end of the 6-week alprazolam treatment (48%) had a diagnosis of "withdrawal", versus 11 of 56 patients (18%) in the alpidem group;
- In the second study, 24 of 40 patients in the lorazepam group (60%) had a diagnosis of "withdrawal" syndrome versus 5 of 45 patients in the alpidem group (11%).

Some patients were previously treated with benzodiazepines and we cannot exclude that withdrawal signs observed following discontinuation of the active treatment were in effect due to the previous drugs.

In these 2 studies, the intensity of withdrawal symptoms was less severe in the alpidem group compared to the 2 benzodiazepines.

Furthermore, the majority of the symptoms aggravated in the alpidem group were non-specific (nausea, headache), unlike those noticed with the 2 benzodiazepines (paresthesia, tremor, agressivity, nightmares etc.).

Conclusion

In these 2 double-blind studies, quantitative analysis of the clinical effects observed following the discontinuation of treatment showed the incidence and intensity of withdrawal signs to be significantly lower in the alpidem group than in the benzodiazepine groups. Qualitative analysis of the symptoms which occurred during the 2-week placebo run-out phase clearly differentiated alpidem from lorazepam and alprazolam. These results confirm those of previous studies, indicating a very low potential for alpidem to induce dependence.

References

1. Clinthorne JK (1986) Arch. Gen. Psychiatry 43: 527–532.
2. Golombok S (1989) Human Psychopharmacol. 4: 15–22.
3. Lader MH and Petursson H (1981) Biol. Psychiatry 16: 1195–1201.
4. Rickels K, Schweizer E, Csanalosi I, Case G and Hack Chung (1988) Arch. Gen. Psychiatry 45: 444–450.
5. Tyrer P (1980) Br. J. Psychiatry 137: 576–577.

Biological Psychiatry, Volume 1. G. Racagni et al., editors.

Independent cellular and ontogenetic expression of mRNAs encoding α polypeptides of the rat $GABA_A$ receptor

Allan J. Tobin, Karl Anderson, Nicholas Brecha, Ming-Yi Chiang, Michel Khrestchatisky, Mable Lai, A. John MacLennan, Richard W. Olsen, Catia Sternini and Niranjala J.K. Tillakaratne

University of California, Los Angeles, CA 90024, U.S.A.

Experiments with injected oocytes and with human non-neural cells engineered to express GABA receptor cDNAs showed that the type of expressed α polypeptide influenced the affinity for GABA and the gating properties of the resulting receptor [1–4]. Sigel et al. [5], for example, have shown that oocytes injected with RNAs encoding α_5 (our α_4), β_2, and γ_2 produce functional GABA receptors, with cooperative responses to GABA and modulation by diazepam and pentobarbital. The replacement of β_2 by β_1 resulted in a decreased sensitivity to GABA, but an increased responsiveness to diazepam, again showing the importance of specific subunit composition in the functional properties of receptors.

The distinctive properties of GABA receptors with differing subunit compositions points to the importance of gene regulation in establishing the response to GABA in a particular neuron. With this in mind, we and others have undertaken to study the distribution of individual GABA receptor mRNAs by in situ hybridization to molecular probes derived from specific cDNAs [6–8]. These experiments have revealed striking differences in the pattern of expression of individual members of the α and β families. In one case at least, the pattern of expression of a particular polypeptide (α_1) resembles that defined by binding a specific class of benzodiazepines, again supporting the functional and pharmacological importance of α subunits.

α_1, α_2 and α_4 mRNAs are differentially expressed along the neuraxis. Overall, α_1 mRNA is more abundant than either α_2 or α_4 mRNAs. In many regions, all three mRNA species are coexpressed in the same structures, but often in different cell types and at different levels.

Structures with high to moderate levels of α_1 mRNA include the main and accessory olfactory bulbs, anterior olfactory nuclei, piriform or primary olfactory cortex, claustrum, globus pallidus, ventral pallidum, medial septal/diagonal band complex, amygdala, hippocampal complex and cerebral cortex. High to moderate levels are also present in some thalamic and pretectal regions, including the subthalamic nucleus, the anteroventral thalamic nucleus, ventroposterior thalamic nuclei, ventrolateral thalamic nucleus, anterior pretectal nucleus, and geniculate nuclei. In contrast, lower levels are present in the hypothalamus, although some nuclei, including the supraoptic nucleus, show moderately high concentrations.

The substantia nigra and inferior colliculus have high levels of α_1 mRNA, as do the cerebellar cortex and the deep cerebellar nuclei. In the pons and medulla α_1 mRNA is present in high to moderate amounts in the cranial motor nuclei, pontine nuclei, pontine reticular nuclei and lateral vestibular nucleus. Structures with low to non-detectable levels of α_1 mRNAs include the nucleus accumbens, caudate-putamen, and other nuclei located within the hypothalamus, thalamus, pons and medulla.

α_2 mRNA is less abundant than α_1 mRNA and has a more limited distribution. The highest levels are in the olfactory bulb, hippocampal formation, and the cranial motor nuclei. High to moderate labeling is found in several structures, including the anterior olfactory nuclei, olfactory tubercle, caudate-putamen, nucleus accumbens, ventral pallidum, piriform cortex, and cerebral cortex.

α_4 mRNA is less abundant than either α_1 or α_2 mRNAs and is mainly found in neurons within the olfactory bulb and hippocampal formation. Moderate to low levels of α_4 mRNA are seen in the anterior olfactory nuclei, piriform cortex, cerebral cortex, and amygdala. Most structures within the hypothalamus, thalamus, prectectum, midbrain, cerebellum, pons and medulla had trace or non-detectable levels of either α_2 or α_4 mRNAs.

The olfactory bulb provides an excellent example of the distinctive cellular distributions of individual α mRNAs within a specific brain region. Overall, there is a high level of all three α mRNAs in olfactory structures. In the main olfactory bulb, α_1 mRNA is strong in the mitral cell layer, and moderate in the external plexiform layer, and all mitral cells appear to contain α_1 mRNA. Our studies did not firmly establish the presence of α_1 mRNA in other interneuronal cell types, which are also present adjacent to or within the mitral cell layer. In the external plexiform layer, most labeled cells are near or adjacent to the glomerular layer, and some cells lie close to the mitral cell layer, suggesting that both internal and external tufted cells contain α_1 mRNA. In the granule cell layer, only a few cells have any α_1 mRNA, while α_2 and α_4 mRNAs are present at high levels. The dense labeling pattern suggests that all granule cells and perhaps other interneuronal cell types located in this layer express α_2 and α_4 mRNAs. In addition, α_2 and α_4 mRNAs are present in the mitral cell and olfactory glomerular layers.

Each of these three α mRNAs is regulated during ontogeny in a distinctive manner. Thus, the relative concentrations of the three mRNA species change dramatically during development, as judged by Northern blotting. From E18 to P7, α_4 mRNA is present at significantly higher concentrations than those of α_1 or α_2 mRNAs. By adulthood, however, α_1 mRNA is clearly the major species.

The persistence of multiple gene families in many cases reflects differing physiological needs in different cells and at different developmental stages. It may also reflect a need for coordinate regulation. In addition to information specifying an amino acid sequence, each gene contains DNA sequences that establish its pattern of expression, specifying both the cell types in which it is to be expressed and its regulation in response to environmental changes.

References

1. Khrestchatisky M, MacLennan AJ, Chiang M-Y, Xu W, Jackson M, Brecha N, Sternini C, Olsen RW and Tobin AJ (1989) Neuron 3: 745–753.
2. Levitan ES, Schofield PR, Burt DR, Rhee LM, Wisden W, Kohler M, Fujita N, Rogriguez H, Stephenson FA, Darlison MG, Barnard EA and Seeburg PH (1988) Nature 335: 76–79.
3. Malherbe P, Sigel E, Baur R, Persohn E, Richards JG and Möhler H (1990) J. Neurosci. 10: 2330–2337.
4. Pritchett DB, Lüddens H and Seeburg PH (1989) Science 245: 1389–1392.
5. Sigel E., Baur R, Trube G, Möhler H and Malherbe P (1990) Neuron 5: 703–711.
6. MacLennan AJ, Brecha N, Khrestchatisky M, Sternini C, Tillakaratne NJK, Chiang M-Y, Anderson K, Lai M and Tobin AJ (1991) Independent cellular and ontogenetic expression of mRNAs encoding three α polypeptides of the rat $GABA_A$ receptor. Neuroscience (in press).
7. Zhang J-H, Sato M and Tohyama M (1991) J. Comp. Neurol. 304: 1–21.
8. Wisden W, Morris BJ, Darlison MG, Hunt SP and Barnard EA (1988) Neuron 1: 937–947.

Biological Psychiatry, Volume 1. G. Racagni et al., editors.

^{3}H-propofol binding, a new tool to study the interaction of general anesthetics with the $GABA_A$ receptor complex

A. Concas, G. Santoro, M.P. Mascia and G. Biggio
Department of Experimental Biology, Chair of Pharmacology, University of Cagliari, Italy

Introduction

Recently, propofol (2,6-diisopropylphenol), a sterically hindered phenol derivative, has been introduced into clinical practice as an intravenous anesthetic agent characterized by its short recovery time either after a single bolus injection or after infusion [1]. The pharmacology of propofol has been broadly reviewed, with regard to its pharmacokinetics and pharmacodynamic properties, but little is known of its neurochemical mechanism of action. Electrophysiological data have indicated a possible interaction of propofol with the GABA receptor complex [2]. In fact, it has been shown that propofol potentiates the GABA-evoked neuronal inhibition both in central neurones and in bovine chromaffin cells. The capability of propofol to potentiate the GABA-induced response is similar to that induced by other general anaesthetics. Accordingly, electrophysiological and biochemical data have clearly shown that nonvolatile and inhalation anaesthetics produce a marked and persistent enhancement in the function of the GABA-coupled chloride channel [3–5].

Thus, to investigate the possible interaction of propofol with the $GABA_A$ receptor complex, we studied the modulatory action of this drug on the biochemical parameters (^{3}H-GABA binding, ^{35}S-TBPS binding, $^{36}Cl^-$ uptake) currently used to evaluate the function of the $GABA_A$ receptor complex [6,7]. Moreover, in an attempt to clarify the molecular mechanism involved in the pharmacological action of this compound more recently we examined the characteristics of its putative binding site in rat brain membranes using the radiolabelled propofol (^{3}H-propofol).

Methods

Male Sprague-Dawley rats (Charles River, Como, Italy) weighing 200–250 g were used. After sacrifice the brains were rapidly removed, the cerebral cortex was dissected out and was used for measurement of ^{3}H-GABA binding, ^{35}S-TBPS binding and $^{36}Cl^-$ uptake [7].

For ^{3}H-propofol binding the tissue was homogenized in 20 vol of ice-cold 0.32 M sucrose in a glass homogenizer fitted with a Teflon pestle. The P_2 pellet was resuspended in 10 vol 50 mM Tris-HCl buffer, pH 7.4 and the incubation was carried out in the presence of ^{3}H-propofol (spec. act. 23.3 Ci/mmol) using 200–250 μg proteins in a total incubation volume of 500 μl. After 7 h at 37°C the incubations were terminated by rapid filtration through glass fiber filter strips (Whatman GF/B) which were rinsed twice with 4 ml of ice-cold Tris-HCl buffer. Non-specific binding was defined as the binding in the presence of 30 μM propofol. Saturation studies were based on 12 different concentrations of ligand (50–3200 nM). The specific activity of ^{3}H-propofol was kept constant at 50 nM and then diluted with unlabelled propofol dissolved in dimethyl sulphoxide.

Results and Discussion

As shown in Table 1 propofol increased ^{3}H-GABA binding, reduced ^{35}S-TBPS binding and enhanced muscimol-stimulated $^{36}Cl^-$ uptake in a concentration-dependent manner.

These data suggest that propofol, like several hypnotics, anticonvulsants and other general anesthetics, enhances the function of the $GABA_A$ receptor complex. However, different sites or mechanism of action for propofol, alphaxalone, pentobarbital, benzodiazepines is suggested by the finding that the concomitant addition of propofol with these drugs produced a simple additive effect on the above-mentioned biochemical parameters [6,7]. The effect of propofol at the level of the $GABA_A$/ionophore receptor complex was completely antagonized by bicuculline, a specific $GABA_A$ receptor antagonist [6,7]. This finding indicates that the action of this compound is strictly dependent by the interaction of GABA with its recognition site. Accordingly, the removal of GABA by extensive washing of membranes completely reversed the effect of propofol on ^{35}S-TBPS binding. Thus, using washed membranes (devoid of GABA) propofol, like diazepam [8] enhanced ^{35}S-TBPS binding in a concentration-dependent manner (maximal enhancement

Table 1. Effect of propofol on ^{3}H-GABA binding, ^{35}S-TBPS binding and $^{36}Cl^-$ uptake in rat brain membranes

Concentration (μM)	^{3}H-GABA binding (% of control)	^{35}S-TBPS binding (% of control)	$^{36}Cl^-$ uptake (% of control)
0.1	–	98 ± 4	100 ± 1
1	114 ± 3	82 ± 5	115 ± 2
3	119 ± 5	61 ± 1	120 ± 1
10	125 ± 6	23 ± 4	137 ± 3
30	132 ± 7	3 ± 4	143 ± 7
100	140 ± 8	–	–
300	159 ± 10	–	–

Data are the mean ± S.E.M. from 4–7 experiments.

+75 ± 9% of control at 10 μM); an effect different from those elicited by alphaxalone and pentobarbital in the same membrane preparation [5].

In order to clarify the molecular mechanism involved in the pharmacological action of propofol we examined the binding of the radio-labelled propofol (^{3}H-propofol) to rat cortical membranes. ^{3}H-propofol binding to a crude synaptosomal preparation was specific (80–90% of specific binding), increased linearly with the proteins concentration, reached equilibrium within 7 h at 37°C. Our studies show that ^{3}H-propofol binds to two population of binding sites in the rat cerebral cortex (high affinity K_d 112 ± 8 mM; B_{max} 7.8 ± 2 pmol/mg protein; low affinity K_d 6.4 μM; B_{max} 55 ± 12 pmol/mg protein). The finding that ^{3}H-propofol binding is completely inhibited by pretreatment of membrane with proteinase K suggests the possible specific interaction of propofol with some protein rather than component of membrane.

References

1. Langley MS and Heel RC (1988) Drugs 35: 334–372.
2. Collins GGS (1988) Br. J. Pharmacol. 95: 939–949.
3. Keane PE and Biziere K (1987) Life Sci. 41: 1437–1448.
4. Moody EJ, Suzdak PD, Paul SM and Skolnick P (1988) J. Neurochem. 51: 1386–1393.
5. Turner DM, Ransom RW, Yang JS-J and Olsen RW (1989) J. Pharmacol. Exp. Ther. 248: 960–966.
6. Concas A, Santoro G, Mascia MP, Serra M, Sanna E and Biggio G (1990) J. Neurochem. 55: 2135–2138.
7. Concas A, Santoro G, Serra M, Sanna E and Biggio G (1991) Brain Res. 542: 225–232.
8. Concas A, Sanna E, Mascia MP, Serra M and Biggio G (1990) Neurosci. Lett. 112: 87–91.

Biological Psychiatry, Volume 1. G. Racagni et al., editors.

Pharmacology of partial agonists at the benzodiazepine receptor

Willy Haefely

Pharma Division, Preclinical Research, F. Hoffmann-La Roche Ltd, CH-4002 Basel, Switzerland

Introduction

The analysis of the mechanism of action of benzodiazepine (BZ) tranquilizers initially revealed their highly selective potentiation of GABAergic synaptic transmission and subsequently led to the identification of the $GABA_A$ receptor ($GABA_A$-R) complex as the molecular site of action of BZ. The specific, high-affinity binding site for BZ, called the benzodiazepine receptor (BZR), is one of several allosteric modulatory sites of the $GABA_A$-R (Fig. 1). BZ were the first drugs found to produce their pharmacological and therapeutic effects through allosteric modulation of a neurotransmitter receptor. The uniqueness of the BZR up to the present day lies in its ability to mediate two opposite effects, namely positive (GABA-facilitating) and negative (GABA-depressant) modulation of the $GABA_A$-R function. BZR ligands with positive modulatory activity (resulting in anxiolytic, anticonvulsant, sedative and myorelaxant effects) are called BZR agonists, those with a negative modulatory activity (anxiogenic, convulsant, stimulant and spasmogenic effects) have been coined inverse agonists of the BZR. The

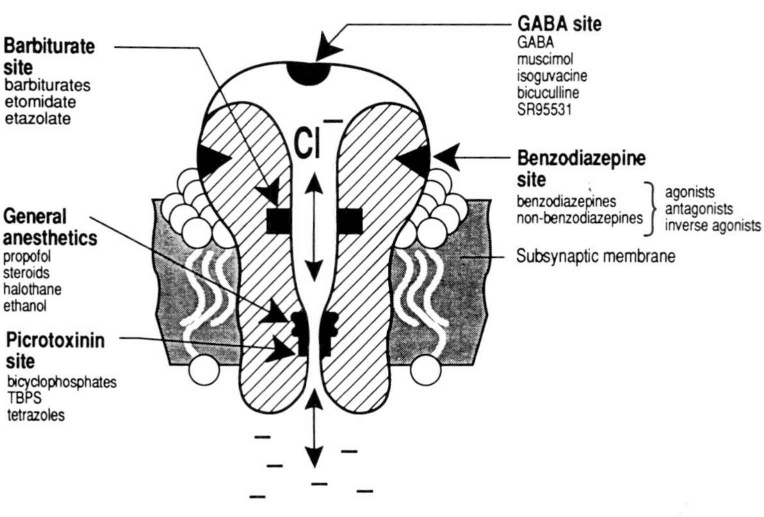

Fig. 1. Schematic drawing of the $GABA_A$ receptor (cut perpendicularly to the neuronal membrane) with its binding sites for GABA and for allosteric modulators.

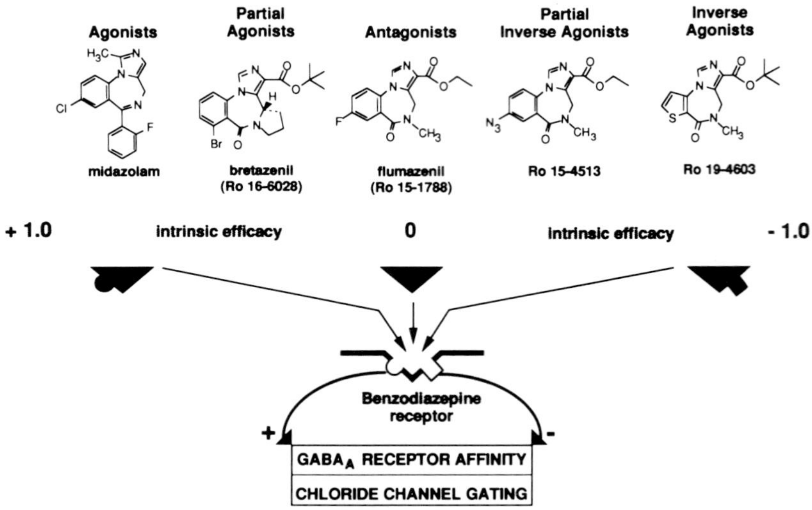

Fig. 2. Spectrum of ligands of the BZR according to their intrinsic efficacy.

BZR also recognizes ligands without modulatory activity which, however, competitively block the effects of agonists and inverse agonists (BZR antagonists) (Fig. 2). The intrinsic property of BZR ligands which determines direction and intensity of allosteric modulation is called intrinsic efficacy according to the basic principles of pharmacology.

From agonist to partial agonist profile of activity

BZR ligands exist that have an intrinsic efficacy in between that of full agonists (+1) and pure antagonists (0); they are called partial or low efficacy agonists (Fig. 2). The pharmacology of partial agonists predicts a number of highly interesting properties for therapy.

Three major factors, besides the dose, determine the fractional effect (E_L/E_{max}) of a receptor ligand (L), i.e. the magnitude of a biological response in percent of the maximal response that can be mediated by the receptor in a given test situation: a) fractional receptor occupancy [LR]/[R], i.e. the percent available receptors that are bound to the ligand. Affinity of the ligand for the receptor is the main determinant of fractional receptor occupancy; b) intrinsic efficacy, an inherent property of a ligand that expresses its ability to activate the receptor when binding to it. Activation is the conformational transition of the receptor from an inactive to a functionally active state. Intrinsic efficacy can be expressed in the simplest way by the ratio of activated receptors to total receptor-ligand complexes [LR*]/[LR]; and c) the receptor density of the biological target (parts of a cell, a cell, a cell population). While all target cells, independent of their receptor density, show the same fractional receptor occupancy at a given ligand concentration, the absolute amount of ligand-receptor complexes, of course, is higher in a target cell with higher receptor density than in one with lower density. The receptor number or density determines the total amount of chloride current flowing through activated $GABA_A$-R.

Fractional receptor occupancy and receptor density can be measured directly in vitro and in vivo using radioligands (positron emission tomography allows this to be done in the intact human brain). [LR*], however, the concentration of activated receptor-ligand complexes, can only be assessed by indirect functional assays (biochemical and electrophysiological chloride flux measurements, neurological and behavioral tests).

Bretazenil (Ro 16-6028) is an imidazo-benzodiazepinone congener of the BZR antagonist flumazenil [1]. Its partial agonist profile of activity is illustrated by fractional receptor occupancy vs. fractional effect curves in various test situations in comparison to full agonists. In vitro on rat cortical membrane vesicles, measuring fractional receptor occupancy (with ^{3}H-flumazenil as radioligand) and potentiation of GABA-stimulated chloride flux, the full agonists triazolam and diazepam produced a half-maximal potentiation at about 25% receptor occupancy, while bretazenil required over 90% occupancy to reach about 25% the maximal effect of diazepam. Correlations between in vivo fractional receptor occupancy (total forebrain) and various pharmacological effects in mice revealed a low occupancy by full agonists for anxiolytic and anticonvulsant effects and somewhat higher occupancy for moderate and severe sedation. Bretazenil required a higher fractional receptor occupancy than full agonists for equivalent anxiolytic and anticonvulsant effects. Severe sedation and motor impairment were not obtained with this compound even at receptor saturating doses.

These data clearly demonstrate the great value of the partial agonists of the BZR as in animals they produce equivalent anxiolytic and similar anticonvulsant effects to full agonists; however, they are unable to produce severe CNS depression. In fact, partial agonists antagonize the latter effects of full agonists.

The profile of activity of bretazenil can be completely imitated by appropriate mixtures of a full BZR agonist and the antagonist flumazenil, in confirmation of the theoretical concept of partial agonism.

Conclusion

Partial agonists at the BZR are highly promising novel agents that retain several highly desired effects of classic BZ but do not produce severe degrees of CNS depression. This selective profile is accompanied by the greatly reduced eliminated liability for tolerance and physical dependence development as well as by the virtual absence of reinforcing property. All these novel properties can parsimoniously be explained by the fact that BZR are less frequently in the activated state when exposed to a partial agonist.

Reference

1. Haefely W, Martin JR and Schoch P (1990) Trends Pharmacol. Sci. 11: 452–456.

Biological Psychiatry, Volume 1. G. Racagni et al., editors.

Clinical abuse liability of partial and full agonist benzodiazepines: A comparison of bretazenil, diazepam and alprazolam

Edward M. Sellers, Usanda Busto and Howard L. Kaplan

Departments of Pharmacology, Medicine and Psychiatry and the Faculty of Pharmacy, University of Toronto and the Clinical Research and Treatment Institute, Addiction Research Foundation, 33 Russell Street, Toronto, Ontario M5S 2S1, Canada

Introduction

The purpose of abuse liability testing is to learn at an early stage of human investigation whether a new drug, once it is made more widely available, will be more or less likely to be abused than already marketed medications. Some full agonist benzodiazepines can serve as reinforcers and, although less so than barbiturates, are abused by certain individuals, particularly individuals who are abusing or who have in the past abused other drugs [1]. Clinical and experimental studies have shown differential abuse patterns among the benzodiazepines [2] suggesting that there are clinically meaningful differences among the benzodiazepines with respect to their abuse potential. New drugs may have differential effects on benzodiazepine receptor subtypes or have lesser intrinsic efficacy than full agonists and may have lesser reinforcing activity or relatively greater aversive activity. Either pharmacologic activity could lead to an even lower abuse liability than seen with full agonist benzodiazepines [3]. Selectivity for central W1 receptors has been proposed to account for the pharmacologic differences between triazolam and zolpidem [3-5].

In pre-clinical studies, partial agonist benzodiazepines may show lesser self-administration [6]; not generalize to full agonists in drug discrimination studies; and fail to produce or produce lesser physical dependence and withdrawal. Continuous administration of triazolam, alprazolam or diazepam for 7 days produced physical dependence in DBA/2J mice which could be unmasked with RO 15-3505. In contrast, no precipitated withdrawal signs were observed following chronic high dose exposure to the benzodiazepine partial agonist bretazenil [7]. Similar inability of flumazenil to precipitate withdrawal after chronic bretazenil has been seen in squirrel monkeys, cats, mice, and rats (Hoffmann-La Roche, on file).

We have recently completed a human study on the abuse liability and pharmacologic properties of the partial benzodiazepine agonist, bretazenil.

Methods

The design used in this study was a novel one in which each of 28 subjects received

10 of 13 possible doses over 10 experimental sessions. The first 7 sessions consisted of placebo and the middle 2 doses of each of 3 active drugs. The subject's clinical responses to the 2 doses of each active drug determined whether he received the highest or lowest dose of that drug in the remaining 3 days of the experiment, depending on his tolerance to sedating drug effects. The drugs and doses used in the study were placebo; alprazolam 0.5, 1, 2 and 4 mg; diazepam 5, 10, 20 and 40 mg; bretazenil 0.5, 1, 2 and 4 mg, administered as 2 capsules and 1 sublingual lozenge.

The subjects included in the study were adult male volunteers ranging in age from 19 to 45 years who were experienced users of two or more CNS depressant drugs and who did not meet DSM III-R criteria for psychoactive substance use disorder. Those who appeared eligible were screened for their ability to detect the positive subjective effects of secobarbital 150 mg orally [8]. On each testing day, the subject completed objective and subjective tests 7 times, including 2 baseline tests before drug administration. The following tests were included: measures of motor sedation and memory impairment, the 10 scales of the Profile of Mood States (POMS) as modified by Johanson and Uhlenhuth; the 7 subscales derived from the Addiction Research Center Inventory (ARCI) by Cole et al. [9]; 13 questions having rating scale answers; and the Disinhibition and Euphoria Behaviour Index (DEBI), a 14-item observer-rated instrument.

Each subject's individually favourite dose (IFD) of each active drug was determined by a factor analysis of 11 measures chosen as likely to reflect "liking" for the drug or subjective effects likely associated with abuse liability. The advantage of this strategy is that it permits comparison among the drugs at the pharmacologically most important doses with respect to the likelihood of abuse.

Results

While bretazenil was found to be pharmacologically similar to diazepam and alprazolam on many measures, e.g. motor sedation and memory impairment, a number of important qualitative differences among the 3 tested drugs were also seen. These differences were most often of the form that the bretazenil dose-response curve was significantly less steep than for the other two drugs.

With respect to diazepam vs. bretazenil abuse liability differences, bretazenil was associated with lower abuse liability on the following: POMS friendliness, elation, and positive mood; Cole/ARCI euphoria, abuse potential, and dysphoria; rating scales of overall liking, effect on the mind, and price demanded to take the drug again; DEBI friendliness and drug satisfaction. Concerning alprazolam vs. bretazenil abuse liability differences, bretazenil was associated with lower abuse liability on the following: POMS friendliness, elation, and positive mood; Cole/ARCI abuse potential.

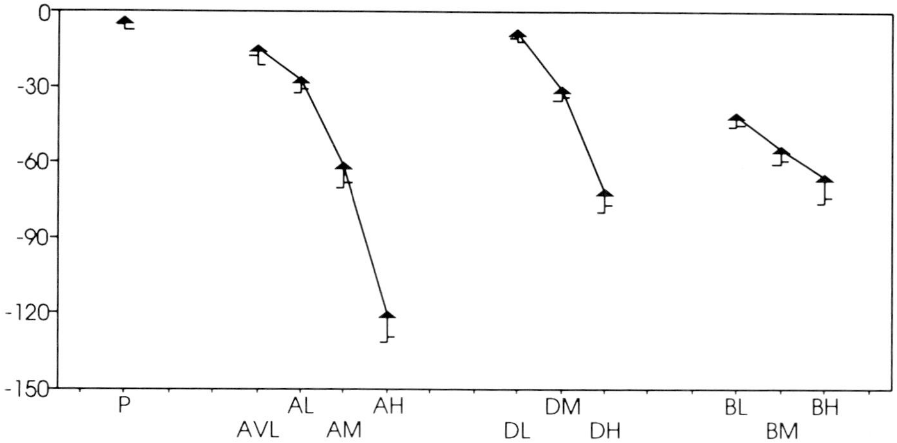

Fig. 1. Area under curve decrement in motor tracking task performance (% of time over road). P = placebo; A = alprazolam; D = diazepam; B = bretazenil. VL = very low; L = low; M = medium; H = high.

Discussion

This study has confirmed the low abuse liability of alprazolam and diazepam as reflected in the small absolute changes in measures such as "liking" and the abuse liability scale. In addition, the study has shown that, while there are numerous similarities among the tested drugs, there are also important differences, since all differences are in the direction of lesser abuse potential for bretazenil. Based on these data we conclude that the partial agonist bretazenil will have lower abuse liability than full agonist benzodiazepines diazepam or alprazolam. In clinical

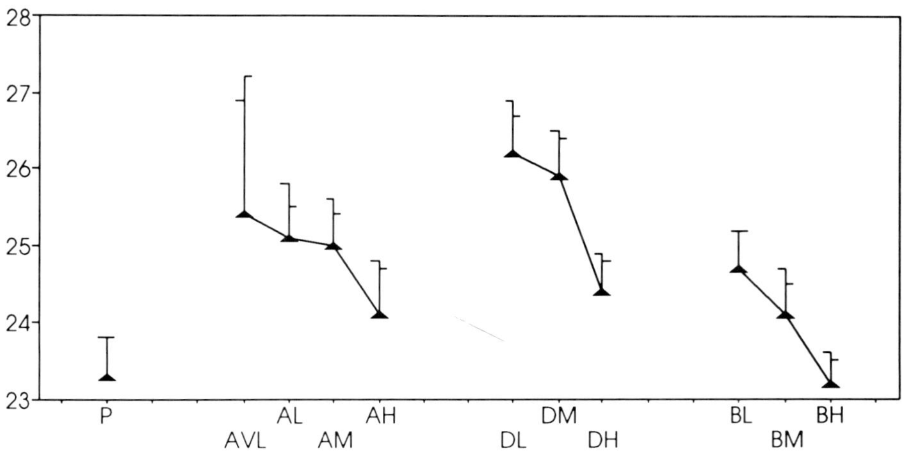

Fig. 2. Peak response on abuse potential scale total score. Placebo < bretazenil < diazepam = alprazolam, $F_{3,111} = 10.26$, $P = 0.0001$, for IFDs. VL = very low; L = low; M = medium; H = high.

practice, it would not be surprising to find bretazenil had minimal or no abuse liability. The clinical importance of this needs to be judged in the context of the low abuse liability of benzodiazepines in general.

References

1. Woods JH, Katz JL and Winger G (1987) Pharmacol. Rev. 39: 251–415.
2. Griffiths RR and Wolf B (1990) J. Clin. Psychopharmacol. 10: 237–243.
3. Sieghart W (1989) Trends Pharmacol. Sci. 10: 407–411.
4. Dennis T, Dubois A, Bcnauid J and Scatton B (1988) J. Pharmacol. Exp. Ther. 237: 649–658.
5. Evans SM, Funderburk R and Griffiths RR (1990) J. Pharmacol. Exp. Ther. 255: 1246–1255.
6. Martin JR, Kuwahara A, Horii I, Moreau J-L, Jenck F, Sepinwall J and Haefely W (1990) Abstr. Soc. Neurosci. 16(2): 1104.
7. Moreau J-L, Jenck F, Pieri L, Schoch P, Martin JR and Haefely WE (1990) Eur. J. Pharmacol. 190: 269–273.
8. Busto U, Somer G, Zawertailo L, Collis R and Sellers EM (1991) Clin. Pharmacol. Ther. 49: 46.
9. Cole JO, Orzack MH, Beabe B, Bird M and Bar-Tel Y (1982) J. Clin. Psychiatry 43: 12.

Biological Psychiatry, Volume 1. G. Racagni et al., editors.

Attack-related treatment of panic disorder with bretazenil – A randomized placebo-controlled clinical trial

Heinz Katschnig, Walter A. Merz, Peter Berger, Detlev Nutzinger, Claude Alf, Max Kutzer and Michaela Amering

Department of Psychiatry, University of Vienna, Währinger Gürtel 18-20, A-1090 Vienna, Austria; and Hoffmann LaRoche, Basle, Switzerland

Introduction

Panic disorder has become a treatable condition. Tricyclic antidepressants, MAO-inhibitors and high potency benzodiazepines are able to prevent the occurrence of panic attacks and to improve agoraphobia if continuously administered. However, if these drugs are discontinued, the relapse rate is high, and there are problems with the long-term use of these compounds. As panic attacks are rapidly arising outbursts of short-lasting severe anxiety, it is sensible to try a p.r.n. treatment of the individual attacks with a potent anxiolytic with rapid onset, short duration of action and with a relatively low sedative activity. This profile of action corresponds to that of bretazenil, an imidazodiazepinone with partial agonistic (mixed agonist/antagonist) activity at the benzodiazepine receptor [1]. As results obtained in an open study [2] suggest that bretazenil is efficacious in suppressing panic attacks, a randomized placebo-controlled clinical trial was designed.

Patients and Methods

Patients

Twenty-four DSM III-R panic disorder outpatients from the department of psychiatry at the University of Vienna took part in this double-blind randomized placebo-controlled clinical trial. In order to qualify for inclusion, patients had to have had at least 3 panic attacks in the 3 weeks preceding baseline and had to fulfil a number of other inclusion and exclusion criteria.

Methods

The study had 2 phases, a titration phase and a treatment phase. During the the titration phase the optimal dose had to be determined. Patients were instructed to start with one tablet (of 0.5 mg bretazenil or placebo), which they had to take either in the case when a panic attack had already started or was felt to be imminent because the patients were about to enter a phobic situation in which they usually experienced a panic attack. During the titration phase the dose could be gradually increased up to 3 tablets per attack or anticipated attack. If in 3 consecutive panic attacks or anticipated panic attacks a dosage of 3 tablets showed no effect, the patient was counted as a dropout. If a certain dosage had proven to be both efficacious and devoid of side-effects on 2 occasions, the patient entered into the treatment phase. During the treatment phase, patients were instructed to use the dose determined during the titration phase on 12 successive occasions.

Results

Dropout rate

One highly significant finding was the large difference in dropout rates between the 2 groups. Whereas in the bretazenil group only 1 of 12 patients did not experience any beneficial effect at the maximum dosage allowed (1.5 mg) and consequently dropped out, 8 of 12 patients dropped out in the placebo group ($P < 0.01$).

Suppression of panic attacks

The suppression of the individual panic attack had to be rated by the patient after each drug intake in a diary on a 4-point scale (1 = unchanged; 2 = slightly lower intensity; 3 = markedly lower intensity; and 4 = (nearly) complete suppression). In the bretazenil group the effect corresponded to nearly complete suppression (mean 3.5 ± 0.9), whereas in the placebo group the effect was not very different from no suppression (1.7 ± 1.2).

Secondary effects

While the trial was probably too short to show a significant effect beyond a successful treatment of the individual panic attacks, there is an interesting trend of improvement in phobic avoidance and also in the frequency of panic attacks in the bretazenil group, where the weekly frequency of panic attacks decreased by 3.1 (± 4.6), while it increased slightly in the placebo group (± 1.0 ± 9.4).

Discussion

Both the wide difference in efficacy-related dropouts and in the main outcome variable "suppression of panic attacks" suggest that the attack-related application of bretazenil could be a useful alternative to continuous administration of psychotropic medication. A larger trial is now underway which will show whether these results found in a relatively small sample can be reproduced. The possible secondary effects, such as reduction of phobic avoidance and frequency of panic attacks, create some interesting questions. Since the pharmacological effect obviously does not act directly on phobic avoidance, it is probably psychological mechanisms which work. On the one hand, if a patient has a drug in his pocket which he knows does work, his anticipatory anxiety is reduced, which may not only increase the threshold for the onset of a panic attack, but may also lead to more "exposure in vivo". Studies are in preparation in order to elucidate these mechanisms.

Despite the apparent advantages of a p.r.n. treatment as opposed to continuous administration of psychotropic medications – the former type of treatment can be called treatment according to the "angina pectoris model", the latter according to the "epilepsy model" [3] – there are certain limitations to the new strategy. One is that most patients who come to outpatients departments do not suffer just from panic attacks but also from anticipatory anxiety, phobic avoidance or depression. In such cases a p.r.n. treatment may be insufficient and chronic administration of antidepressant drugs might be more appropriate.

References

1. Merz WA (1984) Clin. Neuropharmacol. 7: 672.
2. Merz WA and Katschnig H (1990) In: Stefanis CN et al. (eds.) Psychiatry – A World Perspective – Vol. 3. Elsevier, Amsterdam, pp. 385–390.
3. Katschnig H (1989) In: Achté K, Tamminen T and Laaksonen R (eds.) Psychiatr. Fenn. 20 (Suppl.): 112–119.

Biological Psychiatry, Volume 1. G. Racagni et al., editors.

Pharmacological therapy of depression: Achievements and prospects

A. Delini-Stula
Roche International Clinical Research Center, 67382 Lingolsheim, France

Introduction

From a historical perspective, 3 periods characterize the research and the development of antidepressants. In the first period the *presynaptic monoamine neuron* has been considered as target structure both with respect to the search for the origin of depression and the mechanism of action of antidepressants. Two types of antidepressants: monoamine uptake inhibitors and monoamine oxidase inhibitors (IMAO) are representative of this period. In the second period, the research focused its interest primarily on *monoaminergic receptors*, anticipating that they were critically involved in the pathophysiology of depression. This approach led to the design and development of antidepressants directly acting on various pre- or postsynaptically-located receptors. The onset of the third period is recent and it is characterized by the shift in research emphasis to *intracellular transmission events*. From this approach new theoretical concepts of depression and probably quite novel types of antidepressants might emerge.

Epidemiological studies of depression indicate that 20–26% of women and 8–12% of men will suffer from depression during their lifetime. Even though a large number of antidepressants exist, the need for more efficient and safe treatment persists. All research strategies therefore are aimed at the discovery and development of antidepressants which could meet this need. What has been realized and what the future developments seem to indicate will be reviewed in the following discussion.

Monoamine uptake and MAO-inhibitors

Selective inhibitors of monoamine uptake

The classical theory of the origin of depression which assumes a deficit of monoamines (noradrenaline, serotonin and/or dopamine) as the primary cause of the disease, was the general background rationale guiding the development of monoamine uptake and MAO-inhibitors. With time, however, particular roles of noradrenaline (NA), serotonin (5-HT) or dopamine (DA) in depressive states were differently emphasised.

The assumption that one monoamine is more important than another [1] has directed research towards discovery and development of drugs with very selective NA or 5-HT uptake inhibiting properties. Such selective drugs were expected to offer more specific treatment of depressive disorders to allow biochemical identification of particular sub-populations of depressive patients and it was assumed that due to the selectivity and specificity of their action, as well as the novelty of their chemical structures, they would be better tolerated than non-selective and pharmacologically polyvalent acting tricyclic, imipramine-like uptake-inhibitors. At present only one selective HA-uptake inhibitor, e.g. maprotiline, has been introduced onto the world market and its efficacy is established beyond doubt. Maprotiline does not, however, considerably differ in any of its features from imipramine-like drugs, probably because its overall pharmacological spectrum of activity is more or less similar to imipramine [2]. Other elective NA-uptake inhibitors have not yet been introduced onto the market. The possible advantages of this principle of action cannot therefore be estimated. By contrast, present experience with biochemically and pharmacologically selective 5-HT uptake inhibitors indicates that in many respects they can be considered innovative. Even though in terms of their overall antidepressant efficacy they do not seem to differ from other established antidepressants, they do appear to have other advantages. Clinical studies indicate that they may be more specific than conventional antidepressants in the treatment of suicidal patients, compulsive-obsessive disorders, anxiety and panic disorders. They do not affect performance ability or body weight and are devoid of anticholinergic and cardiovascular effects. Last but not least, selective inhibitors of 5-HT uptake offer a research tool in identifying conditions in which serotonin abnormalities might be of particular importance.

There is no doubt today that the classical monoamine-deficiency hypothesis as it was formulated in the mid-1960s does not hold true. Nevertheless, the inhibition of monoamine uptake can be considered an established therapeutic principle in depression. With emphasis being placed on the side-effect profile, drugs of this type are therefore still being searched for.

Selective and reversible MAO-inhibitors

The assumption that monoamine oxidase inhibition is a therapeutic principle of antidepressant action is, as for monoamine-uptake inhibition, based on the classical monoamine deficiency hypothesis of depression. Recent targeted development of reversible and selective MAO-A inhibitors is therefore, from the general point of view, not a conceptual novelty. Nevertheless, these compounds should be considered as remarkable achievements resulting from goal-directed, rational research.

The development of selective MAO-A inhibitors was based on the discovery that the MAO enzyme is present in 2 forms, MAO-A and MAO-B. Endogenous amines such as A, and in some species also DA, are preferentially desaminated by MAO-A, whereas the exogenous amine tyramine is preferentially desaminated by MAO-B. Both facts have led to the assumption that the selectivity of MAO-A inhibition is the key factor in determining the safety of MAO-inhibitors. The combination of selectivity with reversibility of MAO-A inhibiting action alone with the novelty of chemical structure was expected to offer additional advantages of such drugs over classical, irreversible and non-selective IMAO. Present clinical evidence with moclobemide and brofaromine, 2 representative reversible and selective MAO-A inhibitors (RIMA), is largely in agreement with these expectations: a) the tyramine-potentiating effect (responsible for the hypertensive crisis and limiting the use of classical IMAO), is almost absent with moclobemide and much less pronounced with brofaromine [3]; b) cumulation does not seem to occur; and c) the general side-effect profile, in comparison to classical IMAO or tricyclics, is much more favorable. Also, contrary to earlier assumptions, therapeutic efficacy of this new generation of IMAO does not seem to be limited to "atypical depression". They seem to be just as effective as tricyclics in major depressive disorders [4]. The indications for their use may even expand to anxiety, panic disorder and perhaps also to there psychiatric conditions where serotoninergic deficiency is assumed to be of importance.

Monoaminergic receptor agonists and antagonists

The assumption that the abnormalities of monoaminergic receptor function may be the origin of depression emerged from the observation that long-term treatment

Table 1. Conceptually new antidepressants

Site and mode of action	Prototype and development drugs
1. Receptor blockade	
– α_2 (presynaptic)	Idozoxan Septiptilene ORG 3770 Imiloxan
– DA_2 (presynaptic)	Amperozid
– 5-HT_2	Ritanserin
– GABA-A	SR-95103
2. Receptor stimulation	
– α_1	Adrafinil
– 5-HT_{1A}	Gepirone RU-24696
3. "Second" messenger increase (cAMP) (phophodiesterase inhibition)	Rolipram
4. Unknown	Levoprotiline Medifoxamine Rilmazafone

The list is not exhaustive and only few examples of drugs under development are given.

with antidepressants produces functional or biochemical sensitivity changes in monoaminergic receptors. The initial β-receptor "hypersensitivity" hypothesis of depression [5] could in this respect be considered as a turning point in the research and development of new antidepressants. Novel concepts focusing on direct and selective action on monoaminergic receptors were introduced into the strategies of antidepressant research. In Table 1, some of the resulting new antidepressants presently under development are listed. Clinical experience with selective direct agonists or antagonists acting at monoaminergic receptor sites is at present rather scarce. It is not possible therefore to say whether they will fulfill the expectations: more rapid onset of action, greater specificity of antidepressant effect and better tolerability in comparison to conventional or other antidepressants. Initial studies with drugs such as idazoxane (selective α_2-adrenoceptor antagonist) and ipsapirone or gepirone (selective 5-HT_{1A}-agonists; [6,7]) nevertheless indicate that they do possess antidepressant properties.

New trends

The introduction of more refined biochemical, molecular biology and autoradiographic imaging techniques [8] has in recent years contributed much to our knowledge of intracellular transmission processes and of second messenger sys-

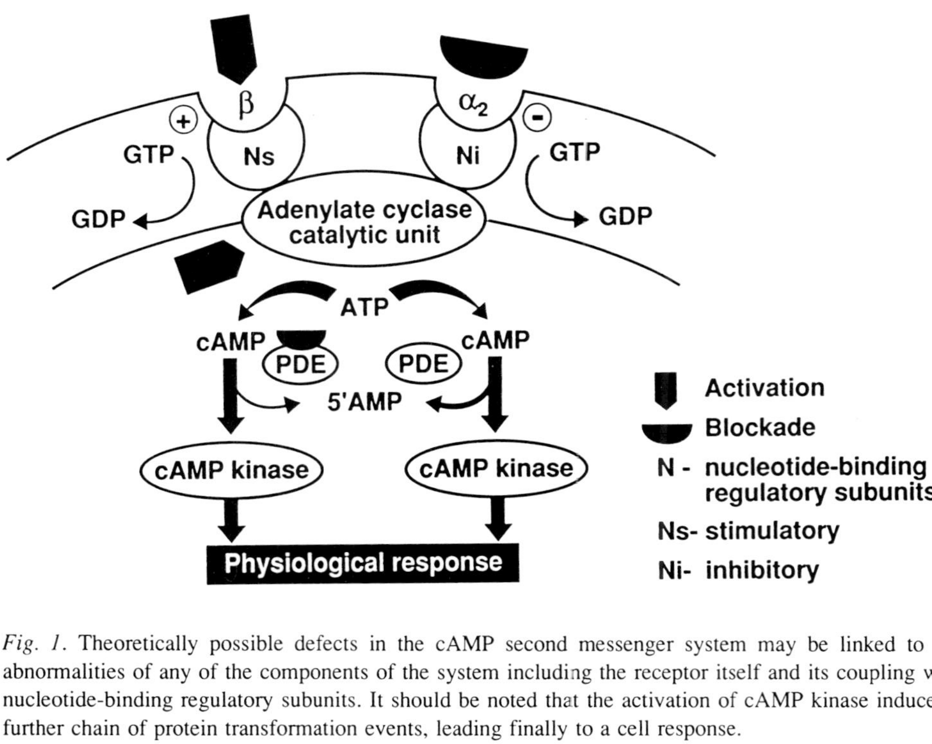

Fig. 1. Theoretically possible defects in the cAMP second messenger system may be linked to the abnormalities of any of the components of the system including the receptor itself and its coupling with nucleotide-binding regulatory subunits. It should be noted that the activation of cAMP kinase induces a further chain of protein transformation events, leading finally to a cell response.

tems coupled with monoaminergic receptors. Their selective manipulation may offer a new approach in the research of antidepressant drugs.

The concept of defective second-messenger function in the etiology of depression was postulated by Wachtel in 1988 [9]. He suggested an increase in cAMP as the possible mechanism of antidepressant action. The concept was based on the observation that rolipram, a phosphodiesterase inhibitor, exerts a clinical antidepressant effect. The possible defects in the receptor-adenylatecyclase coupled transmission and tentative targets for antidepressant action are illustrated in Fig. 1.

The phosphoinositide system, implicated in the action of lithium, is the other second messenger system which also increasingly attracts attention. Recently Banks et al. [10] reported findings indicating abnormalities of [^{3}H]-inositol incorporation into the phosphoinositides of the lymphoblastoid cells derived from bipolar manic-depressive patients. Rolipram and lithium are at present the prototypes of drugs which may exert their therapeutic effects via a direct action on second messenger systems. The clinical efficacy of rolipram is, however, not proved beyond doubt at present. Further research is necessary to validate the second messenger hypothesis as a basis for antidepressant drug development.

Lastly, Table 1 lists some drugs presently under development with yet unidentified modes of action, but with apparently antidepressant effects. Providing that their antidepressant activity can be confirmed, the elucidation of their mechanism of action may open up additional new approaches in this area of research.

References

1. Carlsson A, Corrodi H, Fuxe K and Hökfelt T (1969) Eur. J. Pharmacol. 5: 367–376.
2. Delini-Stula A (1987) In: Simhandl C, Berner P, Loccioni H and Alf C (eds.) Moderne Psychiatrie, Klassifikationsprobleme in der Psychiatrie. Purkerdorf, pp. 131–148.
3. Youdim MBH, Da Prada M and Amrein R (1987) J. Neural Transm. Suppl. 26.
4. Stabl M, Bizière K, Schmid-Burgk W and Amrein R (1989) J. Neural Transm. (28): 77–89.
5. Sulser F (1978) Trends Pharmacol. Sci. 1: 92–94.
6. Heller AH, Beneke M, Kuemmel B, Spencer D and Kurtz NM (1990) Phychopharmacol. Bull. 26 (2): 219–222.
7. Rausch JL, Ruegg R and Moeller FG (1990) Psychopharmacol. Bull. 26 (2): 169–171.
8. Hwang MH, Bredt DS and Snyder SH (1990) Science 249: 802–805.
9. Wachtel H (1988) In: Briley M and Fillion G (eds.) New Concepts in Depression. Mac Millan Press, London, pp. 227–293.
10. Banks RE, Aiton JF, Cramb G and GJ Naylor (1990) J. Affective Disord. 19: 1–8.

Biological Psychiatry, Volume 1. G. Racagni et al., editors.

Pharmacology of β-carbolines

D.N. Stephens, M. Hillmann, R. Huba, H.H. Schneider,*J.D. Turner and L. Turski

Department of Neuropsychopharmacology, Research Laboratories of Schering AG, P.O. Box 65 03 11, W-1000 Berlin, Germany

β-carboline-3-carboxylic acid derivatives bind with high affinity to central benzodiazepine receptors, where, depending on the particular structure, they may act as agonists, inverse agonists or antagonists in modulating the $GABA_A$ receptor. The β-carboline series is to date the only chemical series which possesses ligands covering the entire spectrum from full agonist to full inverse agonist. This series of compounds therefore offers itself for a series of indications, including not only the classical therapies of anxiety, sleep disturbances and epilepsy associated with the benzodiazepines, but also new approaches, such as the use of weak inverse agonists to improve cognitive function.

At present, we have gathered most information about β-carbolines possessing anxiolytic activity in animal models and, in the case of one substance – abecarnil, also in the clinic. Among such compounds we have identified a series of structures possessing partial agonistic activity at the benzodiazepine receptor. These substances, including ZK 91296 [1] and ZK 95962 [2], show good anxiolytic effects in animal models without displaying the sedative and muscle relaxant side-effects associated with benzodiazepines and this separation of effects is usually ascribed to such compounds being less efficacious than full agonists in potentiating the inhibitory effects of GABA on membrane excitability [3]. In keeping with this hypothesis, the anxiolytic effects of such partial agonistic β-carbolines are achieved only at receptor occupations higher than those required by full agonists for similar effects [2].

Recently, we have gained experience in animal pharmacology with a novel β-carboline, abecarnil (ZK 112119). Like partial agonistic β-carbolines, this substance possesses good anxiolytic [4] and anticonvulsant [5] activity without impairing coordination, or inducing muscle relaxation and for this reason, abecarnil was initially characterised as a partial agonist. We noted, however, that several aspects of the pharmacology of abecarnil are inconsistent with a partial agonist characterisation. Thus, abecarnil induces several pharmacological effects in animal models of anxiolytic and anticonvulsant activity at receptor occupancies lower than those at which the benzodiazepine, diazepam, achieves similar effects [4]. Furthermore, abecarnil is not capable of antagonising diazepam in reducing electromyographic activity of rats treated with etorphine. These observations suggest that the selective profile of abecarnil in achieving anxiolytic effects in the absence of muscle relaxant properties may be due to an action at a subpopulation of benzodiazepine receptors. In particular, the absence of effects of abecarnil on muscle relaxation, and the failure to antagonise the muscle relaxant effects of diazepam might suggest that abecarnil has a low affinity for receptors in spinal cord.

This prediction was tested in autoradiographic studies in which the abilities of abecarnil and diazepam to compete with ^{3}H-lormetazepam for binding sites in rat cortex was compared to their affinities in the dorsal horn of monkey spinal cord (Schneider et al., unpublished). In rat cortex, abecarnil showed an approximately 10-fold higher affinity than diazepam for the ^{3}H-lormetazepam-labelled receptors, whereas in spinal cord dorsal horn, the two substances showed similar affinities. Expressed differently, diazepam possessed a similar affinity for rat cortex and monkey spinal cord receptors, whereas the affinity of abecarnil for spinal cord receptors was about 17 times less than for cortical receptors. These results clearly demonstrate that abecarnil shows some selectivity for a subpopulation of benzodiazepine receptors, though the nature of this selectivity is not yet clear.

Recent results from Seeburg's laboratory have suggested that the nature of the α subunit of the benzodiazepine receptor may determine the selectivity of receptor ligands, so that, although benzodiazepines are non-selective (i.e. have similar affinities) for receptors containing α_1, α_2, α_3, α_4 or α_5 subtypes, ligands from other chemical classes, including β-carbolines, show a preference for receptors containing the α_1 subunit. It can be speculated that abecarnil may show some similar sort of selectivity. Of particular interest are receptors made up of α_6 subunits in combination with a β_2 and γ_2 subunit. These receptors have been suggested to be selective for inverse agonists, since they allow the binding of Ro 15-4513, an inverse agonistic imidazodiazepine, but not agonistic benzodiazepines. Although we have not yet investigated the action of abecarnil directly on cells expressing this combination of receptor subunits, we have obtained indirect evidence that abecarnil, in contrast to agonist benzodiazepines, may act at this subtype (Hillmann et al., unpublished). Binding of ^{3}H-Ro 15-4513 to sites in cerebellum can only be partially displaced by benzodiazepines, the failure to displace Ro 15-4513 completely probably reflecting the lack of affinity of benzodiazepines for some of Ro 15-4513's binding sites, including the $\alpha_2\beta_2\gamma_2$ receptor subtype. In contrast to benzodiazepine anxiolytics, abecarnil does displace ^{3}H-Ro 15-4513 from all its binding sites. Thus abecarnil may differ from benzodiazepines, not only in showing a low affinity for spinal cord receptors, but also in possessing affinity for a receptor subtype which is not susceptible to modulation by benzodiazepine anxiolytics.

The extent to which these differences account for the differences between abecarnil and benzodiazepines in their pharmacological effects and apparent lack of dependence potential remains to be evaluated.

References

1. Petersen EN et al. (1984) Psychopharmocology 83: 240–248.
2. Stephens DN et al. (1987) Brain Res. Bull. 19: 309–318.

3. Schneider HH et al. (1989) Modulation of the $GABA_A$ receptor complex. In: Bowery N and Nistico G (eds.) GABA: Basic Research and Clinical Applications. Pythagora Press, Rome.
4. Stephens DN et al. (1990) J. Pharmacol. Exp. Ther. 253: 334–343.
5. Turski L et al. (1990) J. Pharmacol. Exp. Ther. 253: 344–352.

Biological Psychiatry, Volume 1. G. Racagni et al., editors.

Abuse liability of benzodiazepine (BZ) receptor ligands: Abecarnil

Nancy A. Ator[1], Roland R. Griffiths[2] and Christine A. Sannerud[3]
[1]Department of Psychiatry and Behavioral Sciences; and [2]Department of Neuroscience, The Johns Hopkins University School of Medicine, 720 Rutland Avenue, Rm. 621, Baltimore, MD 21205; and [3]National Institute on Drug Abuse, Addiction Research Center, P.O. Box 5180, Baltimore, MD 21224, U.S.A.

Introduction

Recently non-BZ compounds have been synthesized that bind with high affinity to the BZ receptor but produce distinctive and more delimited profiles of biochemical and behavioral effects than BZ. β-carbolines are among such non-BZ structures and fall along a continuum of behavioral efficacy, from full agonist through antagonist to full inverse agonist [1]. Abecarnil is a β-carboline with good bioavailability which displaces tritiated BZ from binding sites in brain with a 10-fold higher affinity than diazepam; but its binding is virtually unaffected by GABA, suggesting a partial or selective agonist effect [2]. Consistent with this interpretation of the neurochemical data, abecarnil has a behavioral profile that includes anxiolytic and anticonvulsant effects but not severe muscle relaxant effects, compared to diazepam [2]. The present studies investigated the discriminative-stimulus, reinforcing and physiological-dependence-producing effects of abecarnil in adult male baboons (Papio cynocephalus) to compare those data with the effects of BZ. Such data have proven useful in the assessment of the abuse liability and dependence potential of psychoactive compounds [cf., 3].

Drug discrimination study

In a drug (D) versus no-drug (ND) discrimination procedure [4], 4 baboons were trained to operate one lever to obtain food pellets after administration of lorazepam (1.8 mg/kg p.o.) and to operate a second lever to obtain food in the ND condition. Three baboons were trained to discriminate pentobarbital (10 mg/kg p.o.) from the ND condition. For the baboons trained to discriminate lorazepam, tests with abecarnil (0.32–32 mg/kg, p.o.) showed reliable abecarnil generalization (i.e., dose-dependent increases in D-lever responding to >80% of total test session responses) in all 4 baboons only in test sessions 3–5 h after abecarnil. The duration of D-lever responding generally decreased by 9–13 h after abecarnil. Response rates generally were not affected by any dose of abecarnil. The discriminative-stimulus effects of abecarnil were blocked by flumazenil, indicating they were mediated at the BZ receptor. For the baboons trained to discriminate pentobarbital, only 1 of the 3 showed complete dose-dependent generalization to abecarnil.

Self-administration study

Three baboons, prepared with chronically indwelling venous catheters, were trained to self-inject cocaine; a standard substitution procedure [5] was used to study abecarnil. A 3 h timeout limited the maximum injections per day (inj/day) to 8; mean cocaine self-injection was 7–8 inj/day. Substitution of the abecarnil vehicle for 15 days resulted in a mean of about 2 inj/day over the last 5 days. Abecarnil (0.032–1.0 mg/kg/inj) was substituted for cocaine for 15-day periods per dose and maintained mean rates of self-injection that were generally similar to or marginally above the vehicle mean. By comparison, triazolam maintained 6–7 inj/day. The highest abecarnil dose (1.0 mg/kg, i.v.) produced sedation and ataxia in 2 baboons.

Chronic administration study

Four baboons were implanted with i.g. catheters for study of the effects of chronic abecarnil and its withdrawal [cf., 6]. Abecarnil vehicle was given by slow infusion for 2 weeks, followed by 6–8 consecutive weeks of abecarnil 100 mg/kg/day, followed by return to vehicle infusion for 4 weeks. Observational sessions were conducted systematically throughout the study. Chronic abecarnil produced few signs of sedation. During the first 4–7 days of abecarnil, 2 baboons showed intention tremor, an effect that was also observed after high doses of BZ. Flumazenil on day 8 of abecarnil produced vomiting in 1 baboon, increases in limb tremor in 2 baboons, and increases in "twitch/jerks" in 3 baboons compared to the previous 7 days of chronic abecarnil and compared to the effects of flumazenil in baboons not receiving chronic drug. There were no myoclonic jerks or seizures. During the 4 weeks of vehicle substitution, there were transitory increases in some mild signs of BZ withdrawal. In general, these signs decreased within baseline ranges by the end of the 4 weeks. The profile of signs observed under conditions of both precipitated and spontaneous withdrawal were indicative of a mild BZ-like withdrawal syndromes [6].

Conclusions

The profile of effects of abecarnil in the present study was novel compared to classic BZ-agonists [3–6] in the baboon because of: a) lack of initial sedative effects; b) low occurrence of withdrawal signs after flumazenil administration or vehicle substitution; c) lower probability of maintaining even modest self-injection i.v.; and d) failure to occasion reliable drug-stimulus generalization in baboons trained to discriminate pentobarbital. The delayed onset of lorazepam-like discriminative-stimulus effects in baboons was unlike that for BZ or other non-BZ ligands tested, except for halazepam, which, unlike abecarnil, is a slowly converted pro-drug. Overall, these results suggest low abuse liability and dependence potential of abecarnil.

Acknowledgements

This research was supported by National Institute on Drug Abuse Grants DA 04133 and DA 01147 and by a contract from Schering AG, Berlin.

References

1. Stephens DN and Jensen LH (eds.) (1987) Brain Res. Bull. 19: 291.
2. Stephens DN, Schneider HH, Kehr W, Andrews JS, Rettig K-J, Turski L, Schmiechen R, Turner JD, Jensen LH, Petersen EN, Honore T and Bondo Hansen J (1990) J. Pharmacol. Exp. Ther. 253: 334.
3. Griffiths RR, Lamb RJ, Ator NA, Roache JD and Brady JV (1985) Neurosci. Biobehav. Rev. 9: 133.
4. Ator NA and Griffiths RR (1989) Drug Dev. Res. 16: 355.
5. Griffiths RR, Lamb RJ, Sannerud CA, Ator NA and Brady JV (1991) Psychopharmacology 103: 154.
6. Griffiths RR and Sannerud CA (1987) In: Meltzer HY (ed.) Psychopharmacology: The Third Generation of Progress. Raven Press, New York, pp. 1535–1541.

Biological Psychiatry, Volume 1. G. Racagni et al., editors.

Partial benzodiazepine agonists: New concepts in the treatment of panic disorder and schizophrenia

Walter A. Merz
Department of Clinical Research, F. Hoffmann-La Roche Ltd, P.O. Box, CH-4002 Basel, Switzerland

Introduction

Partial agonists at the benzodiazepine receptor share with conventional full agonists many of the well known pharmacological and clinical properties of this class of drugs; in particular, anxiolytic, sedative, muscle relaxant and anticonvulsive activity, and an excellent profile of safety. Under these conditions, it is not surprising that partial agonists may substitute full agonists in the conventional usage pattern of the classic benzodiazepines, in particular, if they are able to show an even better margin of tolerance.

An enlargement in the range of useful indications, however, requires clear quantitative and qualitative pharmacological differences as compared with conventional benzodiazepines. This paper will show that new pharmacological properties of the partial agonists may be the clues to the introduction of new fields of use of benzodiazepines and similar GABAergic modulator drugs.

P.R.N. treatment of panic disorder

The old view that benzodiazepines are of only limited value in Panic Disorder is no longer true. Potent benzodiazepines, such as alprazolam, are able to prevent panic attacks and a number of accompanying complications of Panic Disorder. However, the doses and duration of treatment required may typically lead to side-effects and to dependence on some of the drugs used [1]. P.R.N. treatment with a fast-acting, potent, but rapidly eliminated benzodiazepine may avoid long-lasting side-effects as well as dependence. Such considerations, however, must fail because the profile of rapid absorption, high potency, and patient-controlled frequency and/or dosage of the drugs bears an increased risk of drug abuse and, on uncontrolled cumulation of single doses, of an unpredictable severity range of side-effects.

The partial benzodiazepine agonist bretazenil (Ro 16-6028) appears able to overcome the problem of self-directed use of a benzodiazepine in Panic Disorder and other indications showing largely fluctuating severity of anxious mood. This drug is a potent anxiolytic (10 to 100 times more potent than diazepam). It is rapidly absorbed and shows in humans, 5 to 10 min after sublingual administration, quantifiable plasma concentrations and clinically relevant anxlolytic activity. The half-life of elimination from plasma is around 2.5 h. An extensive human pharmacological investigation of the abuse liability of bretazenil in recreational drug users resulted, despite the described "abuse-prone" pharmacokinetic profile of the drug, in the conclusion, "that bretazenil will have lower abuse liability than diazepam or alprazolam and that in clinical practice it would not be surprising to find this was a drug with minimal or no abuse liability" [2], thus confirming the result of self-administration experiments in cynomolgus monkeys. In addition, bretazenil causes, as predicted by animal pharmacology, even after large doses only a limited range of sedation and impairment of performance (see Table 1).

In view of these findings, bretazenil is studied in P.R.N. treatment of Panic Disorder. Current evidence is based on the results of a large open label pilot study and a placebo-controlled double-blind study; in addition, the first phase of a large cross-national multicenter double-blind dose finding study is currently being analyzed.

Due to its simple design, the open label study clearly demonstrates the effectiveness of a P.R.N. dosage schedule in Panic Disorder. The sample of evaluable patients consisted of 89 patients [3]. Including dose titration, a mean total of only 20 doses was administered during a mean treatment period of 57 days. The most frequently used individual dose was 0.5 mg bretazenil. These 20 doses led to a complete suppression of the panic attacks in 56% of the cases and to a marked alleviation of the remaining panic attacks in 35% of the cases. A diminished frequency or total disappearance of panic attacks was observed in 69% of the patients. No treatment was given during the interval between successive panic attacks. Nevertheless, there was also a marked decrease of anticipatory anxiety (complete suppression or marked alleviation in 63% of the cases) and phobic avoidance (complete suppression or marked alleviation of the phobic fear in 55%, slight alleviation in another 23% of the cases). The (mean of) 20 doses led within the (mean of) 57 days to only few and short-lasting adverse reactions, mostly of the usual benzodiazepine type. No withdrawal reactions were observed after treatment with bretazenil. It is concluded that P.R.N. treatment of panic attacks with a partial benzodiazepine agonist may be a treatment with a remarkably good risk/benefit ratio.

Table 1. POMS Fatigue scale: peak response

Dose:	Low	Medium	High
Alprazolam	7.90 (1.06)	9.52 (1.08)	10.69 (1.62)[a]
Diazepam	6.06 (1.04)	8.67 (0.99)	8.84 (1.27)
Bretazenil	7.97 (1.26)	7.76 (1.05)	7.85 (1.29)[b]

(mean and S.E.M.; n = 28; [a]n = 24; [b]n = 27). According to E. Sellers: (this congress; [2]).

Therapy of schizophrenia

There are dozens of publications reporting monotherapy of schizophrenia with benzodiazepines [4]. The common denominator of the few publications showing efficacy to some extent is the extremely high dosage used (e.g. 400 mg/d [5]). It is clear that such dosages can only be considered as experimental doses; in practice, the accompanying adverse effects preclude such a type of treatment.

Pharmacology predicts a shallow dose-response curve for selected effects of partial agonists at the benzodiazepine receptor [6]. In humans, this has been demonstrated by Sellers et al. [2] for impairment of psychomotor skills and sedative effects induced by bretazenil (1, 2 and 4 mg) in comparison with alprazolam (1, 2 and 40 mg). An example for this behavior is given in Table 1. The relative scores of the 3 compared drugs in the POMS Fatigue Scale are of less importance, as the selected dose ranges may be of unequal anxiolytic potency. However, whereas fatigue due to alprazolam or diazepam is clearly dose-dependant, no such relation between dose and sedative effect can be observed for bretazenil: the effect has its maximum already at 1 mg of the partial agonist and shows, up to 4 mg, no further increase.

Under these conditions it appears possible to administer in schizophrenia or other indications doses of bretazenil corresponding in potency to 200–400 mg of diazepam without risk of dramatic adverse effects. In view of the expected good safety and tolerance, an open pilot study in schizophrenia was performed. Seventy-three hospitalized patients (56 males, 17 females) were eligible for analysis of efficacy [6]. The main inclusion criterion was an active phase of schizophrenia, diagnosed according to the DSM III criteria. Six cases showed the disorganized type, 4 the catatonic type, 47 the paranoid type and 16 the undifferentiated type of

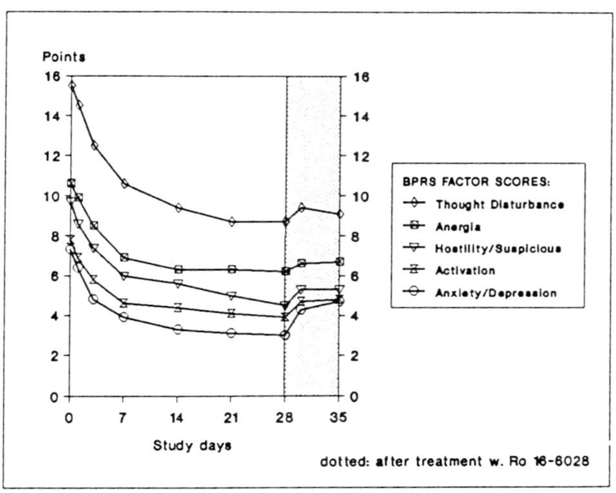

Fig. 1.

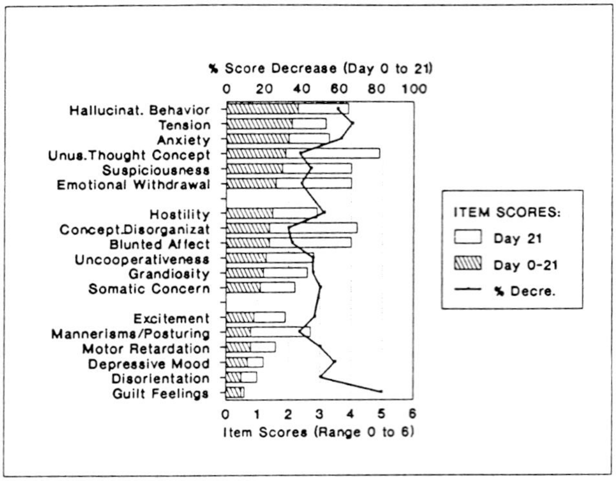

Fig. 2.

schizophrenia. Two patients were, according to the CGI, moderately ill, 13 markedly ill, 41 severely ill and 17 were among the most extreme cases. After a wash-out phase of one week, bretazenil was administered for 4 weeks (1 week titration, 2 weeks maintenance dose, 1 week tapering). This was followed by placebo or, where necessary, by thioridazine. Day of reference for efficacy rating is thus day 21, at the end of the full dosing regimen. During treatment with bretazenil, 11 evaluable patients dropped out of the study (9 because of lacking efficacy, one because of early recovery, and 1 for other reasons). In Figs. 1–3, their data are carried forward for end-point analysis on day 21. The total score of the BPRS (item

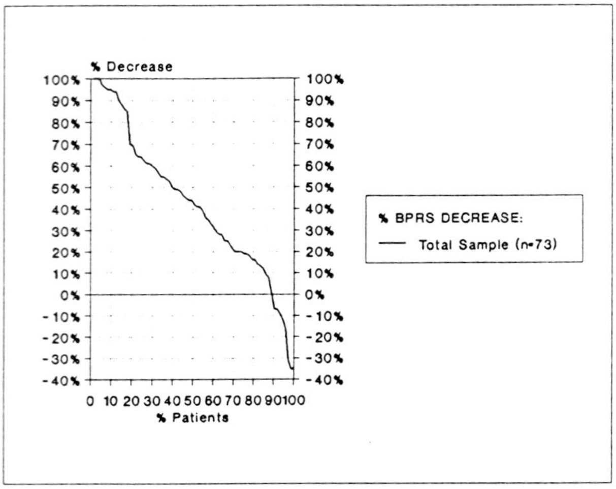

Fig. 3.

range 0 to 6) decreased from 50.9 points at baseline to 27.2 points on day 21. This fall is not only due to a decrease in the factors Anxiety/Depression, Activation, or Hostility/suspiciousness which may at least in part be susceptible to simple anxiolytics. It is also due to the schizophrenic core factors Thought Disturbance and Anergia (Fig. 1). Moreover, the decreasing activity of the illness is consistent in all 18 items of the scale (Fig. 2). Figure 3 demonstrates that the overall success of the treatment is not due to a little group of patients alone, but represents a whole spectrum of responding, ranging from full responders to patients with worsening of their states. Drug treatment was well tolerated by all patients, the spectrum of side-effects corresponding to that of conventional benzodiazepines.

It is clear that the reported data ask for confirmation in placebo-controlled double-blind studies. However, they may at least open an area for new ideas in the drug treatment of schizophrenia.

References

1. Fyer A et al. (1987) Am. J. Psychiatry 144: 303–308.
2. Sellers E (1991) Abuse liability of full and partial agonists in animal and man (this congress).
3. Merz WA and Katschnig H (1990) In: Stefanis CN et al. (eds) Psychiatry: A World Perspective, Vol. 3. Elsevier, Amsterdam, pp. 385–390.
4. Stula-Delini A (1991) Perspectives in the use of partial benzodiazepine agonists in schizophrenia (this congress).
5. Beckmann H and Haas S (1980) Psychopharmacologia 71: 79–82.
6. Richards JG et al. (1991) In: Olsen RW (ed.) GABA and Inhibition in the Brain, W.B. Saunders, New York (in press).
7. Merz WA et al. (1990) Research Report B-116'557, F. Hoffmann-La Roche Ltd., Basel.

Biological Psychiatry, Volume 1. G. Racagni et al., editors.

Problems in the diagnosis and treatment of anxiety disorders

M.H. Lader
Institute of Psychiatry, London, SE5 8AF, U.K.

Anxiety is important because it is found in many mental illnesses as well as constituting a range of syndromes in its own right, the anxiety disorders. Anxiety is a subjective state which is unpleasant and related to the vague perception of a real or imagined threat [1]. It is usually associated with various psychological and somatic symptoms, and often with phobic avoidance behaviour and crescendos of anxiety, the panic attacks [2].

Problems of diagnosis

The main distinction is between anxiety as a reaction to social and personal pressures and the anxiety disorders in which the intensity of the emotion is disproportionate to the extent of the threat. The former is usually understandable and may be adaptive, the latter is unreasonable and maladaptive. Prognostic studies suggest that almost all individuals with reactive anxiety and most patients with anxiety disorders recover quite rapidly.

The vast majority of anxious patients are seen by primary care practitioners, only a small and untypical subgroup being referred to a psychiatrist or a clinical psychologist [3]. Furthermore, general practitioners typically see such patients over the course of many years and consequently regard the disorders in a somewhat different light from specialists who are accustomed to a more cross-sectional view. For example, on one occasion a patient may present with generalized anxiety disorder, on another with a phobic state and yet later become depressed or obsessional. Nevertheless, it is useful both for research and clinical purposes to have a pragmatic classification and this includes: Generalized Anxiety Disorder, Phobic Disorder, Panic Disorder, Acute Stress Reactions, Adjustment Reactions, Post-Traumatic Stress Disorder and Obsessive-Compulsive Disorder [4]. It is also useful to set the acute or semi-acute disorder against the background of the personality profile of the individual.

A common diagnostic problem is the distinction between Anxiety and Depressive Disorders. Compared with those patients attending psychiatric outpatient clinics, many patients presenting to a G.P. show mixed features of anxiety and depression. Careful elucidation of the symptom pattern, precipitating factors, previous history and true course of onset and development of the disorder usually clarifies the diagnosis, but many practitioners in doubt tend nowadays to diagnose depression because of the less contentious management implications.

Treatment of anxiety disorder

General measures are essential to provide a supportive framework in which more specific stratagems can be tried. Reassurance and education, especially about the physical symptoms of anxiety, usually have an immediate effect. The provision of support is important, although one must beware of fostering an unhealthy attitude of dependency. Stressors should be assessed carefully as patients often search desperately for causes for their condition and may identify spurious factors. Counselling is simple, practical and directive and, together with some instruction in anxiety management such as relaxation or respiratory exercises, is usually effective as drug treatment in cases of mild to moderate severity.

In general practice where acute disorders are common, non-specific measures as outlined above are often sufficient and the symptoms subside over a few weeks. In psychiatric practice and in the more severe G.P. patients, drug treatment may be needed to lessen the severity of the symptoms to tolerable levels and to allow the introduction of non-drug treatments [5]. If a benzodiazepine is used, a long-acting one like diazepam or clorazepate is preferable to a short-acting one like lorazepam because the risk of rebound symptoms is much less. Dosage levels should be conservative and the duration of use should not normally exceed 4 weeks. Sedative effects, both subjective and objective, should be sought, in particular memory disturbance, and the dosage lowered if necessary. Paradoxical release of anxiety or hostility may be noted, necessitating stopping the drug. Beyond 4 weeks' use, the risk of dependence rapidly increases.

Beta-adrenergic antagonists such as propranolol may be useful in lessening severe palpitations, tremor and gastro-intestinal upsets, providing such somatic symptoms are pivotal to the wider syndrome [6]. Performance anxiety, e.g. in musicians, is often greatly helped.

Buspirone is an anxiolytic acting on serotonin mechanisms [7]. However, the onset of action is often slow and gradual, there may be initial dysphoria or side-effects such as dizziness and headache, and patients with experience of benzodiazepines often respond poorly. Nevertheless, in the more chronically anxious patient, a gratifying improvement may be seen after 2 weeks or so.

General practitioners often use low dose antipsychotic drugs, but autonomic side-effects and akathisia resemble anxiety symptoms and there is a remote risk of inducing tardive dyskinesia.

Finally, patients with chronic anxiety especially with a phobic or panicky flavour often respond well to tricyclic or other antidepressants. Initial dosage must be very low, e.g. clomipramine 10 mg. MAOIs are also effective but require the usual dietary and drug precautions.

References

1. Lewis A (1970) Int. J. Psychiatry 9: 62–79.
2. Lader MH, Marks IM (1971) Clinical Anxiety. Heinemann, London.
3. France R (1990) In: Wheatley D (ed.) The Anxiolytic Jungle: Where Next? Wiley, Chichester, pp. 79–98.
4. Jablensky A (1985) In: Tuma AT and Maser J (eds.) Anxiety and the Anxiety Disorders. Erlbaum, Hillside, New Jersey, pp. 735–758.
5. Catalan J and Gath DH (1985) Br. Med. J. 290: 1374–1376.
6. Lader M (1988) J. Clin. Psychiatry 6: 213–223.
7. Goa KL and Ward A (1986) Drugs 32: 114–129.

Biological Psychiatry, Volume 1. G. Racagni et al., editors.

Gene structure and characterization of the mitochondrial benzodiazepine receptor

S.O. Casalotti, G. Pelaia, M. Whalin, D.R. Grayson and K.E. Krueger
Fidia-Georgetown Institute for the Neurosciences, Georgetown University Medical School, 3900 Reservoir Rd., Washington DC 20007, U.S.A.

Introduction

The peripheral-type or mitochondrial benzodiazepine receptor (MBR) is an integral membrane protein localized predominantly in the outer mitochondrial membrane. This protein was initially identified for its ability to bind a class of benzodiazepines (e.g. Ro5-4568) and isoquinolines (e.g. PK 11195) [1] and has been shown to have a wide tissue distribution, but its abundance varies greatly with adrenal cortex being the richest source for MBR. Moreover, MBRs have recently been shown to be involved in steroidogenesis [2,3]. This receptor can be irreversibly photolabelled by the isoquinoline PK 14105 which has been instrumental in the purification of an 18 kDa polypeptide [4]. A cDNA clone coding for this protein has been isolated [5] and expressed showing it to bind Ro5-4864 and PK 11195 in a manner similar to the native rat MBR.

In this study a full length cDNA clone encoding the 18 kDa MBR protein was used to screen a rat genomic library in order to identify the MBR gene. We have isolated a clone comprising the whole cDNA sequence and extending several kb in both directions. The characterization of this clone might help in the study of the regulation of MBR expression.

Results and Discussion

A Wistar rat genomic library cloned in λ Dash (Stratagene) was screened at high stringency with the MBR-encoding cDNA clone and 7 positive clones were isolated. Restriction digests of these clones and characterization by Southern blotting revealed the same hybridization patterns for all 7 clones, indicating that they were overlapping representations of the same genomic fragment. A detailed restriction mapping of one such clone using both the MBR cDNA clone and synthetic oligonucleotides as probes revealed that the MBR gene is approximately 3 kb in length and contains in the protein coding region two introns of 641 and 854 bp each (see Fig. 1). Southern blot experiments with restriction-digested rat genomic DNA indicated that a single copy of MBR is present per rat haploid genome.

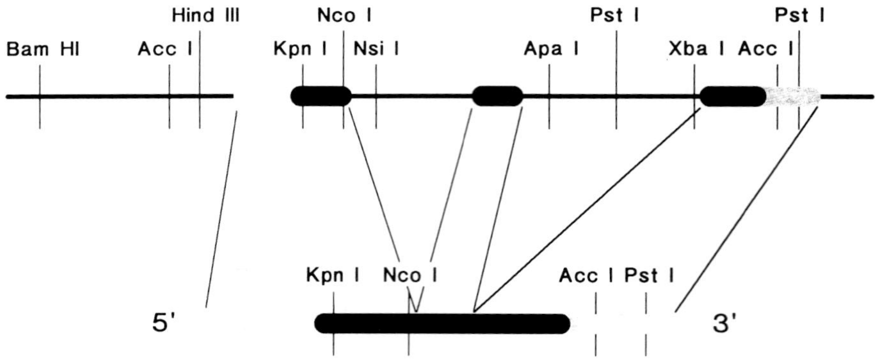

Fig. 1. Structure of rat MBR gene. Exons are indicated by boxes where translated sequence is filled and non-coding sequence is stippled. Locations of significant restriction enzymes sites are labeled and processing of the primary transcript to the mature mRNA is depicted.

The MBR genomic clone was subcloned into Bluescript KSII plasmid and fully sequenced by the Sanger dideoxy nucleotide method. The full exonic DNA sequence was reconfirmed with the exception of one base in the 3' non-coding region. This discrepancy is due to a reading error of the original sequencing of the cDNA clone [5]. The described introns and exons are flanked by the consensus donor/acceptor splicing sequence GT/AG. Both introns are found within the coding sequence corresponding to hydrophobic membrane-spanning domains of the receptor protein.

Primer extension experiments have shown that the untranslated region of RNA upstream of the ATG translation initiation codon extends for about 250 bases. Approximately 1000 bases of the 5' upstream region have been sequenced and shown to contain a putative CAAT box and a long GT repeat sequence, whereas other known regulatory consensus sequences are absent in this region. Our studies are directed at evaluating whether these or other sites have functional significance in the regulation of the expression of MBR.

Acknowledgement

This work was funded in part by National Institutes of Health Grant MH44284.

References

1. LeFur G, Perrier ML, Vaucher N, Imbault F, Flamier A, Uzan A, Renault C, Dubroeucq MC and Gueremy C (1983) Life Sci. 32: 1839–1847.

2. Mukhin AG, Papadopoulos V, Costa E and Krueger KE (1989) Proc. Natl. Acad. Sci. U.S.A. 86: 9813–9816.
3. Papadopoulos V, Muhkin AG, Costa E and Krueger KE (1990) J. Biol. Chem. 265: 3772–3779.
4. Doble A, Ferris O, Burgevin MC, Menager J, Uzan A, Dobreucq, Renault MC, Gueremy C and LeFur G (1987) Mol. Pharmacol. 31: 42–49.
5. Sprengel R, Werner P, Seeburg PH, Muhkin AG, Santi MR, Grayson DR, Guidotti A and Krueger HE (1989) J. Biol. Chem. 264: 20415–20421.

Biological Psychiatry, Volume 1. G. Racagni et al., editors.

Pharmacological, biochemical and endocrinological aspects of peripheral benzodiazepine receptors

Moshe Gavish

Rappaport Family Institute for Research in the Medical Sciences and Department of Pharmacology, Bruce Rappaport Faculty of Medicine, Technion-Israel Institute of Technology, P.O.B. 9649, 31096 Haifa, Israel

Introduction

Benzodiazepines (BZs) have anxiolytic, anticonvulsant, muscle-relaxant and amnesic properties. It has been suggested that these therapeutic effects are mediated via specific BZ receptors located in the central nervous system and coupled with γ-aminobutyric acid (GABA) receptors and chloride ion channels [1]. Another type of BZ receptor, the peripheral BZ receptors (PBR), has been identified in peripheral tissues as well as in the brain of various species [2]. PBR differ from central-type BZ receptors in their lack of coupling to GABA receptors and their ligand specificity. Central-type BZ receptors exhibit high affinity to clonazepam, but not to Ro 5-4864 (4'-chlorodiazepam) or PK 11195 (an isoquinoline carboxamide derivative). The reverse is true with regard to PBR, which exhibit high affinity to Ro 5-4864 and PK 11195, but low affinity to clonazepam.

The present report will deal with several studies on the pharmacological, biochemical and endocrinological level.

Material and Methods

Preparation of membranes and binding studies

The various organs were homogenized separately in 50 volumes of 50 mM Tris-HCl buffer, pH 7.4, using a Brinkmann Polytron (setting 10) for 15 s. The homogenate was centrifuged at 49,000 × g for 15 min. The pellet was suspended in 50 mM ice-cold Tris-HCl buffer, pH 7.4, to achieve 0.5 mg protein/ml and the mixture was used for binding assays.

The specific binding of $[^3H]$PK 11195 or $[^3H]$Ro 5-4864 was assayed as previously described [3]. The maximal numbers of receptors (B_{max}) and the equilibrium dissociation constants (K_d) were determined by Scatchard analysis of saturation curves of $[^3H]$PK 11195 or $[^3H]$Ro 5-4864 binding.

Results and Discussion

PBR in human cerebral cortex, kidney and colon

Recent studies have identified marked quantitative and qualitative differences and heterogeneity between PBR located in calf tissues and PBR located in rat tissues, with reference to their density and distribution within the brain, as well as to their binding affinity for the classical prototype PBR high-affinity BZ ligand Ro 5-4864. The main aim of this study was to compare the specific binding of [^{3}H]PK 11195 and [^{3}H]Ro 5-4864 to various human tissues, in order to elaborate whether PBR binding characteristics located in human tissues are similar to those located in calf or to those located in rat tissues. While [^{3}H]PK 11195 bound with high affinity (about 2 nM) to human cerebral cortex, kidney and colon membranes yielding B_{max} values of 255 ± 23, 1908 ± 28, and 1633 ± 98 fmol/mg protein, respectively; the specific binding of [^{3}H]Ro 5-4864, on the other hand, was barely detectable (nonspecific binding about 90% of the total binding). Furthermore, unlabeled PK 11195 was two orders of magnitude more potent than unlabeled Ro 5-4864 in displacing [^{3}H]PK 11195 specific binding from human cerebral cortex and kidney membranes. These results are in accord with those previously reported for calf tissues, but differ from those reported for rat tissues. These results may have importance for the evolution of these receptors in various species.

Preliminary studies indicate that the affinity differences were not accompanied by alterations in the molecular weight of the sites for PK 11195.

Effect of hypophysectomy and hormone treatment on the induction of PBR in female rat genital axis

A significant reduction of [^{3}H]PK 11195 specific binding was noted in the ovary (60%) within 2 days, and in the oviduct (48%) and uterus (47%) within 8 days, after hypophysectomy of rats.

Administration of 15 IU pregnant mare serum gonadotropin (PMSG) for 2 days to hypophysectomized (Hypox) rats overcame the effect of hypophysectomy and induced a significant increase in [^{3}H]PK 11195 specific binding in the ovary (4-fold), uterus (2.9-fold) and oviduct (2-fold) compared to Hypox rats. Insertion of a diethylstilbestrol (DES)-filled capsule induced a significant increase in [^{3}H]PK 11195 specific binding after 4 days' treatment in the ovary (3.4-fold), oviduct (2-fold) and uterus (3.6-fold) compared to Hypox rats. It appeared that the effect of PMSG and DES on PBR density was due to an increase in B_{max} values, while the K_d values remained unaltered. These observations suggest that the decrease in PBR density following hypophysectomy was caused at least partially by gonadotropin and estrogen deficiency. However, no significant change was observed in PBR density in the kidney following hypophysectomy.

Anholt et al. [4] reported that PBR are located in the mitochondrial outer membrane of brain and various peripheral tissues. The mitochondria are involved in the rate-limiting steps of the steroidogenic activity, which is a gonadotropin-dependent process. After hypophysectomy, there is an increase in follicular degeneration and a decrease in follicular steroidogenic capacity. Therefore, it may be suggested that the decrease in follicular steroidogenic activity and ovarian PBR after hypophysectomy reflects a general decrease in ovarian mitochondrial activity.

Modulatory action of BZs on human term placental steroidogenesis in vitro

The effect of various BZ ligands and PK 11195 on the secretion of progesterone (P_4) and estradiol-17β (E_2) from human term placental explants was studied. Exposure of placental explants to low doses (10^{-8} M) of Ro 5-4864, a BZ ligand which binds with high affinity to PBR, caused a significant ($P < 0.05$) increase in the secretion of P_4 and E_2 into the media (2.4- and 1.4-fold, respectively). On the other hand, high doses (10^{-5} M) of Ro 5-4864 caused a significant ($P < 0.05$) decrease in the secretion of P_4 and E_2 into the media. Also, exposure of explants to diazepam (10^{-7} M) and PK 11195 (10^{-6} M) caused a significant increase in P_4 and E_2 secretion into the media. In contrast, clonazepam, a BZ ligand specific for central BZ receptors, had no effect on the secretion of either steroid. The combination of diazepam (10^{-7} M) or Ro 5-4864 (10^{-8} M) with PK 11195 (10^{-6} M) did not enhance the stimulatory effects obtained with each agent alone. The effects exerted by Ro 5-4864, PK 11195, and diazepam may be mediated via PBR.

PBR density as predictor of pregnancy at in vitro fertilization

In this study we investigated the relationship between PBR density in human ovarian granulosa-lutein (G-L) cells and successful pregnancy with treatment by in vitro fertilization and embryo transfer (IVF-ET). Initially, PBR were identified in human G-L cells collected at IVF-ET. [^{3}H]PK 11195 bound to G-L cells with high affinity in a saturable manner. In women undergoing IVF-ET who conceived, the B_{max} value of [^{3}H]PK 11195 in G-L cells was 900 ± 127 fmol/mg protein, which was 80% higher ($P < 0.01$) than in women who did not conceive. This remarkable increase in PBR density could be used as a fast and convenient predictor of the chance of pregnancy with human IVF-ET treatment.

Acknowledgements

This work was supported by Grant 87-00234 from the U.S.-Israel Binational Science Foundation. We thank Miss Ruth Singer for typing the manuscript.

References

1. Tallman JF, Paul SM, Skolnick P and Gallager DW (1980) Science 207: 274–281.
2. Verma A and Snyder SH (1989) Ann. Rev. Pharmacol. Toxicol. 29: 307–322.
3. Awad M and Gavish M (1987) J. Neurochem. 49: 1407–1414.
4. Anholt RRH, Pedersen PL, De Souza EB and Snyder SH (1986) J. Biol. Chem. 261: 576–583.

Biological Psychiatry, Volume 1. G. Racagni et al., editors.

Hormone-stimulated steroidogenesis is coupled to mitochondrial benzodiazepine receptors

Vassilios Papadopoulos

Department of Anatomy and Cell Biology and Fidia-Georgetown Institute for Neurosciences, Georgetown University School of Medicine, Washington D.C., WA 20007, U.S.A.

A primary point of control in the stimulation of steroidogenesis by hormones is the cholesterol conversion to pregnenolone by the cholesterol side-chain cleavage cytochrome P-450 (P-450_{scc}) and auxiliary electron transferring proteins, enzymes localized on the inner mitochondrial membranes. This enzymatic reaction is not rate-limiting in the synthesis of steroid hormones, but the rate-limiting step is the cholesterol transport from intracellular stores to the inner mitochondrial membrane where steroid production appears to be regulated. The ultimate effect of peptide hormones such as corticotropin (ACTH) or gonadotropins on their target tissues (adrenal, testis and ovary) is an increase in the delivery of cholesterol to P-450_{scc}. In search for regulatory components of the intramitochondrial cholesterol translocation process, we recently considered that the peripheral-type or mitochondrial benzodiazepine receptor (MBR) primarily located on the outer mitochondrial membrane and abundant in steroidogenic cells, may play a role in steroidogenesis.

The addition of several MBR ligands stimulates steroid biosynthesis, in a manner related to their binding affinity, in adrenocortical [1] and Leydig cell systems [2]. Moreover, this drug effect was cycloheximide-resistant and could also be observed in isolated mitochondrial preparations [2]. Furthermore, it was verified that MBR agonists failed to stimulate P-450_{scc} directly [2]. Finally, evidence was provided that MBR activation mediates cholesterol translocation from the outer to the inner mitochondrial membrane [3]. Therefore these findings imply that very likely MBRs are operative in the mitochondrial intermembrane translocation of cholesterol, the rate-determining step in steroid biosynthesis. Moreover, the relationship between MBRs and tropic hormone-stimulated steroidogenesis is supported by studies with flunitrazepam, a MBR ligand acting as weak partial agonist with strong antagonistic activity [4].

Using adrenocortical and testicular Leydig cell lines responsive to the steroidogenic activation by adrenocorticotropin and human choriogonadotropin [1,2,4] flunitrazepam, a benzodiazepine which binds to MBR with high nanomolar affinity and which has a low intrinsic activity, inhibited the steroidogenic activity of these hormones by 30–60% [4]. Specific [^{3}H]flunitrazepam binding in both cell lines was completely displaced by a series of MBR ligands with a rank order of potency related to their MBA affinity. Moreover, these ligands could inhibit the flunitrazepam intrinsic activity on hormone-stimulated steroidogenesis, with a similar rank of potency. These findings clearly indicate that the antagonistic activity of flunitrazepam is mediated through its binding to MBR and suggest that the steroidogenic activity of tropic hormones operates via their indirect action on MBR. The molecular mechanisms involved in this intermediate interaction remain to be clarified, but appear to involve cAMP formation and cAMP-dependent phosphorylation.

It has been well documented that the hormonal stimulation of steroidogenesis is sensitive to cycloheximide inhibition. The site of cycloheximide action appears to include the step of intramitochondrial transport of cholesterol. This supports the belief that a protein with a rapid turnover rate is required for steroidogenesis stimulation by tropic hormones. From the studies reported here, it appears likely that this protein acts via a MBR mediated mechanism; this is indicated by the flunitrazepam inhibition of the intramitochondrial cholesterol transport and steroidogenesis activation elicited by tropic hormones. A number of proteins have been postulated to play such a role. Among them, the polypeptide diazepam binding inhibitor (DBI) has received some attention [5]. DBI was first characterized for its ability to displace benzodiazepines from $GABA_A$ receptors in the brain and to inhibit GABA-activated chloride channel opening [6]. Successively DBI was found to displace ligands from MBA, to be highly expressed in steroidogenic cells [7] and to activate mitochondrial steroidogenesis [5,8]. More recent studies have demonstrated that flunitrazepam antagonizes the DBI stimulation of pregnenolone biosynthesis in adrenocortical mitochondria [8]. Because the inhibitory action of flunitrazepam on both the tropic hormone and DBI stimulates mitochondrial steroidogenesis, it could be surmised that DBI mediates the hormonal activation of mitochondrial steroidogenesis acting as the endogenous modulator of MBR, through a mechanism mediated by the tropic hormone activation of cAMP biosynthesis.

Acknowledgement

I would like to thank Drs. K.E. Krueger and E. Costa for the collaboration and helpful comments during the course of this work.

References

1. Mukhin AG, Papadopoulos V, Costa E and Krueger KE (1989) Proc. Natl. Acad. Sci. U.S.A 86: 9813–9816.
2. Papadopoulos V, Mukhin AG, Costa E and Krueger KE (1990) J. Biol. Chem. 265: 3772–3772.
3. Krueger KE and Papadopoulos V (1990) J. Biol. Chem. 265: 15015–15022.
4. Papadopoulos V, Nowzari FB and Krueger KE (1991) J. Biol. Chem. 266: 3682–3687.
5. Besman MJ, Yanagibashi K, Lee TD, Kawamura M, Hall PF and Shively JE (1989) Proc. Natl. Acad. Sci. U.S.A. 86: 4897–4901.
6. Guidotti A, Forchetti CM, Corda MG, Konkel D, Bennett CD and Costa E (1983) Proc. Natl. Acad. Sci. U.S.A. 80: 3531–3533.
7. Bovolin P, Schlichting J, Miyata J, Ferrarese C, Guidotti A and Alho H (1990) Regul. Pept. 29: 267–281.
8. Papadopoulos V, Berkovich A and Krueger KE (1991) Neuropharmacology (in press).

Biological Psychiatry, Volume 1. G. Racagni et al., editors.

Molecular and functional characterization of peripheral-type benzodiazepine receptors in glial cells

Karl E. Krueger and Vassilios Papadopoulos

Fidia-Georgetown Institute for the Neurosciences and the Department of Anatomy and Cell Biology, Georgetown University School of Medicine, Washington, D.C. 20007, U.S.A.

Introduction

Peripheral-type benzodiazepine receptors have been found to be very highly expressed in steroidogenic cells and primarily associated with mitochondria. In accordance with these findings, mitochondrial benzodiazepine receptors (MBR) were also shown to mediate the rate-limiting step in steroid biosynthesis as evidenced by a stimulation in the conversion of cholesterol to pregnenolone. In light of these findings, we considered whether MBR may have a similar role in the central nervous system.

Recent studies have suggested that steroid biosynthesis occurs in the brain and that this activity is within the glial cells. Previous work has also suggested that MBR within the central nervous system appear to be abundant in glial cells, whereas these receptors are very low in neurons. These parallel observations prompted the current investigations to test whether MBR play a role in glial steroidogenesis.

Results

Two model systems chosen to characterize MBR in glia were primary glial cultures prepared from neonatal rat cerebral cortex and the C6-2B subclone of the rat glioma C6 cell line. Subcellular fractionation of both types of glial cells verified that MBR, determined by specific [^{3}H]PK 11195 binding, primarily cofractionated with the mitochondrial marker enzyme cytochrome c oxidase. The densities of MBR found on these mitochondrial fractions were 25–50 pmol/mg of protein (Table 1). In contrast, mitochondrial fractions prepared from rat brain had much lower levels (1 pmol/mg of protein). The very high abundance of MBR in glial mitochondria is characteristic of other steroidogenic cells.

Molecular characterization of the glial and brain MBR was performed by photolabeling the mitochondria with the MBR photoaffinity probe [^{3}H]PK 14105. In addition, mRNA from the glia and brain were subjected to Northern analysis probed against the cDNA for the 18-kDa MBR protein. The protein and mRNA detected by both types of analysis displayed the same molecular sizes as was found

Table 1. Dissociation constants and binding site densities for [^{3}H]PK 11195 in mitochondrial fractions derived from the indicated sources were determined by Scatchard analysis

Mitochondrial source	B_{max} (pmol/mg protein)	K_d(nM)
Brain	1.1	1.6
Primary glia	48	5.6
C6-2B	27	4.6

with rat adrenals and several other peripheral organs. These findings therefore do not indicate heterogeneity in MBR from central or peripheral tissues.

Recent studies in our laboratory have established that C6-2B cells contain the cytochrome P-450 side-cleavage enzyme which converts cholesterol to pregnenolone. Furthermore, this enzymatic activity is detectable in mitochondrial fractions from these cells. The high-affinity MBR ligands PK 11195 and Ro5-4864 at nanomolar concentrations stimulate pregnenolone synthesis by C6-2B mitochondria, and this potency correlates with their affinity for MBR as demonstrated by their abilities to compete for specific [^{3}H]PK 11195 binding (Fig. 1). In contrast, clonazepam, a benzodiazepine selective for $GABA_A$ receptors, failed to stimulate steroidogenesis.

Discussion

These findings support earlier observations that glial cells have the ability to

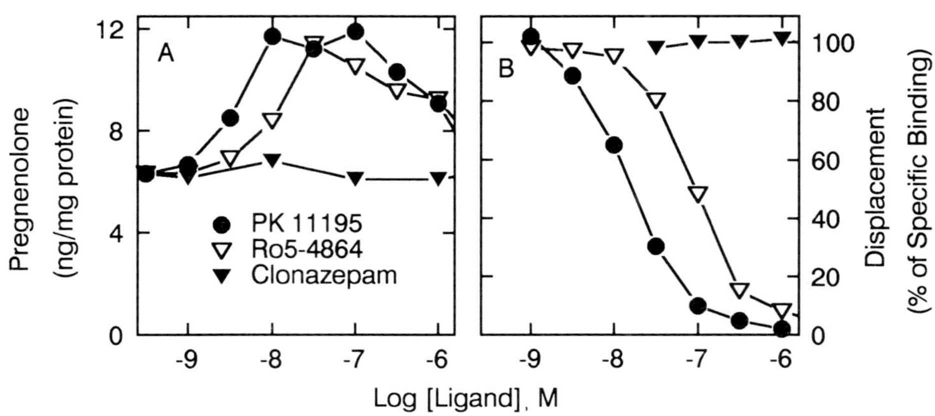

Fig. 1. MBR are coupled to pregnenolone synthesis in C6-2B glioma cells. The ligands PK 11195, Ro5-4864, and clonazepam were tested for their effects on pregnenolone formation in mitochondrial fractions from C6-2B cells (A). Mitochondria were incubated for 20 min at 37° with the indicated concentrations of ligands. Pregnenolone was then extracted and quantified by radioimmunoassay. The right panel (B) shows the ability of the ligands to compete against [^{3}H]PK 11195 specific binding (2 nM) from the mitochondrial fractions.

synthesize steroids. Furthermore, the participation of MBR in glial steroidogenesis implies that these recognition sites may contribute to the pharmacological actions of benzodiazepines by modulating this glial activity. Relevant to these aspects, other investigations have shown importance of DBI in regulating steroidogenesis mediated by its interaction with MBR.

Recent evidence has demonstrated that specific steroids modulate $GABA_A$ receptor chloride conductance in a positive or negative manner. If these specific neurosteroids are synthesized by glial cells, they could modulate $GABA_A$ receptor function. Hence, it could be hypothesized that MBR may play an indirect role in the modulation of GABAergic transmission by virtue of their participation in the steroid biosynthetic pathway. This possibility, therefore, should open a new series of investigations to determine whether anxiolytic drugs have secondary behavioral actions mediated by MBR. It is important to characterize the selective function of drug-induced stimulation of MBR in order to evaluate whether drugs, specifically acting on these mitochondrial receptors, can be used in the treatment of specific anxiety disorders.

Biological Psychiatry, Volume 1. G. Racagni et al., editors.

ω_3 (Peripheral type benzodiazepine) binding sites as in vitro and in vivo markers of brain lesions

Jesus Benavides[1], Sylvie Toulmond[1], Philippe Cornu[2] and Bernard Scatton[1]
[1]Synthélabo Recherche (LERS), Biology Department, 31 Avenue Paul Vaillant-Couturier, 92220 Bagneux; and [2]Hôpital de la Salpétrière, Department of Neurosurgery, Paris, France

It is now well recognized that macrophage invasion and astroglial activation are the almost unavoidable consequences of any kind of experimental or human brain lesion. Macrophages and astrocytes are highly enriched in the so-called peripheral type benzodiazepine binding sites (ω_3 sites according to a novel nomenclature). Although the functional relevance of ω_3 sites has long remained elusive, recent studies have suggested that they may be involved in the immune response and in the control of mitochondrial steps of steroid biosynthesis. These effects are totally unrelated to GABAergic neurotransmission. Indeed, ω_3 sites are associated with a 17 kDa polypeptide which is structurally and functionally unrelated to the α-subunits of the $GABA_A$ receptor complex to which central ω_{1-2} (benzodiazepine) receptors are associated.

The presence of high ω_3 site densities in reactive macrophages and astrocytes provides an explanation for the dramatic increase in their density in experimental brain lesions. Elevated binding densities have been observed in the brain following middle cerebral artery occlusion in cat, rat and mouse, as well as in stroke-prone spontaneously hypertensive rats. Focal increases in this autoradiographic marker are also seen in the brain parenchyma after local or systemic administration of excitotoxic compounds or fluid percussion lesions (a model of brain trauma) in the rat. In every case, a good spatial correspondence has been observed between the histologically defined limits of the ischaemic lesion and the autoradiographic distribution of ω_3 sites. Autoradiographic studies using a photoaffinity ω_3 site radioligand have clearly demonstrated the association of these sites with reactive astrocytes and macrophages supporting the use of ω_3 sites as an index of the glial reaction [1].

The good quantitative correspondence observed, in middle cerebral artery occluded mice, between the extent of brain damage and the increase in ω_3 site densities (as measured in cortical homogenates by a filtration technique) led us to use this marker to quantify the effects of neuroprotective agents in this focal ischaemia model. These studies demonstrated that the reduction of middle cerebral artery occlusion induced-increase in ω_3 site densities in cortical homogenates faithfully reflects the neuroprotective effects as quantified by the histological measurement of the infarcted volume. The easy quantification of ω_3 site densities allowed us to compare in the same study a large series of potential anti-ischaemic agents acting through different mechanisms and to demonstrate that NMDA antagonists constitute the most promising approach for neuroprotection in irreversible focal ischaemia [2].

The question arises as to the mechanisms leading to the increase in ω_3 site densities in all these experimental brain injury models. We have observed that the local injection of interleukin-1 (IL-1), tumor necrosis factor-α (TNF-α) or LPS (a bacterial wall lipopolysaccharide inducing IL-1 and TNF-α release in cultured glial cells) into the brain resulted in a local increase in ω_3 site densities with no change in the density of neuronal markers; the increase in ω_3 site densities reflected the accumulation of macrophages and activated astrocytes around the injection site. Thus, increases in ω_3 site densities following brain lesions may result from the operation of a sequential mechanism involving activation of the microglia, release of IL-1 and TNF-α and subsequent astroglial reaction [3].

The density of cerebral ω_3 sites has also been found to be elevated in various types of human neuropathological processes such as brain infarction, multiple sclerosis, Huntington's chorea and Parkinson's disease.

Tumoral cells are also endowed with high ω_3 site densities. In autoradiographic studies, we have observed up to 12-fold increases in these binding sites in high grade astrocytoma and glioblastoma specimens, whereas low grade gliomas (astrocytomas) or meningiomas exhibited only moderate increases (2 to 3-fold). Up to 20-fold increases in local ω_3 site densities were quantified by autoradiography in brain metastases from lung and kidney origin or in brain melanoma metastasis. As in experimental brain lesions, there exists a good correspondence between the extent of the lesion and the increase in the density of this biochemical marker [4].

These observations prompted us and others to propose the use of positron or γ-ray emitting ω_3 site radioligands for the in vivo imaging of human brain lesions. Despite early unsuccessful attempts due to the use of ^{11}C-Ro5 4864 (a benzodiazepine derivative with low affinity for human ω_3 sites) further studies using ^{11}C-PK 11195 have demonstrated the feasibility of this tomographic approach [5]. Indeed, a 2-fold accumulation of this marker has been observed in high grade glioblastomas as compared with the normal parenchyma. Moreover, we have recently demonstrated that this preferential labelling was partially displaced by i.v. administration of cold PK 11195. These results give further support to the applicability of ω_3 site radioligands for the clinical investigation of ischaemic, autoimmune, traumatic or tumoral neuropathological processes. However, ^{11}C-PK 11195 has a poor brain penetration and an in vivo selectivity much lower than that predicted from in vitro studies in human brain specimens or ex vivo in the rodent. Thus, new ω_3 ligands with a lower in vivo non specific binding are needed to render this tomographic approach entirely satisfactory.

References

1. Benavides J, Capdeville C, Dauphin F, Dubois A, Duverger D, Fage D, Gotti B, MacKenzie ET and Scatton B (1990) Brain Res. 522: 275–289.

2. Gotti B, Benavides J, MacKenzie ET and Scatton B (1990) Brain Res. 522: 290–307.
3. Bourdiol F, Toulmond S, Serrano A, Benavides J and Scatton B (1990) Brain Res. 543: 194–200.
4. Benavides J, Cornu PH, Dennis T, Dubois A, Hauw JJ, MacKenzie ET, Sazdovitch V and Scatton B (1988) Ann. Neurol. 24: 708–712.
5. Junck LMD, Olson JMM, Ciliax BJ, Koeppe RA, Watkins GL, Douglas MJ, McKeever PE, Wieland DM, Kilbourn MR, Starosta-Rubinstein S, Mancini WR, Kuhl DE, Greenber HS and Young AB (1989) Ann. Neurol. 26: 752–758.

Biological Psychiatry, Volume 1. G. Racagni et al., editors.

Lymphocyte peripheral-type benzodiazepine receptors in neuropsychiatric diseases

Luigi Ravizza[1], Paola Rocca[1] and Patrizia Ferrero[2]
[1]Department of Psychiatry; and [2]Department of Neurology, University of Turin, Via Cherasco 11, 10126 Turin, Italy

Diagnostic identification of psychiatric patients according to biological markers has been a constant goal but has met with limited success. A relatively unexplored parameter is the peripheral-type benzodiazepine receptor (pBDZr) located in blood elements. BDZ are well established drugs in the treatment of certain forms of pathological anxiety. BDZ act at specific high-affinity recognition sites in the brain, the central-type BDZ receptors, that are located in a subunit of the GABAa receptor (cBDZr) [1,2]. It is highly possible that abnormalities of cBDZr may underline anxiety disorders, but the study of these receptors in man is difficult. Direct imaging of receptors by emission tomography is promising, but the method is not yet perfect. The potential connections between pBDZr and the central BDZ GABA-mediated activities are far from clear. In vitro GABA does not alter the binding affinity or density of pBDZr and neither do chloride ions. However, systemic administration of drugs with known affinity for the various components of the GABAa receptor has been shown to alter the density of pBDZr in both peripheral tissues and brain. Ligands that can bind to pBDZr with high affinity lack anxiolytic effects but have been reported to induce convulsions and exhibit proconflict actions. Moreover, alterations in pBDZr have been described in several stress paradigms in animals and also in man [3,4].

Presence of pBDZr on PBMC

The density and affinity of pBDZr on peripheral blood mononuclear cells (PBMC) can be quantified in both cells and crude membrane preparations by mean of the binding of ^{3}H-PK11195 [5,6]. Porphyrins, that bind selectively to pBDZr located in mitochondria, consistently inhibit binding of ^{3}H-PK11195 to PBMC membranes, suggesting that the receptor subcellular localization in these cells includes the mitochondrial compartment. PBMC consist of a heterogeneous mixture of lymphocytes with a lower proportion of monocytes. The binding of ^{3}H-PK11195 to each of these cell types and subtypes was investigated in order to determine the localization of pBDZr (Table 1). pBDZr were demonstrated in nearly every cell that we studied although an example was found on a leukemic T-cell-derived cell line (Jurkat) that appears to lack these receptors. pBDZr are not randomly distributed on PBMC: monocytes bear approximately 700,000 sites per cell while the density for lymphocytes falls to approximately 250,000 sites per cell. pBDZr accommodate not only widely prescribed anxiolytic BDZ, such as diazepam, but also endogenous anxiogenic ligands such as DBI or its metabolites [7]. In an attempt to determine if PBMC contain DBI, we used a specific radioimmunoassay which allowed us to detect a diffuse DBI-LI in acidic extracts prepared from these cells. Significant differences in DBI-LI content were observed among the individual cell types. The highest content of immunoreactive DBI was detectable in monocyte extracts while the lowest was in those of T-cells (5-fold less). A role for pBDZr as a target for immunomodulatory activities is worthy of consideration, but nothing is known about the intracellular mechanism(s) implicated in these effects [8]. The distinctly different DBI-LI distribution in PBMC shows an interesting correlation with their abundance in pBDZr, thereby suggesting these two signals might share some physiological interaction in these cells. The recent observation that a DBI peptide metabolite like certain BDZ modulates the production of cytokines by murine macrophages and human monocytes may support this hypothesis [9]. However, as no immunological correlates have hitherto been established for the receptors located in lymphocytes, the physiological significance for the presence of DBI-LI in these cell types remains unknown and a matter of speculation.

Changes of pBDZR in PBMC in pathological anxiety

^{3}H-PK11195 was used to study pBDZr characteristics in PBMC membranes prepared from a relatively large population of patients with subtypes of anxiety disorders, other neuropsychiatric diseases and normal controls. pBDZr were significantly reduced in subgroups with generalized anxiety and obsessive-compulsive disorders (GAD and OCD). Conversely no difference was observed in the other groups and particularly in the one with panic disorder (DAP) (Table 2).

Table 1. Distribution of peripheral benzodiazepine receptors and BDI-LI content in different populations of human peripheral mononuclear cells

Cell type	^{3}H-PK11195 specific binding		DBI-LI
	B_{max} (fmol/10^{6} cells)	K_d (nM)	fmol/10^{6} cells
Monocytes	1186 ± 15.0	6.9 ± 1.0	1456 ± 43
B-lymphocytes	534 ± 11.0	5.3 ± 1.0	593 ± 30
Large granular lymphocytes	506 ± 8.0	4.1 ± 1.0	535 ± 28
T-lymphocytes			
Total T-cells	388 ± 5.2	7.8 ± 0.8	275 ± 10
T-helper/inducer	372 ± 7.0	4.7 ± 0.7	260 ± 30
T-cytotoxic/suppressor	340 ± 15.0	8.3 ± 1.3	294 ± 10

The data shown are mean ± S.E.M. of 3–4 independent determinations.

Table 2. Specific binding of ^{3}H-PK11195 on lymphocyte membranes of controls and neuropsychiatric patients

Groups	No.	Age	B_{max} (pmol/ mg prot)	K_d (nM)
Controls	40	43.5 ± 2.8	10.0 ± 0.5	9.8 ± 0.6
GAD	15	41.1 ± 4.3	5.7 ± 0.4[a]	10.3 ± 0.6
DAP	8	31.8 ± 2.2	9.4 ± 0.5	10.6 ± 0.9
OCD	16	41.2 ± 3.0	7.0 ± 0.8[a]	11.2 ± 1.1
Alzheimer's disease	10	65.1 ± 2.2	9.8 ± 0.6	9.9 ± 0.6
Parkinson's disease	10	64.6 ± 2.8	10.7 ± 0.8	9.3 ± 0.5
Alcoholism	10	44.8 ± 4.3	9.1 ± 0.8	10.1 ± 1.0
Epilepsy	10	45.8 ± 7.8	9.0 ± 1.5	9.5 ± 0.4

[a]$P > 0.01$ if compared with controls and all the other disease groups; the data shown are mean ± S.E.M. of 3–4 independent determinations.

Interestingly, when most of the patients were examined for the characteristics of lymphocyte muscarinic receptors only a subgroup with Alzheimer's disease showed a significantly reduced density of these receptors [10]. This observation suggests that the biochemical abnormality reported in OCD and GAD subgroups might be in some way specific for pBDZr. The present results clearly confirm earlier observations of reduced pBDZr in distinct blood elements from GAD patients [5,11]. Moreover, the possibility that alterations in lymphocyte pBDZr are highly associated with GAD and even distinguish certain forms of pathological anxiety should be considered. Our data also reveal that some differences in binding profile may exist among patients with OCD. Current concepts suggest the separation of the syndrome of panic disorder from other forms of pathological anxiety [12]. Furthermore, recent investigations underline the possibility that OCD may represent clinical heterogeneity [13]. The lack of pBDZr abnormality in DAP may be ascribed to the absence of anxious symptoms during baseline conditions (blood samples were never taken during a panic attack). Within the OCD series, a normal number of pBDZr was observed in a subgroup of subjects who showed an episodic course of illness, less severe symptoms of compulsions and anxiety, while a significant reduction in binding capacity was observed in a subgroup which presented chronic clinical course and more severe anxiety.

Effect of chronic BDZ treatment on pBDZr in anxious patients

There is limited information concerning the effect of treatment with anxiolytic BDZ on pBDZr. Chronic administration of diazepam to experimental animals seems to induce an up-regulation of these sites [14]. Studies in man have been controversial, namely, an up-regulation was reported by Weizman et al. [11] in platelets from GAD patients while no changes were observed by Ferrarese et al. [5]

in lymphocytes from either GAD or normal subjects. However, both these investigators clearly demonstrated that diazepam treatment reversed the reduction in pBDZr number associated with GAD. We carried out a long-term treatment (up to 6 months) with 2'-chloro-desmethyldiazepam in 13 GAD patients and found that their clinical recovery was associated with normal pBDZr density in lymphocytes. Nonetheless, no up-regulatory effect on pBDZr was apparent for this drug either during treatment to the patients or after 1 month withdrawal. Furthermore, there was no change in pBDZr in 8 additional patients with DAP who were under similar therapy. Although serum levels of 2'-chloro-desmethyldiazepam were not determined, it seems reasonable to assume that at the dosages used (3–6 mg/day) they should be much below the drug concentration required to bind to lymphocyte pBDZr (K_i 2.8 μM). Additionally, in few healthy volunteers who agreed to receive an acute higher dose of the drug (5 mg i.v.), we did not observe any change in their lymphocyte pBDZr. The receptor density decline associated with GAD has been tentatively explained as a down-regulation phenomena induced by an overproduction of DBI or its metabolites which allosterically modulate the GABAa receptors [5]. Perhaps BDZ administration to the patients may act in reversing this effect. We recently described a significant reduction of pBDZr in PBMC from patients with hepatic encephalopathy. Very high levels of DBI were found in spinal fluid of these patients, which may reveal the abnormal GABAergic activity generally associated to the disorder [15].

Conclusion

Our data support the view that certain forms of pathological anxiety are associated with profound alterations of pBDZr. ^{3}H-PK11195 binding to PBMC seems therefore a useful addition to the few biological markers available for the study of anxiety disorders in humans. Moreover, the normalization of the binding density in some anxious patients in response to BDZ treatment suggests that it might represent a state dependent marker of the disease. Possible explanations for the reported change in pBDZr include an overproduction of endogenous anxiogenic compounds in affected patients, the most plausible being DBI or its metabolite. The postulated DBI effect should be systemic, merely because pBDZr alterations in the patients are not restricted to PBMC but also occur in platelets. Although no measures are available for anxious subjects, in normal individuals levels of DBI-Li in plasma (1 pmol/ml) are much lower than those effective to bind to pBDZr (K_i 4 μM). Hence, the possibility that DBI may act through modulation of other biological substances should be considered. Furthermore, in view of the finding that an anxiogenic DBI metabolite seems to affect particular immunologic parameters on monocytes [9], it appears necessary to investigate the impact of these responses in isolated cells from patients with abnormal pBDZr activity.

References

1. Olsen R and Venter C (1986) Benzodiazepine/GABA Receptors and Chloride Channels: Structural and Functional Properties. A.R. Liss, New York.
2. Prichett DB, Southeimer H, Shiver BD, Ymer S, Kettenmann H, Schofield PR and Seeburg PH (1989) Nature 338: 582–585.
3. Saano V, Rago L and Raty M (1989) Pharmacol. Ther. 41: 503–514.
4. Snyder SH, Mcenery MW and Verma A (1990) Neurochem. Res. 15: 119–123.
5. Ferrarese C, Apollonio I, Frigo M, Perego M, Piolti R, Trabucchi M and Frattola L (1990) Acta Psychiatr. Scand. 82: 169–173.
6. Ferrero P, Rocca P, Gualerzi A, Benna P, Enrichens F, Mao P, Olivero G, Ravizza L and Bergamasco B (1991) J. Neurol. Sci. 102: 209–219.
7. Guidotti A, Berkovich A, Ferrarese C, Santi MR and Costa E (1988) In: Sauvanet J, Langer SZ and Morselli PL (eds.) Imidasopyridine in Sleep Disorders. Raven Press, New York, pp. 25–28.
8. Zavala F, Tuapin V and Descamps-Latscha B (1990) J. Pharmacol. Exp. Ther. 255: 442–450.
9. Tuapin V, Herbelin A, Descamps–Latscha B and Zavala F (1991) Lymphokine Res. (in press).
10. Ferrero P, Rocca P, Eva C, Benna P, Rebaudengo N, Ravizza L, Genazzani E and Bergamasco B (1991) Brain (in press).
11. Weizman R, Tanne Z, Granek M, Karp L, Golomb M, Tyano S and Gavish M (1987) Eur. J. Pharmacol. 138: 289–292.
12. Klein DF (1984) Psychopharmacologia 5: 397–408.
13. Rasmussen SA and Tsuang MT (1986) Am. J. Psychiatry 143: 317–322.
14. Fares F, Weizman A, Pick CG, Yanai J and Gavish M (1990) Brain Res. 506: 115–119.
15. Rothestein JD, McKhann G, Guarnieri P, Barbaccia ML, Guidotti A and Costa E (1989) Ann. Neurol. 26: 57–62.

Biological Psychiatry, Volume 1. G. Racagni et al., editors.

Neuropharmacology of benzodiazepines in aging

Benedetto Vitiello and Trey Sunderland

Unit on Geriatric Psychopharmacology, Laboratory of Clinical Sciences, National Institute of Mental Health, Bethesda, Maryland, U.S.A.

The elderly are major consumers of benzodiazepines. Of all the benzodiazepines prescriptions, 26% are for patients above 65 years of age [1]. A third of all the long-term users of benzodiazepines, i.e., regular users for more than 1 year, are elderly [2]. A community survey has indicated that the use of benzodiazepines increases with age, particularly in women, and that it is more difficult for the elderly to discontinue chronic use of these drugs [3]. This practice contrasts with reports of decreased prevalence of anxiety disorders with aging [4].

From a pharmacological point of view, the elderly are more sensitive to the effects of benzodiazepines, as assessed by clinical, neuropsychological and biochemical measures. Clinically, an age-related increase in the incidence of adverse reactions following different doses of flurazepam has been well known [5]. Physicians, who use benzodiazepines for sedation prior to gastrointestinal endoscopy, have pointed out that the dose of diazepam or midazolam required for adequate sedation progressively declines with age, reaching a dose, in patients above 70 years, which is up to three times less than in a 30-year-old [6]. Neuropsychological tests have confirmed the effects of benzodiazepines on memory. A single dose of diazepam 2.5 mg p.o. significantly disrupts anterograde memory in old, but not in young subjects [7]. Also, the development of tolerance to the sedative effects of benzodiazepines occurs more slowly in the elderly [8]. From a biochemical point of view, the elderly showed a greater drop in plasma cortisol following diazepam [9].

This increased sensitivity of the elderly to benzodiazepines has been in part explained by the well known pharmacokinetic differences which occur with aging. In particular, the reduced hepatic microsomal oxidation significantly prolongs the half-life of the compounds which are metabolized through hydroxylation, such as diazepam and flurazepam. There is a direct correlation between half-life of diazepam and age [10]. This mechanism, however, does not explain the increased sensitivity of the elderly to benzodiazepines which are not hydroxylated and whose half-life does not increase with age, such as nitrazepam [11]. The decreased binding of benzodiazepines to plasma proteins in the elderly, with a consequent increase in the free unbound drug levels, can in part explain this finding [12,13]. It seems, however, that the increased sensitivity of the elderly to benzodiazepines cannot be entirely ascribed to pharmacokinetic differences and that pharmacodynamic effects, at the level of the receptor or, possibly, of the second messenger, have to be considered.

As an example, changes in the GABAergic system in aging may account for the increased sensitivity to benzodiazepines. The GABA modulation of the benzodiazepine receptors was found to be intact in older rats [14]. Unchanged cerebellar benzodiazepine receptor binding, but increased GABA receptor binding were found in mice [15]. The cortical GABA receptor binding was decreased in rats when measured during the daytime, but unchanged when measured at night [16]. In humans, central GABA levels are decreased or unchanged [17,18] and the central levels of glutamic acid decarboxylase, the GABA synthetic enzyme, decrease with age [19]. Similarly, GABA receptor levels remain normal or decrease [18,20]. Thus, the research data so far available do not allow a satisfactory explanation of the increased sensitivity to benzodiazepines with age and further research is needed.

In summary, there is evidence that the elderly are more sensitive to the effects of benzodiazepines. This phenomenon is not specific or limited to these drugs, since the elderly are well known to display increased sensitivity to several other psychotropics, including anticholinergics and antidopaminergics. Pharmacokinetic changes in aging cannot completely account for these findings. Pharmacodynamic changes must be involved, but the exact biochemical mechanisms are still unclear.

References

1. National Disease and Therapeutic Index (1986) Ambler, NDTI, PA.
2. Mellinger GD et al. (1984) J. Am. Med. Assoc. 251: 375–379.
3. Dunbar GC et al. (1989) Br. J. Psychiatry 155: 836–841.
4. Regier DA et al. (1990) J. Psychiatr. Res. 24: 3–14.
5. Greenblatt DJ et al. (1977) Clin. Pharmacol. Ther. 21: 355–361.
6. Scholer SC et al. (1990) J. Clin. Gastroenterol. 12: 145–147.
7. Pomara N et al. (1989) Psychopharmacol. Bull. 25: 144–148.
8. Kroboth PD et al. (1990) Psychopharmacology 100: 477–484.
9. Pomara N (1991) Biol. Psychiatry 29: 121A.
10. Klotz V et al. (1975) J. Clin. Invest. 55: 347–359.
11. Castleden CM et al. (1977) Br. Med. J. 1: 10–12.
12. Macklon AF et al. (1980) Clin. Sci. 59: 479–483.
13. Fisch HU et al. (1990) Eur. J. Clin. Pharmacol. 38: 229–232.
14. Kochman RI et al. (1986) Neurobiol. Aging 7: 363–365.
15. Ito Y et al. (1988) Brain Res. Bull. 21: 251–255.
16. Niles LP et al. (1988) Prog. Neuro-Psychopharmacol. Biol. Psychiatry 12: 337–344.
17. McGeer EG, McGeer PL (1991) In: Terry RD and Gershon S (eds.) Neurobiology of Aging, Vol. 3. Raven Press, New York, pp. 389–403.
18. Allen SJ et al. (1983) J. Neurochem. 41: 256–265.
19. McGeer EG (1981) Prog. Neuropharmacol. 5: 435–445.
20. Komiskey HL et al. (1988) Brain Res. 458: 37–44.

Biological Psychiatry, Volume 1. G. Racagni et al., editors.

Relationship between anxiety and medical disorders

Roger G. Kathol, Tina Wald, Russell Noyes and Brendan Carroll
Departments of Internal Medicine and Psychiatry, University of Iowa Hospitals and Clinics, Iowa City, IA 52242, U.S.A.

Introduction

Although anxiety is mainly a normal psychological reaction to life events, anxiety symptoms can become pronounced or occur in the absence of a precipitating event and thus interfere with the ability to perform in an optimal manner. This is when a patient is considered to have an anxiety disorder. Several etiologies appear to be related to the development of anxiety symptoms. Some patients develop anxiety de novo. These patients are considered to have a *primary* anxiety disorder. Anxiety symptoms can also occur in conjunction with pre-existing psychiatric or medical illness, i.e. *secondary* anxiety disorder. Some of the psychiatric syndromes which have a high incidence of anxiety associated with them include: alcoholism, depression, somatization disorder and cluster B personality disorders.

Anxiety is one of the leading psychiatric symptoms which requires attention in the primary care setting. There are several ways in which medical illness can influence the development of anxiety symptoms. First, anxiety can occur in response to the distress associated with being told about a medical illness or the distress of the illness itself. Second, anxiety can appear to be present due to the overlap of symptoms between the medical illness and those used to define the anxiety syndrome, i.e. pseudoanxiety. Third, anxiety can occur in response to the CNS effects of the disease itself. Each of these potential causes of anxiety in the medical setting will be discussed in turn.

Association of anxiety with medical illness

Reaction to stress

Those with medical illness who manifest symptoms compatible with an anxiety disorder are relatively few. In a recent study of 128 patients admitted for acute treatment of a medical illness, only 6 (5%) met criteria for generalized anxiety disorder, panic disorder or adjustment disorder with anxious mood [1]. In fact, many more patients on initial admission to the hospital are found to have a syndrome compatible with depression (33%) rather than anxiety although even these depressive symptoms are of relatively short duration and are contributed to substantially by symptoms which could also be attributed to the medical illness.

Pseudoanxiety

In patients with some medical diagnoses such as thyrotoxicosis, hypoglycemia, paroxysmal atrial tachycardia and coronary artery disease, "anxiety" symptoms could be related to the physiologic changes associated with the medical illness. For instance, Beitman et al. [2] has documented that 59% of patients with atypical angina pectoris and 53% with typical angina pectoris will have symptoms compatible with a primary anxiety disorder. Although some of these patients may indeed have an anxiety disorder, the fact remains that angina can cause symptoms of apprehension, tachycardia, palpitations, substernal pressure and/or chest pain, flushing, sweating, shortness of breath and feelings of impending doom. All of these symptoms could be attributed to the medical illness (cardiac ischemia) or primary anxiety disorder. The importance of such a distinction is that for patients with angina pectoris the primary treatment would be anti-anginal agents rather than anti-anxiety agents. Certainly a mistake in this area could be devastating to the ultimate outcome in the patient.

Anxiety related to physiologic effects on the central nervous system

Some medical illnesses could, due to their effect on the central nervous system, induce symptoms of anxiety disorder. Examples include temporal lobe epilepsy, caffeine intoxication, and pheochromocytoma. These disorders suggest that structural CNS changes, exogenous agents and endogenous neurotransmitter alteration can lead to symptoms of anxiety disorder. In these situations the treatment of the anxiety symptoms would be to treat the underlying medical illness. If these can be treated effectively, the anxiety symptoms should resolve as structural, toxic, or metabolic effects resolve.

Diagnosing anxiety in medical patients

Because anxiety disorder is a syndrome which can have a variety of etiologies, the evaluation of a patient with anxiety symptoms is a stepwise process. First, anxiety symptoms which are sufficiently severe to impair the patient's ability to function and are persistent must be identified. Second, demographic and clinical variables associated with *primary* anxiety disorders should be assessed. These include: age of onset before 30 years; history of episodic anxiety; family history of anxiety or alcoholism; typical syndrome presentation; and a history of appropriate response to anti-anxiety agents. When this is the case, primary anxiety disorder is more likely to be the principle etiology of the patient's symptoms.

When the presentation is not typical for primary anxiety disorder, an alternative etiology should be considered and a more aggressive evaluation performed to rule out other causes of the anxiety symptoms. Of course, other psychiatric illnesses should be excluded, such as depression, substance dependence, somatization disorder and cluster B personality disorder. As importantly, medical illness should be excluded as a cause. For instance, if anxiety occurs for the first time in a 60-year old female with no personal or family history of psychiatric illness, a medical etiology is the principle consideration, not primary anxiety disorder. The most common medical conditions which cause anxiety symptoms include thyrotoxicosis, hypoglycemia, pheochromocytoma, caffeine intoxication, paroxysmal atrial tachycardia, coronary artery disease and temporal lobe epilepsy. The workup of an atypical presentation of anxiety should include a medical history, a physical examination and a basic laboratory examination. When abnormalities are identified, the evaluation should be pursued until an adequate explanation for the abnormalities has been identified.

Treatment of anxiety associated with medical illness

A recent treatment study performed at the University of Iowa in 30 cancer patients (15 on alprazolam, 15 on placebo) suggests that the natural history of anxiety symptoms presumably associated to the stress of the illness is one of resolution in a relatively short period of time whether on active medication or placebo, and that anxiety does not return. This study suggests that the medical practitioner in the primary care setting should address the problem of anxiety but regardless of the therapeutic approach taken, symptoms are likely to resolve [3]. If anti-anxiety agents are considered necessary, they should be prescribed for 1–4 weeks since resolution of symptoms is the rule rather than the exception. Of course, if anxiety symptoms are related to physiologic effects of the underlying illness, then treatment for the illness is necessary.

Conclusion

Anxiety symptoms are relatively frequent in the primary care setting. Anxiety disorders, however, which impair functional ability or persist over time, are relatively uncommon. When anxiety disorder is present, it is necessary to determine whether the symptoms are primary or related to the stress of having a medical illness, the overlap of symptoms with the medical illness, or physiologic effects of the illness on the central nervous system. In the latter two situations, treatment of the anxiety symptoms would include treatment of the primary medical illness. When anxiety is associated with the stress of having a medical illness, the anxiety has a natural history of resolution over 1 week even when given placebo. In patients in whom anxiety persists, a 1–4 week course of antianxiety agents can be considered.

References

1. Kathol RG, Wenzel R, Wenzel A and Candill M (1991) Natural history of symptoms of anxiety and depression after admission to the hospital (submitted).
2. Beitman BD, Basha I, Flaker G, DeRosear L, Mukerji V, Trombka L and Katon W (1987) Arch. Int. Med. 147: 1548–1552.
3. Wald T, Kathol RG, Noyes R and Carroll B (1991) Alprazolam and placebo trial for anxiety associated with cancer (submitted).

Biological Psychiatry, Volume 1. G. Racagni et al., editors.

Differential diagnosis of anxiety in later life

Gabe J. Maletta

Anxiety encompasses a variety of disparate psychiatric disorders. They are also known as "primary anxiety states" and include phobic disorders, panic, generalized anxiety, obsessive compulsive disorder, adjustment reactions and post-traumatic stress disorder. One reason for this disparity is because patients with these disorders seem to exhibit the same constellation of signs and symptoms which describe anxiety. These signs and symptoms may be organized into three categories: motor tension, autonomic hyperactivity, and vigilance and scanning. However, anxiety in the elderly is more complex, with anxiety-like symptoms varying in frequency depending on the body systems involved. Also, the symptoms seem to gather into different clusters depending on the problem, i.e. some conditions produce trembling, tachycardia or hyperexcitability, while others produce dread, bewilderment, weakness, sweating or respiratory distress.

Besides primary anxiety, non-primary causes of the signs and symptoms of anxiety also exist. This is particularly true in the elderly. These causes are described as "secondary anxiety states" because the signs and symptoms occur as part of the symptom complex of other conditions, both psychiatric and general medical. The presentation of these signs and symptoms is no different than when they are caused by primary psychiatric disorders, making the search for the principle cause of the anxiety a complex affair.

Anxiety in the elderly is often secondary to an organic condition. The elderly are more likely then the young to have significant health problems, especially chronic multi-system diseases. The abrupt onset of new anxiety symptoms in a patient over the age of 45 should always raise suspicion of a medical etiology, especially if the condition remains resistant to treatment. It is particularly important to find an etiology for the signs and symptoms of anxiety in an elderly patient because medical illnesses with associated anxiety often may be mistaken for primary anxiety disorders. Also in these patients a combination of primary anxiety and a secondary medical cause of anxiety may be coexistent.

Anxiety may be a herald for some occult diseases, e.g. hyperthyroidism, pheochromocytoma, silent MI, diabetic ketoacidosis, VIPomas, mitral valve prolapse and perhaps sleep apnea. Patients with carcinoma, particularly of the pancreas or parathyroid gland, may present initially with anxiety and depression. The changes may develop rapidly, as with parathyroid tumor, or gradually, as with pancreatic cancer.

Anxiety signs and symptoms accompany many diseases, especially chronic illness. This is also called medical co-morbidity. Clinical disorders causing concomitant anxiety symptoms, sometimes even panic disorder, can develop in virtually every body system. Common problems include:

1. *cardiovascular/respiratory* disorders, e.g. asthma, arrhythmias, COPD, pulmonary embolus;
2. *endocrine and metabolic* disorders, e.g. hyperthyroidism and sometimes hypothyroidism, Cushing's syndrome, hypoglycemia, vitamin B_{12} deficiency and other vitamin deficiencies;
3. *neurologic* disorders, e.g. epilepsy, normal pressure hydrocephalus, Parkinson's disease, multiple sclerosis, Huntington's disease and temporal lobe syndrome.

Anxiety may be an important part of some clinical syndromes, e.g. delirium or dementia (especially in the early stages). Anxiety is often seen in a sub-category of demented patients, i.e. those who are prone to agitated or assaultive behavior.

Anxiety symptoms, vague bodily complaints and hypochondriasis are frequently associated, especially in elderly patients. However, one research study of 300 patients over 65 years showed that almost one-half of those complaining of GI symptoms had a physical etiology.

Elderly patients use a significant amount of medication to treat their multiple medical illnesses. Anxiety signs and symptoms as side-effects of medication treatment, both psychotherapeutic and other general medical medications, may occur secondary to either ongoing dosing or to the abrupt withdrawal of chronically used medications.

Ongoing dosing

1. Psychotherapeutic medications, i.e. benzodiazepines, neuroleptics and antidepressants can cause anxiety as a side-effect, especially those with high anticholinergic activity. "Paradoxical anxiety" may appear shortly after placing an already anxious patient on a benzodiazepine and disappears after the drug is discontinued.
2. General medical drugs, e.g. steroids, thyroid medication, sympathomimetics, theophylline.
3. Over-the-counter medications, e.g. cold remedies, eye-drops, aspirin, alerting agents, sleep-aides, gastrointestinal preparations.
4. Social drugs, e.g. coffee, chocolate, cola, cigarettes, tea.

Withdrawal

A particular area of concern in the elderly are the benzodiazepines and sedative hypnotic medications. These may be associated with "rebound anxiety" and insomnia when abruptly discontinued after chronic use.

Narcotics and alcohol also can cause rebound anxiety, as can many illicit drugs including marijuana, cocaine and hallucinogens, including PCP. Abrupt discontinuation of relatively limited alcohol consumption, especially in an elderly patient, can cause anxiety. There are often subsyndromal signs and symptoms of anxiety related to the abrupt decrease in alcohol levels after a bout of heavy drinking. Alcohol use and abrupt withdrawal in the elderly is a relatively unexplored area in terms of initiation or exacerbation of anxiety signs and symptoms.

Most of the common organic causes of anxiety may be ruled out with a comprehensive history including medication history, physical examination and laboratory studies (routine as well as EKG and thyroid function studies, including TSH). Some researchers have reported "frequently finding abnormal liver function tests in elderly anxious patients who secretly drink too much" as a major cause of anxiety in the elderly.

Chronic pain is an important cause of anxiety in the elderly, as is chronic insomnia. It is often difficult to determine in these patients whether the anxiety observed is a primary psychiatric problem, or whether it is secondary to the pain or insomnia, or a combination of both.

Psychosocial stressors such as negative life events may cause anxiety in elderly patients. This is a particularly confusing area because the anxiety may be secondary to the negative life event itself and therefore potentially time-limited; or there may be a failure to adapt to the event, which may exacerbate an existing primary anxiety disorder or even precipitate one. Negative life events with aging include the death of a spouse or other loved one, serious illness in a family member, institutionalization of oneself or a loved one, or victimization by crime.

Anxiety also may be produced in the elderly by increased isolation either environmentally (which includes prolonged bed rest), or pathophysiologically with increasing sensory impairment (hearing and vision loss, including problems with cataracts). Anxiety signs and symptoms may also be caused by fear of abandonment, or of dying, as well as fear of impending death in those patients with a terminal illness. There is an apparent increased vulnerability to morbidity and mortality in elderly patients resulting from psychosocial stress.

Anxiety may be a component in patients with co-morbid psychiatric problems which include a variety of psychiatric states, both psychotic and non-psychotic. A common and important psychiatric co-morbidity situation in the elderly is anxiety and major depression, which causes "clinical overlap" in terms of patient presentation, often a major source of confusion. There is some evidence of genetic as well as clinical differences between patients with pure depression and those with mixed anxiety and depression. Also, when examining co-morbidity data in geriatric patients, it has been reported that 38% presented with mixed anxiety and depression whereas only 2% presented with pure anxiety. Besides anxiety and depression, other common psychiatric co-morbid states involving anxiety in the non-psychotic category include anxiety and dysthymia, anxiety and personality disorders, anxiety and bi-polar disease, and anxiety and alcoholism. Panic disorder and depression should also be considered in this category. In the psychotic category, psychiatric co-morbidities involving anxiety include anxiety and schizophrenia, both acute and chronic, anxiety and psychotic depression, and anxiety and psychotic bi-polar disease.

Understanding the etiology of anxiety as a component of co-morbid psychiatric disease is more difficult, especially when combined with an affective disorder. In such instances the most important information to obtain is: 1) which symptom came first; 2) which symptom is likely to be present without the other; and 3) which symptom is the most important in the opinion of the patient. Further research on anxiety as a co-morbid psychiatric condition is necessary.

References

1. Pasnau R and Bystritsky A (1990) Psychiatr. Med. 8: 163–173.
2. Cohen G (1991) In: Salzman C and Lebowitz B (eds.) Anxiety and General Medical Disorders. Springer, New York, pp. 47–62.
3. Abrams R (1991) In: Sadavoy J, Lazarus L and Jarvik L (eds.) Anxiety and Personality Disorders. American Psychiatric Press, Washington D.C., pp. 369–386.
4. Barbee J and McLaulen J (1990) Psychiatr. Ann. 20: 439–445.
5. Raj A and Sheehan D (1988) Psychiatr. Ann. 18: 176–181.

Biological Psychiatry, Volume 1. G. Racagni et al., editors.

Benzodiazepine treatment of late-life anxiety disorders

George T. Grossberg

Division of Geriatric Psychiatry, St. Louis University School of Medicine, Department of Psychiatry and Human Behavior, 1221 S. Grand Blvd., St. Louis, MO 63104, U.S.A.

Introduction

The epidemiologic catchment area study (ECA) in the United States found anxiety disorders to be the most common psychiatric syndromes in community based elderly with an incidence of 10.1% among those over 75 years of age [1]. These patients are generally diagnosed as having generalized anxiety disorder (GAD) with panic disorder being uncommon [2]. Benzodiazepines, particularly the short to intermediate half-life agents without active metabolites have been the standard treatment for GAD in the elderly [3], with alprazolam perhaps having special utility in late-life panic disorder, which is being increasingly recognized, especially in patients with cardiac symptoms [4].

Methodology and Results

We studied the prevalence of anxiety disorders and benzodiazepine treatment recommendations in two subgroups of geriatric patients: a) nursing home patients referred for geriatric psychiatry consultation; and b) patients in a university hospital referred for psychogeriatric consultation.

Table 1.

Impression	n	%
Primary degenerative dementia – Alzheimer's type with or without behavioral problems	49	22.8
No psychiatric disorder; includes patients with diagnosis of medical/neurological disorder	42	19.5
Major depression	41	19.1
Delirium	31	14.4
Multi-infarct	13	6.0
Adjustment disorder	24	11.2
Personality disorder	8	3.7
Anxiety disorder	5	2.3
Psychotic disorder	0	0
Dysthymia	1	0.5
Other dementias	1	0.5

Table 2.

Diagnosis	Grossberg et al., 1991 (n = 147)
Dementia	33 (22%)
Delirium	20 (14%)
Organic affective disorder	1 (0.5%)
Affective disorder	40 (27%)
Adjustment disorder	38 (26%)
Chronic schizophrenia	3 (2%)
Anxiety disorder	5 (3%)
Personality disorder	2 (1%)
Other	2 (1%)
No psychiatric diagnosis	3 (2%)
Not reported	–

Relative to benzodiazepine treatment, 13% of nursing home patients were on a benzodiazepine while in 24% of hospital consultations, the recommendation for benzodiazepine treatment was made, with most of these patients receiving benzodiazepines for symptomatic treatment of insomnia or adjustment disorders with anxious features.

Table 1 lists the initial diagnostic impressions among nursing home patients referred. Of them, 2.3% were found to have a diagnosis of anxiety disorder (GAD).

Table 2 shows the primary psychiatric diagnoses among 147 patients referred for psychogeriatric consultation in a university hospital. In this study, 3% were diagnosed as having anxiety disorders [5].

References

1. Avant RF (1984) Fam. Pract. Recert. 6(3): 19–26.
2. Barber JG and McLaulin JB (1990) Psychiatr. Ann. 20(8): 439–445.
3. Nakra BRS and Grossberg GT (1986) Compr. Ther. 12(10): 16–22.
4. Beitman BD, Kushner M and Grossberg GT (1991) Int. J. Psychiatry Med. 21(1): 29–35.
5. Grossberg GT, Zimny GH and Nakra BRS (1990) Int. Psychogeriatr. 2(2): 161–168.

Biological Psychiatry, Volume 1. G. Racagni et al., editors.

Patient characteristics in benzodiazepine abuse and therapeutic dependence

Edward M. Sellers, Usoa E. Busto and Myroslava K. Romach

Departments of Medicine, Psychiatry and Pharmacology and Faculty of Pharmacy, University of Toronto and Comorbidity Treatment Research Program, Clinical Research and Treatment Institute, Addiction Research Foundation, 33 Russell Street, Toronto, Ontario M5S 2S1, Canada

Introduction

Benzodiazepines are the most commonly prescribed psychotropic drugs in the world. In the past several decades a number of surveys have been conducted in the United States and Europe to determine the prevalence of long-term benzodiazepine use [1,2]. These surveys failed to show any evidence of significant over-prescribing or misuse of this class of drugs. In fact, the suggestion most recently has been that they may in some circumstances be underprescribed [3]. Nevertheless, the use of benzodiazepines continues to be a source of concern and debate by the medical profession and the general public and the perception remains that these are drugs with high risk especially as newer compounds come on the market. Several factors contribute to this protracted debate, including lack of proper data about actual reasons for long-term benzodiazepine use. In an attempt to learn more about long-term users of benzodiazepines we have studied 3 different populations: alprazolam users in the community; patients presenting to an outpatient treatment program for help in discontinuing their benzodiazepine use and a group of patients admitted for acute detoxication from benzodiazepines.

Community survey study

Current long-term alprazolam users (those using the drug for 3 months or longer) were recruited on 3 separate occasions 1 year apart (1988, 1989, 1990) by identical newspaper advertisements in the Metropolitan Toronto area. All respondents were mailed a questionnaire with a stamped, addressed return envelope. The questionnaire was used to collect information pertaining to age, sex, length of drug use, pattern of use, side-effects, patient attempts to stop use, reported withdrawal symptoms and physician's advice regarding duration of treatment and discontinuation. The combined sample had a response rate of 73% and included 312 respondents.

Results

The mean age was 50.2 ± 5.09 ($\bar{x} \pm$ S.D.) years and the majority of respondents were female (62%). The primary indications for initial alprazolam use were anxiety (76%), panic attacks (46%), depression (36%) and insomnia (29%). The majority of users (66%) had previous psychotropic drug use. Of these subjects, 57% reported previous benzodiazepine use for their symptoms, while 33% had previously been prescribed an antidepressant. The majority of patients used less than 1.0 mg of alprazolam per day with only 20% using 2.6 mg or more per day. Within-patient dose was constant or had been decreased over the period of drug use in all 3 surveys. Across the 3 surveys median deviation of use exceeded 1 year. When first given the drug, while 61% of patients took it as prescribed, many eventually switched to taking alprazolam "as required" for control of their symptoms. Of the pooled respondents, 75% indicated that the effectiveness of the drug was maintained throughout the period of use.

Over two-thirds of respondents (71%) reported having tried at least once to stop taking alprazolam with the median number of stop attempts being 2; 88% reported experiencing discontinuation symptoms.

Outpatient discontinuation study

Study patients were 110 long-term alprazolam (n = 33) or lorazepam (n = 77) users (use > 3 months) who were informed about a treatment-research program by newspaper treatment ads or referred by physicians for a program to help them discontinue their benzodiazepine use. These patients presented for treatment because they felt they no longer required the medication but were having difficulty discontinuing its use on their own. These subjects completed the same questionnaire as the survey population. In addition, as part of their comprehensive assessment, a structured clinical interview for psychiatric diagnoses (SCID, DSM III-R part I and II) was conducted [4]. To assess current symptomatology the Beck Anxiety Inventory [5] and the Clinical Institute Withdrawal Assessment for Benzodiazepines Scale (CIWA-Br revised, [6]) were completed.

Results

The age (mean ± S.D.) of the treatment group was 46 ± 12 years and the sex distribution was equal. The median duration of use of alprazolam was well in excess of 1 year. Median current daily dose was 0.5 mg although the range was from 0.25–4.5 mg. The majority of patients (63%) had previously used psychoactive medications, primarily other benzodiazepines (47%) and antidepressants (23%). The indications for use of alprazolam reported were anxiety (84%), panic attacks (45%), depression (41%) and insomnia (41%). Approximately half of the patients assessed (54%) described continued effectiveness of alprazolam in controlling their symptoms in spite of their long duration of use. Patients tended to switch from taking the medication as prescribed only to using it increasingly "as needed" for their symptoms.

Table 1. Lifetime Axis I mental disorders in patients discontinuing benzodiazepines

Lifetime disorder	Outpatients (%)	Inpatients (%)
Major depression	48.0	38
Panic	29.6	25
Agoraphobia	5.1	0
Social phobia	10.1	7.4
Simple phobia	7.1	7.1
Obsessive-compulsive	4.0	0
Anorexia nervosa	0	3.6
Bulimia nervosa	3.0	3.6
Alcohol abuse/dependence	25	56

On psychiatric evaluation, while all patients met DSM III-R criteria for dependence on lorazepam or alprazolam, 65% also met DSM III-R criteria for another current Axis I psychiatric disorder, primarily an anxiety disorder (Table 1). A substantial number had a personality disorder (39%) but no particular personality structure predominated.

Past psychiatric history revealed a high lifetime prevalence of alcohol abuse/dependence (32%). Despite the incidence of past and current mental disorders, overall anxiety symptomatology, at the time of interview, was low as evidenced by the mean score on the Beck Anxiety Inventory, 11.67 ± 6.4 (cf. mean for healthy controls 15.9 ± 11.8, mean for anxiety disorder group 25.8 ± 11.4 [5]. Daily functioning as measured by the Global Assessment of Functioning Scale (GAF) was not markedly impaired, 67.4 ± 11 (mean ± S.D.).

Inpatient benzodiazepine discontinuation study

Twenty-seven consecutive consenting patients admitted for inpatient rapid detoxication from benzodiazepines were studied using similar methodology for the outpatient study (Table 1). These patients were different from the outpatients in that they use much higher doses (127 mg/day diazepam equivalents) and were somewhat younger. They had a significantly increased frequency of avoidant, dependent and antisocial personality disorder and psychoactive substance use disorder (alcohol, cannabis, stimulants, opioids, cocaine, hallucinogens and polydrugs).

Discussion

These results support the evidence that alprazolam and lorazepam are not widely abused when used in a therapeutic setting [7–9]. These patients tend to be older and have a substantial lifetime history of mental disorders and other psychotropic medication use. Their use is characterized by continuing therapeutic efficacy and increasing use on an "as needed" basis for symptom reduction [10]. Many patients attempt to decrease their daily dose or stop the medication entirely. These patterns of use do not represent abuse or addiction as usually understood. The community and treatment groups were similar with respect to patterns of use, daily dose and indications for use. However, some significant differences were noted. Males presented more frequently than females for treatment. Individuals seeking treatment had less past psychoactive medication use and more frequently reported diminishing therapeutic efficacy. These factors suggest they were self-selected as appropriate to try to stop medication.

References

1. Balter MB et al. (1984) Curr. Med. Res. Opin. 8 (Suppl. 4): 5–18.
2. Mellinger GD et al. (1974) In: Josephson E and Carroll E (eds.) Overview of Psychotherapeutic Diagnosis in Drug Use: Epidemiological and Sociological Approaches. Hemisphere Publishing Corp., pp. 333–365.
3. Uhlenhuth E et al. (1988) J. Clin. Psychopharmacol. 8(3): 161–167.
4. Spitzer RL et al. (1989) Structured Clinical Interview for DSM III-R. New York State Psychiatric Institute, Biometrics Research Department, New York.
5. Beck AT et al. (1988) J. Consult. Clin. Psychol. 56(6): 893–897.
6. Busto U et al. (1989) J. Clin. Psychopharmacol. 9(6): 412–416.
7. Salzman C et al. (1983) Benzodiazepine Dependence, Toxicity, and Abuse. American Psychiatric Association, Washington D.C.
8. Haskell D et al. (1986) Psychopharmacol. Bull. 22(2): 434–438.
9. Romach MK et al. (1990) Clin. Invest. Med. 13(4): B14.
10. Rickels K et al. (1988) Arch. Gen. Psychiatry 45: 444–450.

Biological Psychiatry, Volume 1. G. Racagni et al., editors.

Benzodiazepine abuse potential in normal and anxious individuals

Harriet de Wit and Chris E. Johanson*
Department of Psychiatry, University of Chicago, 5841 S. Maryland Ave, Chicago, IL 60637, U.S.A.

Introduction

Benzodiazepines are among the most widely prescribed psychoactive drugs. Despite their widespread use, however, the incidence of benzodiazepine abuse in the general population is relatively low [1,2]. Benzodiazepine abuse (i.e. non-medical or recreational use) has been documented in individuals with established drug abuse histories, but occurs rarely in individuals without prior drug use histories. The studies described here were designed to explore risk factors for persistent benzodiazepine use among non-drug-abusing individuals. The studies utilized laboratory self-administration procedures which measure an individual's tendency to ingest a drug. Such procedures are considered to be good indicators of the abuse potential of a drug: known drugs of abuse (e.g. cocaine, alcohol) are self-administered under laboratory conditions, whereas non-abused drugs (e.g. chlorpromazine) are not. In the present studies, a self-administration paradigm was used to investigate variables thought to be associated with risk for benzodiazepine abuse. For example, diazepam preference was studied in individuals with high levels of anxiety to test the assumption that the drug's anxiolytic effects would make it preferred in these individuals. Additional studies investigated other subject-related variables or varied the setting in which the drugs were administered.

Methods

Two self-administration choice procedures were used. In the first, subjects were tested on an outpatient basis, experiencing the drugs' effects in their normal daytime environments. In the second, the studies were conducted during the evening in a controlled recreational environment. The outpatient procedure has been shown to be sensitive to the reinforcing effects of amphetamine, a stimulant with known abuse liability, while the laboratory-based procedure has been shown to be sensitive to the reinforcing effects of alcohol.

**Present address*: Uniformed Services University of the Health Sciences, Bethesda, MD 20814, U.S.A.

Table 1. Description and results of outpatient preference studies

Drug	Dose[a] (mg)	Subjects	n	% Drug choice	Ref.
Diazepam	2, 5, 10	Control; healthy volunteers, 21–35 yrs	31	50, 10, 10	3
Diazepam	5, 10	Anxious (low)[b]	11	46,30	4
Diazepam	5, 10	Anxious (moderate)[c]	13	48,9	4
Diazepam	10	Anxious (severe)[d]	14	42	5
Diazepam	5, 10	Older, healthy volunteers, 40–55 yrs	11	47, 38	6
Flurazepam	15, 30	Control, healthy volunteers, 21–35 yrs	12	48, 20	7
Lorazepam	0.5, 1, 2	Control, as above	12	49, 32, 16	8
Amphetamine	5, 10	Control, as above	31	81, 78	9

[a]Each dose refers to a separate experiment comparing drug to placebo. Percent of occasions on which drug was chosen is shown in column on the right;
[b]Anxious (low): scoring high on standardized tests of anxiety;
[c]Anxious (moderate): meeting DSM III criteria for Generalized Anxiety Disorder;
[d]Anxious (severe): similar to moderate group but seeking treatment for their anxiety.

Outpatient studies

Subjects. Participants were healthy male and female volunteers (21–35 years in most studies) with no history of drug or alcohol abuse. They were screened for medical problems and psychiatric problems other than those specified as selection criteria (Table 1).

Procedure. Each experiment consisted of 9 sessions, 4 sampling sessions on which subjects ingested color-coded capsules containing active drug (see Table 1) or placebo and 5 choice sessions in which they chose and ingested whichever capsule they preferred. The primary dependent measure was the number of times subjects chose the active drug. On each session, subjects completed baseline self-report mood questionnaires in the laboratory before taking their capsule. They then left the laboratory, completing additional questionnaires in their normal daily environments. The mood questionnaires were used to assess the drugs' subjective effects.

Neither normal healthy control subjects nor individuals with higher-than-average levels of anxiety preferred benzodiazepines over placebo. Doses of diazepam, flurazepam and lorazepam that were high enough to produce measureable subjective effects (i.e. anxiolytic or sedative-like effects) were chosen *less* often than placebo. Diazepam was not preferred even by highly anxious individuals, even though the drug decreased anxiety ratings as measured by the subjective effects questionnaires. Amphetamine, included as a positive control, was preferred over placebo.

Table 2. Laboratory-based studies

Drug	Dose range	Subjects	n	% Drug choice	Mean dose	Ref.
Diazepam	4–28 mg	Healthy adults, light drinkers[a]	18	66	16 mg	10
Diazepam	4–28 mg	Healthy adults, moderate drinkers[b]	12	100	25 mg	10
Diazepam	4–28 mg	Healthy males, FHP[c]	14	47	25 mg	11
Diazepam	4–28 mg	Healthy males, FHN[d]	13	38	18 mg	11
Diazepam	4–28 mg	Healthy adults, social groups[e]	31	30	19.2 mg	12
Diazepam	4–28 mg	Healthy adults, isolated[f]	30	34	16.8 mg	12
Ethanol	0.1–1.1 g/kg	Healthy adults	12	75	0.8 g/kg	13

[a,b] Light and moderate drinking groups consumed means of 4.8 and 11.8 drinks/week;
[c,d] FHP or FHN: family history (positive or negative) of alcoholism;
[e,f] Subjects tested under group (standard) or socially isolated conditions.

Laboratory-based studies

Subjects. Recruitment and screening was generally as described above. Screening criteria for specific studies are described in Table 2.

Procedure. Studies consisted of 7 evening sessions, 4 sampling sessions in which subjects received drug or placebo and 3 choice sessions in which they chose the substance they preferred. The drugs (diazepam or ethanol) were administered in divided, cumulating doses administered at 15- or 30-min intervals. During choice sessions subjects could take fewer or more doses than the number sampled. Table 2 summarizes the studies and their results.

The only group which consistently preferred diazepam over placebo and reported positive subjective effects was the group of moderate social drinkers. These results are consistent with epidemiological data indicating that only individuals with established drug use histories are at appreciable risk for benzodiazepine abuse. The present results extend this relationship, however, from individuals with diagnosable substance use disorders to moderate, non-problem social drinkers.

Discussion

Preferences for diazepam and other drugs were examined in a variety of subject populations using 2 different procedures. In general, diazepam was not highly preferred either by normal healthy volunteers or by symptomatic (anxious) volunteers, suggesting that these groups would not be at high risk for developing problems with benzodiazepine abuse. Even when diazepam was made available to subjects during the evenings in a recreational environment, only selected subjects (i.e. heavier alcohol drinkers) clearly preferred the drug. The majority of subjects reported only sedative-like subjective effects, without increases in measures of drug-induced euphoria.

Acknowledgements

Supported by Grants DA02812 and MO1RR00055.

References

1. Mellinger GD, Balter MB and Uhlenhuth EH (1984) J. Am. Med. Assoc. 251: 375–379.
2. Woods JH, Katz JL and Winger G (1987) Clin. Pharmacol. Ther. 39: 251–419.
3. Johanson CE and Uhlenhuth EH (1980a) Psychopharmacology 71: 275–279.
4. de Wit H et al. (1986) Arch. Gen. Psychiatry 43: 533–541.
5. McCracken SG et al. (1990) Clin. Pharmacol. Ther. 10: 190–196.
6. de Wit H, Uhlenhuth EH and Johanson CE (1985) Psychopharmacology 87: 186–193.
7. de Wit H, Johanson CE and Uhlenhuth EH (1984a) Drug Alcohol Depend. 13: 31–41.
8. de Wit H et al. (1984b) Pharmacol. Biochem. Behav. 21: 865–869.
9. Johanson CE and Uhlenhuth EH (1980b) Psychopharmacology 71: 269–273.
10. de Wit H, Pierri J and Johanson CE (1989) Psychopharmacology 99: 416–421.
11. de Wit H (1991) Alcohol. Clin. Exp. Res. (in press).
12. Johanson CE and de Wit H (1991) (unpublished data).
13. de Wit H, Pierri J and Johanson CE (1989) Psychopharmacology 98: 113–119.

Biological Psychiatry, Volume 1. G. Racagni et al., editors.

Low-dose therapeutic benzodiazepine dependence: Are there differences between benzodiazepines?

M.H. Lader
Institute of Psychiatry, London, SE5 8AF, U.K.

The first benzodiazepines introduced as anxiolytics were chlordiazepoxide and diazepam, both long-acting compounds. Later, shorter-acting drugs were marketed, lorazepam and, more recently, alprazolam being the most successful. Concern has been expressed about the dependence potential of the benzodiazepines and many prescribers have focused their attention on these short half-life compounds. Is this concern justified?

Pharmacological differences

Traditionally, benzodiazepines have been sub-divided on the basis of the elimination half-life. However, this does not necessarily equate to duration of action. Thus, diazepam with a long elimination half-life and even longer-acting metabolites can actually be short-acting in single dose because of a pronounced redistribution phase; conversely, oxazepam with a half-life of around 12 h may have a prolonged action because of slow absorption. The duration of action is closely related to bodily tissue and fluid concentrations.

Recently, it has become apparent that the receptor affinity and perhaps the intrinsic activity of the benzodiazepine may also influence its profile of activity and not merely the active dosage range. Low potency compounds include chlordiazepoxide and oxazepam, high potency compounds lorazepam, clonazepam, alprazolam and the hypnotic, triazolam. Intermediate potency drugs comprise diazepam, clorazepate and clobazam.

There is a clinical impression that high potency compounds are more likely than low potency compounds to induce adverse effects such as sedation, psychomotor and cognitive impairment and in particular amnesic effects. Clinical reports abound on amnesic episodes following the administration of lorazepam and, more recently, alprazolam. Such anecdotes usually relate to single-dose administration, say for transient jet-lag. More formal comparative studies are rare.

We carried out a study comparing the memory and psychomotor functions of oxazepam, 15 and 30 mg, lorazepam, 1 and 2 mg, and placebo given in single dose to normal volunteers, 9 per group [1]. Lorazepam and oxazepam affected tests of attention, manual motor speed and coding skills in a similar dose-related way. Both drugs caused anterograde impairments of long-term verbal memory but did not alter short-term verbal span or recency. The magnitude of anterograde amnesia produced by the 2 benzodiazepines was not linearly dose-related in that the 2 low doses had similar effects, whereas the high dose of lorazepam produced much more pronounced effects than oxazepam 30 mg. Follow-up studies have confirmed this effect. Similarly, in a laboratory paradigm of aggressive responding, the higher dose of lorazepam was most effective in increasing aggressive behaviour, whereas the subjective effects of oxazepam and lorazepam were quite similar [2].

Withdrawal syndromes

Several features should be distinguished in comparing withdrawal aspects of various benzodiazepines. Firstly pharmacokinetic factors determine the time of onset of withdrawal symptoms, being 24–48 h after stopping a short half-life compound, 7–10 days after a long half-life drug. These differences between short and long half-life drugs become less distinct when the drugs are gradually discontinued.

Secondly, several well-designed and conducted studies document the greater severity of withdrawal phenomena following discontinuation of high potency short-acting compounds than after low-potency long-acting compounds, despite tapering schedules [3,4]. The usual comparisons are between lorazepam and alprazolam on the one hand, and diazepam and clorazepate on the other. Even after short-term use, abrupt discontinuation of short half-life compounds is more troublesome than that of long half-life drugs [5,6].

A recent study from the Rickel's group compared withdrawal severity and acute outcome in 63 patients tapering off short half-life or long half-life benzodiazepines [7]. Ninety percent of the patients experienced a withdrawal reaction that was rarely severe. Most withdrawal symptoms in the short half-life group occurred after a 75% reduction and for the long half-life group after full reduction. However, 42% of short half-life and 32% of long half-life discontinuers were unable to achieve a drug-free state.

Finally, do benzodiazepines vary in their capacity to induce dependence? There are no data directly addressing this difficult issue, but it would be surprising if the high potency short half-life compounds did not induce dependence more frequently than the others because of the higher frequency of rebound phenomena and greater severity and relapse rate on withdrawal after long-term use.

Unfortunately, most comparative studies in this area have confounded potency with half-life by comparing for instance diazepam and lorazepam. Withdrawal studies directed separately towards potency and duration of action would be invaluable.

References

1. Curran HV, Schiwy W and Lader M (1987) Psychopharmology 92: 358–364.
2. Bond A and Lader M (1988) Psychopharmacology 95: 369–373.
3. Tyrer P, Rutherford D and Huggett T (1981) Lancet i: 520–522.
4. Rickels K, Case WG, Schweizer EE, Swenson C and Fridman RB (1986) Psychopharmacol. Bull. 22: 407–415.
5. Fontaine R, Chouinard G and Annable L (1984) Am. J. Psychiatry 141: 848–852.
6. Rickels K, Fox IL, Greenblatt DJ, Sandler KR and Schless A (1988) Am. J. Psychiatry 145: 312–317.
7. Schweizer E, Rickels K, Case WG and Greenblatt DJ (1990) Arch. Gen. Psychiatry 47: 908–915.

Biological Psychiatry, Volume 1. G. Racagni et al., editors.

Management of benzodiazepine discontinuation

Karl Rickels, W. George Case and Edward Schweizer

Department of Psychiatry, University of Pennsylvania, 203 Piersol Building, 3400 Spruce Street, Philadelphia, PA 19104-4283, U.S.A.

Preliminary results are presented of a study assessing the utility of buspirone, imipramine and placebo as adjuvants in the management of drug discontinuation in long-term benzodiazepine (BZ) users.

Patients referred by physicians or responding to newspaper advertising are being screened for inclusion into a taper discontinuation program. They are stabilized on their benzodiazepine, either diazepam, lorazepam or alprazolam, receiving the medication in identical capsules. If patients are on another benzodiazepine, they are shifted to diazepam in equivalent dosages. After this initial 1 to 3 week period, patients enter the double-blind treatment phase in which they receive, under double-blind conditions, either buspirone (10–50 mg/day), imipramine (25–225 mg/day) or placebo. Patients are pretreated for 4 weeks while they continue on their benzodiazepine (BZ). Under the protection of these adjuvant therapies, the BZs are gradually withdrawn over a 4-week taper period. After the patient becomes BZ-free, he/she continues on placebo and on adjuvant study medication for another 2 weeks, at which time adjuvant medication is discontinued and patients are shifted to single-blind placebo for an additional 2 weeks. At that time all placebos are discontinued and the patient is evaluated 1 week later, which is 5 weeks after discontinuation.

Of the 102 patients who were accepted into the program and entered the pre-taper period, 73 patients agreed to enter the taper period 4 weeks later, while 29 patients dropped out during the 4-week pre-taper pretreatment phase. Patients who dropped out during pre-taper differed from patients entering taper in that they were initially more anxious and depressed, had higher neuroticism scores and showed significantly less improvement during the 4-week pre-taper period while being treated with placebo, imipramine or buspirone. Patients not entering taper did not differ in terms of daily dose of benzodiazepine intake or duration of treatment.

The sex distribution was 50% male and female; the mean age was 45 years, and the mean daily BZ intake was 11.8 mg/day for diazepam, 14 mg/day for lorazepam, expressed in diazepam equivalents, and 19.9 mg/day of alprazolam, also expressed in diazepam equivalents ($P < 0.05$). Of the 15 diazepam patients, 10 were on diazepam when they entered our program while 5 were switched from benzodiazepine hypnotics to benzodiazepine. It is of interest to note that of the patients originally on diazepam, 80% were successfully tapered while only 20% of patients shifted from a hypnotic to diazepam did so (Fisher's Exact Test, $P < 0.05$).

Thus it appears that patients dependent on BZ hypnotics need different taper strategies to patients dependent on daytime anxiolytics.

Because of these differences in the diazepam group, the diazepam group was eliminated from the data analysis in which we examined peak severity of withdrawal as a function of type of benzodiazepine, either lorazepam or alprazolam, and of adjuvant treatment agents, either buspirone, imipramine or placebo.

The main results are that for peak withdrawal symptomatology a significant interaction exists with lorazepam, patients having significantly less severe withdrawal symptomatology when treated during taper with buspirone or imipramine than with placebo, while alprazolam patients responded more poorly to imipramine than to placebo, and best to buspirone.

Most interestingly, these differences in withdrawal severity do not transmit into benzodiazepine-free status 5 weeks post-taper termination. Only a trend level ($P < 0.25$) existed for placebo patients to be slightly less successful in their taper attempts (54%) than buspirone (67%) or imipramine (77%) patients. Diagnosis (GAD, PD, MDD, no psychiatric diagnosis) did not affect taper outcome, even if taper success rates were lowest for panic disorder patients (47%) and highest for patients with no psychiatric diagnosis (80%). A larger sample size may well make some of these weak trend differences significant.

As expected from clinical experience, buspirone, irrespective of whether it was added to lorazepam or alprazolam patients, was ineffective as a taper facilitator for patients who had a panic diagnosis, but was quite helpful for patients who had a GAD diagnosis ($P < 0.05$). In contrast, patients on imipramine did equally well, irrespective of whether they had a panic or GAD diagnosis. Placebo patients in contrast did less well in all diagnostic categories.

The results of this preliminary analysis indicate that withdrawal can be significantly affected by adjuvant therapy of buspirone or imipramine with alprazolam patients doing poorest when treated with imipramine and with lorazepam patients doing exceedingly well. Why these different responses of withdrawal severity to imipramine are present, and why decreases in withdrawal severity do not fully transpose to a successful benzodiazepine-free state at the end of taper and 4 weeks later, the authors are unable to explain at present.

Acknowledgement

Research reported in this paper has been supported by USPHS Research Grant MHO8957.

Hypnotics and sleep disorders

Biological Psychiatry, Volume 1. G. Racagni et al., editors.

Response of human sleep and melatonin secretion to changes in photoperiod: Implications for manic-depressive illness

Thomas A. Wehr

Clinical Psychobiology Branch, National Institute of Mental Health, Room 4s-239, Building 10, 9000 Rockville Pike, Bethesda, MD 20892, U.S.A.

Introduction

Most plants and animals go through dramatic seasonal changes during the course of the year. In many cases, these changes are triggered by biological mechanisms that track and respond to seasonal changes in day length, or photoperiod. Animals respond to changes in the photoperiod principally in 2 ways. First, they adjust the duration of their activity phase (if they are diurnal animals) or rest phase (if they are nocturnal animals) to match the continually changing duration of the photoperiod. Second, they display novel types of behavior, accompanied by striking physiological changes, that represent special adaptations to conditions that prevail at a particular time of year. The best studied example of the latter type of response is photoperiodic seasonal reproductive cycles. To ensure that their young are born at a time when environmental conditions are most favorable for survival, most animals confine their reproductive activity to one time of year. The time of year is different in different animals, depending on the length of their gestation period. For example, sheep are conceived in winter, hamsters in spring.

The pineal hormone, melatonin, plays a critical role as a mediator of photoperiodic rhythms in reproduction, body weight, metabolism and thermoregulation. Melatonin is secreted at night. When nights become longer, the duration of nocturnal melatonin secretion becomes correspondingly longer. This change in the duration of nocturnal melatonin secretion serves as a chemical signal that triggers winter-type changes in physiological systems that respond to changes in the photoperiod. These systems appear to possess an interval timer that is capable of measuring the duration of melatonin secretion and triggering appropriate responses when the duration changes in a critical direction and to a critical degree [1].

Although photoperiodism is ubiquitous in biology, no experiments, to my knowledge, have been carried out to determine whether human beings respond to changes in photoperiod. In modern times, the routine use of artificial light may have prevented or attenuated any possible effect of the natural photoperiod on human behavior and physiology. To investigate whether human beings are capable of responding to changes in photoperiod, I exposed 8 individuals to a conventional 16 h (summer) photoperiod for 1 week, then to a short 10 h (winter) photoperiod for 4 weeks [2]. I hypothesized that when the duration of the nightly dark period was lengthened, the duration of the nightly sleep phase and the nightly phase of active melatonin secretion would both lengthen.

Subjects and Methods

The individuals who participated in the study were of European extraction, and their ages ranged from 20–36. During the dark portion of each photoperiod schedule, they remained in a completely dark room on a research unit. They were encouraged to sleep, and no other activities were permitted while they were in the room. During the light portion of each photoperiod schedule, they were free to engage in their usual daytime activities off the ward. At these times, they were exposed to whatever ambient natural and artificial light they encountered.

During each photoperiod schedule, sleep EEG was recorded nightly. At the end of each photoperiod schedule, blood samples were obtained every 30 min during a constant routine protocol in which the individuals remained continuously awake while sitting in very dim (<1 lux) light and eating small isocaloric meals every 2 h. Melatonin levels in the samples were subsequently measured by radioimmunoassay [3].

Differences between durations of sleep and melatonin secretion in the two photoperiods were evaluated with paired *t*-tests. Results are expressed as mean ± S.D.

Results

When the duration of the dark phase was lengthened from 8 to 14 h, the duration of the nightly sleep phase lengthened from 7.7 ± 0.2 to 11.0 ± 0.8 h ($t = 11.754$, $P < 0.001$). When the individuals were transferred from the 8-h dark period to the 14-h dark period, their sleep gradually separated into two components with a waking interval between them. An evening component appeared to be entrained to the onset of the dark period ("sunset"), and a morning component appeared to be entrained to the offset of the dark period ("sunrise"). The duration of nocturnal melatonin secretion also lengthened, from 10.3 ± 0.8 to 12.5 ± 1.8 h ($t = 31.778$, $P < 0.01$).

Discussion

Human beings responded to being transferred from long (summer) days to short (winter) days in a manner similar to animals. Their sleep phase and the duration of their nocturnal melatonin secretion lengthened. In animals, such lengthening of the duration of nocturnal melatonin secretion can serve as a chemical signal that triggers major changes in reproductive function, body weight, metabolism and thermoregulation. To determine whether the change in melatonin secretion observed here would trigger similar physiological changes in human beings, it would be necessary to expose individuals to short photoperiods for several months.

The bimodal pattern of sleep that appeared when human beings were exposed to the short photoperiod is similar to bimodal patterns in nocturnal behavior exhibited by other species in similar experimental conditions. For example, the diurnal Siberian chipmunk, Eutamias sibiricus, displays a strikingly similar bimodal sleep pattern when it is exposed to short photoperiods [4]. Nocturnal animals, such as the whitefooted mouse, Peromyscus leucopus, show bimodal patterns in their nighttime motor activity when they are exposed to short photoperiods [5].

It has previously been shown that melatonin secretion can be suppressed by light [6]. However, the different patterns of melatonin secretion that were observed after exposure to the two photoperiods in the present experiment were not directly caused by light suppression, because no light-dark cycle was applied during the constant routine protocol in which melatonin measurements were obtained. For this reason, changes in the pattern of melatonin secretion that were observed after transfer from long days to short days must reflect changes in the timing of internal processes, such as circadian rhythms that control melatonin secretion. In effect, these processes "remembered" the photoperiod to which the individuals had most recently been exposed. This "history dependence" of the behavior of circadian rhythms has been well-described in animals [1].

Pittendrigh and Daan developed and Illnerová et al. extended a model to describe the mechanism whereby animals modify the duration of their sleep phase and of nocturnal melatonin secretion in response to changes in the photoperiod [7,8]. According to this model, the onset of the sleep phase (in diurnal animals) and the onset of nightly melatonin secretion are controlled by a circadian oscillator that is entrained to sunset. The offset of the sleep phase and the offset of nightly melatonin secretion are controlled by a second circadian oscillator that is entrained to sunrise. As the photoperiod lengthens and shortens during the course of the year, the dawn- and dusk-tracking oscillators cause the duration of sleep and melatonin secretion to shorten and lengthen correspondingly.

This demonstration of a mechanism in human beings that tracks the photoperiod and controls the duration of human sleep might be important for understanding the pathophysiology of manic-depressive illness. Manic and depressive episodes exhibit seasonal patterns in their onsets [9]. Furthermore, manic-depressive illness is characterized by cyclic changes in the duration of sleep [10]. The fact that restriction of sleep (partial sleep deprivation) can improve depression and trigger mania and that resumption of sleep (after sleep deprivation) can trigger depression, suggests that changes in sleep in manic-depressive illness contribute to its pathogenesis [10]. In light of these facts, the photoperiodic mechanism that was shown to regulate the duration of human sleep in the present experiment deserves to be investigated as a possible pathogenic mechanism in manic-depressive illness.

Acknowledgements

I thank Douglas Moul, Holly Giesen and the 4-West nursing staff for invaluable assistance in carrying out the experiment.

References

1. Bartness TJ and Goldman BD (1989) Experientia 45: 939–945.
2. Wehr TA (1991) J. Clin. Endocrinol. Metab. (in press).
3. Fraser S, Cowen P, Franlin M, Franey C and Arendt J (1983) Clin. Chem. 29: 396–397.
4. Dijk DJ (1989) J. Comp. Physiol. 165: 205–215.
5. Pittendrigh CS and Daan S (1976) J. Comp. Physiol. 106: 223–252.
6. Lewy AJ, Wehr TA, Goodwin FK, Newsome DA and Markey SP (1980) Science 210: 1267–1269.
7. Pittendrigh CS and Daan S (1976) J. Comp. Physiol. 106: 333–355.
8. Illnerová H and Vanecek J (1982) J. Comp. Physiol. 145: 539–548.
9. Wehr TA and Rosenthal NE (1989) Am. J. Psychiatry 146: 829–839.
10. Wehr TA (1990) In: Montplaisir J and Godbout R (eds.) Sleep and Biological Rhythms. Oxford University Press, Oxford, pp. 42–86.

Biological Psychiatry, Volume 1. G. Racagni et al., editors.

Delayed sleep phase syndrome: Clinical picture and treatment with light

Norman E. Rosenthal, Christine L. Cameron, Scott H. Johnston, Jean R. Joseph-Vanderpool, Alytia A. Levendosky and Richard Allen

Clinical Psychobiology Branch, National Institute of Mental Health, Building 10, Room 3n-228, 9000 Rockville Pike, Bethesda, MD 20892, U.S.A.

Introduction

Delayed sleep phase syndrome (DSPS) is a condition characterized by an inability to fall asleep in the evening and wake refreshed in the morning at conventional times. Weitzman et al. defined the condition as having the following features: a) chronic inability to fall asleep at a desired clock time; b) symptoms for at least 6 months; c) when not on a strict schedule patients fall asleep without difficulty and, after a sound sleep of normal duration, awaken spontaneously [1]. Their group suggested treating these patients by having them sleep at progressively later clock times on successive days until the desired sleep onset time is reached [2]. In this report we describe the clinical features of DSPS patients, using modern diagnostic criteria. We also summarize the phase shifting effects of modifying the light-dark cycle in these patients. These results have been reported more fully elsewhere [3].

Methods

We recruited patients via the local media and screened them by means of questionnaires, a month of sleep log ratings, wrist-worn activity monitors, SCID-R interviews, clinical polysomnography and physical examinations. We excluded those with other sleep disorders, active psychiatric disturbances or any major medical problems. Inclusion criteria adapted from those of Weitzman et al. were: a) sleep onset later than 1 a.m., at least 4 nights a week over at least 3 years; b) poor morning alertness (7 to 9 a.m.); c) disrupted functioning due to their sleep problem; d) repeated unsuccessful attempts to move their sleep onset and wake times earlier; and e) motivation to change.

We treated 20 DSPS patients in a balanced crossover study. The active treatment was 2,500 lux full-spectrum light for 2 h in the morning (between 6 and 9 a.m.) and dark goggles from 4 p.m. until dusk. The control was 300 lux full-spectrum light for 2 h (between 6 and 9 a.m.) and clear goggles from 4 p.m. until dusk.

Before each treatment condition, expectations were assessed by means of a questionnaire modified from that of Borkovec and Nau [4]. Patients were treated for 2 weeks, were allowed at least 2 weeks of washout to relapse, and were then crossed over to the alternate condition.

Twenty-four-hour temperature profiles and multiple sleep latencies were obtained before and after each treatment. Core body temperature was measured every 5 min using a Vitalog® monitor and thermistor. The timing of the circadian temperature minima was determined by a blind rater. Repeated measures analysis of variance (ANOVA) was performed on the temperature data. Paired *t*-tests were performed on temperature minima. The multiple sleep latencies were scored according to the criteria of Carskadon et al. [5] and analyzed by paired *t*-tests for each time point. The 24-h core body temperature measurements and multiple sleep latency tests, together with a self-report post-treatment questionnaire, were used to evaluate efficacy.

Results

Three hundred and thirty subjects returned the questionnaire. Of the 176 patients who met criteria for DSPS, 69% were women and 31% were men. Mean age of responders (± S.D.) was 34.4 ± 10.4 years; mean age of onset was 11.8 ± 12 years and mean age when sleep schedules became a problem was 16.4 ± 12.4 years. Sleep schedule problems interfered with work functioning in 91% of patients and with interpersonal relations in 82%. Of the 81% who were currently working, 35% had a standard, nine-to-five schedule, while 65% worked at unconventional times. On average, subjects reported falling asleep at 2:15 and 3:06 a.m. on weekdays and weekends respectively. Average wake-up times for week- and weekend days were 9:21 and 10:51 a.m. Subjects reported mean weekday and weekend sleep latencies as 46 and 32 min respectively. Most (84%) described the quality of their sleep as sound. Many participants had used nicotine or caffeine to keep themselves awake in the morning (64%). Many had used sedatives to sleep at night: 30% had used over the counter sleep medication and 24% had used alcohol. Fourteen percent had sought psychotherapy to help with their sleep problem.

Of the 33 patients who were given the SCID-R, 17 met lifetime criteria for one or more psychiatric disorders. In these 17 patients, the following diagnoses were given: major depression 27%, depressive disorder NOS 6%, bipolar disorder 6%, bipolar disorder NOS (bipolar II) 3%, alcohol abuse 24%, non-alcohol substance abuse 15%, anxiety disorder 9%, somatization 9%, dysthymia 6%, and schizophrenia 3%.

Twenty patients completed the light treatment protocol. Subjective reports favored the "active" treatment ($t = 3.51$, df = 13, $P \leq 0.001$). Morning alertness and earlier sleep-time were reported to be significantly improved during the "active" condition as compared to the "control" condition. (Alertness: $t = 4.79$, df = 13, $P < 0.01$; Sleep-time: $t = 3.35$, df = 13; $P \leq 0.01$). There were no significant differences in a priori patient expectations between the two treatments (F = 2.15, df = 11, $P = 0.17$).

Temperature profiles revealed a significant phase advance in the sleep-associated part of the temperature rhythm on the "active" condition (F = 2.39, df = 287, $P \leq 0.001$) but not on the "control" condition (F = 0.92, df = 287, $P = 0.77$). Analysis of the timing of the temperature minima indicated a significantly greater phase advance following the "active" treatment (1 h 25 min, $t = 2.3$; df = 18; $P \leq 0.05$) as compared with the "control" treatment (10 min, $t = 0.49$, df = 15, $P = 0.63$). A significant increase in 9 and 11 a.m. sleep latencies was seen following the "active" condition (9 a.m.: $t = 2.44$, df = 11, $P \leq 0.05$; 11 a.m.: $t = 2.75$, df = 14, $P \leq 0.05$), but not the "control" condition (9 a.m.: $t = 0.98$, df = 11, $P = 0.35$; 11 a.m.: $t = 0.35$, df = 16, $P = 0.73$).

Discussion

Our data on age of onset confirm earlier reports [1,2,6] that DSPS typically develops before adulthood and remains stable over time. Sex ratios in DSPS are inconsistent across studies. The female:male ratio in our study was 11:5. Other studies have reported more males than females [6] and equal numbers of males and females [1]. Differences in the sex distribution of the DSPS population may be an artifact of recruitment methods.

Clinical interviews revealed a high incidence of depression. It has been suggested that some depressed patients have advanced circadian rhythms in relation to the timing of their sleep-wake cycle [6]. Such phase-angle abnormalities might be responsible for inducing depression in DSPS patients. Alternatively, their depression may have a psychological basis, considering the psychosocial difficulties associated with DSPS. Patients are often fatigued from sleep deprivation, yet are required to meet work or family obligations. These patients may appear lazy and unmotivated to employers and co-workers, which may harm their self-esteem.

Consistent with previous research [1,2], substance abuse was common in our population. In DSPS substance abuse usually begins as an attempt to help induce sleep at night. However, most DSPS patients are not helped in the long-run by sedatives or alcohol [7], which may lead to increased intake to achieve the desired effect.

Despite close supervision of compliance, patients found it difficult to give up their old sleep-wake schedule, even after successful phase advance. Many patients enjoyed the privacy of the late evening hours, when they were functioning at their peak and wished to gain morning hours without sacrificing precious evening hours. Some individuals had power struggles with the clinicians, perhaps replaying earlier conflicts with parents over their sleep-wake schedules. Some found it difficult to give up such habits as watching late-night TV programs. These psychological factors should be recognized by clinicians since they can sabotage treatment.

We found that modification of timing of light and darkness can exert a prominent effect on the timing of circadian rhythms in DSPS patients. Our data provide further evidence that a phase response curve (PRC) seen in animals [8] is present in humans as well. By understanding this PRC, appropriately timed bright light and darkness can be used therapeutically in DSPS patients. Improvement in morning alertness generally occurred in the second week of treatment, a lag that might have been predicted by the time required for reentrainment of human circadian rhythms [9]. Our subjects reported that in order to maintain the phase-advancing effect of light, they had to keep using it regularly. This suggests that their circadian rhythms must be continually reset.

References

1. Weitzman E, Czeisler C, Coleman R et al. (1981) Arch. Gen. Psychiatry 38: 737–746.3.
2. Czeisler C, Richardson G, Coleman R et al. (1981) Sleep 4: 1–21.
3. Rosenthal NE, Joseph-Vanderpool JR, Levendosky AA et al. (1990) Sleep 354–361.
4. Borkovec T, Nau S (1972) J. Behav. Ther. Exp. Psychiatry 3: 257–260.
5. Carskadon M, Dement W, Mitler M et al. (1986) Sleep 9: 519–524.
6. Thorpy M, Korman E, Spielman A et al. (1988) J. Adolesc. Health Care 9: 22–27.
7. Wagner D (1990) In: Thorpy MJ (ed.) Handbook of Sleep Disorders. Marcel Dekker, New York, U.S.A., pp. 493–527.
8. Pittendrigh C (1981) In: Aschoff J (ed.) Handbook of Behavioral Neurobiology. Plenum Press, New York and London, pp. 95–124.
9. Wever R (1979) The Circadian System of Man: Results of Experiments Under Temporal Isolation. Springer Verlag, New York, U.S.A.

Biological Psychiatry, Volume 1. G. Racagni et al., editors.

Resetting the sleep-wake cycle of schedule disorders and vitamin B_{12} treatment

Tatsuro Ohta, Yuhei Kayukawa, Tamotsu Okada, Tokihisa Iwata and Masayoshi Terashima

Department of Psychiatry, Nagoya University School of Medicine, Nagoya 466, Japan

Introduction

A definitive method of treatment for the persistent sleep-wake schedule disorders such as delayed sleep phase syndrome [1,2] (DSPS) and non-24-h sleep-wake (hypernychthemeral) syndrome (HNS) has not yet been established. Resetting the sleep-wake time with chronotherapy was easily accomplished in all the DSPS patients we treated [3], but it was not always easy to maintain the reset rhythm because of a gradual delay after treatment. We had little success in treating the hypernychthemeral syndrome with chronotherapy.

We observed that some adolescent patients' sleep-wake schedule disorders were so severe that the patients were unable to attend school or that they resulted in poor school performance and behavioral problems [4,5].

As a pharmacotherapeutic method, we tried to treat these patients with methylcobalamin, the methyl derivative of vitamin B_{12}, to reset their biological clock to fall asleep at a socially acceptable time of night and to be easily aroused in the morning.

Subjects and Methods

Subjects

The subjects in the present study were 10 patients, 5 DSPS (2 females and 3 males) and 5 hypernychthemerals (2 females and 3 males). The patients consisted both of those who came to our clinic spontaneously and those referred by the National Center of Neurology and Psychiatry (Tokyo) on the basis of a multi-center study. Six patients were adolescent and the others were adult. Data on all of our patients has been shown in Table 1.

Methods

The patients were treated with 6 tablets (0.5 mg each) of methylcobalamin orally per day. We evaluated the blood concentration of vitamin B_{12} (VB_{12}) and thyroid

Table 1. Patients treated with methylcobalamin

Case No.	Age (years)	Sex	Age of onset (years)	Blood levels		Thyroid function
				Before (pg/ml)	After (pg/ml)	
DSPS						
1	14	F	12	–	1078	–
2	18	M	15	641	–	N
3	25	M	24	447	–	N
4	29	F	3	355	1445	N
5	33	M	30	648	1261	A
HNS						
6	15	F	12	350	1350	N
7	17	M	15	590	2209	N
8	19	M	18	267	1287	N
9	19	F	17	291	875	N
10	23	M	17	510	970	N

DSPS: delayed sleep phase syndrome; HNS: non-24-hour sleep-wake syndrome; F: female; M: male; N: normal range; A: abnormal range.

function (T3-uptake, T3, T4, TSH, free-T3, free-T4) in 9 of the 10 patients before the administration of methylcobalamin. In the course of the medication, serum concentrations of VB_{12} were measured in 8 patients.

Results

Five adolescent patients (Cases 1,2,6,7,8) who had been unable to attend school returned to their classes after medication with methylcobalamin. Three adult patients (Cases 3,5,10) were able to be easily aroused in the morning after the administration of the vitamin. The wake-up time of 1 adult patient (Case 4) gradually advanced from 2 p.m. to 8 a.m. with the combined treatment of methylcobalamin and triazolam 0.25 mg per day. The average serum concentration level of vitamin B_{12} before treatment was 455.4 ± 148.5 pg/ml ($n = 9$), within the normal range. The average level after treatment was 1342.4 ± 433.7 (Cases 4–10), which was significantly increased ($n = 7$, $P < 0.001$) compared with the average concentration before treatment. The thyroid function was measured in 9 cases, and 8 of them showed normal range results. Only 1 patient (Case 5) showed high T3-uptake (40.8).

Discussion

Non-pharmacotherapy for the persistent sleep-wake schedule disorders has been reported in recent years. Few pharmacotherapy trials, however, have been carried out on the treatment of DSPS [7,8] and HNS [9,10]. In the present study, high doses of methylcobalamin (3,000 μg/day) were used throughout the entire treatment period. Because improvement appeared immediately after the administration of this vitamin, it seems effective to use high doses of VB_{12} for these sleep-wake schedule disorders. The mechanism of the vitamin's efficacy is unknown. None of the patients showed any laboratory data or clinical symptoms indicating either vitamin B_{12} deficiency or hypothyroidism, which is sometimes associated with VB_{12} deficiency and delay of the biological clock.

References

1. Czeisler CA, Richardson GS, Coleman RM et al. (1981) Sleep 4: 1–21.
2. Weitzman ED, Czeisler CA, Coleman RM et al. (1981) Arch. Gen. Psychiatry 38: 737–746.
3. Ohta T, Iwata T, Ozaki N et al. (1988) Jpn. J. Psychiatry Neurol. 42: 175–176.
4. Ohta T, Ando K, Hayakawa T et al. (1990) Prog. Clin. Biol. Res. 341B: 65–72.
5. Thorpy MJ, Korman E, Spielman AJ and Glovinsky PB (1988) J. Adolesc. Health Care 9: 22–27.
6. Rosenthal NE, Joseph-Vanderpool JR, Levendosky AA et al. (1990) Sleep 13: 354–361.
7. Kamgar-Parsi, Wehr TA and Gillin JC (1983) Sleep 6: 257–262.
8. Okawa M, Mishima K, Nanami T et al. (1990) Sleep 13: 15–23.
9. Wollman M, Lavie P and Peled R (1988) Chronobiol. Int. 2: 277–280.
10. Sugita Y, Mikami A, Teshima Y et al. (1988) Jpn. J. Psychiatry Neurol. 42: 177–179.

Biological Psychiatry, Volume 1. G. Racagni et al., editors.

Vitamin B_{12} treatment for sleep-wake rhythm disorder

Masako Okawa[1], Kazuo Mishima[1], Yasuo Hishikawa[1] and Kiyohisa Takahashi[2]
[1]*Department of Neuropsychiatry, Akita University School of Medicine, 1-1-1 Hondo, Akita; and* [2]*Institute of Neurosciences, NCNP, Kodaira, Tokyo, Japan*

Introduction

Recently, vitamin B_{12} (VB_{12}) has been reported to be effective for different types of sleep-wake rhythm disorders. However, the mechanism through which VB_{12} produces the beneficial effect on such sleep disorders is unclear at present. In this study, we present 8 patients suffering from various types of sleep-wake rhythm disorder for many years, who were treated with VB_{12}.

Subjects and Methods

The clinical features of the 8 patients and clinical course of their treatment are summarized in Table 1. Subjects were 8 patients (6 males and 2 females), aged 12–63 years, suffering from various type of sleep-wake rhythm disorder with some complications such as blindness, mental retardation, allergy, chronic nephritis, brain infarction etc. Two of them showed a non-24-h sleep-wake rhythm, 4 showed delayed sleep phase syndrome (DSPS) and 2 showed insomnia. VB_{12} at the daily dose of 1.5 mg t.i.d. was administered p.o. to each patient. Blood level of VB_{12} was examined before and during VB_{12} treatment in 6 of the patients.

Results

VB_{12} treatment was markedly effective for 2 patients with non-24-h sleep-wake rhythm, effective for 1 of the 4 patients with DSPS and the remaining 2 patients with insomnia.

The blood level of VB_{12} in 6 of 7 patients examined was within the normal range before starting the treatment, and was much higher than the normal range during the treatment.

Detailed findings in patients 1 and 7 have been reported elsewhere [1]. Sleep records in patients 2 and 8 are shown in Figs. 1a and 1b. Patient 2 was a 12-year old boy suffering from a non-24-h sleep-wake rhythm since 5 years of age and had difficulty in attending school. At 11 years of age, in early June of 1989, his treatment with VB_{12} was started. However, VB_{12} was not effective in the initial month. Then, in addition to VB_{12}, phototherapy with illumination of 2,500 lux was carried out every morning for 2 h. Since then, his sleep-wake rhythm disorder has

Table 1. Clinical features and vitamin B_{12} treatment

Case No.	Age (years)/ Sex	Sleep-wake disorder and complications	Serum level of VB_{12}[a]		Additional treatment	Effect
			Before[b]	During[b]		
1	17/F	Non-24-h, blind, mental retardation	560	2770		++
2	12/M	Non-24-h, school refusal, allergy	672	2650	Phototherapy	++
3	24/F	DSPS, depression	452		Triazolam	–
4	15/M	DSPS, school refusal, emotional disorder	803	2450		–
5	15/M	DSPS, school refusal	405			+
6	21/M	DSPS, periodic hypersomnia	659	2890	Phototherapy	–
7	56/M	Insomnia, chronic nephritis, brain multi-infarction				–
8	61/M	Insomnia, depression, brain infarction	3150	7200	Social interaction	+

DSPS: delayed sleep phase syndrome; [a]pg/ml; [b]before or during the treatment, ++: markedly effective; +: effective, –: not effective.

markedly improved. However, during a month of withholding the administration of VB_{12}, a non-24-h rhythm reappeared in spite of phototherapy. Since resuming VB_{12} administration in middle of September 1989, his sleep-wake rhythm disorder improved again, and he became able to attend school (Fig. 1a).

Patient 8 was a 61-year-old male suffering from insomnia and depressive state following brain infarction at 58 years of age. He showed signs of agitation, anxiety, and sometimes violent behavior to nurses or other patients. He slept briefly at a different time every day. Sometimes a reversed day-night sleep-wake rhythm was observed. For the treatment of his sleep-wake rhythm disorder and depressive state, phototherapy with illumination of 3,000 lux was carried out, but was ineffective. As increased contacts of attending nurses (social interaction) did not improve his depressive state and sleep disorder, VB_{12} treatment was added. About 10 days after starting the VB_{12} treatment, he slept mainly at night. In addition, his depressive state and behavioral disorder disappeared (Fig. 1b). Blood level of VB_{12} was much higher than the normal range both before and during the treatment, which was probably due to a prior injection of VB_{12} for his neuritis (Table 1).

Conclusions and Comments

From our study, VB_{12} is effective for the treatment of sleep-wake rhythm disorders, especially for a non-24-h sleep-wake rhythm. However, the mechanism through which VB_{12} produces beneficial effects on sleep-wake rhythm disorders is unclear at present. Possible mechanisms are as follows:

a) VB_{12} may change the period of the sleep-wake rhythm;

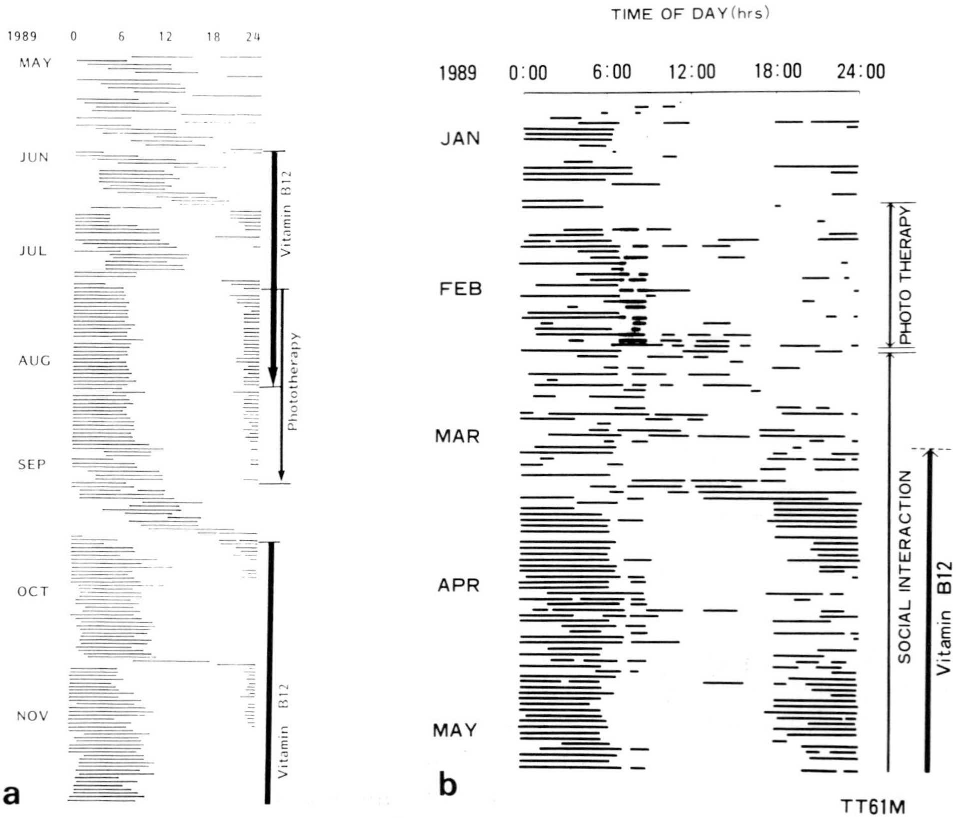

Fig. 1. The sleep-wake records in patients 2 (a) and 8 (b). Black horizontal bars represent sleep (see text).

b) VB_{12} may facilitate the entraining of the endogenous sleep-wake rhythm to the environmental 24-h rhythm. As suggested by the above-described findings, zeitgebers such as bright light or increased contacts of attending nurses seemed to be important;

c) VB_{12} may simply increase the amount of sleep, which was suggested by the findings in patients 7 and 8 with severe insomnia.

Blood level of VB_{12} was in the normal range before the VB_{12} treatment in all patients except patient 8 with prior injection of VB_{12}. Thus, patients whose sleep-wake rhythm disorders responded well to VB_{12} were not in a state of VB_{12} deficiency. In addition, it should be noted that sleep-wake rhythm disorder relapsed several days or a few weeks after discontinuation of the medication. Further study is needed to validate the efficacy of VB_{12} for sleep-wake rhythm disorders.

Reference

1. Okawa M, Mishima K, Hishikawa Y et al. (1990) Sleep 13: 15–23.

Biological Psychiatry, Volume 1. G. Racagni et al., editors.

Pathogenetic considerations on the antidepressant effect of sleep deprivation and the depressiogenic impact of daytime naps

Michael Wiegand[1], Dieter Riemann[2] and Mathias Berger[3]
[1]Psychiatric Clinic of the Technical University, Ismaninger Straße, 22, D-8000 Munich; [2]Central Institute of Mental Health, P.O. Box 5970, D-6800 Mannheim; and [3]Psychiatric University Clinic, Hauptstraße 5, D-7800 Freiburg, Germany

Introduction

The antidepressant effect of sleep deprivation and its possible reversal not only by sleep in the "recovery night" but even by a daytime nap [1] support the global hypothesis that sleep, under certain conditions, can impair mood in depression [2]. The following factors may be involved in the pathogenesis of the depressiogenic impact of daytime naps:

- under a chronobiological perspective, the timing of a nap within the circadian cycle may be relevant to its effect on mood [3];
- the "two-process-model of sleep regulation" [4] allows the prediction that the depressiogenic impact of a nap is related to its duration, its content of slow wave sleep, and the length of preceding wakefulness;
- from the cholinergic-aminergic imbalance hypothesis of depression and the reciprocal interaction model of REM sleep regulation [5] the expectation can be derived that the occurrence of REM sleep during a daytime nap, as a correlate of elevated cholinergic neuronal activity, should be accompanied by a greater propensity of relapse into depression.

The induction of depressive symptomatology by short sleep episodes, as a crucial experiment to test these hypotheses, was systematically examined in the present studies.

Materials and Methods

In 50 drug-free patients suffering from a major depression according to DSM III-R (14 male, 36 female, mean age 46.2 ± 13.2 years, mean Hamilton Depression Rating score (HAMD-21) 27.4 ± 5.5), a total of 85 total sleep deprivations (TSDs) were performed, followed by a nap on the following day at either 9:00, 13:00 or 15:00, recorded by polysomnography. Changes of depressive symptomatology were scored by means of the 6-item version of the Hamilton Depression Scale (HAMD-6 [6]). Response to total sleep deprivation was defined as a 30% reduction in the HAMD-6 score.

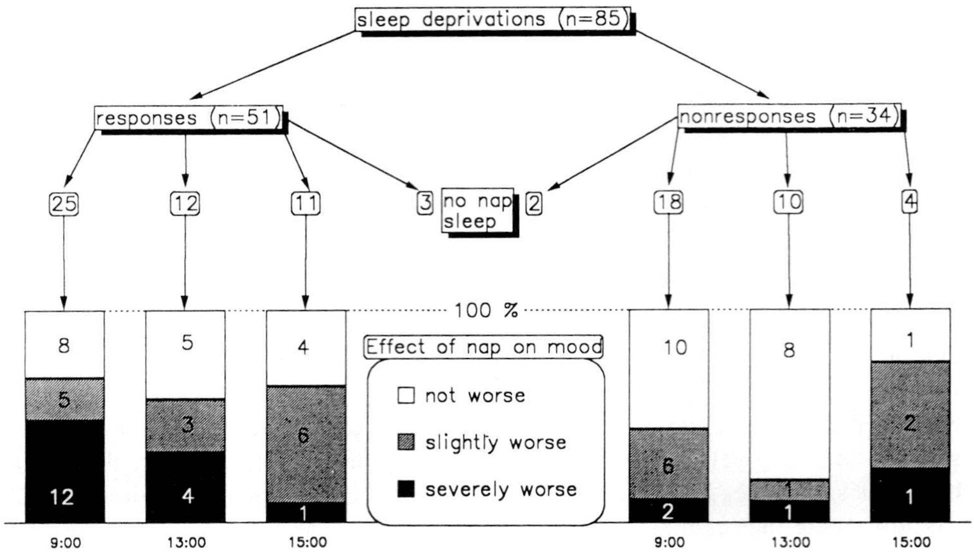

Fig. 1. Effects of sleep deprivations and daytime naps on depressive symptomatology.

Results

Figure 1 summarizes the effects of sleep deprivations and subsequent naps on depressive symptomatology. In responders to TSD, naps at 9:00 had more detrimental effects on mood than naps at 13:00 or 15:00. In non-responders to TSD, severe worsening was rare.

In a global analysis disregarding nap timing, neither the length of a daytime nap, nor the occurrence or the total amount of slow wave sleep were related to its impact on mood. The same held true for REM sleep: naps containing REM sleep did not differ from naps without REM sleep in the impact on depressive symptomatology, and there was no correlation between the amount of REM sleep during a nap and its effect on HAMD-6 scores. In a separate analysis of the 13:00 naps [1], the occurrence of REM sleep and longer nap sleep duration tended to be associated with worsenings.

Discussion

A daytime nap can reinduce depressive symptomatology in depressed patients who had improved by total sleep deprivation. The timing of a nap turned out to be crucial for its clinical effect: morning naps clearly had the most detrimental impact on responders to TSD, whereas afternoon naps were far better tolerated. This finding supports theories which emphasize the role of circadian factors and suggests that there may be a circadian variation of propensity to relapse into depression. However, since afternoon naps were preceded by longer wakefulness than morning naps, the results do not preclude "homeostatic" explanations as provided by Borbély [4] and Wu and Bunney [2]. Yet, the absence of any relationship between the duration of a nap, its content of slow wave sleep and its effect on symptomatology do not support these hypotheses.

Apart from a tendency observed in the 13:00 naps, the occurrence of REM sleep was not generally related to relapses into depression; thus, the prediction derived from the cholinergic-aminergic imbalance model of depression could not be confirmed. This does not necessarily refute the hypothesis that cholinergic overactivity may be involved in relapses into depression caused by a daytime nap. The data rather qualify the role of REM sleep as a reliable indicator of the cholinergic tone. A circadian variation of cholinergic functioning may be involved in the different pathogenic impact of naps at different times of the day, without being necessarily mirrored in variations of REM propensity in short naps.

References

1. Wiegand M, Berger M, Zulley J, Lauer C and von Zerssen D (1987) Biol. Psychiatry 22: 389–392.
2. Wu JC and Bunney WE (1990) Am. J. Psychiatry 147: 14–21.
3. Wehr TA and Wirz-Justice A (1981) In: Xoella WP (ed) Sleep 1980. Karger, Basel, pp. 26–33.
4. Borbély AA (1987) Pharmacopsychiatry 20: 23–29.
5. McCarley RW (1982) Am. J. Psychiatry 139: 565–570.
6. Bech P, Gram LF, Dein E, Jacobson O, Vither J and Bolwig TG (1975) Acta Psychiatr. Scand. 51: 161–170.

Biological Psychiatry, Volume 1. G. Racagni et al., editors.

Therapeutic sleep deprivation and antidepressant medication

S. Kasper, S. Ruhrmann, G. Höflich and H.-J. Möller

Psychiatric Department of the University of Bonn, 5300 Bonn, Sigmund Freudstr. 25, Germany

Introduction

There is an agreement in the literature about the acute antidepressant response of one night of partial or total sleep deprivation (SD) in depressed patients [1] and there is some evidence that repeated SD can be effective for subchronic treatment of major depressed patients [2]. The interaction between SD and antidepressive medication has been studied with regard to the predictive properties of SD for subsequent treatment with antidepressants [3] and whether there is an additive effect between these two [2,4] treatment conditions. Furthermore, there are a few reports in the literature about the effect of SD for the group of patients which have been classified as resistant to antidepressant medication [2].

Response to SD and prediction for subsequent treatment with antidepressants

Different investigators have attempted to predict the outcome of antidepressive treatments based on the initial response of a patient to SD (see Table 1). The published data do not support the notion that those patients who demonstrate a favourable outcome on the first day after SD (day-1 response) have a beneficial response to any antidepressants, irrespective of the mechanism of action [3]. On the other hand, there are two studies (Wirz-Justice et al., 1976; Fähndrich, 1983) which suggest that day-1 responders benefit from a medication which potentiates serotonergic neurotransmission. However, this finding has not been replicated. Psychopathological changes during the sleep deprivation procedure have been documented on the first day (day-1 response) as well as on the second day (day-2 response) after SD. Based on clinical observations Wirz-Justice et al. (1976) have suggested the predictive properties of the day-2 response for subsequent treatment with the noradrenalin reuptake inhibitor, maprotiline, which was confirmed recently by our group using a double-blind design [4]. This finding could be of clinical importance, since it offers the opportunity to decide early in the course of an antidepressant therapy which drug might be most promising for the subsequent therapeutic efficacy.

Although there are significant associations reported in the literature between the response to SD and the subsequent treatment outcome of antidepressants with a

Table 1. Sleep deprivation and antidepressants in depressed patients

	Predictive value[a]	Additive effect[b]
Open Studies		
Pflug and Tölle, 1971	n.d.	Amitryptiline
Loosen et al., 1976	n.d.	Clomipramine
Svendsen, 1976	n.d.	Various antidepressants
Pflug, 1976	n.d.	Amitryptiline
van Scheyen, 1977	n.d.	Various antidepressants
Philipp, 1978	n.d.	Lofepramine ± lithium
Dessauer et al., 1985	n.d.	Various antidepressants
Fähndrich, 1985	n.d.	Amitryptiline
Holsboer-Trachsler et al., 1988	n.d.	Various antidepressants
Wirz-Justice et al., 1976	+	n.d.
Wirz-Justice et al., 1979	(+)	n.d.
Fähndrich, 1983	+	n.d.
Amin, 1978	–	n.d.
Höchli et al., 1986	–	n.d.
Riemann and Berger, 1990	–	n.d.
Double-Blind		
Elsenga and van den Hofdakker, 1983	n.d.	Clomipramine vs. placebo
Baxter et al., 1986	n.d.	Lithium vs. placebo
Kasper et al., 1990b	+	Fluvoxamine vs. maprotiline

[a]predictive value for specific acting antidepressants;
[b]on course of treatment;
n.d. = not determined;
– = response to SD predicts response to specific acting antidepressants;
(+) = response to SD predicts response to antidepressants, irrespective of mechanism of action;
– = response to SD does not predict response to specific acting antidepressants;
References in Kasper (1990a).

specific mechanism of action, it is premature to use this as a distinction between biochemical subtypes within the depressive spectrum, e.g. serotonergic or noradrenergic subtype of depression. This cautiousness is warranted because in the living brain it is likely that interference with one neuronal system gives rise to a series of adjustments in the central nervous system. Furthermore, from a methodological point of view there are several limitations in the interpretation of these studies because they have been carried out in rather small number of patients [5].

Additive effect of SD and antidepressants

The data of the studies in which the antidepressant response to SD was evaluated in samples of depressed patients with and without antidepressive medication are indicative that 55–60% of depressed patients experience a temporary remission of depressive symptomatology on the day after they are kept awake for one night (day-1 response) [6]. Based on the results of these studies, it seems that the acute effect (day-1 response) is not dependent on the length of the washout period and also not on the medication status of patients, e.g. with or without medication or specifically acting antidepressants. This has been documented for total as well as for partial sleep deprivation [6]. However, there is some evidence that the concomitant administration of antidepressants during the SD procedure exerts an additive effect with the possibility of preventing the otherwise occurring relapse, at least partially (see Table 1). Since serotonin is reported to play an important role in the regulation of sleep it seems to be of interest that the latter finding has been documented specifically for antidepressants enhancing the serotonergic neurotransmission [3].

SD in therapy-resistant depression

Pflug and Tölle [7] were the first to report that repeated SD might be efficacious in patients which are resistant to antidepressive medication. Since then there have been a few uncontrolled studies and clinical observations published in the literature which confirmed the experience of the latter authors. In line with these findings we could document in a sample of 103 major depressed patients that the day-1 response to SD is not influenced by the fact of patients responding to previous antidepressant medication or not [2]. Based on the existing knowledge, it can be recommended that repeated SD, administered in addition to antidepressants, can still be beneficial for patients which are refractory to antidepressants alone. Nevertheless, we do not know if there is a superiority of specifically acting antidepressants for this treatment combination.

Conclusions

In conducting studies and interpreting sleep deprivation results researchers are challenged by technical difficulties because it is not possible to perform double-blind studies in sleep-wake manipulations. It therefore seems obvious that several methodological considerations need to be taken into account. These include:

1. the use of standardised clinical assessment scales and blind raters;
2. the control for spontaneous improvement which could also occur without SD;
3. the control for the influence of patient and experimenter expectations on the results.

However, in spite of these methodological drawbacks, it seems worthwhile to further study the interaction between psychopharmacological compounds and SD. A challenging task for future studies will be the prevention of relapse after recovery sleep, since it may well reveal information about the biological mechanism of antidepressive treatment modalities.

References

1. Wu JC and Bunney WE (1990) Am. J. Psychiatry 147: 14–21.
2. Kasper (1990a) In: HJ Möller (ed.) Therapieresistenz unter Antidepressiva-Behandlung. Springer, Berlin, Heidelberg, pp. 149–165.
3. Kasper S, Voll G, Vieira A and Kick H (1990b) Pharmacopsychiatry 23:135–142.
4. Elsenga S and van den Hoofdakker RH (1990) In: WE Bunney Jr., H Hippius, G Laakmann and M Schmauss (eds.) Neuropsychopharmacology Vol. 2, Springer, Berlin, pp. 639–651.
5. Möller H-J and Benkert O (1980) In: S Biefang (ed.) Evaluations-forschung in der Psychiatrie: Fragestellungen und Methoden. Enke, Stuttgart, pp. 54–128.
6. Wehr T (1990) In: J Montplaisir and R Godbout (eds.) Sleep and Biological Rhythms, Basic Mechanisms and Applications to Psychiatry. Oxford University Press, New York, pp. 42–86.
7. Pflug B and Tölle R (1971) Nervenarzt 42: 117–124.

Biological Psychiatry, Volume 1. G. Racagni et al., editors.

REM sleep parameters and psychiatric diagnosis

Carlo Maggini[1], Mario Guazzelli[2] and Antonio Ciapparelli[2]
[1]Clinica Psichiatrica III, Università di Bologna, Bologna; and [2]Clinica Psichiatrica I, Università di Firenze, Florence, Italy

Introduction

Disruption of sleep continuity, loss of delta sleep and changes in REM sleep are common to many psychiatric disorders [1]. However, most available data address the relative specificity of sleep abnormalities found in depression. Special attention has been devoted to REM sleep changes, and REM latency is the most widely studied EEG measure reported in the literature [1]. Since 1972, when short REM latency was considered an indicator of depression [4], the shortening of this parameter has been associated with the severity of the depressive episode [6], presence of endogenous and delusional features, response to tricyclic antidepressants and with vulnerability towards relapse after clinical remission [1]. REM latency measure has also been proposed as a validating criterion for diagnostic and classificatory purposes in psychiatric conditions supposedly affective in nature, despite their clinical presentation [1].

An accepted mechanism underlying REM latency abnormality is consistent with the cholinergic-aminergic imbalance theory of depression, i.e. an absolute or relative overactivity of the central cholinergic system [2].

However, diverging evidence complicates the issue of the specificity of REM latency shortening in depression: the reduction has been found in various psychiatric disorders [3] and even in non-psychiatric conditions [1]. Moreover, several studies and our own experience indicate that tricyclic antidepressant withdrawal, in healthy subjects and in psychiatric patients, is followed by clinical signs consistent with central and/or peripheral cholinergic overactivity [4], which could affect all-night EEG parameters. The significance of this phenomenon, potentially relevant in sleep research in depression, and its course over time have not received systematic attention, and need further study.

In our laboratory, the role of REM latency in depression has been investigated following these experimental approaches: a) we compared REM latency in a large sample of patients with major depression, bipolar disorder, manic and schizophrenia; and b) we designed an investigation, now in progress on the effects of REM latency after tricyclic antidepressant withdrawal in various psychiatric conditions. Very preliminary data concern 9 patients after first 48 h amitriptyline or clomipramine withdrawal.

Methodological approach and analysis of data

REM latency in major depression, bipolar disorder manic and schizophrenia disorder

This study has recently been published (see [3] for details); it was undertaken on 97 inpatients after 14 days of placebo treatment, who meet the DSM III criteria for major depression (depressives) (59 pts; mean age 54 years, Hamilton RSD total score 31; single episode 20, recurrent 39); bipolar disorder manic (manics) (15 pts; mean age 44 years; BPRS total score 38) and schizophrenic disorder (schizophrenics) (24 pts; mean age 38 years; actual relapse duration 6–11 weeks; paranoid type 13, undifferentiated type 6, disorganized type 5) with no positive familiarity for affective disorders and no past or present history of depression.

The second first sleep cycle of 2 consecutive nights was used for the study; REM latency included sleep stages 2, 3 and 4.

REM latency was 55.1 ± 5.2 min in depressives, 60.7 ± 9.1 min in manics, and 52.9 ± 7.6 min in schizophrenics; there were no significance differences between the groups. Delta sleep was 23.6 ± 2.8 min in depressives, 26.1 ± 4.9 min in manics, and 29.2 ± 4.1 min in schizophrenics and REM periods 15.3 ± 1.4, 15.1 ± 2.5 and 14.3 ± 2.1 min, respectively. Very short REM latency (< 20 min) was observed in about 14% of depressives, 7% of manics and 16% of schizophrenics. REM latency was not significantly correlated with REM period in depressives and manics while the correlation was positive ($r = 0.45$, $P < 0.05$) in schizophrenics; a positive, highly significant correlation with delta sleep was found in all groups. These results were confirmed by partial correlation analysis, positive and highly significant ($P < 0.001$) in all groups.

REM latency after tricyclic antidepressant withdrawal

Patients were recruited according to the following criteria: need for therapy, interruption or change after at least three consecutive months of tricyclic antidepressant treatment; no concurrent psychotropic drug use, absence of any medical and neurologic disturbances, informed consent to the study protocol.

Experimental procedure: 2 weeks of controlled tricyclic therapy after admission (same drug and daily dose) followed by a 14-day single blind placebo administration. Clinical examination (videotaped), rating scale administration (Hamilton RSD, AIMS and RESE) and all-night EEG recordings were performed at the end of the 2-week drug treatment and at day 2, 5 and 14 during placebo administration.

Present data concern 9 patients (mean age 36.4 ± 14.4 years), major depressive (5 pts), obsessive-compulsive disorder (3 pts) and borderline personality disorder (1 pt) treated for over 6 months with amitriptyline (5 pts) and clomipramine (4 pts) at a daily dose of 75–150 mg. Within the first 48 h after drug withdrawal the following clinical signs were observed: abdominal pain (2 pts), diarrhea (2 pts), digestive impairment (1 pt), sweating (3 pts), transient (several hours) hypomanic switch (1 pt) and slight-moderate insomnia (5 pts). At baseline, sleep time was 380 min, sleep latency 10 min. Early morning awakening 45 min, awakening number 7.6, Stage 1 18%, Stage 2 47%, delta sleep 22% and REM 12%. REM latency was 104 min. No significant changes were observed after two days of drug withdrawal except for REM latency which fell to 56 min, with a 50% reduction. First sleep cycle parameters, such as cycle length (116 vs. 63 min, $P < 0.005$, Stage 2 (50 vs. 22 min, $P < 0.05$) and delta sleep (53 vs. 30 min $P < 0.05$) were significantly reduced, while REM period (12 vs. 10 min) was unchanged. No differences were observed between depression and other diagnoses and between amitriptyline and clomipramine patients.

Concluding remarks

Our data confirm current reports in the literature showing that in patients with major depression REM latency is consistently shortened [1]. Similar values, however, have been found in manic patients and non-depressed schizophrenics, thus indicating that short REM latency cannot be considered a specific feature of depression. The recent opinion of Buysse and Kupfer [5] that sleep EEG studies have limited usefulness as a clinical diagnostic tool in depression is further supported by this finding.

The preliminary phase of the investigation on the effects of tricyclic antidepressant withdrawal did not allow us to draw any conclusion. We can only mention that clinical signs currently related to central cholinergic overactivity [4] developed within 48 h after abrupt tricyclic antidepressant withdrawal and that at the same time a remarkable reduction of REM latency was observed in all studied patients. The long-term study of tricyclic antidepressant withdrawal effects, now in progress, will provide information on the relevance and course over time of these phenomena in various psychiatric conditions. Should we find similar results throughout the entire withdrawal protocol, questions will then arise on the validity of those investigations on REM latency in depression which use a 14-day washout period from previous therapies mostly tricyclic antidepressant.

REM latency shortening after tricyclic antidepressant withdrawal closely paralleled in these patients the reduction of first sleep cycle delta sleep without any change in the first REM period. These findings, and results of correlation analysis observed in the aforementioned three groups of patients, once again pose doubts on the question of whether REM latency reduction should be primarily considered a measure of REM sleep or of NREM sleep impairment in psychiatric patients.

References

1. Vogel G, Reynolds III CF, Akiskal HS, Lemmi H, Gillin JC, Zarcone V, Joseph KC, Dubè D, Sitaram N and Watson R (1989) In: Kryger MH, Roth T and William WC (eds.) Principles and Practice of Sleep Medicine. W.B. Saunders Co., pp. 413–430.

2. Sitaram N and Gillin JC (1980) Biol. Psychiatry 15: 925–955.
3. Maggini C, Guazzelli M, Pieri M, Lattanzi L, Ciapparelli A, Massimetti G and Rossi G (1986) New Trends Exp. Clin. Psychiatry 2: 93–101.
4. Dilsaver SC (1990) Prog. Neuro-Psychopharmacol. Biol. Psychiatry 14: 137–161.
5. Buysse DJ and Kupfer DJ (1990) J. Nerv. Ment. Dis. 178: 405–414.

Biological Psychiatry, Volume 1. G. Racagni et al., editors.

Reduced REM latency in schizophrenia: Pathophysiological mechanisms

Matcheri S. Keshavan, Charles F. Reynolds, Patricia Houck and Rohan Ganguli
Department of Psychiatry, Western Psychiatric Institute and Clinic, University of Pittsburgh, 3811 O'Hara Street, Pittsburgh, PA 15213, U.S.A.

Introduction

Polysomnographic studies have revealed several abnormalities in schizophrenia. Shortened REM latency is the most frequently reported abnormality; reduced slow wave sleep (SWS), reduced total sleep and impaired sleep continuity are also seen [1]. However, none of these findings have been found to be specific for schizophrenia and only a subgroup of schizophrenic patients seem to manifest these abnormalities.

The most consistent polysomnographic findings in psychiatric research are those in affective disorders, i.e. shortening of REM latency; patients with affective disorders also manifest reduced slow wave sleep [2]. Both these features are nonspecific and are seen in schizophrenia as well. However, there is an important difference: affective disorders are associated with increases in REM sleep amounts, as measured by REM density and REM %. In schizophrenia on the other hand, no consistent changes have been found.

There are, therefore, both similarities and differences between schizophrenia and affective disorders in regard to EEG sleep; clarification of the biological basis for these similarities and differences is likely to further our understanding of the pathophysiology of these disorders.

Sleep EEG in schizophrenia and affective disorders – common mechanisms

Many schizophrenic patients manifest affective symptomatology; there is also a genetic overlap, with many schizophrenic patients having family members with affective disorders and vice versa. It is thus possible that some schizophrenic patients may be biologically similar to affective disorders; such patients may be expected to have sleep findings similar to those in affective disorders. Indeed, there is some preliminary data supporting this. We have seen that schizophrenic patients with family histories of affective disorders have shorter REM latency and a trend for reduced δ sleep in the first NREM period than those without such histories [3].

Cholinergic mechanisms have been invoked as the possible mechanisms underlying shortened REM latency in affective disorders [4]. There is reason to suspect that this system may be similarly involved in schizophrenia as well. Schizophrenic patients have been described to show a rapid (supersensitive) REM sleep induction with the oral muscarinic agonist RS-86 [5] and a reduced prolongation of REM latency with the muscarinic antagonist biperiden [6]. There is also preliminary evidence for increased plasma cholinesterase (ChE) activity in schizophrenia [7]; we have observed an inverse relation between plasma ChE and REM latency in 19 schizophrenic patients.

Sleep EEG differences been schizophrenia and affective disorders

As noted earlier, schizophrenic patients, by contrast with affective disorders, have shortened REM latencies *without* consistent change in the amount of REM sleep. Two explanatory models may serve to clarify this difference.

1. REM latency reduction in schizophrenia may be mainly related to reduced SWS in the first NREM period [9]. SWS decrements in schizophrenia may thus be the primary abnormality and may be related to developmental deficits [10]. If this were true, one should see a significant relation between measures of SWS in NREM Period 1 and REM latency. In our series of 25 schizophrenic patients, we see only a weak relation if any between REM latency and mean % δ sleep ($r = 0.25$; $P < 0.2$); mean δ sleep (min) ($4 = 0.3$; $P < 0.2$), total automated δ counts ($r = 0.27$; N.S.) and δ counts in the first NREM period ($r = 0.20$; N.S.). On the other hand, the REM % sleep had a significant negative relation to REM latency ($r = -0.48$; $P < 0.02$). Thus, NREM mechanisms may contribute only very modestly to reductions in REM latencies in schizophrenia; perhaps REM mechanisms play a role.
2. It is also possible that *both* SWS and REM mechanisms contribute to REM latency in schizophrenia. Kupfer and Ehlers [11] have proposed that there are 2 roads to shortened REM latency: type 1, a "trait" marker mainly related to SWS mechanisms and perhaps to familiar and developmental factors and type 2, an "episode" marker mainly due to REM "pressure" and related to stress and illness severity. There are some data supporting this distinction. In our series of 11 schizophrenic patients, we have seen persistence of shortened REM latency in schizophrenia following acute and chronic neuroleptic treatment [12]; however, Taylor et al. [13] have recently shown that in some schizophrenic patients REM latency returns to normal following treatment. Interestingly, they also found that while shortened REM latency was related to illness severity and negative symptoms before beginning of treatment, such relation was not seen following 3–4 weeks of treatment. This is consistent with the possibility that an episode-related process and a process unrelated to clinical severity could contribute to the shortening of REM latency in schizophrenia.

It is thus possible that REM latency in schizophrenia may not be a singular phenomenon; both "roads" to shortened REM latency, described by Kupfer and

Ehlers, may exist. Kupfer and Ehlers [11] have speculated that separate neurochemical, perhaps peptidergic mechanisms may mediate the type 1 and type 2 deficits in depression; in this model, growth hormone releasing factor (GRF) is thought to underlie SWS mechanisms and corticotropin-releasing factor (CRF) may mediate REM mechanisms. The relation of these neuroendocrine systems to sleep abnormities in schizophrenia remains unclear.

Changes in other better studied neurotransmitter systems may also serve to explain the unique sleep EEG disturbances in schizophrenia. Dopaminergic and noradrenergic mechanisms are widely believed to be overactive during acute episodes of schizophrenia; DA and NE are inhibitory to REM sleep, but the timing of onset of REM sleep is mainly cholinergically mediated [14]. Thus, the NE/DA overactivity in the schizophrenia episodes may counter the possibly cholinergically mediated REM sleep increases [15].

In summary, schizophrenics have a unique profile of sleep EEG findings with shortened REM latency without alterations in REM sleep amounts. While commonalities exist between schizophrenia and affective disorder, important differences also exist, and may elucidate distinct neurobiological mechanisms. Future studies need to examine sleep findings in schizophrenia, paying close attention to: a) family history; b) state vs. trait differences; and c) neurochemical and neuroendocrine correlates.

References

1. Keshavan MS, Reynolds CF and Kupfer DJ (1990) Compr. Psychiatry 30: 34–47.
2. Reynolds CF and Kupfer DJ (1987) Sleep 10: 199–215.
3. Keshavan MS, Reynolds CF, Ganguli R, Brar JS, Houck PR and Kupfer DJ (1990) In: Book of Abstracts. 1990 Annual Meeting. Association of Professional Sleep Societies. Rochester, MN.
4. Sitaram N, Nurnberger J, Gershon ES and Gillian JC (1980) Science 208: 200–202.
5. Reimann D, Fleckenstein P, Hohagen F, Olbrich R and Berger M (1990) In: Book of Abstracts, 1990 Annual Meeting. Association of Professional Sleep Societies. Rochester, MN.
6. Tandon R, Greden JF and Shipley JE (1990) Biol. Psychiatry 27: 96A.
7. Mahadik SP, Mukhojee S, Korenorsky A, Reddy R and Schnuo DB (1989) Biol. Psychiatry 25: 172A.
8. Keshavan M, Reynolds CF, Mahadik SP, Mukhojee S, Korenorsky A, Jarett D and Houck P (1991) Schizophr. Res. 4(3): 334.
9. Hiatt JF, Floyd TC, Katz PH and Feinberg I (1985) Arch. Gen. Psychiatry 42: 797–802.
10. Feinberg I (1982) J. Psychiatr. Res. 17: 319–334.
11. Kupfer DJ and Ehlers CL (1989) Arch. Gen. Psychiatry 46: 945–948.
12. Keshavan MS, Reynolds C, Brar J, Houck P, Campbell K, Ganguli R and McEvoy J (1989) Biol. Psychiatry 25: 181A.
13. Taylor SF, Tandon R, Shipley JE and Eiser AS (1991) Biol. Psychiatry.
14. Shiromani PJ (1989) Sleep Res. 18: 443.
15. Tandon R and Greden JF (1989) Arch. Gen. Psychiatry 46: 745–753.

Biological Psychiatry, Volume 1. G. Racagni et al., editors.

REM latency, eye movement density and slow wave sleep in schizophrenia and depression

Kathleen L. Benson and Vincent P. Zarcone, Jr.

Department of Psychiatry and Behavioral Sciences, Stanford University School of Medicine and VA Medical Center, 3801 Miranda Avenue, Palo Alto, CA 94304, U.S.A.

Introduction

Schizophrenia is characterized by a profound insomnia which is associated with long sleep onset latencies, slow wave sleep deficits, a reduction in the length of the first non-REM cycle (REM latency) and an increase in REM sleep eye movement activity. These abnormalities and others not only characterize sleep in schizophrenia but are also observed in other psychiatric diagnoses such as major depressive disorder. They may also be strongly age-dependent. This paper reviews the principal measures of sleep architecture from the point of view of diagnostic specificity.

Methods

Subjects were either healthy controls (n = 19) or psychiatric inpatients (n = 116) at the Palo Alto VA Medical Center. All subjects were male and their ages ranged from 19 to 66. The controls were screened for psychopathology using the Structured Clinical Interview of Burdock and Hardesty. The patients met Research Diagnostic Criteria for schizophrenia (n = 49), schizoaffective disorder (n = 17) or major depressive disorder (n = 50). All were unmedicated. Subjects were included in analyses if they had 2 consecutive data nights preceded by at least 1 adaptation night. The sleep data were averaged over the 2 polysomnograms. The Rechtschaffen and Kales conventions were applied in visually scoring the records for sleep stages.

Analyses

Data were analyzed by analysis of covariance. Differences in age of onset for schizophrenia and major depressive disorder underscore the need to control for age effects. The results are summarized in Table 1.

Table 1. Sleep measures in 4 diagnostic groups (mean and S.D. in parentheses); Pearson correlation with age (column 5)

	Normals (n = 19)	Schiz. (n = 49)	Schiz.-Aff. (n = 17)	MDD (n = 50)	Correlation (n = 135)
Sleep latency	15.54	70.13	77.89	33.72	−0.16
	(10.44)	(52.26)	(54.66)	(26.45)	$P = 0.062$
Wake after sleep onset	8.44	25.47	33.37	39.09	0.50
	(8.47)	(22.83)	(41.57)	(39.82)	$P < 0.0001$
Total sleep time	446.21	367.24	351.79	384.53	−0.23
	(15.88)	(60.13)	(79.37)	(58.43)	$P = 0.007$
Sleep efficiency (%)	94.47	79.57	76.16	84.29	−0.18
	(2.45)	(11.57)	(17.17)	(10.12)	$P = 0.033$
No. of wakes	6.63	15.13	12.64	18.18	−0.55
	(4.63)	(9.31)	(8.10)	(10.66)	$P < 0.0001$
REM latency	88.24	54.09	58.31	50.38	−0.18
	(41.59)	(20.62)	(25.72)	(19.17)	$P = 0.037$
Stage REM (min)	102.52	80.28	70.17	82.80	−0.33
	(13.63)	(23.30)	(28.54)	(28.25)	$P < 0.0001$
Stage REM (%)	23.29	21.99	20.24	21.77	−0.29
	(3.32)	(4.67)	(5.43)	(6.27)	$P = 0.001$
Stage 1 (min)	30.12	47.95	46.35	60.49	0.53
	(15.40)	(23.50)	(21.49)	(27.95)	$P < 0.0001$
Stage 1 (%)	6.85	13.60	13.71	16.56	0.58
	(3.58)	(7.01)	(5.78)	(7.88)	$P < 0.0001$
Stage 2 (min)	225.92	188.93	180.52	197.17	−0.08
	(30.37)	(39.17)	(48.92)	(42.40)	$P = 0.357$
Stage 2 (%)	51.15	52.58	52.34	52.69	0.15
	(6.06)	(7.67)	(6.90)	(8.85)	$P = 0.077$
Stage 3 (min)	36.23	32.56	34.89	23.64	−0.42
	(19.08)	(22.61)	(18.67)	(20.10)	$P < 0.0001$
Stage 3 (%)	8.16	9.40	10.69	6.08	−0.34
	(4.20)	(6.93)	(5.99)	(4.95)	$P < 0.0001$
Stage 4 (min)	46.10	9.53	11.84	11.34	−0.36
	(25.58)	(17.95)	(18.63)	(20.02)	$P < 0.0001$
Stage 4 (%)	10.53	2.40	3.00	2.88	−0.36
	(6.03)	(4.39)	(4.60)	(5.03)	$P < 0.0001$

Results

With the exception of stage 2 measures, all sleep variables were correlated with age to some degree. The strongest relationships were with the amount of waking and the number of awakenings after sleep onset as well as with measures of stage 1 sleep. The following 5 measures were related only to age and showed no effect of *diagnosis*: wake after sleep onset, stage 1 minutes, stage 3 minutes and percent, and REM percent. The controls differed significantly from all 3 psychiatric groups on the following measures: total sleep, sleep efficiency, REM time, REM latency, stage 1 percent, stage 2 minutes, stage 4 minutes, and stage 4 percent. Sleep latency in the controls was significantly less than in the schizophrenics or schizo-affectives; the controls did not differ from the depressives on this measure. The controls also had fewer wakenings than the schizophrenics or the depressed. Finally, the following measures did not differentiate the 3 psychiatric groups: stage 1 percent, stage 2 minutes and percent, stage 4 minutes and percent, REM latency and the number of awakenings. The schizophrenics and the schizoaffectives had longer sleep latencies and more total wake time than the depressives. The depressives had more total sleep, greater sleep efficiency and more REM time than the schizophrenics or the schizoaffectives. In summary, the only measure that differentiated the schizophrenics and schizoaffectives from both the controls and the depressives was sleep onset latency. Consequently, we should use considerable caution before we attribute diagnostic specificity to sleep measures.

Acknowledgements

These studies were supported by the Medical Research Service of the Department of Veterans Affairs and by Grants MH37252 and MH30854 from the U.S. National Institute of Mental Health.

Biological Psychiatry, Volume 1. G. Racagni et al., editors.

REM latency in insomnia with depression

Edward O. Bixler, Anthony Kales, Alexandros N. Vgontzas, Antonio Vela-Bueno and Rocco L. Manfredi

Department of Psychiatry, Pennsylvania State University College of Medicine, Hershey, PA 17033, U.S.A.

Introduction

During the last decade there has been a growing interest in the application of biomedical tests to psychiatric evaluation. Fifteen years ago, shortened rapid eye movement (REM) latency was proposed as a possible biological marker of depression [1]. Since then, extensive review of psychiatric sleep research has indicated a consensus that as a diagnostic clinical tool, sleep EEG studies of depression have limited function [2–4]. Nonetheless, in one recent study it was reported that polysomnographic results modified substantially the initial diagnosis in 60 of 123 chronic insomniacs; in 27 of these cases, the change in the initial diagnosis was based on the presence or absence of shortened REM latencies [5].

The purpose of our study was 2-fold: to assess the validity (sensitivity and specificity) of shortened REM latency as a diagnostic tool in differentiating depressed from non-depressed insomniacs; and to compare the maximum diagnostic usefulness of REM values to MMPI values in differentiating depressed from non-depressed insomniacs.

Methods

Subjects and Procedures

The study sample consisted of 375 consecutive subjects with a primary complaint of insomnia. Two hundred were recruited for research purposes, while 175 came to the sleep disorders clinic for evaluation and treatment of their insomnia. All of the subjects (mean age 43.2 ± 0.8 years) had a history of chronic (more than six months) difficulty with falling asleep, staying asleep, or both. The control group consisted of 150 healthy, non-medicated subjects (mean age 44.0 ± 1.4 years). Both subjects and controls were interviewed and then required to complete a comprehensive questionnaire and the MMPI. In addition, the clinic insomniacs underwent a comprehensive psychiatric evaluation conducted by two experienced psychiatrists (one of whom was a sleep disorders specialist). Diagnoses were established consensually by the two psychiatrists using DSM III-R criteria.

All subjects were evaluated in the sleep laboratory for one night using standard methods [6]. Throughout the study, subjects were instructed not to nap, not to alter significantly the level of their daily physical activity, and not to use any medications, other than those taken for pre-existing medical conditions.

Data analysis

Because there is no general agreement on the optimal diagnostic REM latency value [7–10], we evaluated three different latencies (<45, <55 and <65 min), respectively. The diagnostic utility of these three REM latency values was evaluated in terms of both sensitivity and specificity [11]. Potential effects of drugs and/or patient selection on sleep were accounted for in the analysis.

Diagnostic information provided by REM measures (REM latency, REM interval, mean duration of REM period, absolute and percent total REM duration and REM duration in the first, second and last thirds of the night, and number of REM periods) was maximized. The measures that were selected by a stepwise logistic regression analysis which included age and sex were empirically optimized by the method of Somoza and Mossman [12]. Further, we similarly established optimized diagnostic criteria based on the valid MMPIs which we contrasted to the optimized criteria for REM variables.

Results

One hundred and seventy-four of the 175 insomniacs evaluated in the clinic had at least one Axis I or Axis II diagnosis. One hundred and thirteen patients had a diagnosis of depression; 29 were diagnosed with major depression, and 84 with dysthymia. Only 13.8% of majorly depressed and 2.4% of dysthymic insomniacs were identified correctly by the sleep laboratory test. The sensitivity of the test increased somewhat with the higher cut-off values (55 and 65 min); 24.1% for majorly depressed vs. 14.3% for dysthymics when REM latency was chosen to be <65 min. The specificity of the test was high for non-depressed insomniacs and healthy controls; however, this specificity was decreased at the higher cut-off values of REM latency. In summary, almost equal numbers of depressed and non-depressed insomniacs were identified as "depressed" by the REM latency testing across the three different latencies (very low sensitivity and moderately high specificity).

The diagnostic utility of REM latency remained inadequate when, instead of clinical DSM III-R diagnoses, we determined depression in the sample of insomniacs and controls by using an elevated t-score (≥70) of MMPI depression scale. Again, almost equal numbers of insomniacs with MMPI D-scale t-scores ≥70 or <70 were identified as "depressed" by the REM latency testing across the three different latencies. The results were no different when we grouped the insomniacs according to their selection (clinic vs. research insomniacs) or drug use (drug-users vs. drug-free).

Finally, the diagnostic utility for depression of REM sleep measures was found to be inferior to the utility of MMPI measures. REM latency did not contribute to the discrimination between depressed and non-depressed insomniacs diagnosed using DSM III-R. Optimized REM values were associated with a sensitivity of 40% and a specificity of 82%, whereas for optimized MMPI values the sensitivity was 75% and the specificity was 62%.

Discussion

This is the first study to evaluate systematically the diagnostic utility of REM latency and REM variables in differentiating depressed from non-depressed insomniacs. Three different cut-off values of REM latency were associated with very low sensitivity and high specificity. The diagnostic accuracy of the test remained low both when DSM III-R criteria or a pathological score (≥70) in MMPI Depression Scale were used to determine the presence of depression. More importantly, the empirically optimized REM variables did not significantly improve the diagnostic performance of the test. In fact, REM latency did not contribute to the successful distinction between depressed and non-depressed insomniacs, a finding that confirms previous reports [13]. Also, optimized REM sleep variables were associated with less diagnostic accuracy than similarly optimized criteria based on MMPI values.

The sensitivity of REM latency or REM variables in this study is somewhat lower than in other studies [7–10]. This can be accounted for by the fact that our population was characterized as outpatient depressed insomniacs, whereas in the majority of other studies, the populations were more severely depressed inpatients.

In conclusion, REM latency or any REM variable is not useful in discriminating depressed insomniacs from non-depressed insomniacs. This population can be assessed and managed effectively in the psychiatrist's office by using his cognitive abilities and skills.

References

1. Kupfer (1976) Biol. Psychiatry 11: 159–174.
2. Campbell SS and Gillin JC (1987) Psychiatr. Ann. 17: 647–653.
3. Wehr TA (1988) Biological Rhythms and Mental Disorders. Guilford Press, New York.
4. Buysse DJ and Kupfer DJ (1990) J. Nerv. Ment. Dis. 178: 405–414.
5. Jacobs EA, Reynolds CR, Kupfer DJ et al. (1988) Am. J. Psychiatry 145: 3.
6. Rechtshaffen A and Kales A (1968) A Manual of Standardized Terminology, Techniques and Scoring System for Sleep Stages of Human Subjects. National Institutes of Health, Publication No. 204, Washington, D.C.
7. Akiskal HS, Lemmi H, Yerevanian B, King D and Bellumini J (1982) Psychiatr. Res. 7: 101–110.
8. Berger M, Doerr P, Lund R, Bronish T and von Zerssen D (1982) Biol. Psychiatry 17: 1217–1242.
9. Feinberg M, Gillin JC, Carroll BJ, Greden JF and Zis AP (1982) Biol. Psychiatry 17: 305–316.
10. Mendlewicz J, Kerhofs M, Hoffman G and Linkowski P (1984) Br. J. Psychiatry 145: 383–388.
11. Baldessarini RJ, Finklestein S and Arana GW (1983) Arch. Gen. Psychiatry 40: 569–573.
12. Somoza E and Mossman D (1990) Biol. Psychiatry 27: 990–1006.
13. Gillin JC, Duncan W, Pettigrew KD, Frankel BL and Snyder F (1979) Arch. Gen. Psychiatry 36: 85–90.

Biological Psychiatry, Volume 1. G. Racagni et al., editors.

Sleep EEG abnormalities in schizophrenia and depression are similar and not diagnostic of either condition

Irwin Feinberg

Psychiatry Service, VA Medical Center, Martinez, CA 94553; and University of California, Davis, CA 95616, U.S.A.

In my career in psychiatry, I have witnessed the rise and fall of several biological tests for the diagnosis and prognosis of mental disorders. Indeed, over 30 years ago, my first publication in a psychiatric journal [1] was a critical analysis of the literature on a biological marker (to use the now fashionable term) thought to have prognostic significance. I found that in spite of considerable research with this test over a period of several years, such basic issues as the reliability of the measurements and the contribution of age to the response had not been addressed.

We have met today to inter one of the more recent failed biological tests of a psychiatric condition: short REM latency (and its associated abnormalities) as a marker of depression. There can be no further doubt, from the work presented at this Symposium by the Pisa and Stanford groups, that short REM latency is not pathognomonic of depression and that it occurs with roughly equal frequency in schizophrenia. Because short REM latencies also occur in other psychiatric and neurological conditions, this non-specific finding is not even generally diagnostic of functional psychosis.

It may be appropriate to ask why it is that we psychiatrists suffer from a repetition compulsion that leads us embrace (often with unseemly passion) biological markers before they have been scientifically validated, only to be disappointed when their validity is disproved. Our loss is more than emotional, because the funds wasted – first in the uncritical application and exploration of the diagnostic test – and later in the controlled studies that lead to ultimate rejection – are often vast. Unfortunately, time does not permit consideration of this interesting question, which touches on the culture of contemporary psychiatric research.

It is certainly the case that the expensive career of short REM latency as a biological marker of depression was unnecessary from the outset. There was never any acceptable evidence presented for its specificity. Let us turn briefly to a parsimonious interpretation of short REM latency in mental illness, an interpretation whose broad outlines were apparent in the 1960s.

"REM latency" is, as I have argued for over twenty years, a misnomer since we are measuring the duration of the first period of NREM sleep (NREMP1). An abbreviated NREMP1 usually occurs in association with a reduction in its deep (Stage 4) sleep component. In addition, REMP1 duration and eye movement density in REMP1 are sometimes increased. Each of these changes is found in the sleep of normal elderly as compared to young adults [2]. Thus, age is obviously a potentially confounding factor, as is now being rediscovered.

In 1969 we noted that "The reduction in stage 4 EEG in the first NREM period may be responsible for certain anomalies of the first sleep cycle occasionally observed in schizophrenic patients. These anomalies include early onset of the first REM period and an increased duration of this period". We went on to state "...these latter findings, rather than representing primary alterations in REM mechanisms, are secondary to decreased pressure of NREM sleep" [3]. We also suggested that these findings might indicate decreased depth of sleep due to anxiety. Recently, we showed how an inverse relation of eye movement activity to depth of sleep (or central arousal level) accounts for virtually all of the known experimental variation in REM density [4].

We have reiterated our interpretations of the biological basis of short REM latency in schizophrenia and depression several times since 1969. For example, Feinberg and Hiatt suggested in 1978 that "it is probable that REM and NREM sleep are in dynamic interaction and for this reason the 2 kinds of sleep ought to be considered together rather than separately" [5]. Thus, the hypothesis that deficient NREM processes underlie the early REM onset in schizophrenia long antedates the restatement of this view [6] in terms of the "two-process" model. In any event, the pertinent (slow wave sleep) component of the "two-process" model was itself antedated by the homeostatic model of δ, which had been advanced 8 years earlier [7].

Acknowledgement

This work was supported by research funds from the Department of Veterans Affairs.

References

1. Feinberg I (1958) Arch. Neurol. Psychiatry 80: 488–501.
2. Feinberg I (1967) J. Psychiatr. Res. 5: 107–144.
3. Feinberg I, Braun M, Koresko RL and Gottlieb F (1969) Arch. Gen. Psychiatry 21: 262–266.
4. Feinberg I, Floyd TC and March JD (1987) EEG Clin. Neurophysiol. 67: 217–221.
5. Feinberg I and Hiatt JF (1978) In: Williams RL and Karacan I (eds.) Sleep Disorders: Diagnosis and Treatment. Wiley, New York, pp. 205–231.
6. Borbely AA and Wirz-Justice A (1982) Hum. Neurobiol. 1: 205–210.
7. Feinberg I (1974) J. Psychiatr. Res. 10: 283–306.

Biological Psychiatry, Volume 1. G. Racagni et al., editors.

Insomnia: Biopsychosocial correlates

Anthony Kales

Department of Psychiatry, Pennsylvania State University College of Medicine, 500 University Drive, Hershey, PA 17033, U.S.A.

Introduction

Insomnia, affecting about one third of the general population, may be secondary to a wide spectrum of psychiatric and medical conditions [1–3]. Transient sleep difficulty commonly develops in response to stressful events, life changes, or health problems. Chronic insomnia (excluding medical conditions) is often the consequence of life-stress factors, inadequate coping mechanisms [4], and internalization of emotions [1,2].

Clinical characteristics

In most patients with chronic insomnia, sleep difficulty begins before the age of 40 years [1,2]. Typically, they obtain varying amounts of sleep, with the most frequent problem being difficulty in falling asleep, either as a single complaint or in combination with difficulty in staying asleep or in early final awakening.

Characteristically, at bedtime insomniacs are tense and anxious and ruminate about unresolved issues of the day and other personal problems [1,2]. Physiologically, they show activation as manifested by increased heart rate, muscle tension, rectal temperature, and peripheral vasoconstriction. During the day, they often feel sleepy, physically and mentally tired, depressed, anxious, and irritable.

Causative factors

Transient or short-term insomnia usually arises due to temporary stresses, "jet lag" or some other situation that results in an irregular schedule of activity and rest [1,2]. In addition, medical conditions, particularly those associated with pain and discomfort, often induce sleep difficulty [1,2,5].

By far the most common etiologic factors in patients with chronic insomnia are the initiating underlying psychological vulnerabilities and disturbances as well as the subsequent behavioral conditioning effects of poor sleep, the fear of sleeplessness and performance anxiety. Minnesota Multiphasic Personality Inventory (MMPI) studies and psychiatric assessments of patients with long-standing insomnia reveal that about 80% have one or more MMPI scales elevated to the pathologic range;

depression, conversion hysteria and psychasthenia are the most frequently elevated scales [6]. In addition, dysthymic disorder and compulsive personality disorder or trait are the predominant DSM III diagnoses [7].

Because chronic insomniacs generally handle stress and conflicts by internalizing emotions, they tend to be emotionally aroused, causing increased autonomic activity at bedtime. Soon, fear of sleeplessness and performance anxiety develop, intensifying emotional arousal and creating a vicious circle. Thus, insomnia is perpetuated [1,2].

Evaluation process

The first step in evaluating insomnia is a complete history that assesses sleep, drug, medical, and emotional factors [1,2,5]. The sleep history consists of defining the specific problem, assessing its development and clinical course, and identifying possible precipitating or exacerbating circumstances [8].

The patient's emotional functioning over his or her entire life should be considered [1,2,8]. It is important to determine whether childhood psychological difficulties, especially those resulting from major family disruptions such as death or divorce, caused the patient to acquire inadequate mechanisms for coping with stress. The patient's mental status must be assessed to identify the presence of psychiatric disturbance, and, in the elderly, organicity [7]. Sleep apnea is rarely a cause in patients presenting with chronic insomnia; it is equally rare among chronic insomniacs and normal controls. Nevertheless, if at all suspected, a thorough history needs to be obtained from the bedpartner. When breath cessations are reported a sleep laboratory recording is in order.

Treatment methods

Insomniacs almost invariably resist treatment efforts because often they are preoccupied with their symptoms and invested in the secondary gain they receive. The key to successful treatment is to develop a multidimensional approach, combining elements from among several modalities [1,2].

Behavioral techniques

The psychiatrist may begin treatment by recommending methods for managing stress and avoiding sleep disturbance caused by commonly used drugs [1,2]. Times to go to bed and to rise should be regularized but not be inflexible. Other behavioral approaches such as stimulus control [9] and attribution techniques [10] may be useful.

Psychotherapy

Areas of psychological conflict should be identified very early in treatment, so that patients are more likely to become actively involved in therapy. The psychiatrist should use an active, directive approach to explore conflict areas rather than a more gradual, uncovering method [1,11].

Insight-oriented psychotherapeutic techniques may be most effective. Therapy provides the patient with a means for understanding and dealing with the suppressed psychological conflicts and emotions that precipitate emotional and physiologic arousal at night.

Pharmacotherapy

Benzodiazepine hypnotics have largely replaced other drugs in the adjunctive pharmacologic treatment of insomnia, primarily owing to their greater margin of safety and degree of effectiveness. Five benzodiazepines are marketed currently in the U.S. as hypnotics: flurazepam, temazepam, triazolam, and quazepam as well as estazolam, which has been recently introduced; significant data is lacking regarding its safety, particularly in terms of long-term use, drug dependence and withdrawal issues. In adults, for the long-term adjunctive drug treatment of chronic insomnia, intermittent use of flurazepam, 15 mg and quazepam, 15 mg is recommended. In the elderly, or whenever a milder short-term hypnotic effect is desired, temazepam 15 mg may be used. Triazolam is not recommended because of frequent and severe adverse reactions including: hyperexcitability states (early morning insomnia and daytime anxiety) [12] and cognitive impairment (memory impairment/amnesia, confusion, delusions, hallucinations and delirium) [13] both during drug administration; and withdrawal difficulties (rebound insomnia) following drug termination [14]. These serious safety concerns and the lack of efficacy of the recommended starting dose (0.25 mg) result in a very narrow benefit-to-risk ratio for triazolam [15].

A small percentage of patients with insomnia may be diagnosed as having major depression [7], a clear-cut indication for the use of antidepressant drugs. Antidepressants with sedative side-effects are generally indicated, with the medication being given at bedtime, when the need for sedation is greatest [1,2,11]. For psychotic patients with insomnia, neuroleptics with sedative effects are preferred [1,2].

References

1. Kales A and Kales JD (1984) Evaluation and Treatment of Insomnia. Oxford University Press, New York.
2. Kales A, Soldatos CR and Kales JD (1987) Ann. Intern. Med. 106: 582–592.
3. Bixler EO, Kales A, Soldatos CR et al. (1979) Am. J. Psychiatry 136: 1257–1262.
4. Healey ES, Kales A, Monroe LJ et al. (1981) Psychosom. Med. 43: 439–451.
5. Berlin RM, Litovitz GL, Diaz MA et al. (1984) Am. J. Psychiatry 141: 582–584.

6. Kales A, Caldwell AB, Soldatos CR et al. (1983) Psychosom. Med. 45: 341–356.
7. Tan TL, Kales JD, Kales A et al. (1984) Am. J. Psychiatry 141: 357–362.
8. Kales A, Soldatos CR and Kales JD (1980) Am. Fam. Physician 22: 101–108.
9. Nicassio P and Bootzin R (1974) J. Abnorm. Psychol. 83: 253–260.
10. Haynes SN, Price MG and Simons JB (1975) J. Behav. Ther. Exp. Psychiatry 6: 279–282.
11. Kales A, Kales JD and Bixler EO (1974) Psychiatr. Ann. 4: 28–44.
12. Kales A, Soldatos CR and Bixler EO (1983) Science 220: 95–97.
13. Bixler EO, Kales A, Manfredi RL, Vgontzas AN, Tyson K and Kales JD (1991) Lancet 337: 827–831.
14. Kales A, Scharf MB and Kales JD (1978) Science 201: 1039–1041.
15. Kales A (1990) N. Engl. J. Med. 323: 486–487.

Biological Psychiatry, Volume 1. G. Racagni et al., editors.

Macro- and micro-structure of sleep in insomniac patients under the influence of a benzodiazepine and a non-benzodiazepine hypnotic

Hartmut Schulz[1,2], Marc Jobert[1] and Peter Jähnig[1]
[1]AFB Arzneimittelforschung GmbH, Berlin; and [2]Freie Universität Berlin, Psychiatric Clinic, Berlin, Germany

Introduction

Polysomnography is today a standard method of evaluating the effect of a hypnotic compound on sleep and of comparing the profile of different hypnotics. But, while the visual analysis of sleep [1] gives only a rough picture of the macro-structure of sleep, computerized analysis is a suitable technique to quantify different aspects of the macro- as well as of the micro-structure of sleep.

The aim of this study was to compare the effect of the benzodiazepine lormetazepam and the cyclopyrrolone zopiclone on the visual observations and computer-analyzed sleep. A central question of this comparison was, whether the 2 compounds differ in their effect on slow-wave activity (SWA). It has been claimed that non-benzodiazepines such as zopliclone may differ in this respect from the benzodiazepines, which are known to reduce SWA in the sleep EEG [2,3]. The following analysis will focus on some aspects of the sleep EEG.

Subjects

Sixteen subjects (12 females, 4 males; mean age ± S.D.: 66.7 ± 5.8 years) with a chronic or subchronic form of psychophysiological insomnia [4] were included. All patients were free of hypnotics, tranquilizers or other CNS-active medication for at least 14 days before the start of the study.

Design

The trial was planned according to a randomized, placebo-controlled, double-blind 3-way crossover design to compare lormetazepam (1 mg), zopiclone (7.5 mg) and placebo. Each treatment was given on 3 consecutive days, 1/2 h before going to bed. The randomized treatment phases took place at weekly intervals (nights 6–8, 13–15 and 20–22). Sleep was polygraphically recorded in the sleep laboratory on trial days 1 (adaptation night), 8, 15 and 22.

Sleep recording

Sleep was recorded for 8 h between 10:30 p.m. and 6:30 a.m. The following EEG derivations were used: C4-A1, C3-A2 and Fz, Cz, Pz and Oz against left mastoid (A1) reference. In addition, horizontal and vertical eye movement (EOG) and muscle tone from the chin region (EMG) were recorded.

Sleep analysis

Sleep was analyzed visually and by the computer. For computer analysis the EEG signal from the central electrode (Cz) was split into 10-s epochs for which power spectra were estimated using Fast Fourier Transformation (FFT). The mean power in 6 frequency bands was computed and compared for the 3 medication conditions. The 6 frequency bands were defined as follows: δ_1: 0.5–2.0 Hz, δ_2: 2.0–4.0 Hz, θ: 4.0–8.0 Hz, α: 8.0–11.5 Hz, β_1: 11.5–15.0 Hz and β_2: >15.0 Hz.

In a first step, the spectral activity in each frequency band under placebo was taken as baseline level and set as 100%. The data for each night under active medication were expressed as percentage of the placebo value. These difference values were averaged over all patients and graphically represented.

Descriptors for the micro-structure of sleep were sleep spindles and K-complexes in the EEG. The number of phasic EEG events was determined by a computer algorithm for those segments of the recording, which were visually analyzed as stage-2 sleep.

Results

EEG power spectrum

Both active medications induced similar EEG changes when compared to placebo. Power was significantly reduced in the δ_2, θ and α frequency band, while it was increased in the 2 β bands ($P < 0.01$). Zopiclone differed from lormetazepam only in the δ_2 band, where the power was more reduced under zopiclone ($P = 0.0365$). For all frequency bands the difference from placebo was more pronounced for zopiclone than for lormetazepam (see Fig. 1).

Sleep spindles and K-complexes

The density of sleep spindles was increased under lormetazepam ($P = 0.0032$) and zopiclone ($P = 0.0001$) compared with placebo, while the density of K-complexes was diminished for both active medications ($P = 0.0009$). With regard to these 2 parameters, the 2 drugs did not differ from each other.

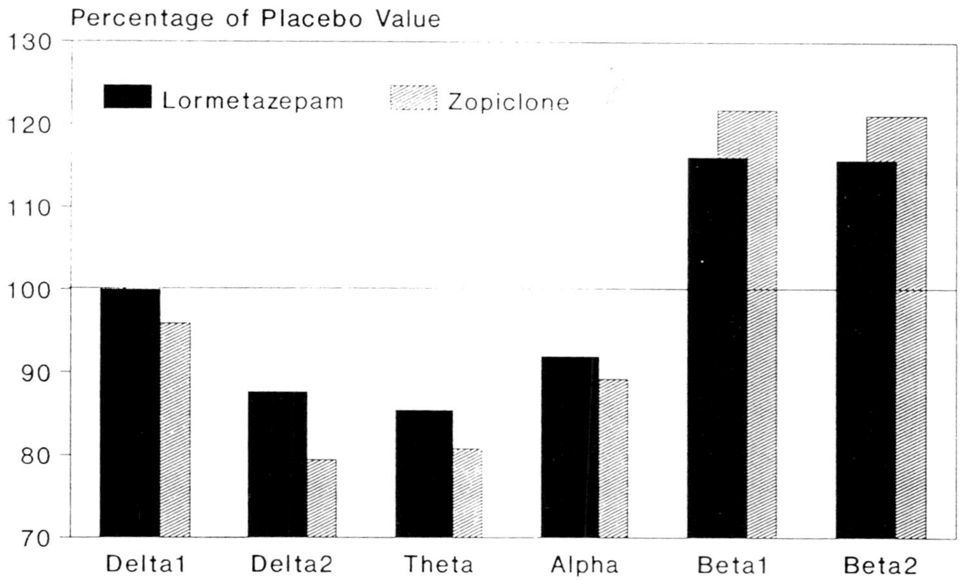

Fig. 1. Effects of lormetazepam (1 mg; black bars) and zopiclone (7.5 mg; shaded bars) on the sleep EEG power densities. The power under medication is expressed for each of the 6 frequency bands as percentage of the respective placebo value, which is indicated by the 100% line.

Discussion

The results presented here are part of a larger analysis of a comparative study between the effect of a benzodiazepine and a non-benzodiazepine on sleep. They demonstrate some advantages of a computerized sleep analysis in comparison to visual analysis. The computerized analysis allows a true quantification of EEG and non-EEG variables.

Both active medications had a very similar effect on the sleep EEG. Activity in the δ_1 (0.5–2.0 Hz) frequency band was not altered by the two hypnotics. This finding corresponds to the result from the visual analysis that SWS sleep was unaltered. Visually analyzed SWS is based on the EEG information in the frequency band 0.5–2.0 Hz. In the other frequency bands both medications induced either decreases in power (δ_2, θ and α) or increases (β_1 and β_2). The effects were very similar for lormetazepam and zopiclone.

If we compare EEG features of the micro-structure of sleep, again both compounds acted similarly by reducing the number of K-complexes and increasing the number of sleep spindles. Thus, one may conclude that the two compounds display great similarities in their effect on the sleep EEG.

References

1. Rechtschaffen A and Kales A (eds.) (1968) A Manual of Standardized Terminology, Techniques and Scoring System for Sleep Stages of Human Subjects. Public Health Service, U.S. Government Printing Office, Washington D.C.
2. Nicholson AN and Stone BM (1983) Pharmacology (Suppl. 2) 27: 92–97
3. Mouret J (1986) Delta sleep enhancement with zopiclone. 8th European Congress of Sleep Research, Szeged, Abstract Vol. p. 242.
4. Diagnostic classification steering committee, Thropy MJ, chairman (1990) International Classification of Sleep Disorders: Diagnostic and Coding Manual. American Sleep Disorders Association, Minnesota.

Biological Psychiatry, Volume 1. G. Racagni et al., editors.

Obstructive sleep apnea syndrome: Clinical, evolutive and epidemiological aspects

E. Lugaresi and E. Sforza
Institute of Neurology, University of Bologna, Italy

The obstructive sleep apnea syndrome (OSAS) involves a complex series of different symptoms and signs but snoring and apnea during sleep are usually the key features defining the condition. The incidence of OSAS is from 22% to 43%, of patients referred to sleep laboratories for daytime sleepiness or snoring. But, the effective incidence of OSAS in the general population is unclear. The convergence of snorers with OSAS patients was confirmed in a study by Cirignotta et al. [1] in 40 everynight snorers in which the AI was over 5 in 50% and over 10 in 33%. A point of great controversy is the validity of self-report in the diagnosis of OSAS. A study on the relative validity of self-reported snoring as a symptom of OSAS found that most men replied affirmatively to the question regarding snoring but this was less apparent for intermittent snoring [2].

To evaluate the relationship between OSAS and subjective symptoms we examined a group of 272 patients referred to us for sleepiness (58 patients) and snoring (214), all diagnosed as OSAS patients by polygraphic study. The patients were asked by questionnaire about snoring, sleepiness, smoking and hypertension between May 1989 and May 1991 (Table 1). In our population females were 13% and men 87%. The mean age of patients was of 49.8 years and their BMI of 30.2. All patients reported habitual snoring: in 15% for less than 5 years, in 21% between 5 and 10 and in 56% for more than 10 years; 8% did not evaluate the onset of snoring. Intermittent snoring was reported in 85% of patients and apnea always in 66% and sometimes in 33%. In the snorer group 67% reported sleepiness during

Table 1. Subjective evaluation of symptoms in OSAS (n = 272)

	Sleepy (58)	Snorers (214)	Total (%)
Snoring	58	214	100
Intermittent snoring	43	188	85
Apnea	36	145	66
Onset of snoring			
<5 years	4	37	15
>5 <10 years	10	48	21
>10 years	37	114	56
Unknown	7	15	8
Sleepiness	58	143	74

monotonous conditions and 19% also during activity. This evaluation showed how the history of patients runs a typical evolution: the patient is a habitual snorer for many years and does not exhibit typical features in the early stage defined as asymptomatic. Then intermittent snoring and sleepiness become evident and finally diurnal hypoventilation and cardiovascular disease appear. However, of 100 patients examined in our center [3], the onset of snoring is reported at about the age of 25, frequently not associated with significant changes in BMI. Then at about 40 intermittent snoring is reported by patients or spouse. The onset of daytime sleepiness is followed by apneas. The interval of time between the onset of sleepiness and referral to a sleep center is 2–5 years.

The subjective and objective history in OSAS patients confirms our hypothesis of a continuum in severity from pure or asymptomatic snoring to the full-blown OSAS [4]. Because many years can elapse between the onset of snoring and complaints of sleepiness a large series of studies are needed to analyse the role of different factors in the progression of the disease and the start of cardiorespiratory risk. Different factors are involved in the transition of snoring in a typical OSAS:
- age at snoring onset
- obesity
- smoking
- anatomical factors
- functional factors

The most frequent factors are age, obesity and smoking.

Age

The early onset of snoring has been stressed in different studies as a factor involved in severe evolution of the syndrome. In our population the predictors of hypoxemia in stage 3 patients are BMI and age at onset of snoring. Thus patients who begin snoring early in life are more prone to develop a severe form of OSAS: a probable role of a greater BMI present at the onset of snoring may be stressed.

Obesity

Obesity plays a role with 2 different effects: a) the mechanical difficulty due to fat deposition in the pharynx; b) and reduced ventilation by the decreased ventilatory drive and mismatched ventilation-perfusion. In our patients a clear correlation between progressive increase of weight and increased intensity of snoring is reported by the spouse.

Table 2. Evolutive factors in OSAS population (n = 272)

	Sleepy (58)	Snorers (214)	Total (%)
Non-smokers	36	151	69
Smokers >10	17	49	24
Smokers >20	5	14	7
Hypertension	13	46	22
Hypertension history	14	61	28

Smoking

The role of smoking has recently been stressed. After adjustment for age and BMI there is an exposure effect to smoking [5]. However the prevalence of snoring among ex-smokers was higher than among non-smokers. In our population examined by the questionnaire (Table 2) 69% were non-smokers and 32% smokers. In the smoker group 24% regularly smoked more than 10 cigarettes and 7% more than 20 a day. In the group smoking more than 10, 29% smoked 20 cigarettes a day. Most patients smoking more than 20 were among the sleepy subjects (snorers: 6.5% sleepy 32.6%) and patients with a severe syndrome. In our opinion, smoking may contribute to severity of the disease, probably by the lung function impairment.

The role of snoring in the incidence of complications is confirmed by studies showing that snoring is a risk factor for cardiovascular diseases and hypertension [6,7]. In our patient group (Table 2) hypertension was reported in 22% of snorers and in 19% of sleepy subjects with an overall incidence of 22% prone whereas a history of transient increase of blood pressure in 28%. Yet, the role of snoring in the genesis of hypertension is controversial. Different studies [8] conducted with oxymeter evaluation have recently shown that obesity and nocturnal hypoxemia are the key factors contributing to diastolic pressure whereas snoring is an independent factor among several risk factors i.e. age, obesity and smoking.

In recent years, the short-term and long-term effects of different therapies in the evolution of the disease and its complications have been investigated. A bias of these different follow-up studies was the evaluation of the therapeutic effects only in selected patients. In our opinion, to evaluate the effect of the therapy it is important to examine the natural evolution of the disease to define the role of anatomical and functional factors as predictive criteria for the progression of the disease and the response to therapy.

References

1. Cirignotta F, D'Alessandro R, Partinen M, Zucconi M, Cristina E, Gerardi R, Cacciatore FM and Lugaresi E (1989) Acta Neurol. Scand. 79: 366–372.
2. Bliwise DL, Nekich JC and Dement WC (1991) Chest 99: 600–608.

3. Lugaresi E, Cirignotta F, Gerardi R and Montagna P (1990) In: Guilleminault C and Partinen M (eds.) Obstructive sleep apnea syndrome: Clinical research and treatment. Raven Press, pp. 25–36.
4. Lugaresi E, Mondini S, Zucconi M, Montagna P and Cirignotta F (1983) Bull. Eur. Physiopathol. Resp. 19: 590–594.
5. Bloom JW, Kaltenborn WT and Quan SF (1988) Chest 93: 678–683.
6. Konskenvuo M, Kaprio J, Partinen M, Langinvainio H, Sarna S and Keikkila K (1985) Lancet i: 893–896.
7. Lugaresi E, Cirignotta F, Coccagna G and Piana C (1980) Sleep 3: 221–224.
8. Stradling JR and Crosby JH (1990) Br. Med. J. 300: 75–78.

Biological Psychiatry, Volume 1. G. Racagni et al., editors.

Oneiric behavior disorder in REM sleep without muscle atonia

Yasuo Hishikawa[1], Tetsuo Shimizu[1], Naoko Tachibana[2], and Yoshiro Sugita[2]
[1]Department of Neuropsychiatry, Akita University School of Medicine; and [2]Department of Neuropsychiatry, Osaka University Medical School, Osaka, Japan

Introduction

Vivid dreams are frequently experienced by man during REM sleep. In addition, skeletal muscle tone is completely abolished, and usually, gross body movements do not appear during REM sleep in both man and animal. However, several researchers have found in cats that, after localized destruction of the bilateral, dorso-lateral parts of the pontine tegmentum, muscle atonia during REM sleep is abolished and cats often exhibit oneiric behavior during REM sleep without muscle atonia [1–3]. Such experimental findings have inspired clinical sleep researchers to look for similar behavior disorder occurring during REM sleep in man. This report is to describe oneiric behavior disorder occurring in REM sleep without muscle atonia in patients with degenerative diseases of the brain and in otherwise healthy elderly patients, which has already been reported elsewhere [4–7].

Subjects and Methods

The subjects consisted of 12 patients suffering from degenerative disease involving the brain stem (olivo-ponto-cerebellar atrophy, Shy-Drager syndrome and progressive supra-nuclear palsy) and of 7 otherwise healthy patients, 4 males and 5 females, aged 61–81 years. All of the patients frequently showed episodes of oneiric behavior disorder characterized by loud sleep talking, shouting and screaming, and by violent behavior, for example, abruptly sitting up on the bed, walking or jumping out of the bed, kicking and hitting the spouse sleeping beside or the wall of the bed room, grasping at and shaking the furniture in the bedroom. Polysomnographic examination of the patients together with simultaneous video-monitoring of their behavior was performed. Other 14 healthy elderly subjects not showing such oneiric behavior disorder were also examined as the controls.

Results

The most remarkable finding in the 2 groups of patients was that tonic activity in the mental muscle was not abolished in the major part of their REM sleep episodes and that they often showed oneiric behavior only in such REM sleep without muscle atonia. REM density (number of REMs per minute) in the period of such REM sleep accompanied by oneiric behavior was significantly larger in the patients with degenerative disease of the brain (24.6 ± 9.2 per min) and in the otherwise healthy elderly patients (19.5 ± 7.7 per min) than in the controls (11.2 ± 5.4 per min). When the patients were awakened from such REM sleep accompanied by oneiric behavior, their oneiric behavior stopped immediately and they soon became well aware of the real situation where they were, and many of them reported that they had been undergoing emotional vivid dreams. The other features of nocturnal sleep, including the percentage of REM sleep in the total sleeping time and the regularity of REM-NREM sleep cycle, did not differ significantly between either group of patients and the control group, except that the percentage of slow wave sleep (stages 3 and 4) in the total sleeping time was markedly decreased in the patients with degenerative brain disease.

Discussion and Conclusion

The present findings suggest that oneiric behavior disorder in our patients is due to enactment of dreams in REM sleep, and that their oneiric behavior appeared because of loss of muscle atonia. Similar oneiric behavior disorder occurring in REM sleep without muscle atonia in man has also been reported by other investigators [8,9]. Recently, it has been found by MRI examination that some elderly patients with such oneiric behavior disorder have minor lesions in the dorsal ponto-mesencephalic region [10]. This finding in man and other previous findings in cat suggest that abolishment of muscle atonia in REM sleep in man is due to some lesion in the pontine tegmentum. The present findings also indicate the importance of increased REM density for inducing oneiric behavior in REM sleep without muscle atonia. Such increased REM density may be induced by elevated activities in some pontine and related suprapontine neural structures.

References

1. Jouvet M and Delorme F (1965) C.R. Soc. Biol. (Paris) 159: 895–899.
2. Henley K and Morrison AR (1974) Acta Neurobiol. Exp. (Warsaw) 34: 215–232.
3. Sastre JP and Jouvet M (1979) Physiol. Behav. 22: 979–989.
4. Shimizu T, Sugita Y, Iijima S, Teshima Y and Hishikawa Y (1981) In: Koella WP (ed.) Sleep 1980. Karger, Basel, pp. 435–437.
5. Shimizu T (1985) Adv. Neurol. Sci. (Tokyo) 29: 154–177.
6. Shimizu T, Inami Y, Sugita Y, Iijima S, Teshima Y, Matsuo R, Yasoshima A, Egawa I, Okawa M, Tashiro T and Hishikawa Y (1990) Jpn. J. Psychiatr. Neurol. 44: 681–692.
7. Tachibana N, Sugita T, Terashima K, Teshima Y, Shimizu T and Hishikawa Y (1991) Biol. Psychiatry (in press).
8. Ishigooka J. Westendorp F, Oguchi T, Takahashi A, Sumiyoshi A and Inami M (1985) Biol. Psychiatry 20: 1003–1008.
9. Schenk CH, Bundie R, Patterson AL and Mahowald MW (1987) J. Am. Med. Assoc. 257: 1786–1789.
10. Culebras A and Moore JT (1989) Neurology 39: 1519–1523.

Biological Psychiatry, Volume 1. G. Racagni et al., editors.

Effects of lecithin and physostigmine on REM sleep in Alzheimer's disease

Hisakazu Furuta, Shoji Yamamori, Keiko Nakagawa, Yoshiki Maeda, Nobuharu Ishiguro, Katsuhiko Ueno, Joh Sano and Nariyoshi Yamaguchi

Department of Neuropsychiatry, Kanazawa University School of Medicine, 13-1 Takaramachi Kanazawa, 920 Japan

Introduction

There is growing evidence that memory disturbances are due to central cholinergic dysfunction in dementia of Alzheimer's type (DAT) [1]. Activation of the central cholinergic system has already been attempted in order to improve memory impairment by the use of lecithin and/or physostigmine [2].

Furthermore, central cholinergic mechanisms are also known to be one of the generators of REM sleep and cortical EEG activities [3,4]. Some reports have appeared on the effects of these agents on REM parameters such as REM sleep latency and % stage REM in normal adults [5]. We examined the effects of oral administration of lecithin and physostigmine on REM sleep in 6 patients with DAT, comparing these REM parameters with those of normal adults.

Methods

Six patients underwent polysomnography (PSG) before and after the administration of 10 g of lecithin and 12 mg of physostigmine per day for an average of 25 days. We compared sleep variables, especially REM variables of the patients with those of 6 age-matched normal control subjects who also underwent PSG. The patient group consisted of two men and four women, ranging in age from 47 to 62 years (mean ± S.D.; 55.5 ± 5.3 years) and the control group of 3 men and 3 women, ranging in age from 53 to 61 years (57.5 ± 3.6 years). We conducted PSG recordings and scored sleep stages in each 20-s epoch according to the protocol of Rechtschaffen and Kales (1968).

EEG power spectral analysis was also performed in the first REM sleep period. EEG spectra were divided into 6 bands, i.e. δ(0.6–3.8 Hz), θ(4–7.8 Hz), α_1(8–9.8 Hz), α_2(10–12.8 Hz), β_1(13–19.8 Hz) and β_2(20–25 Hz).

Results

No significant differences were noted among these 3 groups; control group and patient group before and after administration with regard to non-REM sleep variables except for REM sleep variables. That is, the patient group before administration showed significantly prolonged REM latency compared with the control group, and it was shortened significantly to the level of that of the control group after administration (see Table 1).

There are some reports suggesting that the prolongation of REM latency in DAT is attributable to a disturbance of maintaining sleep. We employed an index, REM latency-W, to exclude the intervening awake time from standard REM latency. As a result, this significant prolongation before and shortening after administration in the patient group remained nearly unchanged excluding awake time (see Table 1).

Sleep architecture revealed another connotative aspect concerning the changes of REM sleep. There were no significant differences or changes in non-REM sleep between the control and patient groups, or between before and after administration, while the patient group before administration showed significantly decreased percentage stage REM compared with the control group, which recovered slightly after administration, preserving significantly less percentage stage REM than that of the control group (see Table 1). The percentages of non-REM sleep showed no significant differences in any stage among these 3 groups.

We also examined the effect of these 2 agents on REM sleep rhythmicity. The duration of the first REM cycle was significantly prolonged in the patient group before administration compared with the control group. After administration, however, it was shortened significantly to the level of the control group (see Table 1).

Table 1. Sleep variables (mean ± S.D.)

	Control (n = 6)	DAT (n = 6)		ANOVA
		Before	After	
Total sleep time (min)	439.2 ± 47.1	485.2 ± 69.2	488.7 ± 58.6	N.S.
Sleep latency (min)	7.1 ± 11.1	6.8 ± 3.1	13.1 ± 11.6	N.S.
Total awake time (min)	78.1 ± 57.3	75.1 ± 35.3	64.6 ± 60.3	N.S.
REM latency (min)	73.6 ± 21.4	116.8 ± 41.9[a]	79.4 ± 15.0	$P < 0.05$
REM latency-W (min)	65.7 ± 14.4	94.6 ± 25.0[b]	73.7 ± 14.0	$P < 0.05$
Stage REM (%)	20.3 ± 4.1	12.7 ± 2.1[c]	15.3 ± 3.4[b]	$P < 0.01$
REM cycles				
1st (min)	93.6 ± 17.7	132.6 ± 34.7[a]	99.2 ± 21.9	$P < 0.05$
2nd (min)	123.9 ± 20.2	113.0 ± 24.3	101.4 ± 50.4	N.S.
3rd (min)	107.1 ± 48.1	110.2 ± 24.6	83.0 ± 19.7	N.S.
4th (min)	100.7 ± 29.9	75.1 ± 40.1	94.7 ± 44.2	N.S.

[a] $P < 0.05$ vs. Control and DAT after (Ryan's t-test);
[b] $P < 0.05$ vs. Control (Ryan's t-test);
[c] $P < 0.01$ vs. Control (Ryan's t-test).

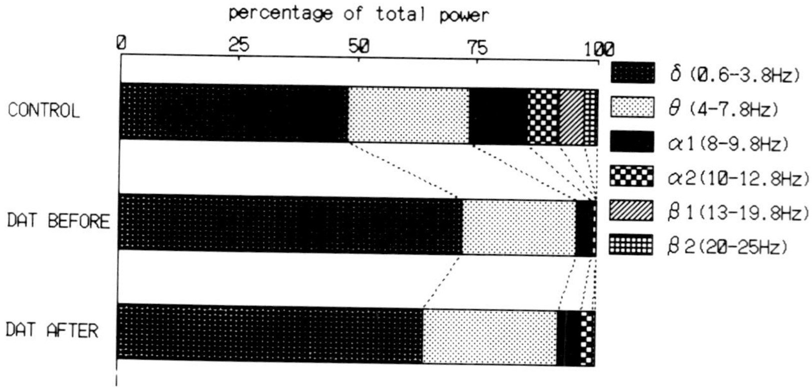

Fig. 1. EEG power spectra in REM sleep.

No significant changes or differences were found in any other of the following cycles.

The results of EEG power spectral analysis are shown in Fig. 1. EEG power spectra are expressed as relative EEG powers (percentages of total EEG powers). Compared with the control group, the DAT group showed increased δ power and decreased power of α_1, α_2, β_1 and β_2 activities before the administration of lecithin and physostigmine. After the administration of lecithin and physostigmine, however, increased power of α_1, α_2 and β_1 activities and decreased δ power were observed.

Discussion

Patients with DAT showed significant changes in REM variables; prolongation of REM latency, increase in percentage of REM sleep and increased duration of the first REM cycle, compared with normal control subjects. After administration, they showed significant improvement in all these REM variables, especially REM latency regardless of sleep disturbance. The REM latency shortening effect in the DAT patients administered lecithin and physostigmine was similar to the results in the normal subjects [5]. Also at the same time, EEG activation in REM sleep was found due to these agents. The above results suggest that the central cholinergic system in DAT patients is depressed. Regarding the clinical effect, no clear improvement was found on the Wechsler Memory Scale, but no deterioration was observed, indicating that these agents may have a transient suppressive effect on the progression of clinical symptoms.

References

1. Perry EK, Perry RH, Blessed G and Tomlinson BE (1977) Lancet i: 189.
2. Thal LJ, Fuld PA, Masur DM and Sharpless NS (1983) Ann. Neurol. 13: 496.
3. Silberman EK, Vivaldi E, Garfield J, McCarley RW and Hobson JA (1980) Brain Res. 191: 215–224.
4. Riekkinen P, Buzsaki G, Riekkinen P Jr, Soininen H and Partanen J (1991) Electroencephalogr. Clin. Neurophysiol. 78: 89–95.
5. Sitaram N, Wyatt RJ, Dawson S and Gillin JC (1976) Science 191: 1281–1283.

Biological Psychiatry, Volume 1. G. Racagni et al., editors.

Sleep-wake rhythm disorder and phototherapy in elderly patients with dementia

Masako Okawa[1], Yasuo Hishikawa[1], Satoshi Hozumi[2] and Hiroshi Hori[2]
[1]Department of Neuropsychiatry, Akita University School of Medicine, 1-1-1 Hondo, Akita; and [2]Kyowa Hospital, Akita, Japan

Introduction

Elderly patients with dementia often suffer from disorders of the sleep-wake rhythm, such as reversed day-night rhythm, insomnia or irregular sleep-wake rhythm and behavioral disorders such as wandering, agitation or delirium. We examined the circadian rhythm in such patients in order to find the aging effects on the biological rhythm and its relation to behavioral disorders. Furthermore, as a trial for treatment of sleep-wake rhythm disorders in these patients with severe dementia, phototherapy was performed.

Subjects and Methods

The subjects consisted of 24 patients with moderate or severe dementia, aged 59–89 years ($M = 76.6 \pm 6.4$ years) and 8 control patients without or with dementia of slight degree, aged 65–81 years ($M = 75.0 \pm 5.4$ years), admitted to a geriatric ward in Kyowa Hospital. The 24 patients were selected because of irregularity of their sleep-wake rhythm with behavioral disorders and/or delirium. Their dementia was due to cerebro-vascular disease (multi-infarct dementia) in 20 of them and senile dementia of Alzheimer's type in the remaining 4 patients.

The sleep-wake state of the patients were frequently judged by nurses for 1–4 months. The oral temperature was recorded at 00:00, 04:00, 10:00 and 16:00 h for 7 consecutive days before and during phototherapy. Serum melatonin was assayed in 21 of the 24 patients with dementia and in the 8 control patients. Blood was sampled 2 times a day, at 00:00 and 12:00 h, on 2 occasions before and during phototherapy.

For treatment of sleep-wake rhythm and behavioral disorders, phototherapy with illumination of 3,000 lux was performed every morning for 2 h between 09:00 and 11:00 h during 1–2 months.

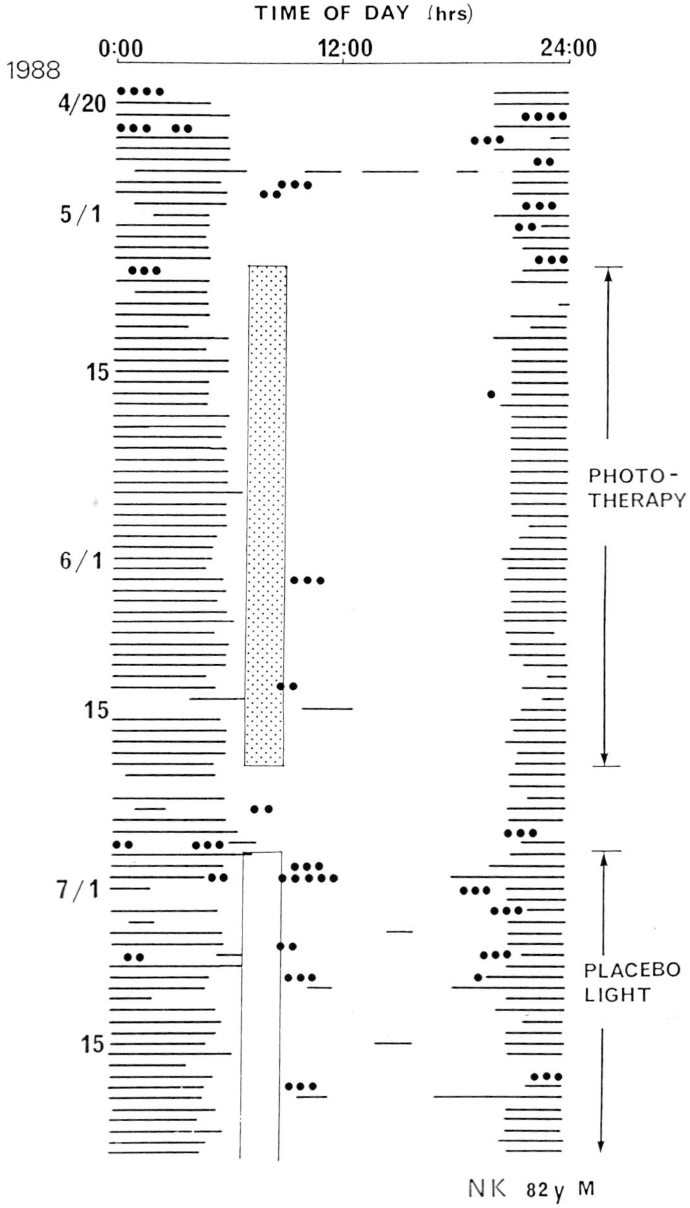

Fig. 1. Illustration of the sleep-wake rhythm and behavioral disorders in an 82-year-old male patient with dementia before and during phototherapy. Black horizontal bars represent sleep. Closed circles indicate episodes of behavioral disorders.

Table 1. Oral temperature in dementia and control group ($\bar{x} \pm$ S.D.)

Group	n	Mean (°C)	Range (°C)	Time of peak temperature (h)
Dementia	24	36.0 ± 0.5^a	2.8 ± 0.7^c	10.9 ± 3.6^b
Control	8	36.5 ± 0.2	1.2 ± 0.4	14.9 ± 2.9

$^aP < 0.05$; $^bP < 0.02$; $^cP < 0.001$ (*t*-test).

Results

Sleep-wake record in a typical case with sleep-wake rhythm disorder and behavioral disorder is illustrated in Fig. 1. All 24 patients showed some type of sleep-wake rhythm disorder; 2 showed a reversed day-night sleep-wake rhythm, 3

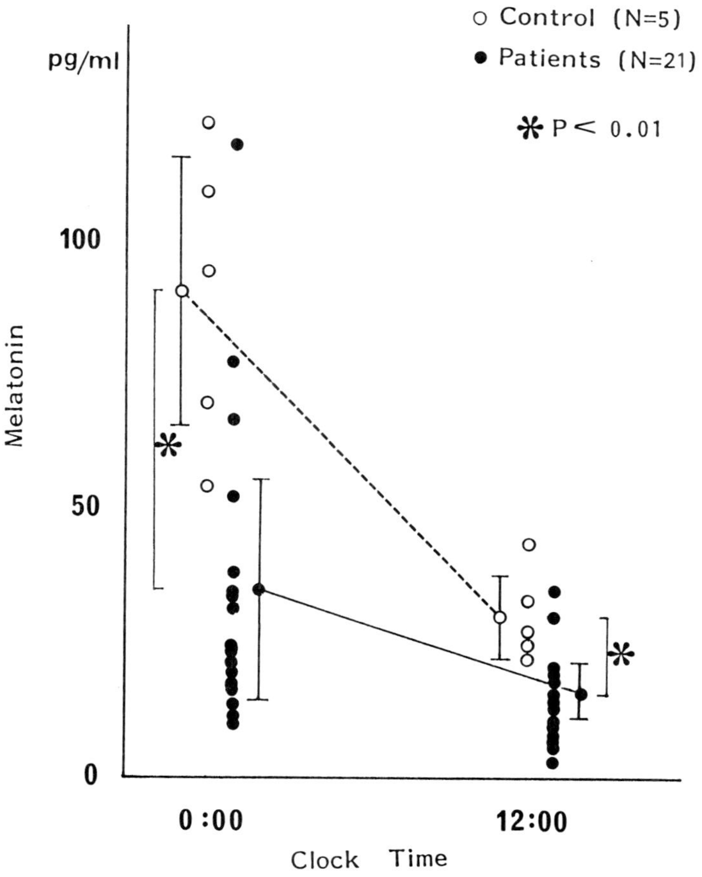

Fig. 2. Diurnal change of serum melatonin in patients with dementia and in controls. Mean melatonin levels at 00:00 and 12:00 were significantly lower than those in controls (see text).

showed insomnia and the remaining 19 patients showed irregular sleep-wake rhythm. The findings on circadian variation of oral temperature were summarized in Table 1. In the control patients, daily variations of oral temperature were relatively small. In contrast, those in the patients with dementia were very large and sometimes an accidental low temperature below 34°C was recorded. Sixteen patients (66.7%) in the dementia group showed an oral temperature rhythm disorder.

Diurnal change of serum melatonin level in 21 patients with dementia and in 5 controls is shown in Fig. 2. Mean melatonin level at 00:00 and 12:00 in the patients with dementia was significantly lower than that in the control patients, i.e. patients with dementia showed reduced amplitude in melatonin secretion rhythm.

For treatment of sleep-wake rhythm disorder, phototherapy was effective in 12 of the 24 patients (50.0%). Illustration of the sleep-wake rhythm and effect of phototherapy in a patient is shown in Fig. 1. Before phototherapy, the patient showed an irregular sleep-wake rhythm and frequent behavioral disorders such as wandering in the daytime and nocturnal delirium. After the beginning of phototherapy, his behavioral disorders almost disappeared and the sleep-wake rhythm improved, although some daytime naps still remained. In order to ascertain the effect of phototherapy, placebo-light therapy was performed; the patients stayed in front of lighting equipment with light-off. During placebo-light therapy, sleep-wake rhythm and behavioral disorder reappeared. However, disordered oral temperature rhythm improved in only 4 of 24 patients (16.7%), and disordered melatonin rhythm did not improve during the phototherapy.

Conclusions

1. Behavioral disorders such as delirium, agitation or wandering in patients with dementia seemed to be closely related to disrupted biological rhythms of sleep-waking, autonomic system (body temperature) and endocrine system (melatonin).
2. For treatment of disturbed sleep-wake rhythm and behavioral disorders, phototherapy was often effective.
3. Bright light did not show significant change in diurnal rhythm of melatonin secretion in these patients during the therapy. This finding indicates that the effect of phototherapy for sleep-wake rhythm disorder is not due to change in serum melatonin.

Biological Psychiatry, Volume 1. G. Racagni et al., editors.

Body temperature and sleep-wake rhythms of healthy elderly subjects

Yoichi Nakazawa, Kensaku Nonaka, Tatayu Kotorii, Naohisa Uchimura and Tetsuro Sakamoto

Department of Neuropsychiatry, School of Medicine Kurume University, 67 Asahi-Machi, 830 Kurume, Japan

Introduction

It is known that the many elderly people are aware of early morning awakening. Gerard et al. (1978) reported that bedtime, sleep onset and morning awakening times of the healthy elderly aged over 65 years were significantly earlier than those of healthy young adults by study using a questionnaire, They also found that sleep onset was significantly earlier in the group older than 75 years than in the group younger than 74 years, whereas no significant difference was observed for morning awakening time. Since it has been suggested that human sleep onset and morning awakening times are highly influenced by body temperature rhythm, we investigated the body temperature rhythm of healthy elderly subjects and examined the effect of age against period, amplitude and phase of the circadian rhythm.

Subjects and Methods

The subjects were 14 healthy elderly people (7 males and 7 females, age 50–87 years, mean age 69.1 ± 9.1 years). Among them, 4 were staff of the special senior citizens' home and the remaining 10 had been admitted to this home. No one complained of insomnia and neither mental nor physical diseases were found by various examinations. Since the sleep of elderly people is apt to change under unusual circumstances, the study was conducted in the places where they were living. They were told to be in bed at their usual time and asked to keep a sleep diary. As for the control group of healthy young adults, 7 healthy male students were studied and their ages ranged from 18 to 24 years (mean age 21.1 ± 2.3 years). They were housed in the Sleep Laboratory of Kurume University Hospital for 2 days and bedtime was established at 23:00 h and awakening time at 07:30 h.

For the recording of rectal temperature, recorder "Memory Mac" (Vain Co., Ltd.) was used and the measurement was successively taken by a thermistor retained in the rectum. The rhythm was analyzed by the least-squares spectrum method.

Results

Comparison of body temperature rhythm between healthy elderly and healthy young adults

When the rhythm of rectal temperature was analyzed, a significant 24-h period was detected in all subjects. Tables 1 and 2 show mean temperature, amplitude, minimal temperature, acrophase and nadir times of respective subjects obtained from analysis. Table 3 shows mean values of elderly and young groups. There was a significant difference in average temperature, amplitude and minimal temperature between these 2 groups. Namely, average temperature was lower, amplitude was smaller and minimal temperature was higher in the elderly group than the young group. Acrophase time was significantly advanced in the elderly group in comparison to the young group, but the difference in nadir time between these 2 groups was insignificant. Moreover, there was a significant inverse correlation between acrophase time and age in the elderly subjects ($r = -0.6229$, $P < 0.05$), but no significant correlation was observed between nadir time and age in the elderly group.

Relationship between sleep onset/morning awakening time and age in the healthy elderly group obtained by sleep diary

Sleep onset and morning awakening times in the elderly subjects are shown in Table 4 and there was a significant inverse correlation between sleep onset time and age ($r = -0.7651$, $P < 0.01$). Namely, the sleep onset time was earlier in older

Table 1. Average temperature, amplitude, acrophase time, minimal temperature and nadir time for 14 elderly subjects

	Sex	Age (years)	Average temp. (°C)	Amplitude (°C)	Acrophase (h)	Min. temp. (°C)	Nadir (h)
N.N.	M	50	37.5	0.4	17:24	36.9	06:07
S.N.	M	59	37.5	0.6	16:30	36.6	03:30
T.A.	M	61	37.3	0.6	16:42	36.9	04:12
M.U.	M	65	37.3	0.6	15:30	36.5	06:29
S.T.	M	65	37.2	0.3	16:06	36.8	00:30
H.E.	F	66	37.6	0.6	15:24	36.9	06:20
T.K.	M	66	37.0	0.3	17:54	36.4	09:00
T.Y.	F	71	37.6	0.5	15:30	36.9	03:30
M.T.	M	72	37.4	0.5	13:36	36.8	23:33
I.A.	F	73	37.2	0.6	14:00	36.4	00:56
F.M.	F	73	37.1	0.4	15:00	36.4	00:30
K.Y.	F	79	37.3	0.4	14:24	36.8	01:00
T.F.	F	80	37.8	0.4	16:30	36.2	04:00
T.O.	F	87	36.4	0.5	14:30	36.6	04:00

Table 2. Average temperature, amplitude, acrophase time, minimal temperature and nadir time for 7 young adults

	Age (years)	Average temp. (°C)	Amplitude (°C)	Acrophase (h)	Min. temp. (°C)	Nadir (h)
J.M.	18	37.6	0.6	18:36	36.4	07:23
F.I.	19	37.2	0.7	17:48	36.2	04:59
Y.M.	20	37.8	0.8	18:42	36.5	04:14
S.T.	21	37.5	0.5	16:54	36.3	05:36
H.I.	22	37.8	0.6	17:12	36.7	03:53
K.K.	24	37.8	0.7	18:12	36.6	04:44
N.H.	24	37.7	0.7	17:00	36.3	03:42

subjects. On the other hand, final awakening time showed only a tendency of correlation with age ($r = -0.5401$, $P < 0.1$).

Discussion

It has been reported that earlier sleep onset and early morning awakening are commonly observed among normal healthy elderly subjects. These facts indicate that the phase of sleep-wake cycle is more advanced than in young adults. On the other hand, the existence of interaction between sleep-wake rhythm and deep temperature rhythm has been suggested by many studies. Namely, sleep onset occurs when body temperature is in a descending phase whereas morning awakening occurs in its ascending phase and sleep is deeper when the decrease in temperature is large. Accordingly, phase-advancement of sleep-wake cycle found among the elderly may possibly be a result of phase-advancement of body temperature rhythm.

The present study demonstrated that acrophase of the elderly group was significantly more advanced than that of the young group. Although nadir time in the elderly group was about 1.5 h advanced compared with the young group, the difference was not significant Moreover, a significant inverse correlation was observed between age and acrophase in the elderly group, although the acrophase of all subjects in the young group was concentrated at between 17:00 and 18:00 h.

Table 3. Mean values of 14 elderly and 7 young adults (X ± S.D.)

	Average temp. (°C)	Amplitude (°C)	Acrophase (h)	Min. temp. (°C)	Nadir (h)
Elderly	37.3 ± 0.2	0.5 ± 0.1	15:39 ± 77	36.7 ± 0.2	03:19 ± 166
Young	37.6 ± 0.2	0.7 ± 0.1	17:48 ± 42	36.4 ± 0.2	04:55 ± 72
P	<0.01	<0.01	<0.01	<0.05	N.S.

Table 4. Sleep onset and morning awakening times of 14 elderly subjects

	Sex	Age (years)	Sleep onset (h)	Awakening (h)
N.N.	M	50	24:00	07:30
S.N.	M	59	23:00	06:00
T.A.	M	61	23:15	07:45
M.U.	M	65	22:00	07:00
S.T.	M	65	21:00	04:50
H.E.	F	66	22:00	07:00
T.K.	M	66	22:50	05:40
T.Y.	F	71	21:30	05:00
M.T.	M	72	22:00	06:15
I.A.	F	73	22:30	05:00
F.M.	F	73	22:00	07:00
K.Y.	F	79	21:00	06:30
T.F.	F	80	20:30	05:00
T.O.	F	87	21:30	05:00

Therefore, it is highly possible that earlier sleep onset and early morning awakening commonly observed among the elderly occur by phase-advancement of body temperature rhythm, although the mechanisms which induce the phase advance of body temperature rhythm are not known.

Moreover, the present study showed that there were significant differences in body temperature rhythm between the healthy elderly and healthy young groups. Namely, average temperature was lower, amplitude was smaller and minimal temperature was higher in the elderly in compared with the young adults. Since it has been reported that the amplitude of temperature rhythm decreases (decrease of the highest body temperature and increase of the lowest body temperature) in both man and animals with advancing age, the results of the present investigation agree with these studies.

Biological Psychiatry, Volume 1. G. Racagni et al., editors.

Chronic insomnia in the elderly

Göran Hajak, Eckart Rüther, Andrea Rodenbeck and Volker Pudel
Department of Psychiatry, University of Göttingen, von-Siebold-Str. 5, 3400 Göttingen, Germany

Normal aging is accompanied by changes in sleep patterns. Total sleep time, sleep efficiency and slow wave sleep stages III and IV decline during night sleep. Wakefulness and brief arousals during the night and frequency of stage shifts increase with age. The sensitivity to environmental stimuli which may provide waking signals increases in elderly individuals [1–6]. These results of polysomnographic recordings contribute to the characterization of sleep in the elderly as being easier to disturb and more fragile than the sleep of younger adults. This suggests a disturbance of the sleep-wake continuity in the elderly and a development of a night-sleep behaviour as seen in insomniacs.

Several studies have examined the subjective sleep complaints of the elderly population in Europe and the U.S.A. The frequency of sleep complaints in Germany is presented here by results of a representative survey in western Germany and a survey on members of a German health insurance, who received a questionnaire by mail.

Of the 109,022 members of the health insurance who sent back the questionnaire, 20.1% reported frequently, or always having difficulties in initiating or maintaining sleep, but only 7.0% of the 1979 individuals of the representative survey reported such a problem. The differences between these results challenge the validity of surveys by telephone calls or mailed questionnaires. Patients with sleep problems, especially women in the health insurance survey, are more likely to present their symptoms in a survey made by a sleep disorder clinic than individuals without sleep disturbances.

However, the number of individuals without difficulties in initiating or maintaining sleep decreases dramatically with age in both populations. The age distribution in the representative survey shows that the elderly are disproportionally dissatisfied with the quality of their sleep compared to younger individuals (Fig. 1).

Although the older persons have remarkably more daytime naps [1,7], the ability to compensate for night-sleep deficits or to accept them as normal is low. Therefore, symptoms of insomnia increase with age, although more people assess their sleeping time as long enough (Fig. 2).

With growing age an increasing number of individuals suffer from sleep problems lasting more than 2 years. This may contribute to the high percentage of chronic insomnia in the elderly with sleep problems (Fig. 3).

Corresponding to the increase of sleep complaints in the general population, the percentage of individuals who never took sleep medication decreases with age. In

Data from a representative survey, western Germany, 1990 (n = 1979, m = 933, f = 1046).

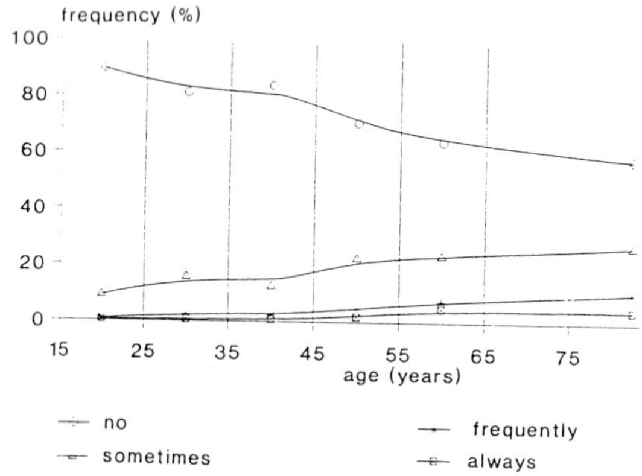

Fig. 1. Difficulties in initiating or maintaining sleep.

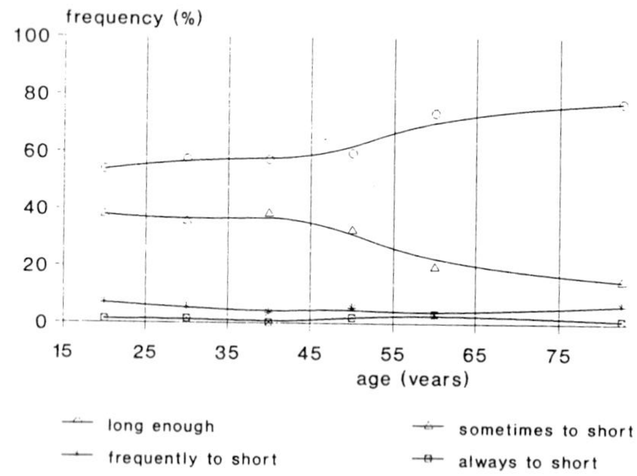

Fig. 2. Subjective assessment of sleeping time.

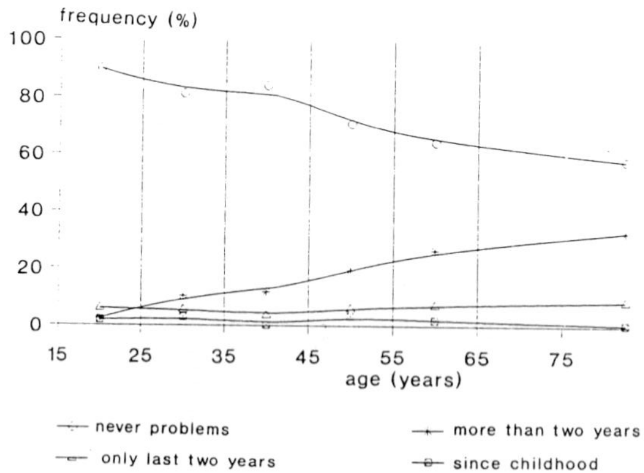

Fig. 3. Duration of sleep complaints.

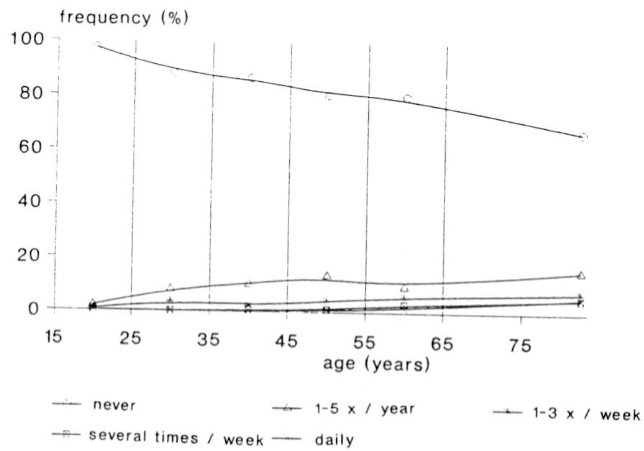

Fig. 4. Frequency of sleep medication intake.

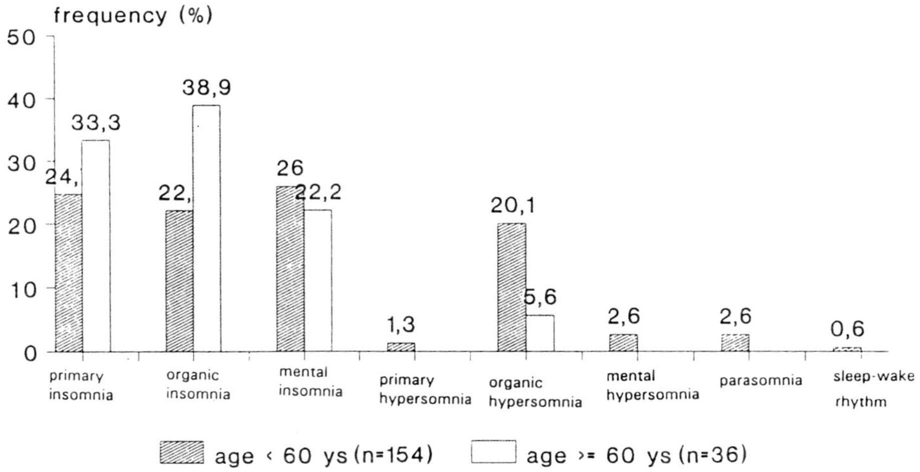

Fig. 5. Diagnoses according to DSM III-R, laboratory of sleep medicine, Univ. of Göttingen, 1990. Age distribution at the age of 60 years (n = 190, m = 114, f = 76).

contrast to much published data, there is no marked increase of chronic sleep medication intake from middle to old age (Fig. 4). It seems that sleep medication is not preferably used to solve sleep problems in elderly Germans.

Of the patients over the age of 60 years which visited the sleep disorders center of the University of Göttingen in 1990, 60.1% had an insomnia secondary to organic diseases or psychiatric illness (Fig. 5). Attempts to treat the underlying disturbance appear as a much more effective means of solving a sleep problem than symptomatic management of the disease. However, 33.3% of the elderly patients suffered from primary insomnia. At present there is limited experience of treatment strategies for this group of patients which cannot be treated by general psychiatry and medication.

In summary, the pronounced sleep disturbances in the elderly appear as a chronic disturbance which can arise as a result of changes in sleep patterns that are age-related, a specific sleep disorder, or a combination of both. Therefore, the physician needs to perform careful diagnostic management and exercise great caution when initiating the therapeutic procedure and prescribing a new medication in elderly insomniacs.

References

1. Carskadon M, Brown E and Dement W (1982) Neurobiol. Aging 3: 321–327.
2. Kahn E, Fischer C and Leiberman L (1970) Compr. Psychiatry 11: 274–278.
3. Prinz P (1977) J. Gerontol. 32: 179–186.

4. Reynolds III CD, Kupfer L, Taska L, Hoch C, Sewitch D and Spiker D (1985) Sleep of Healthy Seniors: A Revisit.
5. Williams R, Karacan I and Hursch C (1974) Electroencephalography (EEG) of Human Sleep: Clinical Applications. J. Wiley and Sons, New York, U.S.A.
6. Zepelin H, McDonald K, Wanzie F and Zammit GK (1980) Sleep Res. 9: 109.
7. Allen SR, Seiler WO, Stahelin HB and Spiegel R (1987) Sleep 10: 140–159.

Biological Psychiatry, Volume 1. G. Racagni et al., editors.

Longitudinal changes in REM sleep in Alzheimer's disease

Christian Guilleminault, Don Bliwise and J.A. Yesavage
Stanford Sleep Research Center, 701 Welch Road, Suite #2226, Palo Alto, CA 94304, U.S.A.

Introduction

Alzheimer's disease (AD) is characterized by widespread cholinergic deficiency in the brain [1]. Rapid eye movement (REM) sleep can be stimulated by direct, local application of cholinergic agonists in animals and by infusion of cholinergic precursors in humans [2]. The distribution of REM sleep in AD could thus be changed and its timing during sleep cycles may also be affected.

In this short report we present longitudinal data obtained on 10 subjects with dementia who are thought to present AD based on clinical, psychiatric and brain imaging data but without confirmation by histology.

The population included 7 men and 3 women with a mean age of 68.6 ± 6.9 years (range 59.82) who were followed over intervals of 22.39 months (mean 30.9 months). Subjects were part of a multi-specialist investigation and follow-up program. Clinical evolution, mental status, clinical neurophysiological variables and brain imaging information were obtained at regular intervals 9–12 months apart. Histologic information may now be available with subject and family consent but was not available at the time of this report.

As part of the follow-up program, sleep monitorings were performed. Informed consent from patients and guardians had been obtained at the beginning of the study. Polygraphic variables EEG (C3/A2-C4-A1), EOG, chin EMG and one-lead ECG were systematically obtained. Respiration was monitored using inductive plethysmography, oral and nasal thermistors and pulse oximetry at entry. Respiration variables were not always obtained or interpretable with progression of dementia and pulse oximetry alone was often substituted for full respiratory monitoring at later recordings. Behavioral observations were made by nurses during the follow-up work-up which required subjects to stay two or more 24-h periods in the facilities. Family and guardians also indicated sleep patterns at the time of monitoring. The Rechtschaffen and Kales International Criteria [3] were used to score sleep recordings.

Results

Mini-Mental State Exam (MMSE) scores when originally studied ranged from 6 to 24 (mean 18.6 ± 6.5). Five of 10 patients had scores of 20 or less, and 5 had MMSE scores in the 22–24 range. Sleep studies showed a progressive increase in nocturnal sleep disturbances, even if short-lived. The most striking findings involved REM sleep. There was a very clear trend (using 2-tailed statistics) for REM sleep percent to increase over time (Time 1: mean = 11.9 ± 6.3%; Time 2: mean = 17.6 ± 5.9%; t = 2.21; $P < 0.06$, 2-tailed). Most of the REM sleep was the tonic type without intense eye movements. In addition there was also a trend for REM sleep latency to decrease in follow-up (Time 1: mean = 106.1 ± 46.5 min; Time 2: mean = 76.5 ± 19.2 min; $P < 0.06$, 2-tailed).

Comments

Even if the results are borderline significant with the 2-tailed test, the findings are clearly in opposition to what is usually predicted. i.e. a decrease in REM sleep percent. These results are similar to those in a case report (with histology) previously reported at Stanford [4]. In the single-patient report, histology had revealed numerous cortical neuritic plaques (NP) and neurofibrillary tangles (NFT). In the brain stem, NP were numerous in the periaqueductal region and NFT in the dorsal raphe nucleus. However, the locus coeruleus was fairly well conserved, with only minimal cell loss. Candal pons and medulla showed no abnormality.

The most likely explanations for the REM sleep phenomena of the sleep patterns involves the specific areas of neuronal loss and their relationship to what is known about the neurophysiology of sleep. The widespread deterioration of the dorsal raphe in the one case with relative sparing of the locus coeruleus is consistent with a preserved inhibitory effect of the dorsal raphe on the more caudally located REM sleep generating areas.

Acknowledgement

Supported by National Institute of Mental Health Grant MH-40041.

References

1. Terry RD and Katzman R (1983) Ann. Neurol. 14: 497–506.
2. Gillin JC and Sitaram N (1984) Psychol. Med. 14: 501–506.
3. Rechtschaffen A and Kales A (eds.) (1968) A Manual of Standardized Terminology, Techniques and Scoring System for Sleep Stages of Human Subjects. BRI/BIS, Los Angeles.
4. Bliwise DL, Nino-Murcia G, Forno LS and Viseskul C (1990) Neurology 40: 1281–1284.

Biological Psychiatry, Volume 1. G. Racagni et al., editors.

Information processing during sleep in brain damaged elderly

Carlo Cipolli[1] and Luigi Murri[2]

[1]Institute of Human Physiology, University of Modena, Via Campi 287, 41100 Modena; and [2]Department of Neurology, University of Pisa, Via Roma 57, 56100 Pisa, Italy

Introduction

Sleep may play an active role in the processing of information (IP) for materials to be retained and re-elaborated for further recall. This view is supported by experiments on the retention of information in animals and humans on the one hand, and by correlational analyses on the age-dependent characteristics of sleep and the effectiveness of waking cognition on the other [1].

Correspondence between the functioning of IP during sleep and in waking may be investigated by studying not only the retention of materials during similar periods of waking and of sleep, but also the correlations between features of dreams (the output of the IP system responsible for dream production) and psychometric assessments of waking cognition. Dream experience is usually not just a sequence of visual images, but a relatively lengthy and coherent narrative of quite plausible and complex events. The sequential and hierarchical organization of a narrative clearly presupposes cognitive resources (in particular, attention and memory) to recruit mnestic sources during sleep and insert these into narrative frames – operations typical of IP [2]. The relations between IP during sleep and in waking have been fairly well explored in children and adults, but not in the aged population, notwithstanding growing interest in the modifications of sleep characteristics along with aging (sleep latency, frequency of interruptions, proportions of NREM and REM sleep). As well known, the elderly are the age group most severely affected by disorders in sleep onset and maintainance, but as several disturbances in sleep and in daytime alertness are associated with the most common neuropsychiatric disorders of later life, such as depression, dementia and Parkinson's disease, it is hard to estimate how much the relationships between sleep characteristics and IP are influenced by aging and how much by such disorders.

In order to investigate the narrative organization of dreams in the focal and non-focal brain-damaged elderly, we carried out three studies, based on the assumption that dream production is negatively influenced by impaired cognition on waking.

Experiment I – Dream experience in patients with acute brain damage

A preliminary assessment was carried out on 3 patients (aged 50 to 64 years) with cerebrovascular lesions, still in the acute phase, who maintained the ability to report dreams (i.e. at least one dream recalled in the 10 days before the sleep recording session), and on 4 normals, with comparable age and education, level of global cognitive functioning and memory abilities. Neuropsychological assessment excluded any lack of visual retention, of capacity for face recognition and of language comprehension. Each subject was awakened from two to three times in REM sleep and reported at least one dream during the night. The reports were analyzed using Mandler and Johnson's story grammar [3], which describe narratives in terms of their conceptual constituents ("statements") and the relationships between these (organizing the narrative into connected "episodes" within an overall "event structure"). Comparison of patients' reports with those of controls showed that in all reports statements were connected into a narrative, rather than just being descriptions of isolated contents. However, the development of the narration, measured in terms of number of statements and number of episodes, was less extended in patients than in normals [4]. Even if sampling constraints and the small number of cases allow only heuristic inferences, these results suggest that in the acute phase of cerebrovascular pathology the functioning of the organizational processes is impaired, even when the capacity of dreaming is not lost.

Experiment II – Dreaming in patients with chronic brain damage

If acute brain damage influences the dream production system, the question arises as to whether this influence is definitive, or whether improvements in cognitive functioning are reflected in dreaming. A follow-up study [5] investigated 32 patients (aged from 42 to 77 years) diagnosed from 2 to 4 years previously for unilateral (vascular or neoplastic) lesions, and compared current dream recall rates with those observed during the acute phase. All 10 subjects previously classified as recallers during the acute phase (that is, with at least one dream report over 10 days) retained capacity for dreaming. Among the 22 previous non-recallers, only 5 remained unable to recall any dream. It is worth stressing that neuropsychological assessment showed diminished visuoperceptive deficits, but not memory deficits in non-recallers. These findings suggest that the dream production system is sensitive to variations in cognitive functioning deriving from the clinical evolution of brain damage.

Experiment III – Dreams in patients with Parkinson's disease

Dream features and cognitive efficiency in waking were compared in patients with Parkinson's disease (PD), varying in age and degree of cognitive impairment [6]. Fifteen patients (aged from 46 to 73 years) with idiopathic PD (in stage II or III of Hoehn and Yahr's scale), without psychiatric symptoms or major medical illnesses and currently treated with levodopa, were each awakened at least twice in REM sleep. Thirteen were able to report at least one dream, and overall frequency of recall (71.4 %) was fully compatible with normative data for the elderly. Multiple regression analysis showed that the length of reports and their organization as narratives varied significantly in relation to global cognitive functioning and, partly, to language comprehension, but not in relation to memory or verbal fluency, age, illness duration or levodopa dose. These findings suggest that some cognitive processes involved in dream production (in particular, declarative and procedural memory systems) may function differently with respect to waking, and that they are not closely related to such factors as age, illness duration and levodopa therapy.

Conclusion

These studies show a substantial correspondence between the functioning of IP in waking and in sleep, as reflected in the organizational characteristics of dreams in patients with both focal (Exp. I) and non-focal (Exp. III) brain pathologies. As dream recall is sensitive to improvement in waking cognition (Exp. II), this correspondence would appear reliable and to offer suggestions as to the nature of the cognitive processes involved in dreaming, through comparison of dream features which supposedly reflect their functioning.

References

1. Lehmann D and Koukkou M (1983) In: Koella WP (ed.) Sleep 1982. Karger, Basel, pp. 46–48.
2. Foulkes D (1982) Sleep 5: 169–187.
3. Mandler JM and Johnson NS (1977) Cognit. Psychol. 9: 111–151.
4. Cipolli C, Maestrini M and Massetani R (1989) In: Horne J (ed.) Sleep '88. Fischer, Stuttgart, pp. 171–176.
5. Murri L, Mancino M, Massetani R, Canapicchi R, Puglioli M and Rossi G (1989) Res. Commun. Psychol. Psychiatr. Behav. 14: 121–142.
6. Cipolli C and Murri L (1991) In: Smirne S and Ferini-Strambi L (eds.) Aging and Sleep. Masson, Milan (in press).

Biological Psychiatry, Volume 1. G. Racagni et al., editors.

Rational approach to the treatment of insomnia

Jean-Michel Gaillard
Institutions Universitaires de Psychiatrie (Genève), Service de la Recherche Biologique et de Psychopharmacologie clinique, 2, Ch. du Petit-Bel-Air, 1225 Chêne-Bourg, Switzerland

The various forms of insomnia, taken together, represent a very frequent condition. Although they usually do not threaten physical health, they constitute an uncomfortable condition with several consequences in terms of daytime fatigue, sleepiness or inability to function normally at work or in the family. Therefore, the treatment of insomnia should be taken seriously and not, as it is still much too often dealt with, simply by the prescription of some drug as soon as the patient has said: "I can't sleep".

The treatment of insomnia should take into consideration the various forms of the disturbance, accompanying conditions such as anxiety and depression, the age of the patient and the therapeutic possibilities presently available: sleep hygiene, behavioural treatment, hypnotic drugs and psychotherapy. The principal forms of insomnia to be taken into consideration fall into the following categories:

- transient insomnia, lasting for a few days or a few weeks, often related to an easily identifiable cause;
- chronic insomnia, lasting for several months or years, often without obvious reasons, with or without overt anxiety;
- insomnia in psychiatric conditions such as major depression or schizophrenia. In this form, some characteristic modifications of the architecture of sleep are often found. It is also more severe than simple chronic insomnia;
- organic insomnia, such as after head trauma or in dementia or other brain organic conditions. This form is often very severe, with major reduction in sleep duration;
- others, such as toxic insomnia in chronic alcoholism, in excessive consumption of coffee or central stimulants, insomnia in somatic illness, alpha-delta sleep etc.

The treatment of insomnia necessitates first a good clinical investigation, addressing the subjective aspects of normal sleep, other phenomena occurring during sleep such as snoring, breathing disturbances or parasomnia, daytime functioning (sleepiness, tiredness, ability to concentrate), the history of the condition as well as the previous treatments the patient has tried. Sleep recordings are usually not indicated in transient insomnia. However, they are very often useful in the other forms of insomnia, although they cannot always be realized in dementia states.

The result of the sleep recordings should always be shown to the patient and discussed with him. This is actually the first step of the treatment, as it is essential that the patient grasps the differences between his own subjective estimation of sleep and objective findings. The evaluation of the degree of sleep fragmentation or the reduction in the duration of sleep is also an important basis for the application of sleep hygiene.

It is a general principle in medicine to suppress the cause of a disease when it is known. This is often the case in transient insomnia; however, most of the time, chronic insomnia presents itself without any recognizable cause. Insomnia in psychiatric conditions is treated along with the condition itself, but can persist long after the depression has disappeared. At present, etiological treatment cannot be considered in organic insomnia. Finally, the suppression of the cause is an obvious measure in toxic insomnia, whereas insomnia in somatic illness depends on the treatment of this illness.

When the suppression of the cause is not possible, transient insomnia is often presented on the best indication for drug treatment. Sleep hygiene is also useful, as well as simple counselling.

The treatment of chronic insomnia is much more difficult and no totally satisfactory solution is presently available. Sleep hygiene is often useful and may be sufficient in itself in milder forms. It is a set of rules presented to the patient to help him to control his own sleep and requiring his active cooperation. The most important rule is restriction of the time spent in bed, as insomniacs often have the tendency to compensate for their lack of sleep by staying longer in bed. The application of sleep hygiene can be accompanied by a sleep agenda the patient fills every morning, allowing him to control his progress.

However, sleep hygiene is not sufficient in the severe forms of chronic insomnia. Relaxation or conditioning therapy can be useful in light forms, especially sleep onset insomnia. Continuous treatment of chronic insomnia with drugs may lead to the problems of drug dependency, withdrawal reactions and sleep rebound insomnia. Therefore, some principles must be followed. First, the drug should be appropriately chosen in consideration of the form of insomnia. The kinetics of the compound is the essential property to consider in this respect: drugs with short half-life should be selected for sleep onset insomnia and it is not a good practice to use them at higher dosage to treat sleep fragmentation. Drugs with intermediate half-life should be used in this case, whereas benzodiazepines with metabolites having long half-life can be useful in insomnia associated with anxiety.

The second principle is that discontinuous treatment should be preferred to continuous treatment in order to avoid dependency, although recently developed hypnotics may be more favourable in their smaller ability to develop drug dependency. Third, the smallest efficient dose should be used, particularly in elderly people. Insomnia in psychiatric conditions often necessitates the prescription of a hypnotic in addition to specific treatment, but sedative antidepressants can be useful. Organic insomnia is usually too severe to respond to sleep hygiene and hypnotics may have to be used as a continuous treatment. Finally, psychotherapy is presently explored in chronic insomnia but no firm conclusion can yet be drawn.

Biological Psychiatry, Volume 1. G. Racagni et al., editors.

Role of ω receptor subtypes in the action of hypnotic drugs

B. Zivkovic, S. Arbilla, D.J. Sanger, H. Depoortere, B. Scatton and S.Z. Langer
Department of Biology, Synthélabo Recherche (LERS), 31 Av. P.V. Couturier, 92220 Bagneux, France

Introduction

It is now well established that the pharmacological effects of benzodiazepines, including sedation and hypnosis, are related to the action of these drugs at specific recognition sites within the $GABA_A$ receptor complex. The activation of these allosteric sites enhances the efficacy of GABA in opening the chloride ion channel associated with this receptor. Such a reinforcement of GABA-mediated inhibition leads to triggering of neuronal mechanisms relevant to the induction and maintenance of sleep [1].

ω Receptor subtypes and selectivity of zolpidem for the ω_1 receptor

The allosteric sites of the $GABA_A$ receptors which are involved in the action of benzodiazepines, traditionally called central benzodiazepine receptors and more recently classified as ω receptors [2], do not represent a uniform population of sites and from the pharmacological point of view 2 subtypes, ω_1 and ω_2, can be distinguished. However, from the molecular point of view the $GABA_A$ receptor component which carries this allosteric site, the α subunit, can be expressed by different neurones in at least 6 variants with different amino acid sequences. Pharmacological studies with transfected $GABA_A$ receptors containing different α subunits indicate that the α_1 subunit corresponds to the ω_1 receptor whereas the other variants may be pharmacologically akin to the ω_2 receptors [3]. However, as receptor subtype characterization strictly depends on the availability of selective agents it is not excluded that such compounds would reveal that the current ω_2 classification is heterogenous.

In addition to benzodiazepines, the emerging hypnotics from other chemical families have been shown to interact with omega receptors. Among these new drugs, cyclopyrrolone zopiclone and the imidazopyridine zolpidem are of particular interest because they have recently entered into wide clinical practice. There is, however, an essential difference between the mechanisms of action of these two drugs. Whereas zopiclone, like benzodiazepines, does not discriminate between the central ω receptor subtypes, zolpidem is highly selective for the ω_1 receptor.Thus, using tritiated benzodiazepines (^{3}H-diazepam or ^{3}H-flumazenil) to non-selectively label ω receptors in membranes of different parts of the central nervous system, it was shown that zolpidem preferentially inhibits the binding of these ligands to those regions which contain the ω_1 receptor subtype, such as the cerebellum and has lower affinity for those regions predominantly containing ω_2 subtypes, such as the spinal cord [2]. Using ^{3}H-zolpidem it was found that in the cerebral cortex the maximum number of binding sites that could be labelled with this ligand represents only two thirds of the total receptor population labelled by ^{3}H-benzodiazepines. More detailed studies using computer-assisted densitometry of receptors in autoradiograms of the baboon cerebral cortex showed that ^{3}H-zolpidem binding sites were localized exclusively in layer IV, whereas ^{3}H-flunitrazepam, in addition to layer IV, also binds to receptors in layer V and VI. Moreover, in the dentate gyrus of the hippocampus, ^{3}H-zolpidem labelled only very few receptors whereas ^{3}H-flunitrazepam heavily labelled this brain region [4]. Finally, studies with transfected receptors demonstrated that zolpidem preferentially binds to the α_1 subunit and is practically devoid of any affinity for the α_5 subunit [5].

The finding that zolpidem selectively binds to the ω_1 receptor subtype suggests that this drug would produce a regionally more restricted increase in GABAergic transmission as compared to the potentiation of the GABA-mediated inhibition induced by benzodiazepines or cyclopyrrolones which are non-selective for ω receptor subtypes.

Involvement of the ω_1 receptor subtype in sedative/hypnotic effects

The finding that zolpidem acts only on a restricted population of receptors which participate in the action of benzodiazepines suggests that this drug would have a pharmacological profile different from that of the former drugs. Indeed, the pharmacological profile of zolpidem is characterized by sedative and hypnotic activity which predominates over the anticonvulsant and anxiolytic action. Moreover, zolpidem appears to be completely devoid of myorelaxant effects [6]. In contrast to zolpidem, benzodiazepines induce sedation only at doses which are greater than those needed for the induction of myorelaxant, anticonvulsant and anxiolytic effects. Therefore, it is tempting to suggest that the hypnotic effects of benzodiazepines and other drugs non-selective for the ω receptor subtypes represent a non-specific depression of the central nervous system function, whereas selective enhancement of GABA-mediated transmission through the ω_1 receptor would induce a more specific hypnotic effect. Indeed, EEG measurements in animals and man indicate that benzodiazepines induce a sleep whose architecture is markedly different from that of physiological sleep, whereas the zolpidem-induced sleep cannot be distinguished from that induced physiologically [6,7]. It is also of interest to note that selective stimulation of the ω_1 receptor produces an increase in deep sleep stages whereas non-selective agents have the opposite effect [8].

Role of ω receptor subtypes in the development of benzodiazepine dependence

The effects of benzodiazepines are attenuated upon repeated administration and abrupt withdrawal of treatment can precipitate abstinence symptoms, indicating the development of tolerance and dependence [9]. Although the mechanisms involved in the development of tolerance and dependence to benzodiazepines are not fully elucidated it can be assumed that these phenomena are related to adaptive changes resulting from prolonged enhancement of $GABA_A$ receptor function and the consequent reinforcement of GABA-mediated inhibition. On the basis of this assumption it may be suggested that the selective enhancement of GABA transmission at a subpopulation of $GABA_A$ receptors will be less likely to induce tolerance and dependence. Indeed, animal studies involving repeated treatment with zolpidem support this hypothesis. Thus, after repeated administration of zolpidem for 10 consecutive days at doses which are 60 times greater than those inducing sedation (2×30 mg/kg, p.o.) no decrease in sedative potency was observed in contrast to the benzodiazepine hypnotics (triazolam, midazolam, nitrazepam) which after repeated administration at pharmacologically equivalent doses showed a 3–7 times lower activity. Moreover, after a similar treatment regimen with zolpidem, the sensitivity of animals to various convulsive challenges was not changed, whereas animals repeatedly treated with benzodiazepine hypnotics were more sensitive to convulsive effects of pentylenetetrazol, isoniazid or β-CCM, indicating that benzodiazepines but not zolpidem induced physical dependence.

Conclusions

Extensive pharmacological studies with zolpidem, a novel imidazopyridine hypnotic which selectively acts at a subpopulation of receptors (ω_1) involved in the action of benzodiazepines, indicate that the ω_1 receptor is relevant to the hypnotic effects of these drugs. Moreover, it is strongly suggested that drugs which selectively act at this ω receptor subtype are less likely to induce the development of tolerance and physical dependence.

References

1. Haefely WE (1989) In: Barnard EA and Costa E (eds.) Allosteric Modulation of Amino Acid Receptors: Therapeutic Implication. Raven Press, New York, pp. 47–69.
2. Langer SZ and Arbilla S (1988) Fundam. Clin. Pharmacol. 2: 159–170.
3. Pritchett DB, Luddens H and Seeburg PH (1989) Science 245: 1389–1392.
4. Benavides J, Depoortere H, Sanger D, Perrault G, Arbilla S, Langer SZ, Zivkovic B and Scatton B (1990) Encéphale 16: 13–22.
5. Pritchett DB and Seeburg PH (1990) J. Neurochem. 54: 1802–1804.

6. Depoortere H, Zivkovic B, Lloyd KG, Sanger DJ, Perrault G, Langer SZ and Bartholini G (1986) J. Pharmacol. Exp. Ther. 237: 649–657.
7. Nicholson AN (1986) Drugs 31: 164–176.
8. Nicholson AN and Pascoe DA (1986) Br. J. Clin. Pharmacol. 21: 205–211.
9. Nutt DJ (1986) Trends Pharmacol. Sci. 7: 457–460.

Biological Psychiatry, Volume 1. G. Racagni et al., editors.

The therapeutic and safety profile of zolpidem

Pierre Attali and Paolo Lucio Morselli
Clinical Research Department, Synthelabo Recherche (LERS), 75622 Paris, France

As described in the previous paper, zolpidem is a new non-benzodiazepine short-acting hypnotic belonging to the imidazopyridine chemical series. It acts at the level of the ϖ_1 receptor subtype within the GABA-chloride channel supramolecular complex.

Following oral intake, zolpidem is very rapidly (T_{max} 30–40 min) absorbed with a bioavailability of about 70% [1]. It is about 92–94% bound to plasma protein and its brain penetration is also very rapid [2]. The clearance is essentially metabolic and less than 1% is recovered as such in urine. The apparent plasma half-life is of 2.0–2.5 h in most subjects. The metabolites are totally inactive. The elimination kinetics is linear and it is most modified during repeated treatment [1,3].

The pharmacodynamic profile and the therapeutic efficacy and safety of zolpidem have been evaluated so far in more than 3,000 subjects in specific studies designed to assess its hypnotic activity and the possible presence of residual daytime effects [3,4].

The hypnotic activity of zolpidem and its effect on sleep architecture have been assessed in 9 studies on 562 healthy volunteers and 6 polysomnographic studies on 124 insomniac patients [3–6,10]. From all these studies, it emerges clearly that zolpidem at the dose of 10 mg significantly decreases sleep onset latency, the number and the duration of nocturnal awakenings, and concomitantly increases total sleep time.

Furthermore, at variance with what was observed with reference to benzodiazepine hypnotics, zolpidem does not alter sleep architecture: it increases only moderately stage 2; it increases, when reduced, stages 3 and 4 (slow wave sleep) and it does not decrease REM sleep. Clinical studies conducted on more than 2,000 insomniac patients have clearly shown [3,4,8–10] that at the dose of 10–20 mg, zolpidem induces from the first night a definite hypnotic effect in all types of insomnia. In elderly subjects an initial dose of 5 mg should be considered.

The possible presence of residual effects occurring the day following the administration of zolpidem has been assessed in 740 healthy volunteers and in 405 insomniac patients according to a double-blind (vs. placebo and/or benzodiazepine) controlled design [3,4,7,10]. The evaluation of residual effects was based on both morning questionnaires and daytime performance tests such as MSLT, CFFT, CRT, DSST and tracking tests. No differences between zolpidem, at doses up to 30 mg, and placebo could be observed in the various tests. On the other hand, sleepiness or reduction in psychomotor or cognitive performances was observed following administration of benzodiazepines such as flunitrazepam and triazolam.

The effects of zolpidem on short-term, retrograde and anterograde memory was specifically assessed in 109 healthy volunteers according to a double-blind (vs. placebo and/or benzodiazepine) controlled design. Zolpidem at doses of 10 and 20 mg had no effect on memory tests. On the other hand, both flunitrazepam and triazolam impaired short-term and anterograde memory.

As stated by previous speakers, dependence potential is one of the major concerns with hypnotics. Dependence may occur when abrupt discontinuation of a hypnotic leads to rebound insomnia and/or withdrawal symptoms, or when its prolonged administration induces tolerance phenomenon. The possible occurrence of rebound insomnia has been assessed analyzing objective (polysomnography) and subjective (questionnaires) parameters in 1,292 insomniac patients treated with doses of 10–30 mg for periods of 15–180 days [11]. No consistent rebound insomnia was observed (as assessed by objective measures and by subjective scales). The occurrence of withdrawal symptoms was also assessed in the same population [10,11]. The percentage and the nature of spontaneously reported adverse events occurring during the "placebo controlled" discontinuation period following zolpidem treatment was comparable to those reported during the same period in patients included in the placebo groups. The percentage of adverse events was 3.2% in the zolpidem group and 2.9% in the placebo group. There were no dose-related effects or duration-effect relationships which could suggest the presence of withdrawal effects.

In addition the adverse events were non-specific, of mild severity and did not differ between both groups. The observations are strongly indicative for the absence of withdrawal signs after the abrupt discontinuation of zolpidem. The hypnotic efficacy of zolpidem was maintained in long-term (6–12 months) studies [3,4,10]. No decrease in efficacy was observed using either objective or subjective parameters. In addition, the zolpidem dose could be decreased in more than 10% of long-term treated patients without any decrease in efficacy, suggesting the absence of tachyphylaxis phenomena.

In conclusion, the data available so far on zolpidem indicate that it may be considered as a new interesting hypnotic with a very favourable benefit/risk ratio. In fact, it does not alter sleep architecture, does not induce residual effects and has no evident effect on memory. It does not induce rebound insomnia, withdrawal symptoms and tolerance phenomena. Thus its dependence potential is low, if it exists. Because of all these features it may be differentiated from presently available hypnotics and it may be proposed as a first choice drug in the therapy of insomniac patients.

References

1. Bianchetti G, Dubruc C, Thiercelin JF et al. (1988) In: Sauvanet JP, Langer SZ and Morselli PL (eds.) Imidazopyridines in Sleep Disorders: A Novel Experimental and Therapeutic Approach (LERS Monogr. Series, 6). Raven Press, New York, pp. 155–164.
2. Garrigou-Gadenne D, Burke JT, Durand A et al. (1989) J. Pharmacol. Exp. Ther. 248: 1283–1288.
3. Sauvanet JP, Langer SZ and Morselli PL (eds.) (1988) Imidazopyridines in Sleep Disorders: A Novel Experimental and Therapeutic Approach (LERS Monogr. Series, 6). Raven Press, New York.
4. Langtry HD and Benfield P (1990) Drugs 40: 291–313.
5. Nicholson AN and Stone BM (1986) Acta Psychiatr. Scand. 74(322): 55–59.
6. Monti JM (1989) Eur. J. Clin. Pharmacol. 36: 461–466.
7. Bensimon G, Foret J, Warot D et al. (1990) Br. J. Clin. Pharmacol. 30: 463–469.
8. Frattola L, Maggioni M, Cesana B et al. (1990) Drugs Exp. Clin. Res. 16: 371–376.
9. Lorizio A, Terzano MG, Parrino L et al. (1990) Curr. Ther. Res. 47: 889–898.
10. Morselli PL (1990) In: Carruba MO and Spano PF (eds.) Farmaci Emergenti nei Disturbi del Sonno: le Imidazopyridine. Edizioni Minerva Medica, Turin, pp. 43–52.
11. Attali P and Morselli PL (1991) (in preparation).

Biological Psychiatry, Volume 1. G. Racagni et al., editors.

Disturbance of cyclic alternating pattern in insomnia: Effect of hypnotics

Mario Giovanni Terzano and Liborio Parrino
Sleep Disorders Center, Department of Neurology, University of Parma, Parma, Italy

Introduction

Sleep is an active process of the nervous system aiming at the achievement of physical and psychological recovery. Various exogenous and endogenous factors may interfere with the basic mechanisms that induce, maintain and regulate sleep and thus determine a subjective complaint of insomnia. However, puzzling inconsistencies generally emerge when we try to distinguish normal sleepers from insomniac patients by means of the traditional polysomnographic parameters [1]. More precise information is supplied by the double modality of arousal organization during non-REM sleep referred to as CAP (cyclic alternating pattern) and non-CAP, respectively [2–4]. Since these complementary patterns correspond to opposite conditions of arousal fluctuations (CAP) and arousal stability (non-CAP), CAP rate, i.e. (total CAP time/total non-REM sleep) $\times$ 100, expresses the measure of arousal instability. In a human model of situational insomnia, we found that the higher the values of CAP rate, the more frequently sleep was judged to be of poor and unsatisfactory quality [5]. The present study based on the pharmacological manipulation of sleep, aims at confirming the exploitation of this parameter in the diagnosis of clinical insomnia.

Material and Methods

Eighteen subjects aged 40–60 years participated in the study. Twelve informed individuals (8 females and 4 males, age: 49.6 $\pm$ 5.1 years) met the criteria for the diagnosis of psychophysiological insomnia [6]. The remaining 6 subjects (3 males and 3 females, age: 47.8 $\pm$ 6.5 years) were paid volunteers with no complaints about sleep. They served as the control group.

Following an adaptation night, all subjects were polygraphically recorded for 500 min during nocturnal sleep. About 20 min before lights-out, each subject could receive alternatively a single dose of either placebo or zolpidem 10 mg. Administration was random and double-blind. The hypnotic agent (zolpidem) was chosen for the lack of significant modifications on the architecture of sleep at the selected dosage of 10 mg [7].

Polysomnograms were scored according to standard criteria [8] and to the published guidelines for CAP and non-CAP [2–4].

After every sleep recording, each subject filled in a multisection questionnaire, integrated by a visual analog scale (VAS). The higher the values of VAS the poorer the subjective judgement of sleep quality.

An ANOVA test with four categories was followed by a Scheffé multiple comparison when F statistics were significant. Data transformations were carried out whenever necessary for homogeneity of variances.

Results

The means and standard deviations for each variable are given in Table 1. The Scheffé test showed significant differences only between the extreme conditions of insomniacs placebo and controls zolpidem for slow wave sleep and total sleep time. A significant difference emerged for total sleep time also between insomniacs placebo and controls placebo. The multiple comparison test allowed a clear-cut discrimination among three different CAP rate subsets:

a) insomniacs placebo (62.2%);

b) controls placebo (38.5%);

c) subjects treated with zolpidem, i.e. insomniacs (26.8%) and controls (31%).

The VAS means differed significantly only within the insomniac group.

Discussion

CAP is the electroencephalographic translation of the active cerebral effort to maintain the depth of sleep against internal or external destabilizing factors. In the present study, CAP rate was significantly higher in untreated insomniacs compared to untreated controls, whereas no other traditional sleep parameter, besides total sleep time, was capable of differentiating the two groups.

An excessive amount of CAP rate likely characterizes the majority of insomnias. Conversely, the excess of CAP rate is attenuated by sleep-promoting conditions such as prolonged sleep deprivation or commonly used sedative-hypnotic compounds. The limited effects on traditional sleep parameters induced by zolpidem both in insomniac patients and in controls allowed us to explore the behaviour of CAP rate in the different contexts. Under placebo, CAP rate was significantly higher in insomniac individuals compared with age-matched normal sleepers, while under medication, the CAP rate means of both groups were referred to the same statistical sub-set. Thus, CAP rate evaluation permitted to differentiate insomniacs and controls and to separate the drug nights from the placebo nights.

The present study reinforced the importance of polysomnography for the diagnosis of insomnia and confirmed the hypnotic properties of zolpidem. Preliminary

Table 1. Means, standard deviations and statistical assessment of polysomnographic and subjective data

	Insomniacs (12 subjects)		Controls (6 subjects)		ANOVA (d.f.: 3, 32)
	1. Placebo	2. Zolpidem	3. Placebo	4. Zolpidem	F statistics
SL (min)	14.5 ± 14.0	8.1 ± 7.1	5.0 ± 6.0	2.0 ± 1.5	$P < 0.06$
WASO (%)[a] (min)	9.2 ± 5.4 (41)	3.6 ± 3.7 (16)	2.0 ± 2.8 (19)	2.0 ± 1.0 (9)	$P < 0.31$
S1 + S2 (%) (min)	60.4 ± 4.4 (268)	53.7 ± 7.7 (235)	56.8 ± 6.7 (274)	57.0 ± 5.0 (270)	$P < 0.80$
S3 + S4 (%) (min)	9.5 ± 5.0[c] (42)	17.6 ± 5.8 (76)	15.9 ± 4.7 (76)	18.0 ± 6.5[c] (83)	$P < 0.004$[c]
REM (%) (min)	20.8 ± 5.0 (92)	25.1 ± 9.6 (109)	23.3 ± 3.5 (112)	23.6 ± 2.6 (112)	$P < 0.48$
Non-REM (%) (min)	69.9 ± 4.7 (310)	71.3 ± 8.2 (311)	72.7 ± 4.4 (350)	75.0 ± 2.6 (353)	$P < 0.37$
TST (min)	402.0 ± 37.9[c]	420.0 ± 49.7	462.0 ± 21.2[c]	465.0 ± 25.2[c]	$P < 0.005$[c]
SPT (min)	443.0 ± 32.4	436.0 ± 44.7	481.0 ± 15.8	474.0 ± 24.2	$P < 0.03$[c]
CAP rate (%) (min)	62.0 ± 3.1[c] (193)	26.8 ± 4.9[c] (83)	38.5 ± 5.6[c] (134)	31.0 ± 2.6[c] (109)	$P < 0.00001$[c]
VAS (mm)[b]	45.0 ± 19[c]	15.6 ± 6.4[c]	25.3 ± 11.6	24.2 ± 15.8	$P < 0.0001$[c]

SL: sleep latency; WASO: wake after sleep onset; S1: stage 1; S2: stage 2; S3: stage 3; S4: stage 4; REM: rapid eye movements sleep; TST: total sleep time; SPT: sleep period time; CAP: cylic alternating pattern; CAP: rate is referred to total non-REM sleep; VAS: visual analog scale. All macrostrucutral percentages are referred to SPT; [a]Arc sin transformation; [b]logarithmic transformation for homogeneity of variance; and [c]significant statistics.

studies with other hypnotic and sedative agents both in insomniacs and controls indicate different grades of drug-induced reduction of CAP rate accompanied by alterations in sleep architecture. We believe that in the near future the fine-grained analysis of CAP rate may provide highly sensitive and consistent information on the pharmacological treatment of sleep complaints.

References

1. Carskadon MA, Dement WC, Mitler MM, Guilleminault C, Zarcone VP and Siegel R (1976) Am. J. Psychiatry 133: 1382–1388.
2. Terzano MG, Mancia D, Salati MR, Costani G, Decembrino A and Parrino L (1985) Sleep 8: 137–145.
3. Terzano MG, Parrino L, Floriti G, Spaggiari MC and Piroli A (1986) Funct. Neurol. 1: 29–41.
4. Terzano MG, Parrino L and Spaggiari MC (1988) Electroencephalogr. Clin. Neurophysiol. 69: 437–447.

5. Terzano MG, Parrino L, Fioriti G, Orofiamma B and Depoortere H (1990) Electroencephalogr. Clin. Neurophysiol. 76: 29–38.
6. Association of Sleep Disorders Centers (1979) Sleep 2: 1–137.
7. Nicholson AN and Pascoe PA (1986) Br. J. Clin. Pharmacol. 21: 205–211.
8. Rechtschaffen A and Kales A (eds.) (1968) Brain Information Service/Brain Research Institute, University of California at Los Angeles.

Biological Psychiatry, Volume 1. G. Racagni et al., editors.

Problems related to long-term use of hypnotics

Jaime M. Monti
Department of Pharmacology and Therapeutics, School of Medicine, Clinics Hospital, Montevideo, 11600 Uruguay

The sleep induced by the benzodiazepine (BZD) hypnotics is characterized by shortened sleep onset latency, decreased number of nocturnal awakenings, reduction in time spent awake, increment in stage 2 NREM sleep, a consistent decrease of slow wave sleep (stages 3 and 4), a dose-dependent REM sleep suppression and improvement of the subjective quality of sleep. Commonly reported side-effects include drowsiness, impairment of intellectual function, dizziness, ataxia and anterograde amnesia.

Long-acting BZDs increase polygraphically measured disposition to fall asleep during daytime (MSLT) and decrease many measures of psychomotor performance. Daytime anxiety has been reported in patients receiving short-term derivatives.

Most BZD hypnotics maintain their effectiveness for 1–2 months (controlled sleep studies). Rebound insomnia has been shown to develop following withdrawal from ultra-short and short-to-intermediate acting BZD hypnotics. In addition, BZD hypnotics can produce psychological and physical dependence [1].

Rebound insomnia

This is characterized by temporary changes from baseline that are opposite to those initially produced by the BZD hypnotic itself. Rebound insomnia can be considered apart from dependence if the BZD has been given for a short period of time. Otherwise, rebound insomnia should be considered as part of the withdrawal reaction [2].

The BZD rebound insomnia includes increased NREM sleep latency, decreased total sleep time, disrupted and fragmented sleep and increased dreaming associated with a REM sleep rebound.

A rebound insomnia has been described for midazolam, triazolam, brotizolam, lormetazepam, lorazepam and flunitrazepam. The rebound insomnia induced by triazolam has been thoroughly studied. It was described in poor sleepers and chronic insomniacs who were given 0.25–0.5 mg triazolam/night during periods ranging from 4–37 nights. The biggest increase in total wake time occurred on the first night of withdrawal and ranged from 10–42%. On the second and subsequent nights total wake time tended to return to baseline levels [3,4].

Rebound insomnia appears to occur more readily following administration of shorter-acting BZDs and according to some authors the rebound phenomenon could lead to increased use or more frequent use of BZD hypnotics [5].

Development of dependence to benzodiazepine hypnotics

The prevalence of BZD use is rather high. Accordingly, it amounts to 9.7%–16% in the general population; 17%–36.9% in psychiatric outpatients and 33.3%–41% in alcoholics.

At least 3 patterns of BZD dependence have been proposed: a) BZD primary low-dose dependency at therapeutic dosage; b) BZD primary high-dose dependency, where patients take 2–5 times the normal therapeutic dosage; although physical dependence has been shown to develop within 6 weeks, in most cases the BZD has been taken for years; in this particular pattern of BZD dependence patients are at risk of developing severe withdrawal reactions; c) BZD secondary dependency or multiple drug abuse. Here, secondary dependency arises in the context of multiple drug abuse and/or alcoholism [6].

Withdrawal syndrome

A withdrawal syndrome follows the abrupt cessation of BZD administration: a) after treatment with standard therapeutic doses or in high-dose BZD dependent patients; b) after substitution of a short-acting BZD for a long-acting one; c) as we have seen, a transient increase of symptoms occurring after stopping a BZD hypnotic that rapidly returns to normal can be more properly called a rebound insomnia; d) from an experimental point of view, a withdrawal syndrome can be precipitated by flumazenil in laboratory animals made physically dependent by subchronic administration of high doses of flurazepam, diazepam, lorazepam or triazolam.

Concerning the onset of the withdrawal syndrome, it has been shown that in patients receiving short or intermediate half-lives BZDs, it develops the day after their discontinuation; when BZDs with long half-lives are given the withdrawal syndrome shows 3–8 days later.

There is no agreement as to the previous duration of BZD administration necessary for a withdrawal syndrome to develop: 6 weeks or longer for Tyrer [7]; 4 months according to Swinson et al. [8] and over 6 months for Uhlenhuth et al. [9].

It seems that short-acting BZD hypnotics have a greater potential for causing a withdrawal reaction as compared to the long-acting ones. Thus, midazolam, triazolam (ultrashort-acting) and lorazepam (short-acting) have a high potential for the development of a withdrawal reaction, while temazepam, lormetazepam and diazepam have a moderate potential and flurazepam a low potential [7]. This could be related to the rapid decline in plasma levels of midazolam, triazolam and lorazepam. Accordingly, short-acting BZDs very frequently undergo biotransformation via conjugation, long-acting metabolites are uncommon and accumulation during multiple dosing is less extensive than with the long-acting group and diminishes as the half-life becomes shorter.

The duration of the withdrawal syndrome depends on the BZD elimination half-life. After discontinuation of therapy with long-acting BZDs the duration of the withdrawal symptoms have been reported to average 10 days. Following withdrawal of BZDs with a short half-life, symptoms have been shown to persist an average of 2–3 days.

Withdrawal symptoms

According to Schöpf [10] the following symptoms can be considered: a) frequent unspecific symptoms including sleep disturbances, anxiety, irritability, muscle pairs, tremor, headache, nausea, loss of appetite, transpiration and blurred vision; b) perceptual changes of a quantitative nature such as hypersensitivity to noise, light, smell and touch; c) perceptual changes of a mainly qualitative nature including kinesthetic, optical, gustatory, acoustic and olfactory symptoms; and d) other and less frequent symptoms such as depersonalization, psychoses and epileptiform crises. Special concern exists about the occurrence of seizures after withdrawal of BZDs. Convulsions can occur in relation to short- or long half-life derivative administration; after relatively short-term administration; in patients who were receiving therapeutic dosages of BZDs and the simultaneous use of alcohol, antidepressants (tricyclics), barbiturates or the presence of fever favours their occurrence.

Abrupt withdrawal and gradual taper of BZDs

The following methods have been found helpful in making BZD withdrawal more acceptable to chronic BZD users: gradual BZD discontinuation; replacement of short half-life with long half-life BZD and the adjunctive use of carbamazepine or buspirone.

During abrupt withdrawal of BZDs the following are predictors of withdrawal severity: BZD short half-life, high daily dose, prolonged administration period, female sex, low education, high initial psychopathology and high neuroticism (Eysenck).

Gradual taper has been tried to decrease withdrawal severity. However, it did not prevent the occurrence of withdrawal symptoms in a relatively large number of patients. Female patients with a diagnosis of depression, high Eysenck neuroticism and mild to moderate alcohol intake had more severe withdrawal reactions following gradual taper. The symptoms included anxiety, insomnia, tremulousness and irritability. Thirty-two percent of long half-life and 42% of short half-life BZD-treated patients were unable to tolerate taper and resumed their daily use of BZDs [11,12].

Available evidence tends to indicate that following long-term administration of the imidazopyridine derivative zolpidem, tolerance does not develop to its sleep-inducing and maintaining effects [13]. In addition, neither rebound insomnia nor dependence have been described during intermediate to long-term administration of the derivative [14,15].

References

1. Monti JM (1988) In: Sauvanet JP, Langer SZ and Morselli PL (eds.) Imidazopyridines in Sleep Disorders. Raven Press, New York, pp. 363–368.
2. Woods JH, Katz JL and Winger G (1987) Pharmacol. Rev. 39: 251–419.
3. Greenblatt DJ, Harmatz JS, Zinny MA and Shader RI (1987) N. Engl. J. Med. 317: 722–728.
4. Gillin JC, Spinweber CL and Johnson LC (1989) J. Clin. Psychopharmacol. 9: 161–172.
5. Kales A, Soldatos CR, Bixler EO, Kales JD and Vela-Bueno A (1988) J. Clin. Psychopharmacol. 8: 340–346.
6. Kleber HD (1990) J. Psychiatr. Res. 24: 57–64.
7. Tyrer P (1988) Pharmacol. Ther. 36: 173–188.
8. Swinson RP, Pecknold JC and Kirby ME (1987) J. Affective Disord. 13: 109–118.
9. Uhlenhuth EH, Balter MB and Lipman RS (1978) Arch. Gen. Psychiatry 35: 650–655.
10. Schopf J (1983) Pharmacopsychiatry 16: 1–8.
11. Rickels K, Schweizer E, Case W and Greenblatt DJ (1990) Arch. Gen. Psychiatry 47: 899–907.
12. Schweizer E, Rickels K, Case G and Greenblatt DJ (1990) Arch. Gen. Psychiatry 47: 908–915.
13. Sauvanet JP, Maarek L, Roger M, Renaudin J, Louvel E and Orofiamma B (1988) In: Sauvanet JP, Langer SZ and Morselli PL (eds.) Imidazopyridines in Sleep Disorders. Raven Press, New York, pp. 339–349.
14. Monti JM (1989) Eur. J. Clin. Pharmacol. 36: 461–466.
15. Herrmann WM, Kubicki S and Wober W (1988) In: Sauvanet JP, Langer SZ and Morselli PL (eds.) Imidazopyridines in Sleep Disorders. Raven Press, New York, pp. 261–278.

Index of authors

Volume 1

Abou-Saleh, M.T. 64
Adams, D. 142
Alf, C. 713
Allen, R. 787
Alling, C. 100, 121
Altamura, A.C. 328
Altamura, C.A. 583
Altshuler, L. 504
Amering, M. 657, 713
Amorosa, H. 418
Anand, A. 515
Anastasiades, P. 654
Anderson, J.L. 206
Anderson, K. 699
Anderson, M.C. 403
Ando, H. 547
Ando, K. 547
Andreasen, N.C. 6, 455
Antonin, K.-H. 406
Arango, V. 118
Aravagiri, M. 590
Arbilla, S. 683, 856
Armitage, R. 52
Armstrong, E. 504
Asnis, G.M. 110, 532
Ator, N.A. 724
Attali, P. 860
Avissar, S. 173
Awouters, F. 535
Axelson, D.A. 213

Baldwin, D. 124
Ballenger, J.C. 657
Ban, T.A. 28
Bareggi, S.R. 328
Baumann, P. 279, 362, 368
Beauclair, L. 560
Bech, P. 288
Becker, T. 372
Beckmann, H. 485
Behrens, S. 431
Bellantuono, C. 441
Belmaker, R.H. 195
Benavides, J. 747
Benkert, O. 43
Benson, K.L. 811
Berg, P. 550
Berger, M. 797
Berger, P. 713
Berger, W. 482
Bernasconi, R. 393
Bertschy, G. 368
Beuger, M. 580
Bieck, P.R. 406
Biegon, A. 103
Biggio, G. 702
Bixler, E.O. 814
Blier, P. 301
Bliwise, D. 849
Boccio, A. 515
Bogerts, B. 507
Bolaños, F. 297
Bolwig, T.G. 602
Bonetti, E.P. 390
Bonin, B. 368
Bono, G. 165
Bouquet, S. 368
Bourgeois, M. 308
Bouvy, P.F. 246
Boval, P. 696
Boyer, W.F. 161, 276, 338
Boyko, O.B. 213
Brecha, N. 699
Briggs, A. 657
Bscheid, I. 544
Buller, R. 657
Bullock, T. 124
Bunney, B.S. 574
Busto, U.E. 709, 767

Calev, A. 257
Cameron, C.L. 787
Campbell, I.C. 149
Caracci, G. 628
Carl, G. 372
Carlsson, A. 467
Carlsson, M. 467
Carroll, B.J. 17, 757

Casacchia, M. 689
Casalotti, S.O. 735
Casanova, M. 504
Cascella, N.G. 523
Case, W.G. 778
Casey, D.E. 587, 605
Cassano, G.B. 136, 657
Checkley, S.A. 149
Chiang, M.-Y. 699
Chouinard, G. 560
Christensson, E. 577
Cialdella, P. 288
Ciapparelli, A. 804
Cini, M. 386
Cipolli, C. 851
Clark, C.R. 635
Clark, D.M. 654
Classen, W. 372
Coccaro, E.F. 106
Coffee, C.E. 260
Cohen, G. 455
Cohen, R. 550
Concas, A. 702
Conley, R.R. 523
Coppen, A.J. 64
Cornu, P. 747
Costa, A. 165
Costall, B. 538
Coward, D.M. 566
Cowen, P.J. 347
Crompton, M.R. 78
Crow, T.J. 511
Cumes-Rayner, D. 639

Damm, K. 222, 225
Da Prada, M. 386, 390
David, S. 507
Davis, J.M. 177
Davis, W. 3
de Kloet, E.R. 217
de Montigny, C. 243, 301
de Paermentier, F. 78
de Souza, E.B. 498
de Vry, J. 431
de Wilde, J. 696
de Wit, H. 771
Deakin, J.F.W. 305
Decaria, C.M. 680
Decina, P. 628
Delini-Stula, A. 716
DeLisi, L.E. 515
den Boer, J.A. 315
Depoortere, H. 856
Distefano, L. 489
Dixon, L.M. 489
Domeney, A.M. 538
Doraiswamy, P.M. 213
Dosser, G. 365
Dostert, P. 386
Dubini, A. 12

Eap, C.B. 362
Ehrhardt, J. 455
Eisner, W. 520
Ekman, R. 580
Ellinwood Jr,, E.H. 213
Ellison, G. 598
Emrich, H.M. 469
Escande, M. 308
Esnaud, H. 294

Falkai, P. 507
Farmer, A. 31
Feighner, J.P. 161, 338
Feinberg, I. 817
Ferrero, P. 750
Figiel, G.S. 213
Finberg, J.P.M. 380
Fineberg, N. 675
First, M. 3
Flaum, M. 455
Fog, R. 275
Frances, A.J. 3
Frank, E. 61, 253
Frattola, L. 696
Freeman, C.P. 661
Frenkel, M. 680
Friese, H.J. 425
Frith, C. 472
Fujita, H. 91
Fukuda, T. 449
Fuller, R.W. 529
Furuta, H. 833

Gaillard, J.-M. 854
Galzin, A.-M. 72
Ganguli, R. 808
Garreau, M. 308, 325, 696
Garvey, M. 657
Gasperini, M. 19
Gattaz, W.F. 431
Gavish, M. 738

Geisler, A. 172, 200, 357
Gelder, M.G. 654
Gelernter, J. 580
Genazzani, A.R. 165
Genda, S. 475
Gerbaldo, H. 43
Gerlach, J. 593, 609
Gjerris, A. 81
Gleders, Y.G. 535
Glenthøj, B. 602
Glover, V. 142
Goldberg, T. 504
Goodman, W.K. 671
Goodnick, P.J. 353
Goodwin, G.M. 197
Gottfries, C.-G. 291
Gozlan, H. 297
Graham, D. 294
Gram, L.F. 359
Grayson, D.R. 735
Greden, J. 520
Green, M. 67, 124
Gregoire, A. 144
Greve, B. 507
Griffiths, R.R. 724
Gross, G. 458
Grossberg, G.T. 765
Gsell, W. 383
Guazzelli, M. 804
Guidotti, A. 580
Guilleminault, C. 849
Guldner, J. 210
Gullion, C.M. 52
Günther, W. 544
Gurklis, J. 580

Haag, C. 544
Hadjez, J. 257
Haefely, W. 705
Haffmans, P.M.J. 246, 413
Häfner, H. 431
Haj-Dahmane, S. 297
Hajak, G. 845
Hamon, M. 297
Hannah, P. 142
Hansen, L. 609
Hashimoto, T. 91
Hatashi, T. 452
Hatta, S. 188
Hebenstreit, G. 383
Heinsen, H. 485
Hemmingsen, R. 602
Henderson, A. 144
Heun, R. 34
Heylen, S.L.E. 535
Hicks-Gray, T. 590
Hillmann, M. 721
Hirschfeld, R.M.A. 646
Hirst, A.D. 149
Hishikawa, Y. 794, 831, 837
Höflich, G. 800
Holan, V. 515
Hollander, E. 680
Hollund, P. 192
Holman, R.B. 268
Holsboer, F. 210, 222, 225
Hopmann, G. 550
Hori, H. 837
Hornykiewicz, O. 489
Horton, R.W. 78
Houben-Gelissen, M. 668
Houck, P. 808
Hozumi, S. 837
Hrdina, P.D. 69
Huba, R. 721
Hubain, P. 332
Huber, G. 458
Humble, M. 282
Humpel, C. 365
Husain, M.M. 213
Hyttel, J. 553

Iio, M. 91
Imperato, A. 566
Inanaga, K. 461
Insel, T.R. 664
Iqbal, N. 532
Ishiguro, N. 833
Ishikawa, T. 91
Ishimaru, M. 501
Iwata, T. 791

Jähnig, P. 823
Jansen, P.A.F. 413
Jellinger, K.A. 383, 485
Jensen, N.-H. 234
Jobert, M. 823
Johannsen, H. 418
Johanson, C.E. 771
Johnson, D.A.W. 556
Johnson, S. 253
Johnston, S.H. 787

Johnstone, E.C. 40
Jolas, T. 297
Joseph-Vanderpool, R.R. 787

Kachi, T. 452
Kahn, R.S. 110, 532
Kales, A. 814, 819
Kaplan, H.L. 709
Kapur, S. 272
Käsbauer, L. 383
Kasper, S. 800
Kathol, R.G. 757
Katona, C.L.E. 78
Katschnig, H. 657, 713
Kavoussi, R.J. 106
Kay, S.R. 532
Kayukawa, Y. 791
Kelley, M.E. 580
Kelly, M.E. 538
Kendell, R.E. 146
Kerkhofs, M. 332
Keshavan, M.S. 808
Kessel, J.B. 526
Khrestchatisky, M. 699
Kidd, E. 297
King, J.M. 78
Kirch, D.G. 621
Kish, S.J. 489
Kishimoto, H. 91
Kitou, H. 452
Klages, U. 544
Kleinman, J. 504
Klerman, G.L. 657
Klompenhouwer, J.L. 146
Koczkas, C. 282
Kofman, O. 195
Kojima, T. 547
Konradi, C. 383
Korn, M. 110
Kornhuber, J. 222, 495
Kosaka, K. 91
Koskinen, T. 563
Kotorii, T. 841
Krishnan, K.R.R. 213
Krueger, K.E. 735, 744
Kumar, R. 144, 149
Kumashiro, S. 501
Kuniyoshi, M. 461
Kupfer, D.J. 37, 55, 61, 253
Kuramaji, A. 501
Kushner, M. 515
Kutzer, M. 713

Lader, M.H. 693, 732, 775
Lai, M. 699
Lanfumey, L. 297
Langer, S.Z. 72, 294, 683, 856
Lauer, C. 210
Lauritzen, L. 234
Laux, G. 372
Legris, P. 308
L'Heritier, C. 696
Leonard, B.E. 311
Lerer, B. 184, 257, 350
Lesch, K.P. 372
Leva, P. 583
Levendosky, A.A. 787
Lewis, A. 489
Li, R. 621
Lichtenberg, P. 184
Lichtermann, D. 34
Liebowitz, M.R. 680
Lieder, F. 365
Linden, M. 129
Linkowski, P. 332
Littlewood, J. 142
Loo, H. 72
Lugaresi, E. 827
Lunde, M. 234
Lurie, S.N. 213

MacLennan, A.J. 699
Maeda, T. 91
Maeda, Y. 833
Maggini, C. 804
Magni, G. 231, 343
Maier, W. 34
Maletta, G.J. 761
Mamelak, M. 489
Mander, A.J. 197
Manfredi, R.L. 814
Mann, J.J. 114, 118, 272
Mann, N. 520
Marcusson, J. 75
Marder, S.R. 590
Marks, M.N. 149
Markstein, R. 566
Marrari, P. 386
Martignoni, E. 165
Mascia, M.P. 702
Matsushima, E. 547
Mauri, M.C. 583

McCrodden, J.M. 378
McDougle, C.J. 671
McFarlane, A.C. 635
McGuffin, P. 31, 434
Medda, P. 136
Mellerup, E.T. 234
Meltzer, H.Y. 538, 570
Memo, M. 596
Mendlewicz, J. 308, 332
Menzel, M. 425
Merskey, H. 228, 231
Merz, W.A. 713, 727
Meshul, C.K. 605
Miller, D. 455
Minami, E. 475
Minges, J. 34
Mishima, K. 794
Missale, C. 596
Molcho, A. 126
Moll, G. 383
Möller, H.-J. 410, 800
Montgomery, D.B. 67, 124, 675
Montgomery, S.A. 67, 124, 343, 675
Monti, J.M. 867
Mørk, A. 172, 192, 200, 357
Morselli, P.L. 325, 691, 696, 860
Morton, S. 693
Mos, J. 668
Mukheriee, S. 624
Müller-Oerlinghausen, B. 375
Munizza, C. 444
Murri, L. 851

Nakagawa, K. 833
Nakajima, K. 547
Nakazawa, Y. 841
Nappi, G. 165
Naylor, R.J. 538
Nemeroff, C.B. 213
Neumann, R. 365
Newman, M.E. 184, 350
Niemegeers, C.J.E. 535
Nishikawa, T. 501
Nissen, G. 416, 425
Nolen, W.A. 246
Nonaka, K. 841
Norberg, B. 282
Nordström, P. 94
Noyes, R. 757
Nutt, D.J. 268
Nutzinger, D. 713
Nyth, A.L. 291

O'Brien, E.M. 378
O'Connor, D.T. 580
O'Leary, D.S. 455
Oberbauer, H. 365
Ohara, M. 452
Ohbayashi, S. 547
Öhman, R. 100, 121
Ohta, T. 791
Okada, T. 791
Okasha, A. 677
Okawa, M. 794, 837
Olivier, B. 668
Olsen, R.W. 699
Opjordsmoen, S. 464
Oreland, L. 121
Ozawa, H. 188

Pandey, G.M. 177
Pandey, S.C. 177
Papadopoulos, V. 742, 744
Parrino, L. 863
Patterson, L. 213
Paykel, E.S. 57, 400
Peacock, L. 609
Pelaia, G. 735
Perel, J. 580
Perrault, G. 686
Pervgi, G. 136
Peters, J.L. 580
Petraglia, F. 165
Philipp, M. 43
Pincus, H.A. 3
Pinder, R.M. 322
Pirfo, E. 444
Pizzi, M. 596
Plenge, P. 234
Poirier, M.F. 72, 308
Posener, J.A. 318
Post, R.M. 49
Prange Jr., A.J. 84
Pudel, V. 845
Puech, A.J. 335
Punzo, F. 444

Raphael, B. 639
Rasenick, M.M. 188
Ravizza, L. 750
Reddy, R. 624
Regnéll, G. 100, 121

Retterstøl, N. 464
Reul, J.M.H.M. 217
Reynolds, C.F. 808
Reynolds, G.P. 491
Rezai, K. 455
Rickels, K. 345, 778
Riedel, R. 544
Riederer, P. 222, 383, 482, 495
Riemann, D. 797
Rigatti-Luchini, S. 231
Riordan, H. 515
Rocca, P. 750
Rodenbeck, A. 845
Roffwarg, H.P. 52
Romach, M.K. 767
Roose, S.P. 240
Rosenthal, N.E. 787
Rossi, M.R. 231
Roth, M. 648, 657
Rothe, B. 210
Rothenberger, A. 418
Rothuizen, J. 217
Roy, A. 97
Ruhrmann, S. 800
Rupprecht, R. 222, 225
Rush, A.J. 9, 52
Rüther, E. 845

Sackeim, H.A. 249, 264
Safadi, G. 560
Saito, T. 188
Sakamoto, T. 841
Sandler, M. 142
Sanger, D.J. 686, 856
Sannerud, C.A. 724
Sano, J. 833
Santoro, G. 702
Saria, A. 365
Saunders, R. 504
Savino, M. 136
Scapicchio, P. 628
Scatton, B. 747, 856
Scharf, M.B. 157
Schatzberg, A.F. 318
Scherschlicht, R. 390
Schilling, W. 393
Schneider, H.H. 721
Schnur, D.B. 624
Schoerlin, M.P. 372
Schreiber, G. 173
Schulsinger, F. 437
Schulz, H. 823
Schulz, R. 406
Schulze, H. 418
Schwartz, J.A. 87
Schweizer, E. 778
Seivewright, N. 133
Sellers, E.M. 709, 767
Sforza, E. 827
Shagass, C. 541
Shapira, B. 184, 257, 350
Shimazono, Y. 547
Shimizu, T. 831
Shipley, J. 520
Silverstone, T. 286
Silvestrini, B. 152
Simeon, J.G. 423
Simonsson, P. 121
Simpson, G.M. 526
Slimovitch, C. 489
Smeraldi, B. 19
Sofic, E. 383
Solyom, C. 657
Souza, F.G.M. 197
Spano, P.F. 596
Speed, N.M. 87
Spengler, D. 222, 225
Stanley, M. 126
Steiger, A. 210
Stein, D. 680
Stephens, D.N. 721
Sternini, C. 699
Stewart, D.E. 146
Stockmeier, C.A. 570
Stolk, J.M. 657
Strizke, P. 515
Strolin Benedetti, M. 386
Studd, J. 144
Suga, H. 452
Suga, I. 501
Sugita, Y. 831
Sunderland, T. 755
Svensson, A. 467
Sydnor-Greenberg, N. 3

Tachibana, N. 831
Takahashi, H. 91
Takahashi, K. 794
Takahata, N. 188
Takatsu, O. 91
Tamminga, C.A. 523
Tandon, R. 520

Terashima, M. 791
Terzano, M.G. 863
Thelander, S. 563
Thomas, D.N. 268
Tibaldi, G. 444
Tillakaratne, N.J.K. 699
Tipton, K.F. 378, 403
Tobin, A.J. 699
Toru, M. 501
Toulmond, S. 747
Träskman-Bendz, L. 100, 121
Trott, G.E. 425
Trungold, S. 680
Tsuru, N. 475
Turek, F. 202
Turner, J.D. 721
Turski, L. 721
Tyrer, P. 133

Uchimura, N. 841
Ueno, K. 833
Underwood, M.D. 118

Vaddadi, K.S. 618
Valerio, A. 596
Vandel, S. 368
van der Poel, G. 668
van Eyl, O. 515
van Hulst, A.M. 146
van Kammen, D.P. 580
van Megen, H.J.G.M. 315
van Praag, H.M. 23, 110, 532
van Putten, T. 590
van Reeth, O. 202
Vela-Bueno, A. 814
Vetulani, J. 181
Vgontzas, A.N. 814
Vinge, E. 121
Vitiello, B. 755
von Bardeleben, U. 210
von Knorring, L. 237

Wachtel, H. 169
Waddington, J.L. 612, 615
Wald, T. 757
Waldmeier, P. 393
Wehr, T.A. 783
Weinberger, D. 504
Weiner, R.D. 260
Weissman, A.D. 498
Westenberg, H.G.M. 315
Wetzler, S. 110, 532
Whalin, M. 735
Wickland, C. 202
Widerlöv, E. 580
Widiger, T. 3
Wieck, A. 149
Wiegand, M. 797
Wiesel, F.-A. 478
Wik, G. 478
Wing, L.L. 621
Winslow, J.T. 664
Winter, P. 43
Wirshing, W.C. 590
Wistedt, B. 282, 563
Wodarz, N. 222
Wyatt, R.J. 621

Yagmur, M.J. 350
Yamaguchi, N. 833
Yamamori, S. 833
Yesavage, J.A. 849
Yokoi, F. 91
Youdim, M.B.H. 397

Zarcone Jr., V.P. 811
Zivkovic, B. 686, 856

Subject index

Volume 1

Abdominal pain, chronic, 231
Abecarnil, 721, 724
Abuse liability testing, 709, 724, 727, 771
α_1-Acid glycoprotein, 311, 362
ACTH (adrenocorticotrophic hormone), 37, 210, 217, 332
Adenylate cyclase activity, 172, 184, 188, 192, 200, 297, 716
Adinazolam, 318
Adolescents, 103, 243, 423, 425
Adrafinil, 716
α-Adrenoceptors, 78, 152, 172, 181
α_2-Adrenoceptor antagonists, 322
ß-Adrenoceptors, 78, 114, 118, 152, 173, 181, 188
ß-Adrenoceptor antagonists, 732
Affective disorders, 40, 87, 91, 106, 169, 400, 504, 808, 811
  see also Specific disorders
Affective Morbidity Index (AMI), 64
Age factor, 217, 328, 386, 587, 612, 615, 661, 755
  and schizophrenia, 431, 458, 511, 515, 583, 811
  and sleep disorders, 811, 817, 819, 827, 837, 841, 845
  see also Elderly patients
Aggressive behavior, 106, 110, 668, 775
Agoraphobia, 282, 646, 648
Akathisia, 590
Akinesia, 590
Alcohol, 237, 276, 550, 761, 771, 867
Alpidem, 683, 686, 689, 691, 693, 696
Alprazolam, 43, 318, 648, 657, 696, 709, 727, 767, 778
Alzheimer's disease, 165, 291, 383, 544, 833, 837, 849
"American nervousness", 129
Amiflamine, 372
Amine hypothesis, 81
Amino acids, 91, 386
Amitriptyline, 12, 12, 136, 288, 322, 328, 332, 362, 400, 804
  in combined therapy, 279, 350, 365, 368
Amoxapine, 126, 328
AMP, cyclic, 142, 169, 181, 195, 200, 225, 716
Amperozide, 570, 570, 577, 716
Amphetamine, 771
Anaesthetics, general, 702
Analgesia, and stress, 152
Angina pectoris, 757
Anorexia nervosa, 276, 680
Anosognosia, 628
Antidepressant drugs, 12, 49, 67, 72, 75, 124, 126, 177, 188, 335, 362, 800
  pharmacokinetics, 311, 328, 338, 368, 375
  treatment response, 328, 343
  see also Specific drugs
Antipsychotic agents, 526
  see also Specific drugs
Anxiety disorders, 133, 305, 400, 423, 750, 767, 778
  classification, 732
  and depression, 9, 761
  diagnosis, 34, 732
  and elderly patients, 691, 761, 765
  and medical illness, 757, 761
  and panic disorders, 34
  and schizophrenia, 478
Anxiolytic drugs *see* Specific drugs and drug classes
Apnea, 827
Apomorphine, 149, 609
Aptazine, 322
Atipemazole, 322
Attention, disturbances of, 635
Aversion, acute, 305

Back pain, chronic, 228
Behavior disorders, 831, 837
Behavioral therapy, 648, 819
Benzodiazepines, 318, 705, 709, 732, 755, 765, 867
  abuse, 709, 724, 767, 771
  comparative studies, 689, 693, 696, 721, 724, 856

dependence, 693, 696, 724, 732, 767, 775, 856, 867
and insomnia, 819, 823, 854, 856, 867
tolerance, 693, 696, 755, 856
withdrawal, 778, 819, 867
Benzofuranylpiperidine, 393
Biological markers
of aggression, 110
of anxiety disorders, 738, 742, 744, 747, 750
of dementia, 165
of depression, 17, 37, 52, 55, 64, 69, 72, 75, 78, 84, 142, 332
of idiopathic pain syndromes, 237
of suicidal behavior, 78, 94, 97, 100, 103, 106, 110, 114, 118, 121, 124, 126, 315
Biperiden, 520
Bipolar disorders, 9, 12, 19, 52, 197, 628, 783, 804
postpartum, 9, 142, 146, 149
Blood pressure
hypertension, 827
reactivity, 639
Body dysmorphic disorder, 680
Body temperature, 206, 787, 837, 841
Borderline personality disorder, 680
Brain, 165, 177, 472, 478, 605, 612, 615
abnormalities in schizophrenia, 485, 504, 507, 511, 515
damage, 547, 747, 831, 851
imaging *see* CT scans; Magnetic resonance imaging; PET; SPECT
receptors, 75, 78, 103, 114, 118, 747
see also Cortex; Hippocampus
Bretazenil, 705, 709, 713, 727
Brofaromine, 246, 372, 393, 403, 406, 410, 413
Bromocriptine, 12
Bufloramine, 136
Bulimia nervosa, 276, 680
Bupropion, 136, 353
Buspirone, 423, 671, 732, 778

Carbamylcholine, 173
ß-Carbolines, 721, 724
Caffeine, 621
Cerebral blood flow, 87, 91, 452, 455, 472, 478, 664
Cerebral metabolic rate for oxygen, 91
Cerebrospinal fluid (CSF), 81, 165, 580
biological markers in, 94, 97, 100, 114, 121, 237, 315, 664
Cericlamine, 297
"Cheese reaction", 403 *see also* Tyramine reaction
Children, 253, 416, 418, 423, 425
see also Adolescents
m-Chlorophenylpiperazine (mCPP), 110, 532, 668, 680
Chloropromazine, 538, 570
Cholesterol transport, 742, 744
Cholinergic system, 520, 526, 797, 833, 849
Cholinesterase, plasma, 808
Chromogranin A, 580
Circadian clock, 202, 206, 332, 783, 787, 791, 797, 837, 841
Citalopram, 75, 276, 279, 282, 288, 291, 294, 328
Classification, 3, 6, 9, 12, 17, 23, 28, 43, 129, 142, 680, 732
Climacteric, 144
Climoxatone, 372
Clomipramine, 136, 184, 279, 288, 328, 328, 664, 675, 680, 804
combined therapy, 279, 347, 350, 368, 390
Clorgyline, 380, 403, 406, 406
Cloxipol, 556
Clozapine, 526, 529, 566, 570, 574, 593, 598, 605
Cognitive therapy, 648, 654
Composite Diagnostic Evaluation (CODE) System, 28
Compulsive behaviors, 661
see also Obsessive compulsive disorders
Concentration, disturbances of, 635
Conduct disorders, 423
Contingent Negative Variation, 550
Cortex, of brain, 268, 297, 315, 472, 485, 491, 504, 507, 507, 612
Corticosteroid receptors, 210, 217
Corticosterone, 217
Corticotropin releasing hormone (CRH), 37, 49, 165, 210, 225
Cortisol response, 106, 110, 114, 121, 142, 152, 165, 210, 213, 217, 237, 332, 532, 583
Cross National Collaborative Panic Study, 43, 648
CT (computerized tomography) scans, 452, 455, 511

Cycloheximide, 742
Cyclopyrrolones, 823, 856

Delta-sleep-inducing-peptide, 580
Delusional psychoses, 464, 498
Dementia, 161, 165, 291, 383, 833, 837, 849
  see also Alzheimer's disease
Denbufylline, 169
Depersonalization, 680
Depolarization blockade, 574, 605
Depression, 55, 57, 78, 110, 129, 213, 222, 544, 624, 716, 767
  agitated delusional, 12
  akinetic, 556, 556, 583
  and anxiety, 9, 761
  atypical, 400
  biological markers, 17, 37, 52, 55, 64, 69, 72, 75, 78, 84, 142, 332
  bipolar *see* Bipolar disorders
  classification, 12, 17, 23, 28, 43
  diagnosis, 31, 34, 37, 43, 129, 133, 136
  endogenous, 12, 17
  major, 9, 31, 34, 43, 52, 136
  minor, 9, 43, 129
  "neurotic", 136
  NOS, 9, 43
  and obsessive compulsive disorders, 661, 671
  pharmacogenic, 583
  post-psychotic, 556, 583
  and psychotic features, 12, 40
  pure familial depressive disorder, 64
  recurrent, 9, 49, 52, 57, 61, 67
  retarded anhedonic, 12
  revealed, 556, 583
  and schizophrenia, 556, 583
  and sleep disorders, 37, 52, 206, 210, 332, 783, 787, 797, 800, 804, 811, 814, 817
  unipolar *see* Unipolar disorders
"Depressive personality", 136
Desipramine, 12, 126, 136, 240, 276, 279, 328, 328, 671
Desmethylclomipramine, 279
Desmethylimipramine, 240
Desoxycorticosterone, 210
Dexamethasone suppression test, 17, 64, 121, 142, 213, 222, 237, 397
Dextromethorphane, 362
Diabetes mellitus, 624
Diagnosis
  affective disorders, 40
  anxiety disorders, 34, 732
  depression, 31, 34, 37, 43, 129, 133, 136
  schizophrenia, 31, 40
  specificity of, 31
Diagnostic systems *see* DSM-III; DSM-IV; ICD-10
Diazepam, 362, 686, 699, 709, 750, 755, 771, 775, 778, 867
Diazepam binding inhibitor (DBI), 580, 742, 750
Dibenzepine, 365
Disruptive behavior, 423
Distractability, 635
Dopamine agonists, 566
  partial, 523, 566, 593, 609
  see also Specific drugs
Dopamine hypothesis of schizophrenia, 489
Dopaminergic system
  and affective disorders, 40, 149
  in dementia, 383
  and depression, 272
  and obsessive compulsive disorders, 671
  in Parkinson's disease, 383, 485
  and schizophrenia, 40, 431, 461, 467, 485, 489, 491, 495, 501, 523, 526, 538, 553, 566, 570, 574, 593, 596, 602, 609, 621
Dothiepin, 328, 635
Doxepin, 328
Dreams, 831, 851
DSM-III, 3, 6, 9, 31, 43, 129, 136, 237
DSM-IV, 3, 6, 9, 646
Dynorphin, 49
Dyskinesia
  acute, 609
  tardive *see* Tardive dyskinesia
Dysthymia, 9, 129, 133, 136
Dystonia, 593, 598

Eating disorders, 276, 680
Ebiratide, 210
EEDQ, 181
EEG, computerized, 544
Efamol, 618
Efavit, 618
Elderly patients
  and anxiety disorders, 691, 755, 761, 765
  and depression, 12, 161, 243, 291, 328, 413, 761

and sleep disorders, 761, 817, 819, 831, 837, 841, 845, 851
see also Age factor; Dementia
Electroconvulsive treatment (ECT), 181, 188, 249, 257, 260, 264, 268, 272, 301, 332, 449
Electrodermal activity, 64
Endocoids, endogenous, 311, 362
Energy metabolism, 206
Enkephalin, 49
Epidemiology, 57, 231, 434, 437, 827
Epilepsy, 547
Epinephrine, 152
Ergolines, 566
Estazolam, 819
Estradiol, 144, 397, 431
Estrogen, 142, 144, 149, 397, 431
Etoperidone, 161
Euphoria, postnatal, 142
Euthyroid sick syndrome, 84
Event-related potentials, 550, 635
Eye movements, 547 *see also* REM

Facial recognition task, 475
Familial factors, 19, 31, 34, 43, 64, 434, 437, 441, 624, 677, 808
Fatal toxicity index, 126
Fatigue, 129, 206
Fatty acids, essential (EFA), 618
Femoxetine, 279
Fenfluramine, 12, 106, 237, 279, 350
Fengabine, 325
Fetish, 276
Fight or flight reaction *see* Stress response
Flumazenil, 683, 686, 686, 705, 724
Flunitrazepam, 742, 856
6-Fluoronoradrenaline, 181
Fluoxetine, 276
and depression, 49, 61, 67, 124, 126, 136, 240, 279, 328, 350, 353, 368, 390
and obsessive compulsive disorder, 276, 664, 680
Fluparoxan, 322
Flupenthixol, 556
Fluphenazine, 570, 583, 590, 598
Fluperlapine, 570
Flurazepam, 755, 771, 819, 867
Fluvoxamine, 136, 240, 276, 279, 328, 350, 368, 664, 671, 675, 680

$GABA_A$ receptor complex, 580, 683, 686, 699, 702, 705, 744, 856
GABAergic drugs, 325
GABAergic system, 325, 485, 491, 580, 705, 755
Gender, 431, 455, 458, 464
General neurotic syndrome, 133
Genetic factors, 31, 43, 434, 437, 511, 556, 596, 612, 624, 661, 664, 699, 735
Gepirone, 301, 347, 716
Geriatrics *see* Elderly patients
Glucocorticoid receptors, 217, 222, 225
Glucose metabolism, 478, 624
Glutamate hypothesis of schizophrenia, 495
Glutamergic system, 485, 491, 495, 501
G proteins, 173, 188, 192
Growth hormone, 37, 149, 210, 332, 332, 332, 523

Haloperidol, 347, 498, 560, 563, 570, 574, 580, 583, 590, 598, 602, 605, 621, 624, 671
Headache, chronic, 228
5-HIAA (5-hydroxyindoleacetic acid), 94, 97, 100, 106, 114, 237, 315, 664
Hippocampus, 268, 297, 485, 491, 507
Hispanic Health and Nutrition Examination Survey (HHANES), 231
Histamine blockers, 322
HIV infection, 544
Homovanillic acid (HVA), 97, 100, 121, 383, 383, 491, 501
HP-370, 570
5-HT *see* Serotonin
Huntington's chorea, 747
Hydrocortisone, 397
5-Hydroxyindoleacetic acid *see* 5-HIAA
4-Hydroxy-3-methoxyphenylglycol (HMPG), 100, 121, 406
5-Hydroxytryptamine *see* Serotonin
Hyperactivity, 423, 425
Hypercortisolemia, 84, 217, 222, 237, 305, 332
Hypernychthemeral syndrome, 791, 794, 837
Hypertension, 827
Hyperthyroidism, 84
Hyperthyroxinemia, 84
Hypnotics *see* Specific drugs
Hypochondriasis, 680
Hypofrontality, 455, 478, 491
Hypomania, postnatal, 142

Hypotension, orthostatic, 246, 413
Hypothalamic D_2 receptor function, 149
Hypothalamic-pituitary-adrenocortical (HPA) axis, 165, 210, 213, 217, 222, 225
Hypothalamus-pituitary-thyroid (HPT) axis, 84
Hypothyroidism, 84, 213

ICD-10 (International Classification of Diseases), 3, 6, 646
Idiopathic pain syndrome, 237
Idozoxan, 268, 268, 322, 716
Imidazopyridines, 683, 686, 856, 860
Imiloxan, 322, 716
Imipramine, 12, 49, 61, 67, 72, 75, 136, 177, 181, 237, 240, 276, 294, 328, 359, 400, 410, 778, 797
  combined therapy, 253, 279, 350, 357, 368
  in panic disorder, 43, 648, 654, 657
Impulsivity disorders, 680
Influenza epidemics, 437, 664
Information processing, in sleep, 851
Inositol, 197
Insomnia, 157, 761, 767, 794, 814, 819, 823, 837, 845, 854, 860, 863
  rebound, 819, 860, 867
Insulin resistance, 624
International Pilot Study of Schizophrenia, 437
Iproniazid, 400
Ipsapirone, 297
Isocarboxazide, 246
Isoproterenol, 173, 173, 181, 200
Iterative strategy, 17

"Jet-lag" paradigm, 202
Jitteriness syndrome, 282

K-complexes, 823
Kindling phenomenon, 602

Lactate infusion, 12
Lecithin, 833
Levoprotiline, 716
Linoleic acid, 618
Linolenic acid, 618
Lithium, 12, 19, 49, 64, 172, 173, 192, 192, 197, 200, 213
  applications, 40, 136, 146, 276, 556, 671
  combined therapy, 243, 286, 301, 328, 347, 350, 353, 357, 671
Litoxetine, 294, 308
Lorazepam, 693, 696, 767, 771, 775, 778, 867
Lormetazepam, 823, 867
Loxapine, 570
Lymphocytes, 750

Magnesium ions, 192
Magnetic resonance imaging, 455, 511, 515
Maprotiline, 49, 67, 124, 126, 240, 276, 328, 350, 800
Marital problems, 253
mCPP, 110, 532, 668, 680
Mecholyl test, 449
Medifoxamine, 716
Melancholic patients, 97
Melatonin secretion, 783, 837
Melperone, 570
Menopause, 144
Mental alertness, 152
Mental pain hypothesis, 152
Mephenytoin, 362
Meta-analysis, of citalopram, 288
Metergoline, 664, 668
Methadone, 362
Methycobalamin, 791
α-Methylmilacemide, 378
Methylphenidate, 423, 425
Metoclopramide, 347
Metyrapone, 222
Mianserin, 124, 126, 322, 328
Midazolam, 755, 867
Milacemide, 378
Minocycline, 195
Mirtazapine, 322
Mitochondrial benzodiazepine receptors, 735, 738, 742, 744, 747, 750
MK-801, 495, 495, 501
Moclobemide, 136, 246, 328, 362, 372, 380, 386, 390, 403, 406, 425
Monoamine oxidase (MAO) activity, 237, 378, 383, 386, 397
Monoamine oxidase (MAO) hypothesis, 425
Monoamine oxidase inhibitors
  MAO-A, reversible (RIMA), 372, 380, 386, 390, 403, 406, 716
  MAO-A, selective, 403
  MAO-B, 386
  MAOI, 9, 12, 61, 126, 136, 246, 286, 301, 311, 315, 380, 390, 400, 406, 716

see also Specific drugs
Mood disorders, 9, 19, 64, 87
Morbidity risks, 19, 34
Motor loop, 485
Multiple sclerosis, 747
Muscle atonia, 831

Narcolepsy, 489
Neurasthenia, 129
Neurodegenerative disorders, 383
Neuroleptics, 441, 444, 461, 491, 535, 556, 580, 587, 590, 598, 602, 609, 612, 615, 618, 624, 671, 808
atypical, 566, 593, 605
see also Specific drugs
Neuropeptides, 580, 742, 750
Neuropeptide Y, 580
Nicotine, 621
Nicotinic acid, 618
NIMH Psychobiology Study, 57
Nitrazepam, 755
Nitroquazone, 169
Nomifensine, 246, 328
Noradrenaline, 165, 181, 268, 380, 635
Noradrenergic system, 121, 165, 383
Norepinephrine system, 272
Nortriptyline, 12, 67, 136, 279
Nosology, 17, 23, 28, 43

Obesity, 827
Obsessive compulsive disorders, 243, 276, 423, 661, 664, 671, 675, 677, 750
related disorders, 680
Obstructive sleep apnea syndrome, 827
Ocaperidone, 535
Odansetron, 538
Oestradiol *see* Estradiol
Oestrogen *see* Estrogen
Oncogenes, 49
Oneiric behavior disorder, 831
Onychophagia, 680
ORG 3770, 716
Oxaprotiline, 240
Oxazepam, 775
Oxygen extraction rate (OER), 91

P3, latency, 635
Pain, chronic, 228, 231, 234, 237, 305, 761
Panic disorder, 12, 110, 133, 305, 646, 654, 750
pharmacotherapy, 43, 243, 276, 282, 648, 657, 713, 727, 767, 778
Papez loop, 485
Paranoid disorders, 464, 498
Paraphilias, 276
Pargyline, 397
Parkinsonism, 526, 560, 563, 628
Parkinson's disease, 383, 485, 535, 747, 851
Paroxetine, 67, 72, 75, 234, 294
Pediatrics *see* Children
Peripheral-type benzodiazepine receptors *see* Mitochondrial benzodiazepine receptors
Personality disorders, 648, 767
PET (positron emission tomography), 91, 472, 478, 664
Phencyclidine (PCP), 467, 498
Phenelzine, 61, 246, 390, 400, 406, 406
Phenothiazides, 177
Phentolamine, 322
Phosphodiesterase inhibitors, 169
Phosphoinositide (PI) system, 177, 181, 197, 716
Photoperiod, effects of, 783
Phototherapy, 787, 794, 837
Physostigmine, 833
Pimozide, 40
Piperoxan, 322
Pittsburgh Study of Maintenance Therapies in Recurrent Depression, 253
Pituitary, in depression, 213
Platelets, 72, 103, 121, 177, 184, 234, 237, 315
Polypeptides, 580, 699, 742, 750
Positron emission tomography *see* PET
Post-imperative negative variation, 550
Postnatal depression, 144
Postnatal mental disturbance, 142
Postnatal psychosis, 144, 146, 149
-3PPP, 523
Pregnancy prediction, 738
Pregnenolone, 742, 744
Premenstrual syndrome, 103, 144, 276
Procyclidine, 560
Progabide, 325
Progesterone, 142, 397
Prolactin response, 106, 114, 210, 237, 301, 332, 332, 347, 350, 532, 566
Propofol, 702
Propranolol, 732
Prostaglandins, 618
Protein kinase C, 181

Prothiaden, 635
Protriptyline, 328
Pseudoanxiety, 757
Pseudo-neurasthenia, 129
Psychopathology, of depression, 23
Psychopharmacology, 23, 28, 40
Psychosocial factors, 253, 423, 761
Psychostimulants, 423
Psychosurgery, 664
Psychotherapy, 61, 253, 648, 648, 654, 819
Psychotic disorders, in DSM-IV, 6, 464
Puerperal psychosis *see* Postnatal psychosis

Quazepam, 819

Raclopride, 570, 598
Reactive psychoses, 464
ω-Receptors, 683, 686, 747, 856
Relaxation training, 654, 854
REM latency, 37, 52, 157, 210, 237, 520, 804, 808, 811, 814, 817, 833
REM sleep, 157, 210, 811, 831, 833, 849
Remoxipride, 593
Research Diagnostic Criteria (RDC), 43
Responsive Search Score, 547
Rilmazafone, 716
RIMA *see* Monoamine oxidase inhibitors
Risk aversiveness, 680
Risperidone, 535, 570
Ritanserin, 136, 305, 535, 716
mRNA expression, 699
Ro 19-6327, 386
Rolipram, 169, 716
Rubidium, 200

Schedule for Affective Disorders and Schizophrenia (SADS-LA), 34
Schizo-affective disorders, 149, 498, 811
Schizophrenia, 121, 431, 434, 437, 449, 452, 458, 467, 469, 472, 475, 485, 489, 491, 495, 498, 501, 526, 529, 532, 535, 541, 547, 550, 556, 570, 583, 618, 624, 628
  atypical, 449, 452
  classification, 6, 23
  diagnosis, 31, 40
  pharmacotherapy, 40, 276, 441, 444, 523, 526, 560, 580, 590, 727
  positive and negative symptoms, 6, 458, 461, 478, 511, 511, 520, 526, 544
  and sleep disorders, 520, 804, 808, 811, 817
  structural brain abnormalities, 485, 504, 507, 511, 515
  typical, 449, 452
Schizophreniform psychoses, 464
Second messenger dysbalance hypothesis, 169
Second messenger system, 177, 181, 184, 192, 197, 716
Selegiline, 403, 406
Septiptiline, 322, 716
Serotonin agonists, 301
Serotonin hypothesis of suicide, 94
Serotonin panic hypothesis, 282
Serotonin reuptake inhibitors, 136, 275, 276, 279, 282, 286, 288, 291, 294, 311, 315, 664, 668, 671, 675
  combined therapy, 240, 279, 390, 535, 671
  long-term therapy, 67, 286, 301
  in schizophrenia, 276, 526, 529, 535, 538
Serotonin system, 106, 237, 272, 383
  and depression, 69, 72, 75, 243, 301, 315, 347
  and obsessive compulsive disorders, 668, 671, 675, 680
  receptors, 72, 75, 103, 106, 114, 121, 184, 297, 315, 529
  and schizophrenia, 529, 532, 570
  and suicidal behavior, 97, 103, 106, 110, 114, 118, 121
  transporter, 72, 75, 294
Sertindole, 553
Sertraline, 67, 279, 675
Sex *see* Gender
Sexual problems, 152, 276, 677, 680
sigma system, 498
Sleep deprivation, 797, 800
Sleep disorders, 52, 237, 246, 489, 827, 831, 845, 849
  cyclic alternating pattern (CAP), 863
  delayed sleep phase syndrome, 787, 791
  in depression, 37, 52, 206, 210, 332, 783, 787, 797, 800, 804, 811, 814, 817
  and schizophrenia, 520, 804, 808, 811, 817
  sleep-wake rhythm disorders, 791, 794, 837, 841
  see also Insomnia
Sleep hygiene, 854
Sleep spindles, 823
Slow wave sleep, 136, 635, 808, 811, 823

Smoking behavior, 621, 827
Snoring, 827
Sodium lactate response, 654
Somatic complaints,unspecified, 129
Somatization, 161, 228
Somatoform pain syndrome, 237
Somatostatin, 37, 49
Sparteine/debrisoquine oxidation polymorphism, 359
SPECT (single proton emission computed tomography), 87, 452, 455
Speech disorders, 472, 511
Statistical considerations, 338
Steroid hormones, 397
Steroidogenesis, 735, 738, 742, 744
Stress disorder, post-traumatic, 635, 639
Stress response, 49, 152, 165, 217, 305, 757, 819
Study design, 338
Stuttering, 418
Substance use, 276, 498, 544, 767, 787, 867
  see also Alcohol
Suicidal behavior, 124, 437, 498
  biological markers, 78, 94, 97, 100, 103, 106, 110, 114, 118, 121, 124, 126, 315
Sulpiride, 593
Surrender stress response, 152
Sydenham's chorea, 664
Sympathetic alarm response *see* Stress response
Sympathetic system, and stress, 152, 165
Systemic lupus erythematosus, 17

Talexipole, 461
Tardive dyskinesia, 587, 593, 598, 602, 609, 612, 615, 618, 621, 624, 628
Targeted strategy, 441
Temazepam, 819, 867
Temperature *see* Body temperature
Terguride, 566, 593
Testosterone, 210, 397
Tetracycline derivatives, 195
Thalamic filter dysfunction hypothesis of schizophrenia, 495
Therapeutic monitoring, of antidepressants, 375
Thermoregulation, 206
Thioridazine, 362
Thyroid panel, 84
Thyroid stimulating hormone (TSH), 37, 84
Thyrotropin-releasing hormone (TRH), 37, 49, 84, 347
Thyroxine (T4), 84
Tiapride, 418
Tiospirone, 570
α-Tocopherol, 618
Toloxatone, 372
Tourette's syndrome, 661, 664, 668, 671, 680
Toxicity, of antidepressants, 126
Tranylcypromine, 246, 406, 410
Trazodone, 126, 152, 157, 279, 328
Treatment response, 12, 40
  see also Specific drugs
Triangulation strategy, 17
Triazolam, 202, 819, 867, 867
Triazolobenzodiazepines, 318
Trichotillomania, 680
Tricyclic antidepressants, 9, 43, 72, 126, 136, 177, 181, 237, 294, 311, 359, 362, 556, 635, 732, 804
  combined therapy, 240, 243, 246, 249, 253, 279, 286, 328, 347, 350, 357
  comparative studies, 288, 318, 322, 325
  maintenance therapy, 49, 61, 188, 301, 301
  in non-responsive depression, 49, 240, 243, 246, 249, 253, 286, 347, 350
  side-effects, 72
  treatment response, 12, 19, 52, 328
Triiodothyronine (T3), 84
L-Tryptophan, 286, 301, 350, 675
Tumor cells, 747
Twin studies, 31
Tyramine, 142, 390, 403, 406
  reaction, 380, 390, 403, 406

Unipolar disorders, 12, 19, 28, 34, 57, 91, 197

Venlafaxine, 343, 797
Ventricular enlargement, 452, 455, 455, 485, 507, 511, 515
Viloxazine, 328
Vitamin B_{12}, 791, 794
Vitamin E, 618

Yohimbine, 322

Zimelidine, 67, 240, 328
Zolpidem, 683, 856, 860, 863
Zopiclone, 823, 856
Zuclopenthixol, 560, 563, 602